Children at risk for schizophrenia

Children at risk for schizophrenia

A longitudinal perspective

Edited by
NORMAN F. WATT, E. JAMES ANTHONY,
LYMAN C. WYNNE, AND JON E. ROLF

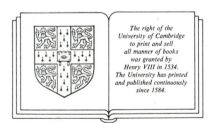

The right of the
University of Cambridge
to print and sell
all manner of books
was granted by
Henry VIII in 1534.
The University has printed
and published continuously
since 1584.

CAMBRIDGE UNIVERSITY PRESS
Cambridge
London   New York   New Rochelle
Melbourne   Sydney

Published by the Press Syndicate of the University of Cambridge
The Pitt Building, Trumpington Street, Cambridge CB2 1RP
32 East 57th Street, New York, NY 10022, USA
296 Beaconsfield Parade, Middle Park, Melbourne 3206, Australia

First published 1984

Printed in the United States of America

Library of Congress Cataloging in Publication Data
Main entry under title:
Children at risk for schizophrenia.
Includes bibliographical references and index.
1. Child psychopathology – Longitudinal studies.
2. Schizophrenia – Prevention – Longitudinal studies.
I. Watt, Norman F. [DNLM: 1. Schizophrenia, Childhood.
2. Longitudinal studies. WM 203 C535]
RJ499.C489 1984   618.92′8982′00722   83-10152
ISBN 0 521 24888 4

Shortly following the Plenary Conference of the Risk Research Consortium in March of 1980, the Steering Committee presented a plaque to Manfred Bleuler on behalf of all its members. On the plaque was engraved the following inscription:

Presented by the International Risk Research Consortium to Professor Manfred Bleuler

In recognition of his pioneer services in the field of schizophrenia risk research. He has shown us the way through distinguished empirical investigations, penetrating clinical case studies and humane dedication to his patients.

Steering Committee:	E. James Anthony, M.D.
	Michael J. Goldstein, Ph.D.
	Jon Rolf, Ph.D.
	Norman F. Watt, Ph.D.

1980

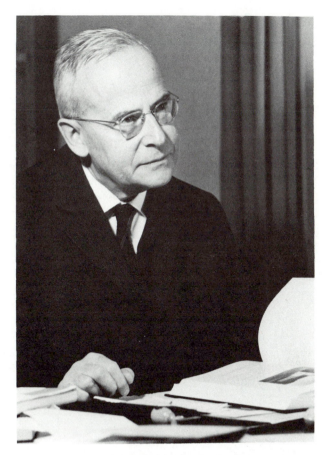

Professor Bleuler has published scholarly investigations of schizophrenic disorder, like most of us. Unlike most of us, he has also treated his schizophrenic subjects clinically, delivered their babies, and cared for their children. This book is dedicated in honor of Manfred Bleuler, for there is nowhere a more faithful champion of schizophrenic people.

Contents

Contents   xi

Contributors

Manhal Al-Khayyal
University of California at Los Angeles

E. James Anthony
Edison Child Development Research Center,
Washington University School of Medicine

Joan Rosenbaum Asarnow
University of California at Los Angeles

Robert F. Asarnow
University of California at Los Angeles

Judith Auerbach
The Hebrew University, Jerusalem

Alfred L. Baldwin
University of Rochester

Clara P. Baldwin
University of Rochester

Ralph Barocas
George Mason University

Hector Bird
University of Puerto Rico School of Medicine

Manfred Bleuler
Burghölzli Clinic, Zurich

Lynne Bond
University of Vermont

Charles M. Burack
University of Chicago

Loretta Cass
Edison Child Development Research Center,
Washington University School of Medicine

J. M. Cleghorn
McMaster University, Hamilton, Ontario

Robert E. Cole
University of Rochester Medical Center

Barbara Cornblatt
New York State Psychiatric Institute and
Columbia University

Janis Crowther
Kent State University

Robert Cudeck
Social Science Research Institute, University of
Southern California

Cyril Dalais
Joint Child Health and Education Project,
Quatre Bornes, Mauritius

Vernon Devine
University of Minnesota and Hennepin
County Mental Health Center

Jeri A. Doane
University of California at Los Angeles

Regina M. Driscoll
St. Paul Children's Hospital

Rosanne Edenhart-Pepe
Edison Child Development Research Center,
Washington University School of Medicine

L. Erlenmeyer-Kimling
New York State Psychiatric Institute and
Columbia University

Barbara Fish
Neuropsychiatric Institute, University of
California at Los Angeles

Lawrence Fisher
Veterans Administration Medical Center,
Fresno, California

David Friedman
New York State Psychiatric Institute and
Columbia University

xii

Norman Garmezy
University of Minnesota

Michael J. Goldstein
University of California at Los Angeles

Deborah Greenwald
Tufts University

John J. Griffith
*Social Science Research Institute, University of
Southern California*

Ted W. Grubb
*Pikes Peak Board of Cooperative Services,
Colorado Springs*

David Harder
Tufts University

Ulla Hilldoff
New York State Psychiatric Institute

Matti O. Huttunen
University of Helsinki

Cynthia L. Janes
*Edison Child Development Research Center,
Washington University School of Medicine*

James E. Jones
University of Rochester Medical Center

Lennart Kaij
University of Lund, Malmö, Sweden

Clarice Kestenbaum
*St. Lukes Hospital Center and Columbia
University*

Robert H. Klein
Yale University Psychiatric Institute

Ronald F. Kokes
*Veterans Administration Medical Center,
Fresno, California*

Paula M. Konen
*Edison Child Development Research Center,
Washington University School of Medicine*

Richard R. J. Lewine
*Illinois State Psychiatric Institute and
Pritzker School of Medicine, the University
of Chicago*

Julia M. Lewis
*Center for the Family in Transition, Corte
Madera, California*

Duncan J. MacCrimmon
McMaster University, Hamilton, Ontario

Manon McGinnis
*Edison Child Development Research Center,
Washington University School of Medicine*

Thomas F. McNeil
University of Lund, Malmö, Sweden

Joseph Marcus
*Department of Psychiatry, University of
Chicago*

Yvonne Marcuse
*New York State Psychiatric Institute and
Columbia University*

Sarnoff A. Mednick
*Social Science Research Institute, University of
Southern California*

Stephen Munson
University of Rochester Medical Center

John M. Neale
State University of New York at Stony Brook

Carl Gustaf Nilsson
University of Helsinki

Keith H. Nuechterlein
*Neuropsychiatric Institute, University of
California at Los Angeles*

Patricia Perkins
University of Rochester Medical Center

Susan Phipps-Yonas
University of Minnesota

Robert Prentky
Massachusetts Treatment Center, Bridgewater

John D. Rainer
*New York State Psychiatric Institute and
Columbia University*

Barry Ritzler
University of Southern Mississippi

Eliot H. Rodnick
University of California at Los Angeles

Jon E. Rolf
*Behavioral Sciences Research Branch,
National Institute of Mental Health, and
the University of Vermont*

Jacques Rutschmann
*New York State Psychiatric Institute and
Columbia University*

Leonard F. Salzman
University of Rochester Medical Center

Arnold J. Sameroff
Illinois Institute for Developmental Disabilities, University of Illinois at Chicago Circle

Fini Schulsinger
Psychological Institute, Copenhagen

Hanne Schulsinger
Institute of Clinical Psychology, University of Copenhagen

Paul Schwartzman
University of Rochester Medical Center

Ronald Seifer
Illinois Institute for Developmental Disabilities, University of Illinois at Chicago Circle

Margaret T. Singer
University of California at Berkeley

Richard A. Steffy
University of Waterloo, Ontario

John S. Strauss
Yale University Medical School

Sharon A. Talovic
Social Science Research Institute, University of Southern California

Linda Teri
University of Oregon

Katherine Van Dusen
Social Science Research Institute, University of Southern California

Herbert G. Vaughan, Jr.
Albert Einstein College of Medicine

Peter H. Venables
University of York, England

Norman F. Watt
University of Denver

David G. Weeks
Edison Child Development Research Center, Washington University School of Medicine

Sheldon Weintraub
State University of New York at Stony Brook

Leland Wilkinson
University of Illinois at Chicago Circle

Ken C. Winters
State University of New York at Stony Brook

Julien Worland
Edison Child Development Research Center, Washington University School of Medicine

Gunnel Wrede
Swedish School of Social Work and Local Administration, and University of Helsinki

Lyman C. Wynne
University of Rochester Medical Center

Pamela Yu
Texas Research Institute of Mental Services, Houston

Foreword

MANFRED BLEULER

To help children threatened by schizophrenic or affective disorders is indeed a great task. There are all too many of these children whom we would like to help, but how can we help them? So far we don't really know how and that is a bitter disappointment. Sadness and resignation threaten those of us who see the great task, realizing that we may not be up to it.

Today we have reason for renewed hope: Whole groups of investigators have set themselves the task to ferret out those harmful life experiences that transform vulnerable persons into ill ones. This objective is to be reached by observing the life circumstances and development of numerous children at risk over many years. These studies seek to establish which conditions allow children at risk to remain well and which lead them into illness. If successful, then we can proceed to undertake preventive measures against those threats that contribute to the onset of psychosis.

Much painstaking research in this direction has been undertaken previously, without achieving decisive success. Eighty years ago psychiatrists endeavored carefully to associate individual symptoms of disease such as hallucinations, delusions, thought blocking, and others with the life experiences of the patients. They did recognize the psychological precursors of individual symptoms but not those of the general syndrome. The next step in this line of research was the finding that certain personal peculiarities are frequent among those destined to become schizophrenic later, as well as among their relatives. The "schizoid personality" was described as predisposing to schizophrenic disorder. It remained unclear whether the schizoid personality of a family member represented a threat only for that individual or also for others in the family. Today only few people realize that the schizoid personality was characterized primarily by difficulties in interpersonal relationships with the closest relatives. More recent research that has flourished especially in the United States placed the relationship difficulties as such into the center of investigation, rather than the personality of the individual experiencing those difficulties, as earlier European researchers had done. This shift signified a great advance: It is easier to conceive of ways to change and improve a relationship than to change the character of a schizoid person. The concept of the schizoid personality type came, therefore, to be perceived as static, whereas the disturbances in family relationships were more fluid and dynamic. The latter stimulates further investigations. How do the disturbances in family relations come about? How can they be prevented or mitigated so as to diminish their pathogenic impact? Clear answers to these questions are not yet at hand, but they are eagerly awaited.

For one of my generation who is privileged to witness the development of the investigations in the Risk Research Consortium from the vantage point of a small country (Switzerland), the sheer magnitude of the undertaking seems almost incredible. During the major part of my life and in my sphere of knowledge, psychiatric research could be pursued only by individuals in their spare time and at their own expense. On the basis of this experience I would not have dreamed what has become reality today, namely, that a collaboration among so many investigators could come about, extending across the boundaries of professional disciplines, of theoretical persuasions, and of nations, in a common effort that can reach fruition only after many years.

The uniqueness of this research organization is matched by the magnificence of its objectives. If it should prove possible to prevent the onset of schizophrenic and affective disorders, the fate of more than 1% of all human beings, as well as that of their families, would be changed for the better. There are probably many environmental influences that predispose to psychosis, but at the same time contribute to other unfavorable personality developments. For this reason alone the results of this research could have great significance far beyond the problems of schizophrenic disorders.

A grand and novel inquiry with long-range perspective brings with it also great inherent dangers, otherwise it would not be novel and grand. Which are the principal dangers that can be foreseen? It is easy to see a danger of failing to achieve the goal of the research, at least as it is formulated by most people today. It is conceivable that no specific pathogens will be discovered that play a decisive role in the etiology of schizophrenic and affective disorders. This could come about because of the inadequacy of the research to uncover them or because they do not exist. However, such an ultimate result need not necessarily be considered a disappointment. It would point to a fundamental lawfulness in human development, namely, that the unique pattern of interaction between the person's innate developmental tendencies and diverse life experiences is decisive for the development of psychosis as well as for the development of personality. This would make apparent that there is no specific prophylaxis against schizophrenic disorders. Such recognition, however, would put the correct focus on the importance of emotional health for all human beings and of proper consideration for the unique course of each individual's life. Even if no specific psychological interventions for the prevention of psychosis should evolve from this work, it would, nevertheless, provide a powerful impetus for mental health in general, especially regarding the formative years of childhood and adolescence. Viewed in this way, it can hardly be considered dangerous if the new research efforts should not achieve the goals envisioned; they would simply yield other unexpected benefits.

I see a second danger in the possibility that the new research may restrict itself too much by studying only phenomena that can be readily counted, measured, or made objective, that it may lose sight of essential human qualities that are difficult to quantify. An example is the love of a mother for her child. It cannot be measured by the number of kisses that the child receives within a certain unit of time. One loving kiss can mean more than 100 kisses bestowed out of stereotyped habit. There are many contemporary studies that have failed because of vain attempts to measure what cannot be measured. I am hopeful that the investigators in this consortium will not succumb to this danger. I have, after all, witnessed how critically they reexamine their work at every step. They will count, measure, and statistically evaluate everything that can be calibrated in those ways, but I would urge them to guard against overvaluing quantitative analysis and to scrutinize the significance of the objective findings with intuition and empathy. Single findings should not cause them to neglect the view of the total life experience.

If one didn't know the members of the Risk Research Consortium, one could be concerned about a third danger inherent in their work: that in observing they could forget to help, that in their commitment to science, humanity would be neglected. The experience of their warmth and openness banishes any fear that they might only observe passively when a child might be helped. Active intervention will make the scientific interpretation of their observations more difficult, but not impossible. To intervene and to observe the impact of the intervention may have greater scientific value than to chronicle passively the decline into psychosis.

In short, the longitudinal investigation – lasting decades – of the fate of children at risk for psychosis is a task of gigantic scope well worth the great investment required. I consider the investigators who have taken on this commitment capable of facing all the dangers inherent in this momentous undertaking. With confident anticipation I wish them well in their endeavors.

Acknowledgments

This book is the culmination of much concerted effort expended over most of a decade by many people. Much of the credit for initiating the Risk Research Consortium belongs to Norman Garmezy, who was the pioneering protagonist responsible for most of the early organizational work, and to Loren Mosher, our inside supporter at the National Institute of Mental Health. Flexible financial support, including a subsidy to reduce the cost of purchasing this book, has been provided by the William T. Grant Foundation. Recent support has also been obtained for the consortium's activities from the National Institute of Mental Health. The active cooperation of the Cambridge University Press and Susan Milmoe, in particular, will be visible to all readers of these pages. Less obvious but most important are the contributions of Linda Wilbanks, who typed or edited most of the manuscript, prepared the bibliography, and coordinated the entire publishing venture from beginning to end. In a just world this book would be cited under her name instead of ours.

The Editors

Introduction

NORMAN F. WATT

Researchers seeking the origins of schizophrenia have traditionally concentrated their attention on systematically analyzing experimental observations of the behavior of schizophrenic patients. Although this research has yielded a few potential etiological clues, attempts to evaluate the significance of differences found between normal and schizophrenic subjects have been stymied by a major and seemingly insuperable methodological problem: the impossibility of determining whether abnormalities observed in people already diagnosed as manifestly schizophrenic reflect a cause or a consequence of illness. To circumvent the problem, a cadre of enterprising researchers have turned to a promising and relatively new research strategy: to study individuals deemed particularly vulnerable to schizophrenia from their early years of childhood through the period of maximum risk for psychological disorder in adulthood. These investigators hope to identify preexisting biochemical, physiological, psychological, or life-history characteristics that consistently differentiate those who ultimately develop schizophrenia from those who do not. At the same time this approach might allow the development and application of techniques that could be effective in preventing or mitigating the severity of manifest schizophrenia and other forms of serious psychopathology.

This research tactic, usually called the *high-risk method*, is a natural outgrowth of the vast body of previous research that has implicated both genetic and environmental factors in the etiology of schizophrenia. Between 1962 and the present, more and more scientists of various theoretical persuasions have grasped the notion that the high-risk strategy offers a unique opportunity to test etiological hypotheses of any type.

These studies all use the prospective high-risk method. Thus, excluded from this volume are prospective studies of normal development, such as the Berkeley growth studies, clinical retrospective studies of adult schizophrenic patients, follow-back studies utilizing records, and follow-up studies in adulthood of subjects seen as children. The important value of those other longitudinal studies to the current generation of prospective studies is widely acknowledged by high-risk investigators. The contributions of various studies and the advantages and disadvantages of the methods employed have been comprehensively reviewed by Garmezy (1974).

1

Since the pioneering efforts of S. A. Mednick and Schulsinger (1968) began in 1962 there has been a gradually expanding interest in this type of research. For example, in 1968 the National Institute of Mental Health supported five longitudinal prospective high-risk projects at a total cost of $40,000. Just 5 years later, and 10 years after the initiation of the Mednick and Schulsinger project in Copenhagen, there were 11 NIMH-supported high-risk grants totaling $880,912. Over this same period several other organizations had begun to support work in this area: the World Health Organization in Geneva, the Grant Foundation in New York City, and the Scottish Rite Foundation in Boston. Using a broader definition, including as high-risk studies not just those using the longitudinal prospective method, Garmezy was able to identify 20 projects by the end of 1973. In fact, this is probably a conservative estimate as multiple projects, sometimes with different investigators in the same center, were listed by Garmezy as single studies.

Soon after its inception in 1968 the Center for Studies of Schizophrenia at the National Institute of Mental Health (NIMH) established high-risk research as an area warranting high programmatic priority. Several administrative mechanisms were used to attract interest to this area. First, Norman Garmezy was contracted to review the existing literature relevant to the topic. Next, in collaboration with Lyman Wynne's Adult Psychiatry Branch at the NIMH Intermural Program, a conference was held in June, 1969, which focused on methodological issues in research with groups at high risk for the development of schizophrenia. The report of this meeting (Mosher & Wynne, 1970) announced widely the establishment of this area as a high priority for research support by NIMH. Based on recommendations made at the 1969 meeting, plans were made to hold another meeting in 3 years to reassess developments in the area. Thus, a second meeting, involving 17 investigators, 15 consultants, and 8 other participants, was planned for October, 1972. The next chapter in this book summarizes the preparations and the results of that important meeting. During the intervening 3 years, it became clear that the difficulties inherent in prospective high-risk research had been underestimated and certain unanticipated problems (for example, ethical and legal ones) had begun to assume importance. In turn, several steps were taken to deal with these emergent issues.

The Risk Research Consortium was organized formally in May, 1973, in order to foster closer communication, research consultation, and active collaboration on training and longitudinal research in schizophrenia and related emotional disorders. With financial support from the Grant Foundation, the Consortium has sponsored two or three research meetings each year, usually small and limited in attendance, in order to promote active interchange among investigators. The members of the consortium share in common an interest in studying individuals at high risk for schizophrenia and related disorders. Their specific research objectives vary widely, but generally are aimed at identifying early characteristics that differentiate those who ultimately develop schizophrenia from those who do not. This approach offers opportunities also for *preventing* the development of manifest schizophrenia and other forms of serious psychopathology, through early identification and clinical intervention.

The Risk Research Consortium can be seen in the light of a successful experiment in cooperative science. Several key NIMH staff persons played a catalytic role in fostering a unique collaborative approach to coordinating the research efforts of a variety of investigative teams, studying one of the most difficult problem areas in the field of mental health. The common objective was to plan and conduct prospective longitudinal studies of children with different types and degrees of environmental and genetic risk for psychopathology. There was little precedence or evidence for the adequacy of existing methodology for the task at hand. It was hoped that, by combining the talents of a number of independently funded investigators, the group would be able to create the technology necessary to measure the individual vulnerabilities and competencies of children at risk as they matured and coped with the idiosyncracies in themselves and in their parents. In a broader sense, the goals of the consortium were to test the possibility of a cooperative approach to describing the causes of schizophrenia based on prospective observations, to predict breakdown and recovery in vulnerable individuals, and to validate the concepts of developmental competence and risk for psychopathology.

It is typical in the scientific community for investigators to compete with one another for funding, to withhold unpublished data until the precedence of a publication date is assured, and to be reluctant to share successful methods with other investigators because it would restrict the competitive advantage over other investigators in other laboratories. We might paraphrase a well-known motto as the theme of the Risk Research Consortium: Where scientific competition is, there shall the spirit of cooperation be. Most of the persons who would become involved in the consortium operated, at the start, more in the competitive than in the cooperative model. Trust had to be established, and the value of sharing both successful and unsuccessful techniques (as well as unpublished data) had to be discovered. Were it not for the enormity of the task involved in prospective research in schizophrenia, as well as the catalytic role of Loren Mosher and other NIMH staff, the spirit of collaboration would not have taken hold and led to a decade of mutual assistance and discovery by members of the growing consortium.

A further asset of the cooperative science concept is that the Risk Research Consortium has served an extremely important function as a social-support system for those investigators embarking on longitudinal research. Longitudinal research demands a great deal of patience and delay of gratification. This is especially true when one is dealing with a longitudinal cohort of the offspring of psychotic parents living in the community.

The interdisciplinary nature of the Risk Research Consortium is unique. The organization began as a loose federation of independently funded research centers and investigators, with its members representing a number of professional backgrounds. These include child psychiatry, clinical psychology, adult psychiatry, experimental psychology, physiological psychology, child clinical psychology, pediatrics, behavior genetics, family therapy, sociology, and others. During both the large and small gatherings of the consortium every effort has been made to invite as consultants persons with backgrounds from diverse scientific disciplines that could aid the methodological progress of the consortium.

Owing to the diversity of its membership, there is a large training component inherent in all of the consortium's activities. Reciprocal training can be expected when persons from different disciplines attack the same problem area together. In most of the research groups there is also a constant mixture of senior and junior investigators, as well as the graduate student staff who are so essential for cost economy. This offers a great deal of opportunity for apprenticing the junior people to the senior ones in the professional aspects of conducting research in the community. Because these multidisciplinary team members have been trained during different decades, there is also generational training wherein junior members are able to give to their senior colleagues the advantage of their most recent training in computer technology, theory integration, and that always necessary component of youthful ambition – to attempt the impossible.

We are called on increasingly to serve as spokespersons for the scientific community on such topics as schizophrenic development, family relations, the high-risk method, longitudinal research procedures, and preventive intervention for mental health. These issues have significant national priority that will increase rather than diminish. The Risk Research Consortium has served the function of collective impressario and chronicler of advances in this vitally important area of scientific research. The members of the consortium speak with one voice in saying that this organization has been of great value for our research work, our professional careers, and the cause of mental health.

Many of the prospective projects launched in the early 1970s by members of the consortium are now maturing, as are the research subjects they have studied in childhood and adolescence. Children at risk for schizophrenia have been followed from a variety of points in development for periods up to 19 years now, at an aggregate cost of $11.5 million and hundreds of years of cumulative professional research effort. The aggregate total of subjects at risk for schizophrenia that have been studied by members of the consortium approximates 1,200 with 1,400 normal controls and about 750 children of parents with other psychiatric disorders. It was, therefore, considered timely, at this important midpoint in the lives of our research subjects, to organize a plenary conference of the consortium members for the purpose of presenting comprehensive progress reports on our research projects thus far. With financial support from the Grant Foundation and NIMH that conference was held on March 11–13, 1980, in San Juan, Puerto Rico. Most of the papers presented at that meeting have been carefully edited for publication in this book.

We begin with a summary of the Dorado Beach Conference in 1972 that set the directions for much of the research that has followed since then. Thereafter we present reports from the projects roughly in the chronological order of their inception. Part IX pools reports from six different projects that began in the infancy or very early childhood of their subjects' lives. Part X presents the work of Manfred Bleuler, to whom this book is dedicated. The chapters in the last part review and synthesize the reports from various topical points of view, attempting to assess what we have learned collectively from the first two decades of high-risk research in schizophrenia.

This is our first effort to publish results from all the projects in one place. There is an enormous amount of material for the reader to digest. But there is more to come later as the children we are following pass through their adult years and the period of maximum risk for schizophrenic disorder.

1 An early crossroad in research on risk for schizophrenia: the Dorado Beach Conference

NORMAN GARMEZY AND SUSAN PHIPPS-YONAS

This chapter is tinged with the historical, assuming that one can presume to label historical that which transpired only a short decade ago. For centuries the mental disorder we now know as schizophrenia has denied its most fundamental secrets to researchers and clinicians alike. Although this is still the case, new developments in our understanding of the disorder presage a future breakthrough. The foci for the individual research efforts in schizophrenia have been numerous; this volume reviews the newest area, *risk research*, or the ongoing developmental study of infants and children who presumably are predisposed to the disorder.

Risk research in schizophrenia has a brief history (Garmezy & Streitman, 1974), a portion of which can be told quickly. Although the 1920s saw earlier small-scale efforts to study children born of disordered mothers, Bender's (1937) monograph, which consisted essentially of tabulations based on descriptive clinical reports, was the first systematic effort to evaluate the effects of different forms of parental psychiatric disorders on the offspring. The research of Fish (1957), who followed in the path of her mentor, added to the previous clinical observations an intensive longitudinal quality, by focusing on a small number of infants who were seemingly vulnerable to schizophrenia on three counts: (1) disordered family background; (2) maternal psychopathology; and (3) neonatal signs of neurointegrative deficiencies.

Undoubtedly, the seminal contribution to this research area is the pioneering programmatic effort, initiated by S. A. Mednick and F. Schulsinger (1968) in Denmark, to study prospectively a substantial number of children born to schizophrenic mothers together with control offspring of normal mothers.

These early beginnings provided the impetus for the many investigations that have followed. It has been estimated that from the original group of 12 children Fish evaluated, approximately 1,000 children of schizophrenic parents, together with more than 500 children at risk for other psychopathologies have undergone study. To these numbers we can add more than 1,000 normal control children, some of whom have been matched on various demographic, familial, and cognitive attributes, whereas others have been randomly selected (Garmezy, 1981). This volume updates the status of the many ongoing risk research programs which these children and their families have served so valiantly. In a sense, it constitutes an interim report from the major investigative teams.

6

DORADO BEACH, 1972: CONFERENCE ON CHILDREN AT RISK FOR SCHIZOPHRENIA

Instrumental in its contribution to the expansion of risk research was a conference held a decade ago – our historical referent. Its supportive parent was Dr. Loren Mosher, then Director of the newly formed Center for Studies of Schizophrenia at the National Institute of Mental Health. Mosher had fostered a monographic length report on the status of high-risk research (Garmezy & Streitman, 1974; Garmezy, 1974) and then strongly supported a grant request from the senior author to hold a 5-day Conference on Research on Risk for Schizophrenia. That application carried a request for 2 years' support of visitations among risk research groups to do several things: enlarge the research enterprise; extend the possibilities of collaboration; generate mini-conferences for the research groups; and provide outside consultant support to the groups.

Out of the conference grew the *Consortium of Risk Research Groups in Schizophrenia.* This volume, a product of the consortium, stands as testimony to the generativity and wisdom of NIMH in sponsoring developmental studies uncontaminated by the tradition-bound retrospective methodologies that typified the early efforts to examine the longitudinal skein of schizophrenia.

The pages that follow in this chapter review that extraordinary conference. But why a recital of the contents of a conference held a decade ago? We believe that the questions posed at the conference provide a context for many of the answers that are now available and for the many unresolved issues that remain. As high-risk research expands into other areas of psychopathology (e.g., J. Becker, 1977; Beardslee, Bemporad, Keller, & Klerman, 1983; Weissman, 1979; Orvaschel, Weissman, & Kidd, 1980), the lessons learned at Dorado Beach bear repetition.

The conference was supported by NIMH with supplemental funding by the William T. Grant Foundation. Three major objectives were served:

1. The identification of an outstanding interdisciplinary group of investigators, selected for their expertness in areas relevant to risk research, irrespective of their specific research involvements;
2. The opportunity to catalogue and discuss many of the problems that were then beginning to emerge in studies of risk;
3. The presentation of early findings of the risk investigations that seemed to deserve further study.

Twelve research groups were represented at the conference, ten from ongoing projects in the United States and two from abroad. The panel of consultants numbered 17, covering a wide band of disciplines: developmental psychology, personality study, sociology, law, child and adult psychiatry, clinical psychology, neurophysiology, pediatric neurology, psychiatric genetics, developmental endocrinology, biochemistry, pediatrics, neonatology, psychophysiology, and obstetrics.

Also present were investigators and administrators of NIMH and the Grant Foundation. Publications of the participants were circulated as were prepared position papers. The latter were read at the conference followed by discussant panels made up of the consultants to the conference.

Six major topics were covered: (1) basic issues in risk research; (2) theoretical models of risk; (3) research strategies; (4) independent and dependent variables; (5) selection of subject populations; (6) ethical issues in risk research. The discussions are summarized in turn here with the first two combined due to the similarity of the issues discussed.

BASIC ISSUES AND THEORETICAL MODELS IN RISK RESEARCH

Researchers' theoretical perspectives obviously influence the types of basic questions they raise and the approaches their work takes. One major issue posed at the conference focused on questions concerning the nature of schizophrenia: How is it defined? How do we know when a person is schizophrenic? To what extent do changes in clinical psychiatric concepts affect psychiatric researchers?

Conference participants emphasized differential diagnosis and the importance of process–reactive, paranoid–nonparanoid, and acute–chronic distinctions. Many urged that the discrepancies between American nosology and the more conservative European systems of classification be recognized.

That warning was appropriate. Consider the radical shift in American diagnoses that took place with the appearance of the third revision of the American Psychiatric Association's *Diagnostic and Statistical Manual of Mental Disorders* (DSM III, 1980). Schizoaffective and schizophreniform disorders have removed a portion of schizophrenia's constituency as it existed in DSM II, and there have been even more powerful changes in the nomenclature and inclusion criteria for the affective disorders.

These changes have caught risk research groups in midstream and a rediagnosis of their parental cohorts is in order. Some projects already have reclassified their subjects thereby producing a marked shift in the size of the samples of potentially schizophrenic and potentially affectively disordered individuals.

Another basic lesson culled from the presentations of many participants was the need for caution in positing that a single disease entity is under study; many different disorders may be involved. If the latter holds, investigators should expect to find greater variability in the response patterns of targeted children. It should be noted that the more specific criteria that characterize schizophrenia in DSM III may help to reduce such variability.

The issue of continuity versus discontinuity in development is of fundamental concern to psychopathologists (Rutter, 1972, 1980). As was discussed at the conference, it has special significance for risk researchers because evidence for continuity would favor a selection of variables that would lean heavily on the literature of adult schizophrenia. Within such a framework, vulnerable children might be a bridging group between the behavior of normal children and disordered and/or remitting adult patients in terms of precursor indicators for disorder (R. F. Asarnow et al. 1977, 1978; R. F. Asarnow and Asarnow, 1982).

Differences expressed at the conference represented long-standing views of proponents on both sides of this issue. One advocate of a developmental-stage orientation indicated that because psychophysiology, forms of learning, and social behavior are so different at each stage of development, successful extrapolation from earlier behavior to adulthood is very unlikely. This individual favored research on behaviors salient at each developmental period. Opponents of this view noted evidence of stability of traits from age 3 through adulthood when one looks to heterotypic continuities (different behaviors reflecting the same underlying traits) rather than homotypic continuities (similar behaviors continuous over time).

A second noteworthy point introduced in these discussions was that it is the process of development that is critical rather than isolated variables, however changing or unchanging these may be.

A third theoretical issue which came up involved models of development. Simple mechanistic, linear hypotheses should be rejected, it was argued, in favor of transactional models of growth. There was probably the most general consensus on this point, with everyone recognizing the necessity for examining biological, behavioral, and social variables in conjunction with each other rather than as isolated aspects of the risk child's functioning. Trait and situation interact to form maladaptive response patterns just as they do in the development of adaptive personality patterns.

RESEARCH STRATEGIES

An entire session of the conference was devoted to the topic of research strategies, and much of the discussion focused on the question of cross-sectional versus longitudinal designs. Although the former clearly have an important role to play in identifying critical variables for longer-term investigations, in the search for the final criterion of schizophrenia or nonschizophrenia, longitudinal research has obvious advantages. It was noted by an infancy researcher that discontinuities of development are so marked in the first year that answers taken at a single period in time would be relatively useless in comparing high-risk and normal infants. Similarly it was argued by another that isolated measures of parent–child interaction at one particular age may be of limited significance because parenting tasks vary greatly as a child matures. The importance of differential life experiences at different ages and the possibility of children's "turn-arounds" in adaptation can be seen in some of the research programs. Such important reversals can be noted only in a longitudinal study. But accompanying the methodological virtues are known vices. A long time intervenes between the beginning and the end of a longitudinal study of children at risk for severe psychopathology. Not only do variables erode but so do investigators.

An important factor in evaluating the power of a longitudinal design is the recognition that although it effectively measures change, it does not specify causal relationships. Typically, the manner in which causal relationships are established is through the introduction and manipulation of independent variables, but this raises major ethical issues that will be considered in a later section. On a related note, however, a point was made by several conference participants that a variable need not have etiologic significance nor need it be traceable or continuous through development to be an important empirical precursor for a later clinical state. Discovery of a variable possessing such differential power would still provide an advance of considerable scientific merit. This observation raises an interesting point about scientific contributions in the field of risk research. Even if risk researchers look at variables that do not pay off in terms of bearing a relationship to schizophrenia, they can add to a general body of basic scientific knowledge, *provided* their choices of variables and methodology are sound.

One participant who had made major contributions to longitudinal study advised a "shotgun" approach, involving many different strategies and measures. Noting that a "rifle" approach would be more appropriate later on, he suggested that an initial broader strategy is preferable, provided one remains wary of chance effects. However, one of the problems that heightens chance variation is the size of a sample and, unfortunately, small Ns are a reality in risk research. Advice to seek larger numbers of subjects is splendid in theory but very difficult to execute. Efforts to coordinate the work of different researchers, such as have been carried out by the consortium are certainly a step in the right direction.

A developmental psychologist suggested a rather different research strategy which he referred to as the "risk-emergent" approach. In this approach, timing of the emergence of a behavior or a physiological condition would determine the selection of the dependent variable. It was his contention that such a design would have an advantage over others, which examined more typical kinds of dependent variables, while overlooking the fact that children of a given age may be at different developmental stages with regard to the manifestation of a particular behavior. Parental contributions to later pathological development, this participant warned, may reflect the actions of an infant "off schedule" in some manner that adversely affects its parents, their caretaking relationship, and the quality of the social interaction between parent and infant.

A sociologist present at the conference pressed the design advantages of large random stratified samples to increase the number of case subgroups which could be followed from birth. To compensate for the small number of schizophrenics anticipated on a probability basis, he suggested including schizoid and other related types to increase the subject pool – a recommendation that he based on field studies suggesting that perhaps half of all psychotics were actually so diagnosed and were known to clinical services. Such an approach, he contended, would reduce the biases inherent in the more typical selection procedure of requiring a diagnosis of schizophrenia in a biological parent which, although providing a tenfold increase in "hits," in the offspring fails to account for 90% of patients diagnosed as schizophrenic. It was this individual's impression that when children of brain-damaged parents, welfare parents, very low socioeconomic and single schizophrenic parents are compared, the rates of schizophrenia in these children will not be markedly different. If this observation is correct, it would not be necessary to have a large random sample design. What would be required as risk controls (in addition to normal controls) would be multiple-risk groups in which the inclusion criteria reflected the hypothesized contributions to heightened risk for schizophrenia. To some extent this has been attempted, although not in the systematic fashion advocated. In many programs the contrasting group has been the children of affectively disordered parents. In other cases control children matched for socioeconomic status of the family have ensured the inclusion of low SES samples.

Related to the sociologist's statements was the criticism that selection based on genetic considerations ignores the environmental component presumed to operate in a diathesis–stress formulation of schizophrenia. Disapproval was expressed by several participants that environmental factors have played little, if any, role in selection. Although family dynamics have been investigated in a number of research programs, the concerns about a creeping stereotypy in the mode of selection for risk seem appropriate.

ON SELECTING INDEPENDENT AND DEPENDENT VARIABLES

When David Rosenthal was asked what variables risk researchers should look at, he quipped: "The usual ones – cognitive, emotional, social, neurological, maturational, motor, integrative, sexual, familial, peer group." As the work reported in this volume attests, ongoing risk studies have followed this advice (see Garmezy, 1975b, pp. 186–191).

Variables have been chosen typically on the basis of (1) symptomatic-descriptive behaviors; or (2) laboratory findings with adult schizophrenic patients; or (3) those findings assumed to reflect schizotypic behaviors or trait dispositions thought to be precursors of clinical schizophrenia. The difficulties inherent in each approach were evident to the participants. These included the influence of nuisance factors such as the effects on behavior produced by institutionalization and medication, the absence of base rate data for the general normal population, and the difficulty of defining operationally constructs based on adult behavior when applied to children. Such realities are pressing ones even for advocates of a continuity hypothesis for schizophrenia.

One risk group chose a developmental–adaptational model in screening variables for use. Their choices were to search out screening techniques that would tap "cognitive ability, problem-solving skills, cognitive styles, attention, self-control behaviors, moral judgments and maturity, cooperative behaviors, and social skills" – categories which, in fact, have formed the basis for variable selection by many of the researchers.

A developmentalist moved in on the issue of construct validity, emphasizing the need to sample behaviors across a variety of situations. Important clues to risk factors depend on the selection of variables studied, especially if they capture inherent features of the risk children that are invariant over situation and time. This element of *pervasiveness*, or *ubiquity*, of a response pattern means that it reveals transsituational generalization and such hyperstability often contraindicates maturity, flexibility, and adaptiveness. In cases of childhood psychopathology such pervasiveness often suggest poor prognosis (Rutter & Garmezy, 1983).

The importance of blind assessments to avoid rater bias was also advanced. This requirement of ignorance of the subject's status is particularly important in risk studies where the number of available subjects is small.

We will avoid cataloguing all the suggestions for variables that were set forth at the conference, concentrating instead on several specific areas in an attempt to demonstrate the range of the discussions. One important category was maternal status variables. Participants called for measures of both trait and state factors: age, parity, physical and emotional condition throughout pregnancy, particular stresses of labor and delivery, nutritional status, smoking and drinking habits, health in general, history of prior breakdown, ages of children at home, pattern and severity of psychopathology, and personality prior to pregnancy.

One investigator urged that the risk investigator be present at delivery, whereas a physician recommended that risk researchers studying neonates employ their own obstetrical staff. It is crucial, he stated, that the obstetrician and pediatrician have experience with the specific disorder under study so as to prevent their anxiety from affecting the mother and infant, and that the same team care for all subjects. In his view a properly controlled study would show no relationship between perinatal complications and schizophrenia.

Other obstetrical experts at the conference shared reservations about the usefulness of any general category of so-called pregnancy complications. Such complications are not additive, they noted, given the heterogeneous types of difficulties noted in the risk literature. Illness during pregnancy, placental insufficiency, cesarian section, and so on (there are literally hundreds of similar variables) should be viewed as stressors, exercising differential effects on fetal development as a function of the time of their occurrence. These experts argued that it was very unlikely that such conditions were either necessary or sufficient causes of schizophrenia.

Although some participants advocated study of the biological characteristics of genetically vulnerable infants, one neurobiological researcher expressed the view that in the absence of biochemical markers for schizophrenia in the already deviant population, it would be pointless to engage in a "fishing expedition" for biochemical variants in the infants.

A psychophysiologist expressed the related view that there was little hope that psychophysiological studies of children could provide a direct road into the interpretation of basic physiological deficits in schizophrenia. He noted that because indices of psychophysiological functioning lack construct validity and are markedly affected by the situational context, one must be cautious in ascribing their manifestations to a fundamental deficit state. Systematic investigations of environment–subject interaction are called for, but, in his opinion, risk research is far from ready for the costly studies that would measure psychophysiological reactions as a function of subjects' perceptions of task demands.

In considering neurophysiological and psychophysiological variables another researcher urged strongly that work focus on the behavioral correlates of such responsiveness: attention, cognitive styles, and strategies.

Other foci suggested were intellectual and cognitive competencies, including verbal and nonverbal intelligence, the ability to generalize and abstract, short- and long-term memory, learning ability, and the functional use of language. Modes of coping such as persistence, curiosity, information-seeking, exploratory-style, impulse control, and responsiveness to situation and task also were emphasized along with the concerns that the measures possess *ecological validity* and that adequate developmental norms be available. In addition assessments of social competence as indexed by parents, peers, and teachers, embracing factors such as aggression, attention-getting, anxiety, dependency, depression, and popularity were recommended.

Teachers received more praise than is usual for their reliability in rendering judgments about a child's behavior. It was noted that because clinicians often make biased evaluations of children of disturbed parents, teachers may well do the same. Both as a caution and an ethic teachers should not be informed of the child's status in risk projects.

Another theme worthy of study was seen to be the patterns of interaction within high-risk families. In the chapters that follow the reader will be able to observe the extent to which such studies have yielded significant results both in terms of the social adaptiveness/maladaptiveness of children in different types of intrafamilial environments, and the extent to which such child behaviors resemble those which have been reported as likely precursors to a schizophrenic disorder. Efforts to learn about the families, it was urged, should embrace a combination of home visits, standardized interviews, and a broad spectrum of experimental procedures during which family members engage in interaction and problem-solving tasks. In such studies mother–target child and mother–sib comparisons may reflect the consistency of the mother's interactions with her children. Scoring and coding of behavior in these complex situations are necessarily elaborate and require marked sophistication in the investigator.

An important element in such studies is that they move researchers toward a transactional model. The family should be seen, it was advised, as a composite in which role relationships and assignments are important both in personality development and in magnitude of risk potential for the offspring.

A developmental psychologist described three characteristics that consistently appear conjointly in personality studies of young children and may be an early homologue of an introversion–extraversion dimension: (1) an intensity, enthusiasm, or "squeal" factor which may be related to arousal level; (2) an interpersonal activity factor that includes both positive and negative interactions; and (3) an assertiveness in dealing with other children. These are important variables, it was suggested, for risk researchers to consider. This view was reinforced by the emphasis others gave to the utility of measurements of temperament and of the intensity, duration, appropriateness, and variability of positive and negative affect.

One participant observed that global terms such as "maturity," "competence," and "adjustment" are vague and jargonistic. The attitudinal and social value meanings they convey can detract from the search for more differentiated variables.

At the conclusion of the discussion of variables a new element entered the discussion; this was a focus on the positive and adaptive characteristics that permit most children to escape psychopathology despite inordinate amounts of stress and deprivation. Other echoes of this theme were expressed: "Why do some children with a schizophrenic parent grow up to be normal?" Perhaps that "why" should be substituted with a "how," for that query implicates the construct of coping responses, their type and their origins. Recent events make it clear that if the 1970s are identified with an expansion of risk research, the 1980s may see the growth of studies of personal and environmental factors that conduce to the development of resistance to psychopathology in children, despite evidence of predispositional and stressful forces in their lives that would seem to make them candidates for later breakdown.

Studies of this sort are simply the reverse side of the coin of vulnerability research. The issues and variables discussed in the preceding sections also serve as the beginning points for the study of stress-resistant children.

SUBJECT POPULATIONS

Predicting breakdown in high-risk children and the even more specific status of subsequent schizophrenia poses a problem of inordinate difficulty. Given the low base rate for the disorder, numerous prediction failures are almost assured. From an accuracy-of-prediction standpoint a far lower proportion of incorrect predictions would occur were we to anticipate that no child of a schizophrenic parent would become schizophrenic. However, were one to see children of dual mated parents, as several participants advocated, the prediction of positive findings would improve markedly. One should expect a three to fivefold increase in schizophrenia in the children of such couples compared to the children of one schizophrenic parent. (See the later commentary by Erlenmeyer-Kimling and her colleagues describing the results of research with such contrasting groups.)

It was suggested too that researchers include in their studies the children of schizophrenic fathers. Also recommended were the offspring of various parental combinations: normal, definitely schizophrenic, possibly schizophrenic, not schizophrenic but psychotic, normal but related to a definite schizophrenic parent, that is, samples with different familial genetic loadings.

Cataloguing these various pairings from the comfort of an armchair is an engaging experience, but for those actively involved in the scientific enterprise of locating subjects and securing pedigree data the logistical difficulties posed have a nightmarish quality. For example, many individuals with a "schizophrenic" spectrum disorder are not hospitalized and have never had a psychiatric contact. Furthermore, for the researcher who wishes to study infants at risk the probability that a woman destined to become schizophrenic will have had her first breakdown prior to delivering her first child is low.

One investigator well-versed in studying mothers who give birth to a baby in the course of a psychotic episode commented on the need to assess the quality of the environment provided by the father or a surrogate caretaker as well as his (or her) mental health status. He pointed out that some families are cemented by parental psychosis whereas others break apart (B. Anthony, 1969b). Some healthy parents protectively intervene for their children; others ignore their spouse's deviance or even flee from it.

Other risk populations were discussed: premature infants, infants whose birth involved obstetrical complications, infants of families with a history of diabetes, epilepsy, or von Recklinghausen's disease, children with physical disabilities or handicaps, children who maintained dyssocial relations with peers, teachers and/or family, and so on.

Evaluation of differential risk would consider the histories of the different groups while focusing on the question: "Are these factors together with the nature of the intrafamilial environment conducive to the differential development of forms of psychopathology more severe in one group when compared with others?"

Sociologists reminded conference participants of other elements of risk: minority group membership, very large family size, poverty, poor quality family life, and so forth.

The question of the most appropriate age at which to study children elicited considerable debate. Some participants argued for the choice of neonates, viewing them as "the last stage in ontogenesis when the intrinsic biological constitution . . . can be assessed." Other participants felt that 2- and 3-year-olds or even older children provided a better source for exploring risk factors.

There were adherents too of the view that late childhood and adolescence were particularly worthy periods for studying risk. They noted that the cumulative quality of pathological development through childhood makes behavioral deviations more evident in the 12- to 16-year-old group. The onset of puberty with its concomitant biological and psychological demands adds to the likelihood of stress potentiation. Furthermore it was argued that the use of an older age group reduces the length of the longitudinal inquiry necessary for determining a terminal criterion of breakdown versus nonbreakdown while at the same time allowing an examination of a premorbid period closer in time to such breakdowns.

One developmentalist wisely recommended that the questions being asked should determine the age group studied. If an investigator's primary emphasis is the identification of offspring of schizophrenics who are truly at risk, then the focus belongs in the adolescent years. If, on the other hand, one is interested in the range of difficulties encountered by such children and the patterns of adaptation they use in meeting such stressors, then he or she should begin the study at an earlier age in the lives of the index children.

The issue of sex differences arose in the conference discussions as well. Data on male and female children should be analyzed separately, it was advised. Although several investigators reported male–female differences, a voice of dissent was raised by a sociologist who contended that sex, as a predictor variable, is highly overrated and that most observed differences arise out of stereotypic role notions promulgated by teachers and parents as to what is appropriate behavior for boys and girls. (Although this may be true, it seems inappropriate to negate the potential significance of sex differences in risk research simply because observed differences reflect environmental as well as biological variations.)

Other investigators urged that risk children be classified not only on the basis of age and sex, but also in terms of social class, history of institutionalization or foster placement, and early versus late breakdown of their mothers.

A discussion of the difficulties of follow-up in selected cases of risk arose in the context of status variables. Because chronic schizophrenic patients have such disruptive life experiences and fragmented family ties, those parents who can be followed may be unrepresentative of the pool of schizophrenics.

The issue of generalization took another significant turn: what of those who refuse to participate? Studies have indicated that persons who refuse differ systematically from those who agree to be studied. There is strong evidence too for differences between treated and untreated samples. Does the fact of participation itself add to the unrepresentativeness of the sample of persons under review because of differences reflected in voluntarism?

As for control groups, special emphasis was given to comparing children at genetic risk for schizophrenia with persons who are at risk for other disorders by virtue of different genetic or biochemical indicators. It was recommended also that a variety of deviant groups be compared with the so-called potential schizophrenic group. Matched controls based on age, race, intelligence and social class were additional factors suggested. Because so many factors previously considered precursors of schizophrenia have been shown to be associated with other disorders as well, it was deemed crucial that controls permit specification of factors unique to schizophrenia. This observation, however accurate, raises the unresolved problem: "Wherein does the search for specificity lie?"

Finally, whereas earlier data analyses dwelt on mean differences between risk and control groups, more recent analyses have searched for "outlier" subjects within the risk group. There are indications that such markedly different children more closely approximate the 10% figure of actualized risk in children with a single parent who has received a diagnosis of schizophrenia.

ETHICAL ISSUES

Professor William Curran of the Harvard Law School and the Harvard School of Public Health acted as consultant on the issue of ethical considerations in risk research. For a detailed treatment of his views readers are referred to his final report, *A Review of Legal Precedents and Medical Ethics Involved in Intervention with Children at Risk for Schizophrenia*, submitted in July, 1973 to the Center for Studies of Schizophrenia at NIMH.

Curran remarked that in some ways risk researchers are fortunate. They are not involved in administering or witholding drugs, in removing or transplanting an organ, in issues of abortion, artificial insemination, sterilization, or brain death. Instead, he noted, they must be concerned with the matters of *informed consent, privacy*, and *confidentiality*, and to that triad, one should add the problem of *identifying* and *labeling* a child who is at risk.

Despite the "benign" nature, in Curran's view, of most risk investigations, they do tap three sensitive areas: (1) they are essentially psychiatric studies (but not entirely so); (2) they examine children, the group theoretically most protected by society; and (3) they usually are long-term prospective studies which involve unusual obligations over extended periods of time for the families that elect to participate.

The problem of labeling a child as "at risk" can produce, in the words of one participant, a "reverse Pygmalion effect." Furthermore, the possibility of an overly heavy concentration of lower-class families and minority groups is an added problem that may not be due entirely to the epidemiology of schizophrenia, but rather to the disproportionate number of poor people who are sent to state hospitals during a psychotic episode. A growing militancy in these groups against being labeled and studied adds to the ethical problems. Another consideration described by Curran is the use of captive groups such as current and ex-mental patients, inmates of correctional institutions, and schoolchildren. Protecting the civil rights of such groups has become a major concern of human rights organizations.

Another issue which was discussed centered on the legal or moral competence of schizophrenic patients to give informed consent to their involvement in research. Can such parents give approval to the study of their children? To what extent do such studies heighten the anxiety of parents? If parents are unable to give consent validly, who will protect the children? Does the participation of children in risk studies meet the NIH guideline that such consent to research must be of *direct benefit* to the participating children themselves? Curran expressed the view that even in the absence of direct benefit, research should be permitted if it does not harm the children.

Of the many practical and ethical issues facing the risk researcher, these were described as most salient:

1. Although access to clinical information for aggregating data typically does not require the consent of the individual patient, the use of case records to contact individuals is a breach of confidentiality and privacy which can interfere with the patient's relationship with other physicians.
2. Equivalent problems exist with regard to children's school records, achievement-test scores, and teacher evaluations. If students are to be tested individually, parental informed consent clearly is required. Schools possess a limited right to open themselves to investigators. Classrooms are not completely public, and a pupil's participation in a research project within school boundaries is best limited to those studies that serve some educational purpose.
3. Access to a researcher's data should be restricted. Records might best be labeled "psychiatric" to ensure this provision. Because many risk studies are of a long-term nature, a question is posed as to whom should data that have been gathered be made available: An attending physician? Clinicians interested in preventive work? Adults considering adoption of a high-risk child?

These are all complex problems, but there was basic concurrence that school officials, particularly teachers, should be kept blind to an individual child's risk status so as to avoid jeopardizing the child's normal development in the school setting.

In addition to the issue of whether mental patients may give informed consent, Curran raised the question as to whether the children too should be consulted in the process. The complications stemming from such a seemingly neutral act were evident in a sensitive reminder by one investigator that children of psychotic mothers differ in the extent to which they have been informed about the illness and in their means for coping with such knowledge. Judgments about revelation of such information must be made on an individual case basis.

Curran suggested that the greatest danger in this area arises when no consent is sought, or when subterfuge emphasizing treatment, is used. Partial deception, in particular, must be avoided. It was urged that risk researchers look to the spirit rather than the letter of the law; under certain circumstances, a subject might be better protected by ignorance of potentially harmful information. Realistic appraisals of these difficult decisions must be made by individual investigators who have consulted with their peers. The issue of the researcher's responsibility to withhold specific information should be conditioned by the reliability and validity of the material, its traumatic import, and its possible utility for the individual subject. The likelihood that a child's strengths and potential for adaptation may become evident rather than weaknesses and vulnerabilities is an important factor that modifies the nature of information-giving.

One participant suggested that treatment of the participating subjects may be undesirable, bearing the element of coerciveness, although making referrals available to former patients and their families may reduce such coercive implications.

There was general agreement with the observation that follow-up inquiries are an important and legitimate part of medicine, to which patients tend to respond positively rather than negatively.

A related question concerned the amount of effort one should expend in pursuing subjects for follow-up. If an active response to an inquiry is demanded of research participants, an erosion of the subject pool follows. Should investigators write, call, or appear on a subjects' doorsteps? Good judgment and sensitivity on the part of the experimenter are demanded in resolving these problems equitably.

There is no better way to close this report of what proved to be a very significant conference than to quote the words of John Romano, who contributed much to the discussion of ethics.

In the main, those of us who will be engaged in studies of vulnerability or invulnerability to psychopathology of children born to parents, one or both of whom are, or have been, mentally ill, must afford our subjects the dignity and compassion which will earn us their trust. We must assure them and ourselves (1) that the information to be obtained in our studies sufficiently warrants whatever inherent risks there may be to the subject; (2) that the investigation be conducted by properly qualified persons; (3) that all the criteria for the informed consent be satisfied with particular care for the children, and (4) that the welfare, safety, and comfort of the subject remain a paramount concern so that should the subject require special aid, we should be alert and equipped to respond to his needs.

In the research programs that follow, an ethical, able group of investigators have sought to maintain these criteria set forth by one of psychiatry's most distinguished leaders. As for the content of these programs, they also give indications of the extent to which the risk researchers at the conference profited by the vigorous discussions and suggestions advanced by their colleagues and the invited consultants.

PART I

The Danish High-Risk Project: 1962–1982

Around the turn of this century Adolph Meyer remarked that we have no greater need than for a well-documented life history of a schizophrenic. We have lots of those now, almost all of them retrospective, and we know very little more now than Meyer knew then about the causes and premorbid course of schizophrenic disorders. The strategic dilemma in this task is obvious: Schizophrenia occurs in the lifetime of only 1 or 2 persons out of every 100, and it is very rarely manifest before adolescence. Hence we have been forced to depend on recollections by those afflicted and by their acquaintances and relatives. It is transparent and well documented that such recollections are subject to subtle distortions through selective retention and various psychological defenses; moreover they present the serious scientific shortcoming of being incomplete and unsystematic.

Patently, the solution to this problem is to observe and describe schizophrenic people before they are manifestly schizophrenic, but that is more easily said than done. Sarnoff Mednick has a talent for audaciously creative research designs. Noting the actuarial fact that 10 ± 4% of the offspring of schizophrenics become schizophrenic themselves, he reasoned that the awesome magnitude of such a scientific fishing expedition could be reduced tenfold by studying the children of schizophrenic parents. An initial effort to mount such a project in Michigan foundered in the late 1950s, whereupon Mednick crossed the ocean to the tiny kingdom of Denmark, which possessed an elaborate national archive system for tracing families and individuals. The Danes are less zealous than Americans about protecting individual rights and privacy, or more circumspect about balancing those important protections against the benefits of scientific knowledge. Hence in 1961 the pioneering high-risk project that couldn't work in Michigan was launched successfully in Copenhagan, Denmark.

Mednick forged a close collaborative alliance with Fini Schulsinger, a Danish psychiatrist. That collaboration has been both durable, remaining quite active to this day, and fertile, giving rise to the landmark cross-fostering studies of Kety and Rosenthal and, more recently, to longitudinal studies of alcoholism and criminality. The Mauritius Project, with significant sponsorship by the World Health Organization, was another spinoff from the original Danish High-Risk Project. Part I presents comprehensive reports from both of these ground-breaking ventures.

19

2 The Danish High-Risk Project: recent methods and findings

S. A. MEDNICK, R. CUDECK, J. J. GRIFFITH,
S. A. TALOVIC, AND F. SCHULSINGER

It is by now clear to most investigators that the retrospective study of the origins of psychopathology has certain inherent methodological problems which are difficult to overcome (S. A. Mednick & McNeil, 1968). Many of these limitations can be minimized or overcome by the use of a prospective longitudinal design, which involves the identification of a subject sample prior to psychiatric breakdown and includes periodic reassessment of these individuals on a well-specified set of variables considered to be of theoretical importance. Although the ideal sample would include an entire birth cohort, practical considerations make additional sample selection necessary – particularly when investigating a disorder with a low prevalence in the general population, such as schizophrenia. It was thus for reasons of "efficiency" that a group of children at high risk were originally selected for the prospective longitudinal study of the etiology of schizophrenia.

HISTORY

The research program for the Danish High-Risk Study of Schizophrenia was first formulated in 1960 (S. A. Mednick, 1960) and implemented in Copenhagen in 1962. In 1962, we intensively examined 207 children of mothers whose schizophrenic disorders would be diagnosed as typical and severe both in Europe and the United States. We also assessed 104 low-risk control children who had had no member of their immediate family hospitalized for mental illness for three generations. This was determined by reference to the National Psychiatric Register of the Demographic Institute, Aarhus, which maintains a central file for every psychiatric hospitalization in Denmark going back to 1916. Table 1 presents the characteristics of the high-risk and low-risk groups at the time of their initial assessment in 1962. We attempted to match for their having been reared in a children's home. The average age of the sample was 15.1 years; they ranged from 9 to 20 years of age.

Table 2 presents a list of the procedures and examinations employed for all subjects. During the examination, the examiners did not know whether a subject was a high-risk (HR) or low-risk (LR) individual.

21

Table 1. *Characteristics of the experimental and control samples*

	Control	Experimental
Number of cases	104	207
Number of boys	59	121
Number of girls	45	86
Mean age[a]	15.1	15.1
Mean social class[b]	2.3	2.2
Mean years education	7.3	7.0
Percentage of group in children's homes (5 years or more)[c]	14%	16%
Mean number of years in children's homes (5 years or more)[c]	8.5	9.4
Percentage of group with rural residence[d]	22%	26%

[a]Defined as age to the nearest whole year.

[b]The scale runs from 0 (low) to 6 (high).

[c]We only considered experience in children's homes of 5 years or greater duration. Many of the experimental children had been to children's homes for brief periods while their mothers were hospitalized. These experiences were seen as quite different from the experience of children who actually had to make a children's home their home until they could go out and earn their own living.

[d]A rural residence was defined as living in a town with a population of 2,500 persons or fewer.

Table 2. *List of experimental measures at 1962 high-risk assessment*

Psychophysiology
    A. Conditioning–extinction–generalization
    B. Response to mild and loud sounds
Wechsler Intelligence Scale for Children (Danish adaption)
Personality inventory
Word association test
Continuous Association Test
    A. 30 words
    B. 1 min of associating to each word
Adjective checklist used by examiners to describe subjects
Psychiatric interview
Interview with parent or rearing agent
School report from teacher
Midwife's report on subject's pregnancy and delivery

INITIAL FINDINGS: THE SICK, WELL, AND CONTROL
GROUP COMPARISONS

Following the intensive examination in 1962, an alarm network was established in Denmark so that most hospital and all psychiatric admissions for anyone in this sample would be reported to us. The number of reports of serious psychiatric or social breakdowns reached 20 in 1967. Very brief summaries of their case descriptions are provided by S. A. Mednick (1970) and Mednick and Schulsinger (1973). We then looked back to the 1962 initial assessment data in order to find characteristics that distinguished those who suffered breakdowns (the Sick group) from carefully matched HR (the Well group) and LR (the Control group) controls. The most important characteristics distinguishing the Sick group from the other two groups are as follows:

1. The Sick group lost contact with their mothers much earlier in their lives than did the other two groups. Average age at separation for the Sick group was 4.0 years, whereas the combined average age for the Well and Control groups was 8.25 years. For the Sick group, mother's absence was, in every case, due to psychiatric hospitalization.

2. Rather than confirming the classic textbook picture of the preschizophrenic child, the teachers' reports indicated that Sick group subjects tended to be highly disturbing in class. The Sick subjects were significantly more often described as being disciplinary problems, domineering, aggressive, creating conflicts, and disrupting the classroom with their talking.

3. On the Continuous Association Test, Sick subjects exhibited a strong and significant tendency to produce a whole series of interrelated but contextually somewhat irrelevant responses. They also tended to drift away from the stimulus word during the response period significantly more than the Well subjects.

4. A number of psychophysiological anomalies characterized the electrodermal responses (EDR) of the Sick group: markedly fast latency of response, little evidence in the response latency measure of habituation, resistance to experimental extinction of the conditioned EDR, and a remarkably fast rate of recovery following response peak.

5. The Sick group evidenced considerably more pregnancy and birth complications. An interesting sidelight with respect to these perinatal events is the fact that the HR group that had not suffered breakdown (the Well group) presented fewer perinatal difficulties than did the LR control group. This suggested to us that perhaps there is a special interaction between the genetic predisposition for schizophrenia and pregnancy and delivery complications. It was almost as if in order for a HR subject to fare well, a complication-free pregnancy was needed. In the paper reporting the findings (S. A. Mednick, 1970), mention was made of the fact that there was a marked correspondence between the pregnancy and birth complications and the deviant electrodermal behavior. Almost all of the electrodermal differences between the groups could be explained by these perinatal difficulties in the Sick group. The perinatal difficulties in the LR group were not as strongly associated with these extreme electrodermal effects. This further suggested that the pregnancy and delivery complications trigger some characteristics that may be genetically predisposed.

Table 3. *1972 Follow-up results with 1962 samples*

	High risk (N = 207)	Low risk (N = 104)
Full assessment complete	173	91
Home interview only (social worker)	10	6
Not yet contacted		
(Parent objected or the subject		
could not be located)	6	2
Living abroad	6	0
Deceased[a]	6	0
Subject refused	6	5

[a]Ten of the high-risk subjects have died in the course of the follow-up. Of the 10, 6 died before the assessment began; 4 took part in the assessment.

THE THEORY

A minitheory (S. A. Mednick, 1958) has guided (but not dominated) this longitudinal project. It suggested that the syndrome of schizophrenia is an evasion of life, learned on the basis of physiological predispositions. When exposure to an unkind environment is combined with possession of an autonomic nervous system (ANS) that responds too often and too much *and* an abnormally fast rate of autonomic recovery, this gives rise to an aptitude for learning evasive avoidance responses. If an individual is to become schizophrenic, he must possess both the ANS responsiveness *and* recovery characteristics. If an individual is rapidly, exaggeratedly, and untiringly emotionally reactive, he may become anxious or even psychotic, but will not tend to learn schizophrenic responses, unless his rate of recovery tends to be very fast. It also seems likely that an extraordinarily reactive ANS will only require moderately fast recovery, whereas an extraordinarily fast rate of recovery will only require moderate reactiveness. Both very high reactiveness and very fast recovery will result in a strong predisposition for avoidance learning and hence for schizophrenia.

1972 DIAGNOSTIC ASSESSMENT

From an earlier study by Niels Reisby (1967) at the Copenhagen Psychological Institute, we could estimate that at the average age of 25 years, that is in 1972, we should be able to diagnose approximately half of the eventual schizophrenics in the group. Thus, at that time we initiated an intensive assessment of the HR and LR samples. The central goal of this reassessment was to establish a reliable diagnosis and evaluate their current life status.

The 1972 assessment consisted of psychophysiological and cognitive tests, a social interview, and, most importantly, a battery of diagnostic devices. The diag-

Table 4. *Identifying characteristics of high and low risk subjects participating in full interview (1972)*

	High risk	Low risk
Number – full interview	173	91
Mean age at 1962 assessment	14.9	15.1
Mean social class	2.1	2.4
Number of males	97	53
Number of females	76	38

nostic devices included a 3.25 hour clinical interview by an experienced diagnostician, a full Minnesota Multiphasic Personality Inventory (MMPI), and psychiatric hospitalization diagnoses and records where they existed. Both the Current and Past Psychopathology Scales, or CAPPS, and Present Status Examination, or PSE (9th edition) were completed by the interviewer. Computer diagnoses were obtained from the PSE and CAPPS materials. Details of the assessment have been published (Mednick, Schulsinger, & Schulsinger, 1975; Schulsinger, 1976).

Table 3 presents information on the results of our follow-up contacts with the subjects. Ten of the high-risk subjects have died in the course of the follow-up: seven by suicide, two by accidental causes, and one by natural cause. None of the low-risk subjects has died. This is a dramatic difference which we shall explore further. Of the ten, six died before the assessment began; four took part in the assessment. Thus, of the 201 high-risk subjects available for the assessment, 91% took some part in the interview (10 only had a home interview by the social worker). Of the low-risk subjects 91 took part in the full interview, and 6 took part in the home interview. Thus, 93% of the Low-Risk group has taken some part in the interview.

Table 4 presents identifying information on those who completed the full interview. The groups are well matched with each other and with the total original sample in respect to age, sex, and social class.

Diagnosis

The diagnosis of schizophrenia made by the interviewer is based on the presence of Bleuler's primary symptoms (thought disorder, autism, ambivalence, and emotional blunting), as well as Bleuler's secondary symptoms (delusions and hallucinations). For a diagnosis of schizophrenia it was not necessary that all of these symptoms be observed at the time of the interview; they might also be drawn from the case history. In two separate papers (Mednick et al., 1975; Schulsinger, 1976) detailed descriptions of the tests of the reliability of the diagnoses have been reported. For our purposes here, it is sufficient to say that across the two computer-derived diagnoses, the MMPI (analyzed blindly by Irving Gottesman), and the clinical diagnosis, as well as independent diagnoses arrived at by two Danish psychiatrists listening to the audiotape of the entire interview for ten subjects, excellent diagnostic agreement was achieved. (We wish to thank Lise Hauge and Raben Rosenberg for their work on the reliability tests.)

RESULTS OF 1972 ASSESSMENT: DISTINGUISHING PREMORBID
CHARACTERISTICS OF THOSE DIAGNOSED SCHIZOPHRENIC

Fifteen of the HR subjects received a diagnosis of "schizophrenia" by consensus on two of the following methods: PSE, CAPPS, and clinical diagnosis. Two other HR subjects were diagnosed schizophrenic from hospital records; they were among the subjects who died before the assessment.

In an initial overview of the data, we noted that the high-risk subjects who later became schizophrenic were significantly characterized by the following premorbid factors (in comparison with the other high-risk subjects):

1. Their mothers evidenced a more severe course of illness.
2. The schizophrenics had been separated from their parents and many had been placed in children's homes quite early in their lives.
3. The perinatal difficulties for the schizophrenic group were greater than for the other groups.
4. The schoolteachers reported that the schizophrenics were extremely disturbing to the class, easily angered, violent, and aggressive.
5. The autonomic-nervous-system recovery rate as measured in 1962 was found to predict to later schizophrenia. This was especially true for persons suffering symptoms of hallucinations and delusions and thought disorder.

Pregnancy and birth complications

Parnas, Schulsinger, Teasdale, Schulsinger, Feldman, and Mednick (1982) reviewed midwife reports with a view to assessing possible relationships between pregnancy and birth complications (PBCs) and later schizophrenic breakdown.

Because previous work has shown that the low frequency of any single PBC in a relatively small group makes statistical analysis difficult, and because a variety of PBCs may result in similar effects, a method was developed that would express the general danger of each individual's pregnancy and delivery in a small number of aggregate scores. Each possible type of PBC was assigned a weight reflecting its severity in accordance with obstetrical research and clinical opinion. The summary scores derived from these weights are: (1) number of complications; (2) degree of severity of complications; and (3) weighted sum complications (the sum of the weights of observed PBCs).

The results revealed that the schizophrenics had a significantly higher number of complications, severity of complications, and weighted sum complications than the other HR and the LR subjects.

Several severe complications were uncommon in the HR and LR groups, but occurred in schizophrenics. Three (18%) of schizophrenics had their delivery hampered by abnormal fetal positions. Abnormal fetal positions were not observed in the LR group; they were present in eight (5%) of the HR group. Two of the schizophrenic group (12%) were born with their umbilical cords around their necks; this condition was observed in three of the HR group (2%) and two of the LR group (2%). Uncommon difficulties occurring in other members of the schizophrenic group included: asphyxia, placenta abnormalities, prematurity, and pelvic contractions.

Maternal characteristics

Talovic, Mednick, Schulsinger, and Falloon (1980) analyzed the psychiatric hospital records of the members of HR children to determine whether any of the maternal characteristics were predictive of later breakdown in their children. They found two variables that appeared to discriminate independently those children who suffered schizophrenic breakdown from those who did not: (1) one of the psychotic episodes of the mother was precipitated by and occurred within 6 months of childbirth ($\phi = .54$, $R^2 = .29$); and (2) the mother was unstable in her relations with men ($\phi = .29$, R^2 increment$= .09$). These two variables account for 38% of the schizophrenic/nonschizophrenic diagnostic variance in a multiple regression equation.

Talovic et al. (1980) demonstrated that early parental separation, which might be associated with puerperal psychosis, was not the factor responsible for this relationship; the childbirth that preceded the mother's psychotic episode often involved only the siblings of the index child. It also appeared that, even though mothers who suffered from puerperal psychosis tended to become ill earlier than other mothers, age of onset did not account for all of the prognostic significance of the puerperal psychosis variable.

Mother's instability in relations with men proved to be related to three other factors: antisocial behavior, irregular work history, and drug or alcohol addiction.

Talovic et al. (1980) noted that: "The independence of these two factors (mother's puerperal psychosis and instability in relations with men) ($r = .01$) suggests that perhaps they are each 'explaining' separate subgroups of the schizophrenic children. It will be interesting to explore the possibility that these subgroups have differing symptom and outcome characteristics which might meaningfully relate to the maternal symptoms."

Another approach we are taking involves a search for personal characteristics or life experiences that increase the resistance of high-risk children to severe psychopathology. For example, we are asking, "What characteristics of the schizophrenic mother might protect her children from a schizophrenic outcome?" One research direction we are taking focuses on the high-risk individuals diagnosed as *borderline*. Borderlines represent a group of patients clinically similar to schizophrenics, but not as seriously disordered and able to function in society. The borderline patient is resistant to an eventual schizophrenic outcome. The question of interest thus becomes: "Would borderline individuals have been schizophrenic had not certain protective factors intervened?" We are examining our data bank to determine antecedent factors that differentiate the borderline from the schizophrenic.

Preliminary analyses indicate that borderline schizophrenics have mothers who became schizophrenic at a later age than the mothers of schizophrenics. In addition, the mothers of borderlines tended to be diagnosed paranoid schizophrenic, rather than simple or hebephrenic. The mothers of the schizophrenics tended to be treated with radical interventions such as lobotomy and have suffered a surprising amount of postpartum psychosis; not so for the mothers of the borderlines. Some of these facts suggest that the mothers of the borderlines were less seriously schizophrenic than the mothers of the schizophrenics. Perhaps these more seriously ill mothers transmit a more influential genetic factor to their children. On the other hand, the amount of familial mental illness differentiates mothers of borderlines from those of normals and neurotics, suggesting that the genetic influence is greater for borderlines than for normals and neurotics. It is not a new hypothesis that the genetic influence is greatest for schizophrenics, least for normals and nuerotics, with borderlines falling between.

The rearing environment of the borderlines also seems to have been less pathogenic than that of the schizophrenics. The mothers of the borderlines tended *not* to be drug or alcohol addicts, unstable in work, unstable with men, aggressive, or apathetic (as were the mothers of the schizophrenics). They were emotionally attached and married to the fathers of their child. All of this suggests a more stable rearing environment for the borderline offspring. Moreover, on these same factors, the mothers of the borderlines resembled closely the mothers of normals and neurotics, suggesting that (with respect to these maternal factors) the rearing environment of the borderlines was as stable as that of the normals and neurotics.

Thus, we may tentatively conclude that the borderlines may be less genetically predisposed to schizophrenia than schizophrenics and more predisposed than normals and neurotics; in addition, the rearing environment of the borderlines seems to have been more stable than that of the schizophrenics.

School report data

John, Mednick, and Schulsinger (1982) examined teachers' reports on those HR subjects for whom a 1972 consensus diagnosis of schizophrenia was available. In every case, the teacher chosen to complete the report had known the subject for either 3 or 4 years. A Bayesian approach was employed to determine whether there were specific school-report items forming the basis for decision rules that could be used to identify those individuals with an especially high risk of later being diagnosed schizophrenic or borderline.

The findings were consistent with earlier, preliminary reports relating 1962 reports of school behavior to membership in the 1967 Sick group. School behavior predictive of later schizophrenic breakdown was different from that predictive of later diagnosis as borderline or no mental illness. In addition, the patterns of items predictive for males in the schizophrenic and borderline groups were different from those for females. The male preschizophrenic was generally characterized as behaving inappropriately in school and as constituting a discplinary problem for the teacher. He was viewed as anxious, lonely, and restrained. The male later diagnosed as borderline was seen by the teacher as isolated and distant. Both the female preschizophrenic and preborderline were described as anhedonic, withdrawn, disengaged, and isolated. The female preschizophrenic, however, was seen as being poorly controlled, whereas the female preborderline was characterized as overly restrained.

INTELLECTUAL AND COGNITIVE FUNCTIONING

Verbal associative disturbances

In order to determine whether premorbid verbal associative disturbance was characteristic of those high-risk subjects who later experienced breakdown, we analyzed the single-word and Continuous Association Test behaviors of these individuals, which were assessed in 1962. Griffith, Mednick, Schulsinger, and Diderichsen (1980) found that the high-risk individuals who later became schizophrenic did not manifest premorbidly more deviant associative responses than the other high-risk subjects. In fact, they did not produce premorbidly a significantly greater number of deviant responses than the low-risk subjects.

Griffith et al. (1980) "considered the possibility that this lack of observable associative disturbance prior to onset of schizophrenia was due to the subjects' awareness of the peculiarity of their thoughts, which they might have hidden by screening of inappropriate responses. However . . . they did not exhibit longer latencies to a greater extent than the high-risk subjects who did not become schiziphrenic" (p. 129).

Because of the unexpected nature of these findings, work is now underway in Copenhagen on an analysis of the content of the associations of the schizophrenic–nonschizophrenic subjects. In addition, an analysis of the associations by sex is planned.

Intelligence test performance

Walker, Hoppes, Mednick, and Schulsinger (1981) examined the premorbid intellectual functioning of the HR subjects as measured by the Wechsler Intelligence Scale for Children. HR subjects who were diagnosed as schizophrenic during the 1972 assessment did not differ significantly in Full-Scale IQ from same-sex nonschizophrenic HR subjects.

Verbal–Performance differences in IQ were substantially greater for the schizophrenic subjects, although the difference between the schizophrenic and nonschizophrenic females was not significant ($p < .10$). The patterns, however, were reversed for the schizophrenic males and females: The females showed higher Performance IQs, whereas the males exhibited higher Verbal IQs. The authors noted that the pattern observed was contrary to what would be expected on the basis of general male/female intellectual differences, and related this finding to other reported sex differences in schizophrenics. They outlined possible hypotheses based upon hemispheric asymmetrics in the two sexes.

DIMENSIONS OF CLINICAL STATUS AND LONGITUDINAL
SYNDROMES

In this section we will describe some of our more recent thinking and illustrate this
with the results of relevant data analyses. We will try to make the following points:

1. We find ourselves dissatisfied with traditional, dichotomous diagnostic systems.
2. We will suggest, instead, utilizing life syndrome diagnoses expressed as dimensions rather than dichotomies. The syndromes are also longitudinal, including
   antecedent conditions as well as dimensions to represent current clinical state.
3. We will make recommendations regarding methods of scale construction to measure dimensions of clinical status.
4. We will describe methods designed to deal with the problems of analyzing longitudinal data banks.

Problems in diagnosis

All of the foregoing research has utilized diagnostic divisions emphasizing discrete
categories of pathology. Some of the more recent work from the Danish High-
Risk Project has questioned the usefulness of categorizing individuals di-
chotomously as schizophrenic or not schizophrenic. This level of differentiation is
increasingly being viewed as inadequate.

This is equally true of the old divisions into paranoid, hebaphrenic, catatonic,
and simple, which have virtually been discarded. Carpenter, Bartko, Carpenter,
and Strauss (1976) found almost no symptomatic discrimination between these
traditional subtypes in the IPSS study. Others have expressed almost total dissatisfaction with the subtypes (Katz, Cole, & Lowery, 1964; Brill & Glass, 1965;
Munoz, Kulak, Marten, & Tuason, 1972). As Stephens (1978) has pointed out,
the diagnosis of schizophrenia has no invariant predictive value. Outcome is apparently no better related to a narrow Scandinavian diagnosis than to the typical
broad Bleulerian–American diagnosis (Hawk, Carpenter, & Strauss, 1975).
Strauss and Carpenter (1978) question the operational usefulness of the diagnosis
of schizophrenia. It does not, in itself, suggest etiology, treatment, or prognosis at
any useful level of precision. Certainly the diagnosis no longer implies universally
poor outcome. Strauss and Carpenter suggest that the diagnosis, schizophrenia,
may be putting under one heading several semi-independent or independent
disorders that have varying prognoses. In addition, current diagnostic systems
often make somewhat arbitrary distinctions between very similar disorders. When
individuals are shoehorned into categories, differences between the mildest
schizophrenic and the most severely ill borderline patient may not be meaningful.

Dimensions of clinical status

We would suggest, along with Strauss and Carpenter (1978) that it might be worth
attempting to define systematically these disorders in terms of continuously distributed variables. (Interestingly, as early as 1968 Bannister advocated such a

methodology.) As contributing measures to these continuously distributed variables, we would suggest clinical status characteristics and measurable aspects of the course of the illness, such as age of onset, work history, history of social functioning, and duration of symptoms. It seems reasonable that combinations of such variables must create subtypes of schizophrenia or define new ways of categorizing mental illness in terms of relatively independent dimensions. Since the dimensions are continuous, the interaction of these variables will, in theory, produce an infinite number of subtypes. An individual's "diagnosis" will then be defined by an intersect of the relevant dimensions. Strauss and Carpenter (1978) propose this diagnostic approach because it will yield more useful prognoses, will "imply the need for different specific treatments," and will be preceded by "somewhat different determinants."

Longitudinal syndromes

In the Danish High-Risk Project we have been attempting to define the schizophrenias by specific "longitudinal syndromes." For example, we have found that ANS variables are related to schizophrenia only in men who are characterized by more withdrawn and hallucinatory forms of schizophrenia (Mednick, Schulsinger, Teasdale, Schulsinger, Venables, & Rock, 1978). In a recent analysis by Talvoic (1980) we have seen that a pattern of high scores on schizoid, anhedonic, inexpressive, passive dimensions of clinical status in the HR children is related to symptoms of "dull affect" in their schizophrenic mother. We are attracted to this type of more limited relationship between specific antecedent factors and specific dimensions of clinical status. Whether some of these specific longitudinal syndromes can be collected in higher-order categories remains to be seen. The usefulness of such an approach to diagnosis is noted by Procci (1976). As he points out, diagnosis of schizoaffective psychosis, for example, is most accurately made when it is based not only upon the current symptom picture, but also upon premorbid social functioning, response to lithium-carbonate therapy, and family history. Prognosis also is most valid when based upon these multiple indices. Indeed, the approach has roots in the divisions into good and poor premorbid and into process–reactive types.

Methodological considerations

The description of the clinical status of our high-risk subjects by sets of reliable dimensions will require special statistical techniques permitting the relating of complex antecedent events differentially to the clinical status dimensions. We will describe methods we have utilized and illustrate these with the results of some analyses.

High-risk studies generate life-span data in remarkable quantity. A problem common to this type of research is the reduction of the data into a few meaningful dimensions, or scales, representing cogent aspects of the subjects' characteristics and experiences. In 1976 we made a first attempt to develop such dimensions.

This attempt involved factor analysis of diagnostic information. This analysis yielded five clinical status factors which were then related to antecedent events. Some illustrative analyses using these five factors are presented at the end of this section.

While these five factors yield interesting results when related differentially to antecedent events and characteristics, they represent only a limited range of the clinical status of the high-risk subjects. For this reason, a more ambitious and technically sophisticated attempt at constructing dimensions of clinical status was undertaken by Cudeck, Mednick, Schulsinger, and Schulsinger as described in Chapter 3 of this book.

METHODS OF LONGITUDINAL ANALYSIS

In this section we will present an example of our attempts to relate antecedent life experiences to clinical dimension outcomes. It is important, therefore, to summarize the methods by which these antecedent variables are related to the outcome, namely, "path analysis." The study presented as an example of the use of path analysis (Walker, Cudeck, Mednick, & Schulsinger, 1981) was a forerunner to the one presented later (Beuhring, Cudeck, Mednick, Walker, & Schulsinger, 1982). The latter study built upon the model produced by the Walker study but included an additional antecedent variable.

Complexity of statistical relationships

It is a part of our task in risk research to relate early life events and characteristics to later outcomes. As stated earlier, our variables are often quite numerous and complex (and well they should be to study human lives). We are aware that these life circumstances often influence life outcomes in a complex interactive manner. For example, in our own Danish research in schizophrenia, we are operating with variables that span the lifetimes of the individuals involved. We begin with the seriousness of the schizophrenia of the mother, examine perinatal factors, the intactness of the home, and consider all this in the light of socioeconomic status during rearing, autonomic nervous system functioning, and gender. We know that many of these independent variables are intercorrelated. For example, the earlier the onset of illness of the mother, the more separation from the mother the child experiences. Other, less obvious intercorrelations also exist in these data. Therefore, multiple analyses of individual independent variables in relationship to the dependent variable, schizophrenic outcome, run the risk of emphasizing a few common findings.

It is clear that stressing a few of these relationships ignores the fact that there is a wider fabric of interdependencies which should be explored. Thus, one difficulty with exploratory longitudinal studies is that the number of interrelated facets of behavior is quite large. Examining these factors two or three at a time is simply not an effective or satisfactory research strategy.

Problems with using single variables. At the same time, it is well known that individual measures of any given phenomenon, such as intelligence or psychopathology, are limited. They are limited for two reasons, both of which have serious consequences for the validity of analyses from longitudinal studies. The first reason is simply that psychological and behavioral variables are measured with error. Indeed, the cornerstone of psychometric theory is that measurement error is inherent in *every* test score (Lord & Novick, 1968; Nunnally, 1967). It is an interesting sociocultural phenomenon that researchers laboring in a given substantive field frequently retain a healthy skepticism about their own measures, but covet those from other fields that they suppose are more reliable. Witness, for example, the frequent, almost uncritical use of biological measures by psychologists who would normally demand the most rigorous proof of the reliability of a psychological measure. The point is not that one type of variable is "better" than another, but rather that both are measured with error and should be treated accordingly (Cliff, 1982).

The second limitation of single measures of a phenomenon has to do with the problem of validity. As a general rule, because we cannot be completely confident that our pet measure of thought disorder captures the essence of that construct, a necessary condition for the validity of a measure is that it correlate with other variables purporting to measure the same thing (Campbell & Fiske, 1959). For example, the reason the Stanford–Binet IQ is often accepted as a measure of intelligence is because it correlates with school performance, success on the job, and other types of behavior that are believed to be related to intelligence. Again, an interesting sociocultural commentary on research in the behavioral sciences is that we frequently demand the most strenuous standards of convergent validity for variables in some areas (e.g., the measurement of intelligence), but accept with an almost cavalier attitude the variables in others (e.g., diagnoses of psychopathology for treatment based on a single interview). The standard should be, instead, that we require the evidence of convergence between independently obtained measurements before we are satisfied that the construct has been adequately assessed.

Analysis of covariance structures. Obviously the ideal method of analyzing data from a longitudinal project would somehow include in the system several measures of each variable. Then the unreliability of any individual variable would be minimized. In addition, one could have confidence that the psychological constructs of interest are depicted more accurately. Furthermore, ideally one would include in the analysis as many aspects of the phenomenom as are potentially involved. Of course, no statistical technique could ever manage such an analysis if it were carried to the extreme. However, recent developments in statistical methods have made it possible to pursue this goal to a limited extent.

The general method to perform such an analysis has come to be called *analysis of covariance structures.* Jöreskog (1978) is generally credited with the most important contributions in this area, although several others have played major roles in its development. This name is derived from the fact that the method seeks to analyze the correlation or covariance among a group of variables into a more fundamental structure. Special cases of this general model are multiple regression, path analysis, and factor analysis. The strength of the method is that mixtures of these distinct approaches are now available together. That is, since our interest is in longitudinal designs, regression-type models are clearly important. Because we seek to describe complex relationships among a number of variables which may directly or indirectly influence an outcome such as schizophrenia, elements of path analysis may be desirable. And since we desire to minimize individual variables and emphasize convergent validity among several measures, many aspects of factor analysis theory are relevant. Inasmuch as the statistical work is still in its infancy and can be complicated, there are, as yet, no completely satisfactory introductions to the technique. However, the recent work of Bentler (1980), Kenney (1979), Maruyama and McGarvey (1980), and Nesselroade and Baltes (1979) should provide a good beginning. Examples using this method in the context of high-risk research will be discussed later.

The advantages of using the analysis of covariance structures approach can be only briefly discussed here. Suffice it to say that this method provides a first step in analyzing data from high-risk studies that seeks to operationalize many of the ideals of multiple-measurement research. The primary strength of the method is that it emphasizes the statistical relations among latent variables rather than measured variables. *Measured variables* are the typical bill of fare of all research work and may consist of test scores, rating scales, or behavior measures. *Latent variables*, on the other hand, are composites of measured variables. For example, a latent variable for social class (SES) might be constructed which uses several measured variables such as income, amount of education, occupational status, and a rating of neighborhood quality. By themselves, any of these four variables might be criticized as too limited a measure of the more global construct of SES. However, when the four are considered together, the composite they form together may be a very effective measurement system of SES.

In multiple regression analysis, which is perhaps the principal statistical model used in longitudinal research, the relationships between measured variables are examined. As we have seen, the success of such an analysis is dependent upon the reliability and validity of the variables used. Frequently, even the best variables can be criticized on these grounds. By contrast, in the analysis of covariance structures the relationships one studies are between latent variables. Therefore, the imperfections in any one variable can be minimized. For this and many other reasons, we recommend the method as an extremely useful tool in the analysis of data from high-risk projects.

EXAMPLES OF LONGITUDINAL ANALYSIS

In the Danish High-Risk Project we sought to determine the independent and joint influences of the following antecedent constructs on the child's subsequent clinical picture: amount of mother absence, amount of father absence, and institutional child care. Table 5 presents the latent variables that are considered in this

Table 5. *Observed variables associated with each latent construct*

Latent variable	Observed variables
Amount of mother absence	Mother's absence, Year 1
	Mother's absence, Year 2
	Mother's absence, Years 3–5
	Mother's absence, Years 6–10
Amount of father absence	Father's absence, Year 1
	Father's absence, Year 2
	Father's absence, Years 3–5
	Father's absence, Years 6–10
Institutionalization	During Year 1
	During Year 2
	During Years 3–5
	During Years 6–10
Clinical Construct 1	Psychopathy
	Social impairment
Clinical Construct 2	Paranoia
	Autism
Clinical Construct 3	Borderline schizophrenic features
	Hallucination symptoms
Clinical Construct 4	Hebephrenic symptoms
Clinical Construct 5	Thought disorder

study (Walker et al., 1981). Also presented are the measured variables that define the latent variables. Each latent variable is defined by two or more variables from the 1962 or 1972 data.

The relationships among these latent variables was investigated using the model shown in the diagram of Figure 1. As is the convention, the latent variables are shown as circles, and the measured variables are symbolized by boxes.

The path analysis yielded 12 path coefficients that were statistically significant. Significance was determined by comparing the coefficient with its standard error. Coefficients with absolute values greater than 1.96 times the standard error are considered significant. Significant coefficients and their probabilities are indicated in Figure 1. Nonsignificant path coefficients and path arrows are excluded for clarity. The results of the analyses are indicated by the solid lines in the path diagram for the male subjects and by broken lines for females. The paths indicate that maternal separation is more likely to result in institutionalization than is paternal separation. It is also clear that institutionalization bodes ill for the psychiatric status of the high-risk male. The path coefficient of .80 to thought disorder is rather impressive. Except for the mediation of institutionalization, this causal chain (maternal absence → institutionalization → schizophrenic clinical symptoms) is similar to results we have presented in previous publications (Mednick et al., 1975;

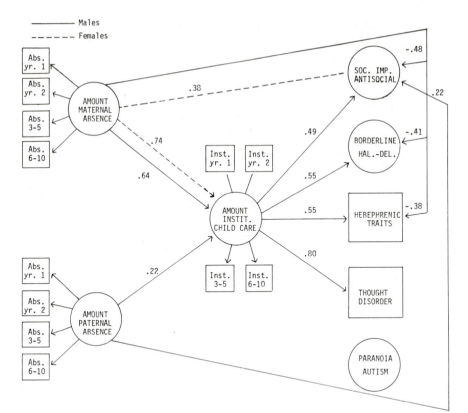

Figure 1. Path diagram for the prediction of clinical symptoms from amount of maternal absence, paternal absence, and institutional child care. (Walker, Cudeck, Mednick, & Schulsinger, 1981). Circles represent constructs (latent variables); boxes represent measured variables defining the constructs; arrows between the constructs illustrate statistically significant path coefficients.

Mednick et al., 1978). As was indicated, the earlier result was puzzling because it suggested that being removed from a severely schizophrenic mother was damaging to the high-risk child. This analysis makes clear that it is damaging because it most often results in institutionalization.

Note the male path arrows that lead directly from maternal absence to the clinical syndromes. These arrows pertain to those high-risk males who are separated from their schizophrenic mothers but do not go to children's homes. They are cared for by their fathers, grandmothers, or other relatives. These are negative and moderately strong relationships. The more these males experienced separation from their mothers (but not being sent to institutions), the less severe their psychopathology. Thus the experience of rearing by an agent less severely pathological than the schizophrenic mother is associated with distinctly better outcomes for the male children.

Father's absence shows a direct relationship with only one symptom, antisocial tendencies, in male offspring. Furthermore, the path coefficient is positive, indicating that father absence is related to increased antisocial traits.

Finally, it is apparent that there are fewer significant relationships for females, in fact, only two. Maternal absence bears a positive relationship with the daughter's antisocial tendencies and also with institutionalization. Thus, as with males, maternal absence is strongly predictive of institutionalization for females. In contrast to the males, there are no significant paths between father's absence and institutionalization or the presence of clinical symptoms in females. Thus it appears that the absence of a father is less damaging for females than for males.

The technique of path analysis has provided a good analytic approach to the problem of evaluating direct and indirect effects of parental absence and institutional child care. Institutionalization has been found to be an important mediating variable in the effects of parental absence on high risk males. Moreover, by focusing on dimensions of clinical status instead of a dichotomous diagnosis, we were able to ascertain which indices of maladjustment are related to the environmental variables in question.

As noted earlier, Beuhring et al. (1982) add an antecedent variable to the model deriving from the above study. This variable is obstetric complication (OC). This study investigated the general hypothesis that schizophrenia develops when a predisposing genetic liability is activated or exacerbated by specific environmental stressors. Since there is some support for the genetic component of the hypothesis (Gottesman, 1979; Gottesman & Shields, 1972; Zerbin-Rudin, 1972), and since retrospective studies suggest that somatic and familial stresses may also play a role (McNeil & Kaij, 1978), Beuhring et al. (1982) chose to investigate the following environmental stressors which may trigger or exacerbate a genetic predisposition of the Danish subjects to schizophrenia: obstetric complications, parental absence, and institutional child care.

Using the findings in Figure 1 as a reference point, we will present two additional analyses conducted in Beuhring et al. (1982). In the first analysis, obstetric complications were the sole predictor of the clinical syndromes. The second analysis simultaneously incorporated obstetric complications, parental absence, and institutional child care as predictors of those syndromes. The differences between these models were used to examine the interaction of biological and rearing–environment factors in the prediction of schizophrenic symptoms.

Obstetric complications as a predictor

Figure 2 summarizes the results for the prediction of clinical syndromes from obstetric complications alone. It can be seen that OCs are useful predictors of later psychopathology in high-risk males, but not females. For the males, OCs were significantly related to social impairment/antisocial traits, borderline schizophrenia/hallucinations–delusions, and to hebephrenic traits.

Just as the percentage of variance accounted for in multiple regression analyses indicates how successfully the independent variables predict the dependent variable, so the percentage of variance accounted for in the present analysis demon-

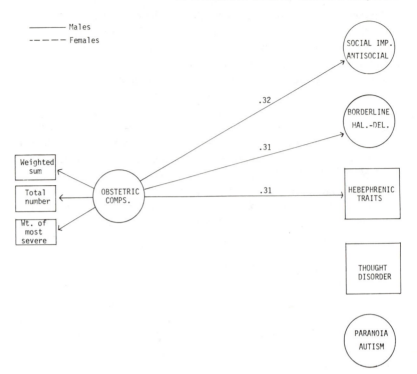

Figure 2. Path diagram for the prediction of clinical symptoms from obstetric complications.

strates the strength of the relationships between OCs and clinical syndromes. The first panel of Table 6 lists the percentage of variance predicted in each clinical syndrome using a history of obstetric complications as the only antecedent construct. As can be seen, almost no variation in the data for females on psychopathological symptoms is accounted for by OCs. For males, 9 to 10% of the variance in social impairment/antisocial tendencies, borderline schizophrenia/hallucinations–delusions, and hebephrenic traits is significantly predicted by a history of obstetric complications.

Figure 3 shows the independent and joint effects of obstetric complications, maternal absence, paternal absence, and institutional child care. As before, the significant coefficients are illustrated by solid lines for the males and broken lines for the females.

Amount of separation from the parents accounted for 71% of the variance in the amount of institutionalization experienced by high-risk offspring, whether male or female. This relationship was most directly attributable to amount of maternal absence, as indicated by the positive coefficients for the paths from maternal absence to institutional child care. Note that paternal absence no longer predicted directly to institutionalization of the males, as it did in the Walker et al. (1981) study. (A small correlation between the constructs of paternal absence and obstet-

Table 6. *Percentage of variance in clinical symptoms accounted for by amount of parental absence, institutional child care, and/or obstetric complications*

			Predictors			
	Obstetric complications alone		Parental absence and institutional child care[a]		Obstetric complications, parental absence, and institutional child care jointly	
Clinical symptoms	Males (%)	Females (%)	Males (%)	Females (%)	Males (%)	Females (%)
Social impairment/antisocial tendencies	10	1	12	5	21	4
Borderline schizophrenia/ hallucinations–delusions	9	1	13	8	20	8
Hebephrenic traits	9	0	9	1	16	1
Thought disorder	4	1	22	3	24	4
Paranoia/autism	1	1	3	4	3	3

[a]From study by Walker et al. (1981).

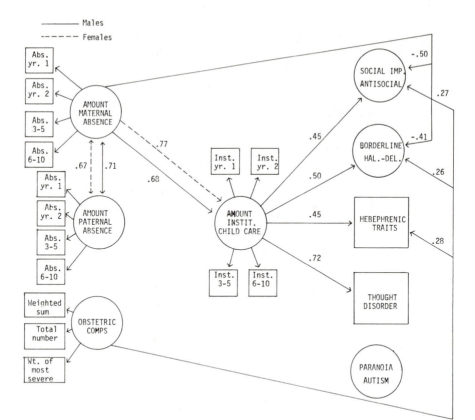

Figure 3. Path diagram for the prediction of clinical symptoms from amount of maternal absence, paternal absence, institutional child care, and obstetric complications.

ric complications may account for this altered finding.) Amount of paternal absence was only indirectly related to institutionalization of the male and female offspring via its correlation with amount of maternal absence.

These results suggest that high-risk children were often institutionalized after separation from their mother because her absence left them without a caretaking parent. This is consistent with the hypothesis that amount of maternal absence would strongly predict the amount of institutional child care provided to her offspring. Obstetric complications did not add to this prediction. There was essentially no relationship between obstetric complications and amount of institutionalization (the correlation between these constructs was .07 for the males and .06 for the females). This suggests that OC-related deficits and resulting behavior problems were not an important additional factor in deciding whether to place or retain a high-risk child in an institution.

In addition, amount of maternal absence was no longer significantly related to increases in social impairment/antisocial tendencies among the female offspring.

Paternal absence no longer predicted directly to increases in these tendencies among high-risk males.

The main pattern of findings reported by Walker et al. (1981) was not appreciably changed, however, by including obstetric complications as an additional antecedent variable. None of the correlations between obstetric complications and maternal absence, paternal absence, or institutional child care was sizable or statistically significant. Moreover, the magnitude of the coefficients for the direct paths from obstetric complications to three clinical syndromes in the males was approximately the same whether or not the child-rearing variables were included as predictors. This indicates that the increased risk for schizophrenia that is associated with a history of OCs is independent of the amount of parental absence or institutionalization experienced by the high-risk offspring.

It is noteworthy that obstetric complications were not related to type of rearing history. Thus it appears that at least two distinct classes of environmental stress, somatic and child-rearing, may serve as antecedents to schizophrenia in high-risk offspring. Beuhring et al. (1982) note that this outcome lends support to the idea that schizophrenia is not the result of a single detrimental factor but rather that many forms of stress may interact with genetic predisposition to eventuate in psychopathology.

A principal question raised by these findings is: Why do obstetric complications, parental absence, and institutional child care have a far greater impact on high-risk males than on females? Our results suggest that high-risk females are relatively impervious to the effects of environmental stress, at least as it is represented by these somatic and child-rearing variables.

One explanation is that males may be exposed to comparatively greater stress in a given familial or institutional setting. Schizophrenic mothers may be generally more harsh or more inconsistent in their treatment of sons than daughters. Although there is little research regarding caretaking behaviors of schizophrenic mothers, there is some evidence that normal parents are less protective and indulgent with male children (Block, 1978) and that the annoyance threshold for male deviance is lower than that for female deviance (Eme, 1979). In a similar vein, the institutional treatment of males may be qualitatively different from that experienced by females. Interviews with the individuals who were directors of the Danish institutions when these high-risk children were residents lend support to this hypothesis. The evidence for consistently more harsh treatment of males is not overwhelming, however. Moreover, the fact that only high-risk males were differentially affected by the type of substitute care provided after parental separation also argues against sex differences in exposure to stress as the sole explanation of our results.

An alternate explanation for the pattern of findings is that high-risk males may be constitutionally more vulnerable than females to *any* form of environmental stress. Greater male susceptibility to a host of pre-, peri-, and postnatal biological insults is well documented (Braine, Heimer, Wortis, & Freedman, 1966; Garai & Scheinfeld, 1968; Gottfried, 1973). In a review of the literature on childhood psychopathology, Eme (1979) concluded that males may be more vulnerable to psychological stressors as well. This hypothesis is consistent with our finding that only among males did the effects of maternal absence depend on the type of substitute care. Also consistent with that hypothesis are studies noting that male offspring of schizophrenic mothers (Higgins, 1974) and psychotic mothers or fathers (Rutter, 1970) are more likely to be adversely affected by rearing with a deviant parent. That is, males may be constitutionally more vulnerable to the effects of psychological as well as somatic stressors.

This explanation is not incompatible with the one offered earlier. Differential exposure and greater constitutional vulnerability may each contribute to the apparently greater impact of environmental stress on high-risk males, at least as it is represented by obstetric complications, parental absence, and institutional child care.

The potential utility of multiple indicators is highlighted by the findings for three of the syndromes defined in our study: borderline schizophrenia/ hallucinations–delusions, social impairment/antisocial tendencies, and hebephrenic traits. Both obstetric complications and institutional child care after separation predicted increased manifestations of these syndromes in high-risk males. Joint consideration of the environmental predictors may also suggest preventative courses of action. Separation from the schizophrenic mother, if accompanied by foster parenting or rearing with a relative, was associated with decreased manifestations of the same syndromes. Although these findings are still tentative, their overall pattern supports the contention that the "net result of a dynamic combination of genetic and environmental sources of liabilities and assets determines whether an individual with the necessary, but not sufficient, genetic predisposition crosses a threshold to clinical schizophrenia" (Gottesman & Shields, 1972).

3 A multidimensional approach to the identification of schizophrenia

ROBERT CUDECK, SARNOFF A. MEDNICK,
FINI SCHULSINGER, AND HANNE SCHULSINGER

The finding that wide agreement exists among researchers concerning the general characteristics of schizophrenia has been documented in several places (e.g., Carpenter, Strauss, & Bartko, 1974). However, specific elements of the disorder are under constant debate (Spitzer, Endicott, Cohen, & Fleiss, 1974). Broad characterizations of schizophrenia appear to pervade clinical and research practice; explicit behaviors or background factors are seldom featured, yet the definition and diagnosis of schizophrenia is a fundamental issue. To a large degree, the more clearly the concept can be identified, the more likely become effectual treatment and prevention.

Recently, several investigators have come to question the usefulness of traditional systems of diagnosis. Carpenter, Bartko, Carpenter, and Strauss (1976), for example, report that the classical subtypes of catatonic, hebephrenic, paranoid, and simple schizophrenia may not be differentiable at all on the basis of symptomatology. In another study, the same research team concluded flatly that "the ability of characteristic symptoms to define schizophrenia has been greatly overestimated" (Hawk et al., 1975, p. 347). Stephens (1978) agrees, noting that application of the schizophrenia diagnosis mostly depends upon the conception which individual practitioners hold.

The effect of this lack of reliable diagnosis is far reaching. Research in schizophrenia rests on the assumption that it is a condition that can be validly identified. The true picture is, unfortunately, not optimistic, for the disorder has proven to be an elusive concept when precision is required. Several factors combine to make identification of cases difficult. First, the clinical topography of schizophrenia varies cross-sectionally from person to person, from male to female and from old to young, and longitudinally for any given individual. Second, because there are a great many theories emphasizing different aspects of the disorder, the "salient" components of even a single case will vary depending upon the perspective of the individual clinician. Third, because most investigations are retrospective studies, results are often confounded by effects on subjects of hospitalization, powerful psychotropic drugs, and so on. Thus the objective identification of schizophrenia is frequently clouded to such an extent that practitioners must rely on subjective judgment in most instances. "Schizophrenia" only occurs whenever a quorum of

43

qualified people agree. The capriciousness of such a state of affairs is succinctly illustrated by the talk of the three umpires:

Said the first, "Balls and strikes, I call 'em as I see 'em."
The second, "Balls and strikes, I call 'em as they are."
The third one, older, shook his head, "Balls and strikes, they ain't nothin' *until* I call 'em!"
[Quoted in Gerard, 1973, p. 70].

On the other hand, a growing body of evidence is accumulating which suggests that schizophrenia is more than an arbitrary label. Recent indications about the heritability of the disorder (Gottesman & Shields, 1972, 1973, 1976; Kety, Rosenthal, Wender, & Schulsinger, 1974) imply that an organic basis may be implicated, in some cases at least. The likelihood that the diagnosis of schizophrenia is completely misapplied becomes improbable as this kind of genetic, biochemical, and other physiological data accumulates (Kolata, 1978). Meehl has suggested: "There is a sufficient amount of etiological and pragmatic homogeneity belonging to a given diagnostic group, i.e., schizophrenia, that assignment of a patient to this group has probability implications which it is unsound to ignore" (quoted in Dohrenwend & Dohrenwend, 1974, p. 427).

It appears that a valid "schizophrenic pattern" of abnormal behavior actually exists, although the exact boundaries that delimit the condition are not known, and although the behavioral pattern is quite variable between persons and over time.

Diagnostic models

Following such theoreticians as J. S. Strauss (1973), research into the diagnosis of schizophrenia can be characterized as following one of two models. The first, the *typological* approach, holds that schizophrenia, as well as other kinds of abnormality, are distinct entities. The role of diagnostic research is to establish behavioral and symptom boundaries for each category and to define systems of diagnosis for classifying persons into the categories. It is important to stress that the categories are viewed as nonoverlapping, so to cover a wide range of abnormal behavior many types need to be defined. This fact frequently leads to disagreements regarding the exact categories that should be advocated. Some researchers propose that the classes should be constructed theoretically, whereas others are willing to define them on an empirical basis (e.g., Skinner, 1979).

This approach is the keystone of nearly all modern-day psychiatry, and has motivated an extensive literature in diagnosis. As an example, Menninger (reviewed in Strauss, 1973) actually compiled a list of various typologies which ran to over 70 pages in length!

A second diagnostic model is based on a *dimensional* approach (Strauss, 1973; Torgerson, 1965). From this perspective, psychological impairment is depicted as a continuum, and investigators attempt to define classes of individuals as located together in a multidimensional space. This model relies heavily upon quantitative methods to define relationships among individuals and seeks quantitative relationships between critical events and their later effects. "Research strategies derived from dimensional models," writes Strauss (1973, p. 448), "investigate such relationships as how an increase in variable A affects variable B, rather than asking, as strategies derived from the typological model would, whether variable A causes variable B." A large amount of work has been done using the dimensional model. Phillips and Draguns (1971) reviewed many studies falling under this research procedure.

The perspective espoused here followed the dimensional model. It appears to be the most approriate strategy theoretically, for deviance is nearly universally characterized as a continuous phenomenon. However, with the dimensional model, it is critical that appropriate variables be used with the right population. If a reduced space method such as factor analysis is to be meaningful, it is important that persons be sampled to correctly represent the general population of interest. The correct variables must also be used in order to represent adequately the range of pathology in the sample. Very few factor analytic studies appear to be much aware of this requirement (Phillips & Draguns, 1971).

Research strategy

This chapter describes the analysis of current functioning of subjects in the Danish High-Risk Project. H. Schulsinger (1976) reported how a consensus diagnosis was reached for each individual and also gave the frequencies of occurrence of each diagnostic group. In contrast, the present research employed a dimensional model and made extensive use of factor analysis. This task is one which parallels that taken by many other studies reported in the literature, since it used data collected after breakdown on an existing psychiatric sample. However, no attempt was made to replicate the classical psychiatric categories, although the correspondence between the two was of considerable interest.

This study is significant for several reasons. The dimensional description of psychopathology is an important first step to employing current functioning in conjunction with antecedent data by means of sophisticated statistical methods. These methods perform most optimally when the data are continuous, normally distributed variates. Findings also may be germane to defining schizophrenic subtypes empirically, an especially important issue since classical subtypes apparently even lack verisimilitude (Hawk et al., 1975). It is not inconceivable that the current designation of "schizophrenia" may turn out to be composed of distinct classes of phenomena – and that each may have a unique etiology.

METHOD

Subjects

The subjects used in this study were 311 Danish children who have been examined periodically since 1962. At that time, they ranged in age from 10 to 20 years. Two hundred and seven of them had mothers who were diagnosed as severe schizophrenics (the High-Risk group). Matched to this index group were 104

Table 1. *Diagnosis, sex, and group by subsample*

	Sample A (N = 179)	Sample B (N = 85)	Total (N = 264)
Schizophrenia and paranoia	9	7	16
Borderline schizophrenia	39	20	59
Psychopathy	6	3	9
Personality disorder	22	9	31
Neurotic	45	18	63
Nonspecific conditions	16	8	24
No mental illness	33	19	52
No consensus diagnosis	9	1	10
Totals			
Males	104	47	151
Females	75	38	113
High-risk	116	56	172
Low-risk	63	29	92

control subjects whose parents and grandparents had had no record of psychiatric difficulties (the Low-Risk group).

In 1972, ten years after the original assessment, 264 of the original 311 subjects were contacted again (H. Schulsinger, 1976). Each subject underwent an extensive examination designed to yield a clinical diagnosis. Part of the examination consisted of two standardized interviews, the *Present State Examination*, or PSE (9th ed., Wing, Cooper, & Sartorious, 1974), and the *Current and Past Psychopathology Scales*, or CAPPS (Endicott & Spitzer, 1972). These instruments are structured interviews. They were selected because they are fairly objective, were in international use at that time, and because their results would be easily comparable for any other researchers using them. A third series of items consisted of a large psychiatric interview constructed especially for the project. Henceforth, this latter portion will be designated as the *Interview*.

A consensus diagnosis was reached for each subject when two of the three sources of information agreed as to the most probable classification.

For this analysis, the available subjects were divided randomly into two groups, sizes of which were roughly two-thirds and one-third of the total number of subjects, and the data from each were examined separately. This practice allowed any findings which emerged from work with the first group (Sample A) to be cross-validated on the second (Sample B). Table 1 shows the distributions of diagnoses, the breakdown by sex, and also by group membership (high- or low-risk) for these subgroups.

Measures

The three sources of information described above were the raw data for the analyses to be reported. Each instrument was composed of behavioral or symptom ratings. By convention, the generic term *item* will be used in reference to these ratings. Each battery of items was originally designed to give information about psychological functioning and was intended for diagnostic research. However, in this study, the various distinctive formats of the batteries were modified freely to fit the present requirements.

CAPPS. The CAPPS (Endicott & Spitzer, 1972) consists of 164 items. They are divided into time periods, those that apply to current functioning of a subject, and others that deal with past history. Some work on the psychometric properties of the instrument has been reported and is relevant here. Interrater reliabilities of the complete set of items ranged from .68 to 1.0 for four experienced CAPPS raters (Endicott & Spitzer, 1972, p. 682).

Twenty-six summary scales have been defined for the CAPPS based on factor analysis of the raw items. However, when computed on the present sample, the internal consistency of the items in these scales was frequently very poor. Since this sample represents a broad range of psychopathology, it was surprising that the replication was rather unsuccessful. Because the interrater reliabilities of individual items were high, all the items from the CAPPS were retained for later use; but the scales which have been suggested for them were not used at all.

PSE. The PSE (Wing et al., 1974) attempts to mimic the clinical process of using critical symptoms for diagnosis. The PSE is highly structured. When enough information is obtained to make certain that a symptom is present, optional items available for clarification can be bypassed. This philosophy, although perhaps efficient for raters, translated into a large amount of missing data. From an initial pool of 140 items, only 73 were available on the total sample, and many of these had extremely low frequencies of occurrence. Here also, scales of a sort have been published, but their usefulness appeared to be minimal for the present purposes and were not used.

On the positive side, the interrater reliabilities were generally very good for individual items. Wing et al. (1974, pp. 59–61) used kappas to evaluate reliability and found average agreement to be .77, which is satisfactory.

Since so few items were retained from the PSE, it was decided to combine the PSE with the CAPPS as a single battery of data with 237 items. The distinction between current and past functioning was also maintained in the combined battery.

Interview. The clinical interview contained 370 items, which were generally complete for all subjects. The interview items cover somewhat more content than either the CAPPS or PSE, although there is a good deal of overlap. No direct information has been given regarding interrater reliability for these items. However, H. Schulsinger (1976, p. 380) reported that on CAPPS items, which have possible scores of 1 to 6, her agreement with a second rater was quite good. Using percentage agreement, she found 91% of the ratings to be either identical, or differing by only 1 point. It was inferred from this that the ratings on the Interview items were probably consistent enough to be used for this research.

Statistical procedures

The analyses used in this research consisted of several stages. First an item analysis was carried out, the purpose of which was to construct more reliable variables for later use. Next, a series of factor analyses was undertaken. This step examined the interrelationships among the variables, and provided a basis for reducing the number of variables. It should be noted that three levels of scores were used (Loevinger, 1971). Original behavior ratings have already been referred to as items. Scores from a cluster of homogeneous items were called *scales*. The sum of the scale scores which resulted from the factor analysis were called *factor scores*. Then a discriminant analysis was performed as a validity check. The intention of this step was to determine whether the new variables could separate the subjects into groups similar to consensus diagnoses. Lastly, the entire process was performed separately with both Samples A and B to replicate each step.

Item analysis. Scales were defined by first identifying groups of items that were intercorrelated, attempting to maximize coefficient alpha (Cronbach, 1951) by emphasizing biserial correlations between items and scale totals. This method is related to other approaches to aggregating items into scales, such as factor analysis (Henrysson, 1962), but generally produces superior results (Hase & Goldberg, 1967; Nunnally, 1967, pp. 255–258).

First, an initial core of candidate items was defined on a rational basis, and alpha was computed for them. Those items in the set with poor item–total correlations or which decreased alpha were dropped. Then others were selected from the item pool that had large item-total correlations with those currently in the core. Alphas were again computed for the combined group, and those with low item–total correlations or which decreased alpha were deleted. The process was continued until no further items could be found which increased alpha. In order to ensure that no artificial dependence was built into the scales, individual items were not used in more than one scale.

In addition to these purely statistical considerations, an attempt was made to select all items within a set to be homogeneous in content. This subjective decision was critical to the final pool. For decisions at this stage, two raters were used.

Final scale scores were taken as the sum of the standardized items, rather than their simple sum. This approach was taken because the items were based on different metrics. Some were of the binary type, such as "Trait X applies to this person or Trait X does not apply to this person." Many were rated on a 3-point scale, such as "Behavior X not present, Behavior X sometimes present, or Behavior X frequently present." Still other items were scored on a 5-point or 7-point scale. Since the variance of a composite variable is the sum of the variances and covariances of the items that make up the composite, the practice of summing the standardized item scores ensured that each item in the scale would be given the same weight in the composite, regardless of original metric.

Principal components. After all scales were completed, the principal components (Gorsuch, 1974, p. 90) of the entire set were calculated. This step examined the relationships among the scales and sought to reduce them to a more parsimonious group. The method of principal components was chosen because a reduced set of scores for each subject was desired ultimately. Theoretically, components describe the variance among a set of variables better than other alternatives such as common factor analysis.

Interbattery factor analysis. The original items used in this study came from two distinct data sets. Those from the CAPPS–PSE have been described in previous research, whereas the Interview items were examined here for the first time. In essence, the two batteries represent two distinct methods of assessing psychopathology. The relationship between them is an important consideration. Frequently, in exploratory analyses using two data sets in a single analysis, factors are produced that are heavily represented by variables from one of the two methods. These *method* factors arise because scales obtained from one battery often tend to correlate more highly with each other than with any scales from the other battery (Skinner, 1977). Thus, the principal components obtained from examining all the scales although ignoring the batteries from which they arise may be biased toward representing one of the methods, instead of a general underlying dimension of psychopathology.

Recently, Browne (1979) has proposed a technique for investigating the extent to which factors occur in each of two batteries, controlling for unique method effects from either. These *interbattery* factors are not subject to powerful specific effects due to different methods, because the multiple correlations of the factors on the batteries are constrained to be equal. The interbattery factors describe the relationships between scales in each battery, while controlling the battery-specific effects.

Moreover, using a second method of analysis will provide information about the stability of the factors across different varieties of factor analysis. If the factors that emerge from two different techniques coincide, this finding will tend to increase confidence in the final solution (Harris, 1967).

Discriminant analysis. According to Armstrong and Soelberg (1968), "In order to judge the validity of a factor analytic study, it may be helpful to specify at least one dependent variable which the factor analysis was designed to help explain or predict" (p. 364). If the proposed factors can measure psychopathology in these subjects similarly to the way in which the various diagnoses categorize them, then there should be good correspondence between the approaches. A method was sought here like the Campbell and Fiske (1959) procedure for convergent and discriminant validity. If factor scores can distinguish between diagnostic groups, that finding would suggest that the factors are doing much the same job as the diagnoses. The factors resulting from the previously described analyses were used as measurement variables in a discriminant analysis (Cooley & Lohnes, 1971; Tatsuoka, 1971) to distinguish the subjects that belonged to different diagnostic groups. Although classification per se was not the goal here, using the diagnoses in this manner helped to index the extent to which the factors successfully described psychopathology in the sample. If the factors are able to produce this discrimination, it would suggest that they are valid descriptors of psychopathology, at least to the extent that diagnosis itself is.

Cross-validation. The above analyses first were undertaken using only the subjects in Sample A. To test the generalizability of the results, the entire process was repeated using data from the subjects of Sample B. Frequently, solutions from individual analyses are quite unstable, and may, therefore, be unrepresentative of global effects. This is especially true in the present instance, with relatively few subjects and a great many items to analyze. Consequently, any relationships found in Sample A that did not replicate in Sample B were viewed critically.

A large number of trial-and-error computations were required in the item analysis. This activity virtually ensured that the scales obtained from Sample A would appear to be more reliable (internally consistent) than they actually were. However, successfully cross-validating the items in Sample B would suggest that the final scales are stable in the general population.

In the factor analysis stage, four independent solutions were produced. Each subsample was used in both the components analysis and the interbattery factor analysis. To ensure that something other than random processes was operating in these data, a high degree of correspondence was required among the various solutions.

ITEM ANALYSIS

Composition of the scales

Altogether, 35 scales were developed from the original items, 14 from the CAPPS–PSE, and 21 from the Interview battery. The items which make up each scale, the scale names, and their shortened forms are listed in Table 2. An attempt was made in the CAPPS–PSE scales to retain the distinction, sought by the authors of the CAPPS (Endicott & Spitzer, 1972), between current symptoms and symptoms that were known to have occurred in the past histories of the subjects. They were designated, respectively, "Current" and "Past" scales in the CAPPS–PSE battery, and in the shortened names are prefaced by a "C" or "P." The Interview scale names begin with an "I."

In Table 3, the number of items in each scale, the scale variance, and Cronbach's (1951) alpha for both subsamples are presented. On the average, the scales from the CAPPS–PSE contained 7.8 items, produced a variance of 30, and had alphas of .83. One of the smallest scales in this set was number 3, Severe substance abuse, which had an alpha of .76 in Sample A, but only .41 in Sample B. This scale may not be useful for later use since it cross-validated so poorly. Of the 237 CAPPS–PSE items available, 109 were used in these scales.

The Interview scales averaged 11.7 items in length, had variances of 56.4, and

Table 2. *Scale composition for multivariate analysis of clinical symptoms*

1. *Current: Schizophrenia: residual impairment (C SCHIZIMP)*
   PSE Social impairment due to psychosis
   PSE Blunted affect
   C-C Denial of illness
   C-C Overall severity of illness

2. *Current: Depression with secondary anxiety (C DEPRESANX)*
   PSE Worrying
   PSE Subjective feeling of nervous tension
   PSE Neglect due to brooding
   PSE Loss of interest
   PSE Depressed mood
   PSE Hopelessness
   PSE Suicidal plans or acts
   C-C Anxiety
   C-C Depression
   C-C Suicide attempt, self-mutilation
   C-C Daily routine, leisure time impairment
   C-C Agitation, excitement

3. *Current: Severe substance abuse (C SUBABUS)*
   PSE Fugues, blackouts, amnesia
   C-C Alcohol abuse
   C-C Narcotics and/or drug use
   C-C Disorientation, memory lapses

4. *Current: Somatic concerns (C SOMATIC)*
   PSE Subject's evaluation of present health
   PSE Tension pains
   PSE Muscular tension
   PSE Restlessness
   PSE Hypochondriasis
   PSE Free-floating autonomic anxiety
   PSE Anxious foreboding with autonomic signs
   C-C Somatic concerns
   C-C Psychophysiological reactions to stress

5. *Current: Thought disorder (C THDISORD)*
   PSE Subjectively inefficient thinking
   PSE Poor concentration
   PSE Derealization
   PSE Evasiveness
   PSE Distractibility
   PSE Perplexity or puzzlement
   PSE Incoherence of speech
   C-C Silliness
   C-C Speech disorganization

Table 2 (*cont.*)

6. *Current: Retarded depression (C RETARDEPR)*
     PSE Tiredness or exhaustion
     PSE Lack of self-confidence with other people
     PSE Delayed sleep
     PSE Subjective anergia and retardation
     PSE Lost emotions
     PSE Slowness and underactivity
     PSE Observed depression
     PSE Slow speech
     C-C Guilt
     C-C Retardation, lack of emotion
7. *Current: Delusions and hallucinations – level of severity (C DELUSHALL)*
     PSE Systematization of delusions and hallucinations
     PSE Overall rating of preoccupation with hallucinations and delusions
     PSE Acting out delusions and hallucinations
     C-C Hallucinations with dissociation
     C-C Visual hallucinations
8. *Past: Agitated depression (P AGITDEPRES)*
     C-P Tiredness
     C-P Insomnia
     C-P Brooding
     C-P Depression
     C-P Guilt feelings
     C-P Thoughts of suicide
     C-P Signs of anxiety
     ·C-P Loss of interest
     C-P Agitation
9. *Past: Psychopathic tendencies (P PSYCHOPATH)*
     C-P Childhood antisocial traits
     C-P Non-academic school difficulties
     C-P No occupational goals, aimlessness
     C-P Problems with drug usage
     C-P Alcohol abuse
     C-P Illegal acts
     C-P Antisocial traits
     C-P Impulsivity
     C-P Poor judgment
     C-P Self-defeating behavior
     C-P Lacking responsibility
10. *Past: Poor social, sexual relations (P SOCLSEXRL)*
     C-P Poor adolescent friendship pattern
     C-P Adolescent sexual maladjustment
     C-P Adult sexual maladjustment
     C-P Poor friendships
     C-P Emotionally distant
     C-P Inadequate pleasure capacity

Table 2 (*cont.*)

11. *Past: Delusional ideation with perceptual distortions (P DELUSIDEA)*
    C-P Suspiciousness
    C-P Preoccupied with religion
    C-P Grandiosity
    C-P Ideas of reference
    C-P Delusions
    C-P Depersonalization, derealization
    C-P Illusions
    C-P Hallucinations

12. *Past: Asthenic personality disorder (P ASTHENIC)*
    C-P Childhood neurotic traits
    C-P Decline in responsibility on job
    C-P Made no efforts to improve position
    C-P Irrational fears, phobia
    C-P Inhibited
    C-P Ineffectual adapting to stress
    C-P Sensitive, feelings easily hurt
    C-P Dependency
    C-P Clings
    C-P Passive aggressive

13. *Past: Severity of disturbance (hospitalization) (P SEVHOSP)*
    C-P Received outpatient treatment
    C-P Psychiatric hospitalization
    C-P Total time of psychiatric hospitalization
    C-P Number of hospitalizations
    C-P Rating of overall severity

14. *Past: Violent behavior (P VIOLENT)*
    C-P Poor stability on job
    C-P No control over affect
    C-P Stubborn, obstinate
    C-P Hostility or anger
    C-P Physically violent
    C-P Poor family relationships
    C-P Blames others

15. *Social avoidance (I SOCAVOID)*
    Goes out alone
    Prefers to eat alone
    Does not face unpleasant situations
    Avoids meeting friends
    Does not sit near interviewer
    Avoids eye contact
    Avoids touchy subjects
    Hides face during interview
    Puts hands to mouth
    Frequently misunderstands questions

Table 2 (*cont.*)

Needs prodding to answer
Unable to communicate with interviewer
Frequently glances at watch
Anxious to terminate interview

16. *Severe shyness (I SHYNESS)*
Shy, bashful, reserved
Quiet
Restrictive affect-control
Self-conscious
Withdrawn
Sensitive, reactive withdrawal
Ambivalent and defensive
Schizoid personality
Shyness
Seclusiveness
Detached reaction to disturbance

17. *Hypersensitive (I HYPERSENS)*
Sensitive or easily hurt
Easily upset, worked up, or beside himself
Very unsure of himself
Reserved toward adults and strangers
Dependent, afraid of being alone
Different, not like other children
Was teased by friends
Emotions easily touched
Insecure
Anxious, timid
Dysphoria, abnormal feelings of discontent
Afraid of being thought stupid
Introjects
Not self-assertive
Shows signs of phobia
Depressive symptoms in early life
Inhibited in early life
Upset for long periods of time

18. *Passive (I PASSIVE)*
Poor conversational involvement
Undercommunicative
Inert
Apathetic contact
Passive
Inactive
Lacking spontaneity
Indifferent, passive contact

Table 2 (*cont.*)

19. *Paranoia (I PARANOIA)*
    Projection
    Distrustful attitude
    Guarded
    Watchful, suspicious
    Oversensitive
    Tendency for misinterpretation
    Blames the environment

20. *Low impulse control (I LOIMPLSCON)*
    Acts out
    Inadequate ethical and moral attitude
    Intolerance of frustration
    Failure of impulse control
    Domineering alloplastic orientation
    Doesn't profit from experiences
    Instability in object relations
    Lacks responsibility
    Evades difficult situations
    No evidence of control in life

21. *Emotionally overcontrolled, inexpressive (I INEXPRESS)*
    No verbal modulation
    Few gestures
    Inadequate affective involvement
    Underemotional
    Affect-isolation
    Displays symptoms of inhibition
    Expressionless face and gestures
    Lacks empathy
    Poor direct contact
    Abnormal range of emotionality
    Humorless
    Not responsive or empathetic toward examiner

22. *Unkempt (I UNKEMPT)*
    Not well-dressed
    Not tidy or well cared for
    Dressed sloppily
    Poorly dressed
    Unkempt
    Unkempt hair
    "Hippie" clothing

23. *Inhibited communication (I INHIBCOMM)*
    Inhibited in conversation
    Not spontaneous
    Unable to find the right word

Table 2 (*cont.*)

Incomplete answers to questions
Underelaboration
Not verbally fluent
Poorly formulated language
Slow response to questions
Thinking not goal-directed
Poor tempo in speech
Weak voice

24. *Immaturity (I IMMATURITY)*
Emotionally immature
Low ego-maturity
Inadequate independent identity
Signs of dependency during examination
Symptoms of dependency in early life
Submissive, insecure
Symptoms of insecurity in early life
Reassurance-seeking, clinging
Displays symptoms of abandonment and helplessness
Unable to find practical solutions to problems

25. *Poor goal-directedness, underachievement (I UNDERACHEI)*
Poor goal-directedness
Narrow scope of interests
Low drive level
Education or employment below ability
Limited self-realization
Achievement inappropriate to ability
Poor coping; unable to pursue plans

26. *Egocentric (I EGOCENTRIC)*
Persistence in one type of response
Speech is "un-interrupted"
Overcompensated self-esteem
Extremely egocentric
Early symptoms of egocentrism
Early symptoms of narcissism
Manipulative
Not easy to like
Unsympathetic

27. *Obsessive–compulsive (I OBSESSCOMP)*
Obsessive–compulsive behavior
Overtalkative
Verbal wandering
Overelaboration
Overly specifies people or events
Histrionic, exaggerated verbalization
Infantile, self-centered

Table 2 (*cont.*)

Engages in undoing
Displays overt neurotic conflict
Symptoms of neurosis in early life
Displays neurotic symptoms
Symptoms of anxiety neurosis in early life
Current symptoms of anxiety neurosis
Symptoms of obsession–compulsion in early life
Displays symptoms of obsession–compulsion
Symptoms of character neurosis in early life
Displays symptoms of character neurosis

28. *Overt hostility (I HOSTILITY)*

Frequently disobedient
Hyperactive
Bad moods
Changing moods
Gets excited easily, hot-tempered
Quarrelsome, cantankerous, contrary
Does not avoid trouble or quarrels
Narcissistic, self-centered
Irritable
Instinctual conflicts openly expressed
No avoidance of aggression in early life
No current avoidance of aggression
Symptoms of overt hatred and bitterness
Lacks close relationships
Lacks intimate relationships
Outbursts of aggression
Openly expresses hostility

29. *Autism (I AUTISM)*

Mind wanders when listening
Poor memory
Interrupted flow of speech
Wide attention, distractibility
Fused, condensed verbalization
Unmodulated facial expression
Inadequate facial expression
Uncooperative
Uncooperative in early life
Moderate autism
Evidence of poor reality testing in early life
Shows current evidence of poor reality testing
Autistic blocking
Eccentric
Autistic thinking

Table 2 (*cont.*)

30. *Anhedonic, depressed (I ANHEDONIC)*
    Unvaried serious expression
    Variable mood and emotions
    Slightly depressed, lowered mood
    Emotional impoverishment
    Lacks cheerfulness and good humor
    Sullen, sour attitude
    Anhedonia
    Symptoms of depression
    Poor facial color
    Unattractive

31. *Schizophrenia: chronic (I SCHIZCHRON)*
    Poor reality testing
    Withdrawn and avoidant in early life
    No primary gain
    No secondary gain
    Subject difficult to follow
    Emotional bluntness

32. *Schizophrenia (I SCHIZFORM)*
    Dissatisfied with life
    Poor defenses
    Unstable neurotic defenses
    Fluctuation of defenses
    Episodes of depersonalization
    Micropsychotic episodes – delusions
    Micropsychotic episodes – hallucinations
    Pan-anxiety
    Breakdowns of defenses

33. *Distorted self-concept (I DISSELFCON)*
    Poor self-concept and identity
    Unrealistic self-esteem
    Low acceptance of gender role
    Poor performance of gender role
    Distorted body image
    Inconsistent self-esteem
    Inadequate sexual identity
    Distorted body image
    Diffuse anxiety

34. *Social phobia (I SOCALPHOB)*
    Restricted vocabulary
    Reassurance seeking during examination
    Evidence of reassurance seeking in early life
    Pallid contact
    Inconsistent contact
    Communication is difficult

Table 2 (*cont.*)

Detachment
Poor eye contact
Abnormal eye contact
Evidence of symbiotic relationships in early life
Stereotypic, conventional reactions
Conspicuous avoidance
Narcissistic, one-way communication
Poor use of language
· Evasive answers

35. *Thought disorder (I THDISORD)*
Illogical explanations
Answers are difficult to follow
Answers are unrelated to questions
Poor hierarchical organization
Overgeneralization
Underspecifies people or events
Train of speech drifts or shifts
Sequential thoughts are unrelated
Transitions between ideas are impaired
Employs "approximate speech"
Answers degenerate over time
Literalizes abstract ideas
Loose tangential associations
Pseudo-intellectual verbalizations

---

produced alphas of .83 in Sample A and .81 in Sample B. These scales accounted for 246 of the 370 Interview items. Taken as a whole, with the exception of Severe substance abuse noted above, the scales are sufficiently consistent to be used in further research (Nunnally, 1967, pp. 259–260). The alphas are generally high in Sample A, and more important, were clearly replicated in Sample B.

Final item–total correlations. If items in a scale are homogeneous with respect to the entire pool, then those belonging to a scale should correlate most highly with the one in which they are a member. The number of item–total correlations which are largest for items in its scale is an index of the success of the item analysis. Of the 355 items used in all scales, 92% of those in Sample A and 80% in Sample B correlated most highly with the scale to which they were assigned. Using the criterion that the item correlate highest or second highest with its appropriate scale, 97% of the items in Sample A, and 88% of the items in Sample B met this goal.

To summarize, the statistical results of the item analysis suggested that these scales were both internally consistent and representative of the population on which they were derived. However, it was also significant that they described a broad range of clinical psychopathlogy, which was immediately recognizable. In both batteries,

Table 3. *Scale variances and alphas for the clinical symptom measures in Sample A and Sample B*

	Number of items	Variance		Alpha	
		Sample A	Sample B	Sample A	Sample B
CAPPS–PSE scales					
1. C SCHIZIMP	4	8.1	8.5	.72	.84
2. C DEPRESANX	12	74.1	77.9	.92	.93
3. C SUBABUS	4	9.2	.6	.76	.41
4. C SOMATIC	9	24.0	30.0	.73	.81
5. C THDISORD	9	34.6	32.8	.85	.83
6. C RETARDEPR	10	34.1	31.1	.80	.81
7. C DELUSHALL	5	18.2	17.0	.93	.95
8. P AGITDEPRES	9	36.0	42.3	.85	.89
9. P PSYCHOPATH	11	60.8	63.6	.91	.92
10. P SOCLSEXRL	6	20.4	21.9	.86	.88
11. P DELUSIDEA	8	35.4	38.9	.84	.83
12. P ASTHENICN	10	27.8	26.6	.74	.75
13. P SEVHOSP	5	16.0	17.8	.86	.91
14. P VIOLENT	7	19.2	16.3	.79	.79
Mean	7.8	29.9	30.4	.83	.83
Interview scales					
15. I SOCAVIOD	14	77.0	70.0	.93	.90
16. I SHYNESS	11	47.9	39.6	.82	.78
17. I HYPERSENS	19	78.6	74.2	.79	.73
18. I PASSIVE	8	38.6	34.9	.84	.86
19. I PARANOIA	10	62.3	85.5	.83	.83
20. I LOIMPLSCON	10	61.2	133.4	.85	.88
21. I INEXPRESS	12	118.9	126.5	.85	.77
22. I UNKEMPT	7	10.2	11.0	.81	.89
23. I INHIBCOMM	11	58.1	43.5	.86	.76
24. I IMMATURITY	12	70.7	78.0	.85	.89
25. I UNDERACHEI	9	30.3	39.6	.84	.89
26. I EGOCENTRIC	9	32.7	27.1	.78	.74
27. I OBSESSCOMP	17	69.4	55.0	.79	.71
28. I HOSTILITY	17	55.9	39.7	.76	.69
29. I AUTISM	15	79.8	64.8	.84	.82
30. I ANHEDONIC	11	39.1	38.2	.76	.74
31. I SCHIZCHRON	6	31.2	40.5	.81	.81
32. I SCHIZFORM	9	24.2	26.2	.79	.81
33. I DISSELFCON	9	29.3	26.0	.83	.80
34. I SOCALPHOB	16	79.5	86.7	.86	.87
35. I THDISORD	14	88.8	91.6	.91	.91
Mean	11.7	56.4	58.7	.83	.81

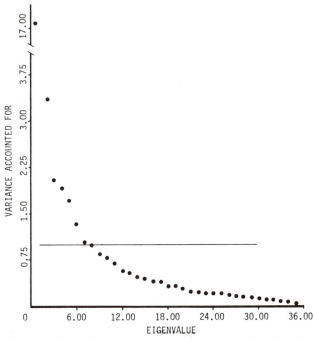

Figure 1. Eigenvalues from correlation matrix of data from Sample A.

scales were obtained that measured extremely abnormal behavior such as thought disorder, and also less severe conditions such as neurosis and depression. Both batteries also produced scales which assessed psychopathy, and the CAPPS–PSE battery produced a general severity scale (Scale 13, P SEVHOSP).

Although these scales were constructed by attempting to make them statistically independent, theoretically, at least, there is some overlap between them, both within each battery and between batteries. The overall structure of the scales was next examined to investigate this overlap among the scales.

Principal components analysis

The matrix of correlations among the 35 scales for Sample A was then calculated and was decomposed according to procedures for principal components outlined in Gorsuch (1974). Several different rotations were used in the course of examining the data, but there was little difference among most of the final solutions. Therefore a modified varimax transformation following Jackson and Skinner (1975) will be reported.

In deciding the number of components to retain, several criteria have been recommended. As a rule, the clearest solutions are those that receive support from two or three of these criteria. For the data from Sample A, seven components were retained. The rationale for this decision is discussed later. It relied heavily upon the distribution of the eigenvalues shown in Figure 1.

Ratio of variables to factors. A general rule of thumb is that three or four variables must have high loadings on any component that is to be considered well defined. Consequently, for 35 variables, eight or nine components is the maximum that could be expected, and this could occur only if the variables were evenly distributed across the factors.

Scree test. The Scree Test (Cattell, 1966) is a rule that defines the correct number of factors as those corresponding to only the largest eigenvalues. From Figure 1 it can be seen that breaks in the distribution of the magnitude of the eigenvalues occurred between Factors II and III, between V and VI, and between VI and VII. The number of "large" eigenvalues conceivably could be taken as either 2, 5, or 6. In addition, it is frequently useful to rotate one factor more than is expected to be retained ultimately, discarding the last after rotation if necessary. For these data, six components accounted for 70% of the variance in the correlation matrix, and seven accounted for 73%. Seven were judged most appropriate by this rule.

Kaiser–Guttman criterion. Perhaps the most frequently used rule for determining the number of factors is to extract as many factors as there are eigenvalues larger than unity (Guttman, 1954; Kaiser, 1970). As can be seen in the figure, seven eigenvalues exceeded 1.

Interpretability criterion. It has been suggested in several places (e.g., Kim & Mueller, 1978) that a criterion of great importance is the substantive interpretability of factor solutions. This stresses the reasonableness of the results in light of current understanding in a field, and depends on a given researcher's subjective evaluation of the factors. Most standard references on factor analysis suggest examining a number of dimensionalities which are plausible by the first three criteria. Solutions to the present data were computed using six through nine factors, but seven seemed especially clear.

The seven rotated components for Sample A are shown in Table 4. The variables and components have been rearranged to facilitate interpretation. Components I through V each had at least four variables with loadings exceeding .50. Factors VI and VII were not as clear, although the salient variables of each appeared theoretically related.

As a whole, the solution was readily interpretable, and the following labels were assigned:

Factor I – Major Mental Illness
Factor II – Interpersonal Communication Disorder
Factor III – Psychopathy, Inadequate Personality
Factor IV – Aggression
Factor V – Severe Depression
Factor VI – Hypersensitive, Avoidant
Factor VII – Neurosis

Table 4. *Rotated principal components for Sample A data*

| | | \multicolumn{7}{c}{Components} | | | | | | |
		I	II	III	IV	V	VI	VII
1.	C THDISORD	|86|	14	08	02	16	−06	17
2.	P DELUSIDEA	|82|	14	23	09	28	03	−11
3.	C DELUSHALL	|76|	16	16	−08	35	02	−07
4.	I THDISORD	|70|	37	20	25	−10	−05	13
5.	P SEVHOSP	|65|	17	16	27	28	13	−05
6.	I DISSELFCON	|59|	33	06	25	26	19	16
7.	C DEPRESANX	|49|	10	20	16	65	01	26
8.	C SCHIZIMP	|44|	40	25	36	31	04	36
9.	I INHIBCOMM	04	|84|	15	−12	12	06	−04
10.	I SOCALPHOB	28	|82|	04	26	−07	03	07
11.	I INEXPRESS	10	|80|	12	30	09	08	10
12.	I PASSIVE	−25	|78|	12	−26	16	−10	−21
13.	I SHYNESS	18	|77|	−04	13	25	23	−08
14.	I SCHIZCHRON	46	|63|	22	30	27	06	−06
15.	I AUTISM	51	|60|	11	21	19	01	01
16.	P SOCLSEXRL	34	|52|	08	38	20	28	−15
17.	P PSYCHOPATH	18	08	|85|	26	10	03	−04
18.	I LOIMPLSCON	19	12	|81|	33	12	05	04
19.	I UNKEMPT	09	13	|63|	−15	−02	15	−02
20.	I UNDERACHEI	33	45	|60|	09	29	14	−02
21.	C SUBABUSE	10	−05	|52|	01	12	−20	24
22.	I IMMATURITY	37	37	|39|	19	27	27	28
23.	I HOSTILITY	04	−03	09	|87|	20	−06	−16
24.	P VIOLENT	19	06	42	|69|	34	07	−01
25.	I EGOCENTRIC	26	43	−05	|64|	−13	04	27
26.	I PARANOIA	32	36	07	|62|	23	07	07
27.	C RETARDEPRES	18	24	10	02	|77|	01	−01
28.	P AGITDEPRES	39	20	18	24	|70|	27	12
29.	I ANHEDONIC	17	47	14	22	|56|	02	06
30.	I SCHIZFORM	43	34	21	19	|50|	00	12
31.	I HYPERSENS	12	03	13	16	47	|62|	31
32.	I SOCALAVOID	15	33	05	−03	−16	|62|	−22
33.	P ASTHENIC	19	32	42	20	30	|42|	35
34.	I OBSESSCOMP	02	−23	−04	03	08	13	|82|
35.	C SOMATIC	22	03	23	12	34	−03	|59|

The correlations from Sample B were next analyzed. Seven components also appeared to adequately describe these data. The components from Sample B were then extracted and matched to be as congruent as possible to the components from Sample A (Cliff, 1966). These matched factors are displayed in Table 5. Table 6 gives the correlations between the Sample A components and the matched components of Sample B.

Table 5. *Matched principal components for Sample B data*

	Components						
	I	II	III	IV	V	VI	VII
1. C THDISORD	|67|	25	47	21	25	−09	05
2. P DELUSIDEA	|82|	32	22	17	02	03	07
3. C DELUSHALL	|86|	19	14	05	14	04	06
4. I THDISORD	|69|	33	25	34	20	09	13
5. P SEVHOSP	|34|	27	32	22	43	18	43
6. I DISSELFCON	|52|	43	22	21	43	10	09
7. C DEPRESANX	|40|	32	17	18	69	11	03
8. C SCHIZIMP	|58|	43	45	12	27	03	16
9. I INHIBCOMM	15	|72|	29	00	33	04	−14
10. I SOCALPHOB	43	|71|	12	27	12	12	−10
11. I INEXPRESS	21	|73|	11	37	13	−01	12
12. I PASSIVE	−34	|69|	11	−06	27	04	−34
13. I SHYNESS	16	|78|	−18	25	17	20	10
14. I SCHIZCHRON	58	|55|	28	33	16	−01	17
15. I AUTISM	54	|64|	32	07	17	−06	15
16. P SOCLSEXRL	26	|57|	01	45	25	02	16
17. P PSYCHOPATH	29	13	|80|	31	04	−02	−02
18. I LOIMPLSCON	44	14	|61|	46	20	−06	01
19. I UNKEMPT	22	36	|59|	−36	−24	25	19
20. I UNDERACHEI	42	40	|56|	04	45	−03	−06
21. C SUBABUSE	23	22	|79|	−04	−16	−05	29
22. I IMMATURITY	47	13	|48|	24	39	−03	05
23. I HOSTILITY	14	25	28	|59|	28	35	17
24. P VIOLENT	24	04	47	|71|	29	09	03
25. I EGOCENTRIC	46	38	−09	|48|	−17	11	33
26. I PARANOIA	23	41	02	|56|	26	13	−07
27. C RETARDEPRES	28	46	08	−12	|70|	12	08
28. P AGITDEPRES	31	25	16	30	|59|	37	27
29. I ANHEDONIC	23	48	02	10	|55|	13	23
30. I SCHIZFORM	51	37	13	47	|40|	09	13
31. I HYPERSENS	00	12	−02	24	51	|54|	32
32. I SOCALAVOID	15	10	09	02	−21	|83|	−36
33. P ASTHENIC	23	24	46	37	51	|20|	17
34. I OBSESSCOMP	16	−13	−12	37	−01	22	|75|
35. C SOMATIC	46	−04	11	39	58	18	|09|

Factors I through V were very closely matched in sample B, the corresponding correlations being .88, .89, .85, .80, and .81. Factors VI and VII were not as clearly replicated. However, the magnitudes of the correlations even for these were far above chance levels of significance.

As with the item analysis above, these results showed excellent congruence

Table 6. *Correlations between Sample A components (rows) and Sample B matched components (columns)*

Sample A components	Sample B matched components						
	I	II	III	IV	V	VI	VII
I	88	−06	07	06	10	−27	10
II	−12	89	−26	−14	−01	−22	−46
III	05	−32	85	−10	−09	−30	−13
IV	09	−09	−05	80	06	−01	20
V	02	−06	−14	−02	81	−01	15
VI	−26	−19	−24	01	06	69	00
VII	10	−48	−10	19	16	−01	59

between the two subsamples. In addition, the seven components appeared substantially recognizable clinically and achieved a high degree of discrimination from one another. Only Factors II, Interpersonal Communication Disorder, and VII, Neurosis, showed questionable independence and this is understandable from a clinical point of view. These results are similar to other factor analyses reported elsewhere, but the methods followed here are more stringent than are commonly used.

INTERBATTERY FACTORS

A complementary approach to principal components for two data sets is interbattery factor analysis. The method was first discussed by L. R. Tucker (1958), but has been most elegantly developed by Browne (1979). Interbattery factors emphasize elements common to two sets of data, while holding unique aspects of either set constant. Therefore, factors that might be largely made up of variables from only one set are minimized. Principal components analysis with two batteries of data produces solutions that are unsatisfactory at minimizing battery specific effects.

Although the derivation of interbattery analysis is independent of other methods, it turns out to have a close relationship to canonical correlation. Rao (1973) showed that the number of interbattery factors is equal to the number of nonzero canonical correlations. Thus to determine the number of interbattery factors, one must examine the magnitude of the canonical correlations. These are given in Table 7 for both samples.

It is apparent from the table that the two batteries are substantially related in Sample A. The first 10 canonical *R*s were statistically significant; however, as in factor analysis, statistical significance alone is not the only criterion for determining the correct number to retain. In addition, it is desirable that the canonical correlations be of substantial size and also that the interbattery factors be clear.

Using these criteria, nine of the interbattery factors for the data from Sample A

Table 7. *Canonical correlations between CAPPS–PSE and INTERVIEW batteries*

Canonical variate	Sample A	Sample B
1	.95	.98
2	.86	.95
3	.81	.92
4	.75	.85
5	.69	.83
6	.62	.73
7	.61	.72
8	.53	.72
9	.51	.61
10	.36	.56
11	.34	.53
12	.28	.46
13	.26	.41
14	.16	.26

were extracted, and rotated by the Varimax procedure. After rotation, two factors did not retain any loadings larger than .4; thus seven factors were finally accepted. The interbattery solutions for both samples were highly similar to the components analysis. It should be emphasized, however, that the interpretation of the interbattery factors is a very different thing. Interbattery factors are equally related to the two sets of variables, whereas components analysis makes no such provision for equating contributions between sets. This finding suggests that each set of variables described nearly the same dimensions of psychopathology.

In Table 8 the correlations between interbattery factors for both subsamples are displayed. Factor VII was rather unsuccessfully replicated in the interbattery factors, just as it was in the components analysis. However, taken as a whole, the interbattery results were virtually identical in each sample.

To summarize, in four distinct analyses, using two independent samples and two different methods, nearly the same factors obtained. This lends a great deal of confidence to the reliability of the solution.

DISCRIMINANT ANALYSIS

In order to validate the above analysis we used the factor scores to distinguish among the formal diagnoses applied to each subject in the 1972 assessment (H. Schulsinger, 1976). Discriminant analysis (Cooley & Lohnes, 1971, Chap. 9) was used for this purpose. In the following discussion, the term "groups" will often be used as a shorthand notation for the diagnostic groups previously defined.

Table 8. *Correlations between Sample A interbattery factors (rows) and Sample B matched interbattery factors (columns)*

Sample A interbattery factors	Matched interbattery factors for Sample B						
	I	II	III	IV	V	VI	VII
I	85	13	12	08	20	−23	08
II	02	81	−30	−10	06	−11	−09
III	12	−33	85	03	−10	−12	−02
IV	08	−03	04	85	−06	06	22
V	14	07	−13	−13	78	17	16
VI	−23	−07	−10	06	21	73	44
VII	−01	−18	−07	17	11	38	53

The goal of discriminant analysis can be viewed as twofold. One step is to test for possible differences between the groups on some set of variables. If differences do exist, the second step is to examine the nature of the differences. The statistical problem is to find an optimal combination of the measurement variables that maximizes differences between groups, while keeping the within-group discrepancies at a minimum. Tatsuoka (1971, pp. 177–183) discusses one solution to this problem which is based on canonical correlation. The two sets of canonical matrices are the measurement variables (in this instance, factor scores) and the group membership variables. If the measurement variables significantly discriminate among the diagnoses, then one or more of the canonical correlations between the two sets of variables will be large.

The measurement variables here were "pseudo-factor" scores, defined with reference to Table 4. The scores are pseudo-scores in the sense that they were obtained by merely adding only the salient variables of a factor together, rather than weighting all variables by the elements of the pattern matrix. This method has been called an "approximation procedure for factor scores" by Gorsuch (1974, p. 236), and is generally recommended when data reduction is the goal. Group membership was recorded by dummy membership codes for the eight diagnostic categories, resulting in seven variables.

As usual, the analysis first was carried out for Sample A and replicated with Sample B. Cooley and Lohnes (1971, p. 250) recommend rotating the discriminant function coefficients to increase interpretability, which does not alter the essential properties of the solution. The rotated coefficients from Sample A were again matched with those from Sample B. The results are in Table 9. It can be seen there that in both samples several of the canonical correlations were very large, suggesting good discrimination between the groups. The canonical Rs were somewhat stronger in Sample B, however. Table 9 also contains the correlations between the rotated discriminant coefficients of Sample A and those of Sample B, matched to the first matrix. The match was excellent, with all discriminant func-

Table 9. *Discriminant coefficients for Samples A and B*

	Discriminant functions					
Factor scores	I	II	III	IV	V	VI
Sample A						
I MAJORMENT	1.41	−.17	−.07	−.07	−.14	−.41
II COMMDISOR	−.07	−.08	.00	−.19	1.06	−.16
III PSYPATHY	−.11	1.13	−.05	−.15	−.08	−.11
IV AGGRESS	−.07	.04	−.79	.19	.15	.21
V SEVDEPRESS	−.46	−.18	−.09	−.22	−.24	1.08
VI HYPERSENS	−.04	−.15	−.09	1.05	−.17	−.14
VII NEUROSIS	−.29	−.01	.90	.20	.51	.39
Canonical R	.79	.63	.55	.32	.27	.12
Sample B						
I MAJORMENT	1.75	−.36	−.01	−.03	−.13	−.59
II COMMDISOR	−.15	−.11	−.16	−.22	.88	−.06
III PSYPATHY	−.46	1.16	−.05	−.19	−.09	.19
IV AGGRESS	.02	.16	−.67	.25	.39	−.02
V SEVDEPRESS	−.77	−.05	−.22	−.37	−.46	1.32
VI HYPERSENS	−.07	−.19	−.23	.93	−.29	−.09
VII NEUROSIS	−.11	.14	1.04	.19	.64	.18
Canonical R	.88	.74	.63	.41	.34	.21

Correlations between discriminant functions of Sample A and Sample B

Sample A discriminant coefficients	Sample B matched discriminant coefficients					
	I	II	III	IV	V	VI
I	97	−37	−06	02	−14	−72
II	−29	97	01	−25	−07	01
III	−06	01	97	−04	25	07
IV	02	−26	−02	99	−19	−28
V	−11	−09	27	−19	94	−21
VI	−64	00	08	−31	−21	93

tions essentially identical in both samples. Therefore, the first question of whether true differences exist between the groups on the measurement variables was answered affirmatively.

The second question, concerning the nature of the differences, was explored by calculating the group *centroids*, means, on each discriminant function, shown in Table 10. There the scores have been standardized to mean 50 and standard deviation 10 to facilitate interpretation. The group Schizophrenia and Paranoia had extremely high scores on the first discriminant function (Sample A = 130,

Table 10. *Discriminant function centroids for Samples A and B*

Diagnoses	Discriminant functions					
	I	II	III	IV	V	VI
Sample A						
Schizophrenic & paranoid	130	56	45	49	54	49
Borderline schizophrenic	49	49	43	49	57	49
Psychopathy	36	75	48	50	46	44
Personality disorder	48	50	49	58	49	50
Neurotic	48	48	57	52	49	54
Nonspecific	45	42	57	46	50	46
No mental illness	44	46	54	48	42	48
No consensus diagnosis	60	61	34	42	63	53
Sample B						
Schizophrenic & paranoid	107	57	47	48	51	50
Borderline schizophrenic	51	47	39	47	60	56
Psychopathy	45	84	35	32	57	67
Personality disorder	39	53	48	52	53	49
Neurotic	48	48	59	54	45	49
Nonspecific	49	45	55	47	51	41
No mental illness	39	45	57	53	42	44
No consensus diagnosis	62	61	43	67	72	78

Sample B = 107). In Table 9 the factor score with the largest weight on the first principal component was named Thought Disorder. The first function thus appeared to be a schizophrenia–thought disorder dimension. The second function in Table 10 produced the largest scores for the psychopathy group (Sample A = 75, Sample B = 84), and in Table 9 the discriminant coefficient for Psychopathy was high in each subsample. The second function was labeled Psychopathy. The third function appeared to describe the Neurotic group. The fourth through sixth functions were less related to any of the diagnostic groups in any clear way, a finding supported by the presence of smaller canonical correlations.

SUMMARY

In the investigation of the causes and prevention of schizophrenia, diagnosis of the disorder plays a central role. Two basic models have been proposed to characterize the process of diagnosis. The typological view asserts that the various forms of abnormal behavior are distinct entities and that it is advantageous to categorize patients into nonoverlapping types on the basis of symptoms and background factors. On the other hand, a dimensional approach emphasizes that abnormal behavior is a continuous phenomenon. Here stress is placed upon the degree to which a symptom is present or on the frequency of a given behavior. This research made use of the dimensional model to define a series of scales of abnormal behavior. Its purpose was to describe the current functioning of a sample of individuals at high risk for schizophrenia. Although related in spirit to projects that seek to assign a traditional diagnosis to a sample of individuals, this work attempted to incorporate data on present symptomatology into a multidimensional model using factor-analytic methods. This work will permit further analyses that seek to find quantitative relationships between premorbid events and current abnormal functioning.

The data used were interview items gathered in the context of a prospective, longitudinal study of 311 Danish subjects, 207 of which have schizophrenic mothers. Altogether, 674 items in three batteries were available. Using procedures of scale construction from item analysis, these items yielded 35 scales, with an average internal consistency reliability of .82. The total sample was split into two subsamples to replicate these findings. These reliabilities were successfully cross-validated in the second subsample also.

The nature of the relationships among these 35 variables was next investigated using two types of factor analyses. Both principal-components and interbattery factor analysis were used. It was found that seven factors satisfactorily accounted for the correlations among the variables. The factors produced an adequate simple structure, and the results were independently replicated in the second subsample.

To examine the validity of these findings, a discriminant analysis was performed using the factors to discriminate among the traditional diagnoses which have been given the members of the sample. This analysis demonstrated that virtually the same information contained in the diagnoses was expressed in factors. As before, these findings were successfully replicated in the second subsample.

These results imply that schizophrenia can profitably be characterized by several dimensions of psychopathology. Specifically, schizophrenia is primarily depicted as the combination of very poor cognitive functioning, very high patterns of avoidance, and low depression levels. Although these findings are not unique to this study, they confirm the hypothesis that the disorder can be characterized dimensionally. In addition, this work lays the foundation for future research between antecedent data from this sample and their relation to these factors.

4   A controlled study of primary prevention: the Mauritius Project

SARNOFF A. MEDNICK, PETER H. VENABLES,
FINI SCHULSINGER, CYRIL DALAIS, AND
KATHERINE VAN DUSEN

One of the critical long-term objectives of high-risk studies is to contribute to research on primary prevention. In this chapter we describe an intervention project instituted in 1972 in the island–nation of Mauritius. The risk criterion was physiological deviance (fast autonomic nervous system recovery) that was related theoretically (Mednick & Schulsinger, 1968) and empirically (Mednick et al., 1978) to a predisposition for schizophrenia.

The project began when the subjects were 3 years of age; it will take some years before the target outcome of schizophrenia is observed. In the meantime we are studying intermediate, age-appropriate outcomes. In later childhood we recorded the children's school performance. The children are now about to enter adolescence, and we are preparing for a prospective study of their delinquency.

In 1960, at a conference in Ann Arbor, we stated our view of the objectives of high-risk research. We planned "to test and interview a group of normal children in the Detroit area. From these tests and interviews we shall predict which of these children will become schizophrenic. . . . We have decided to select a group in which the prevalence rates are considerably elevated. [We sought] individuals who have one or two parents who have been schizophrenic. . . . If our predictions prove to be supported, we are then in a position to do research which is aimed at the prevention of schizophrenia. We might observe a normal population with our tests, detect those individuals who are potential schizophrenics and then explore the possibility of intervention" (Mednick, 1960, p. 69).

The first step in implementing the general plan was the longitudinal study of children of schiziophrenics. Optimally, such study can provide two useful outcomes. First, it can elucidate a pattern of premorbid variables that distinguishes the high-risk individual who later becomes schizophrenic. The pattern must then

The Mauritius Project is currently being supported by the Welcome Trust, Peter H. Venables, Principal Investigator, and the Mauritian Ministries of Health and Education. The original establishment of the cohort was supported by grants from the World Health Organization, the British Medical Research Council, and the Danish Organization for Aid to Developing Nations. The Mauritian government has consistently been a critical support to our work. We wish to especially thank the former Prime Minister, Sir S. Ramgoolam, and other ministerial long-term friends of the project. We also wish to thank the new Prime Minister, Jugnauth, for his continued support of the project.

71

be tested in an unselected population for its predictive utility. If it proves successful in a general population, we have a means of early detection of predisposed
individuals in the society. This would be a first step in a specific program of
primary prevention. Second, the pattern of variables distinguishing the predisposed individual may suggest a theory of etiology that, in turn, may lead to
developing modes of experimental intervention. Goldstein (1975), for example,
reported a type of communication disturbance that marks the parents of adolescents at especially high risk for schizophrenia; perhaps corrective training in family
communication could be tested as a mode of intervention. As another example, in
the Copenhagen High-Risk Project, 17 of the children of schizophrenics have
themselves become schizophrenic. In contrast to a variety of control groups, almost all of these schizophrenics were separated from their parents or substitute
parents very early in life (Beuhring et al., 1982). This result might also tempt an
intervention researcher to test the efficacy of superior foster care as a means of
helping to prevent schizophrenia. High-risk research thus offers the promise of
providing a means of early detection and of suggesting ideas for modes of
intervention.

INFORMATION FROM THE DANISH HIGH-RISK PROJECT

In our view one way to conduct a prevention program is to make it a part of
ongoing research in the longitudinal study of schizophrenia. It is critical that the
prevention program be centered around a body of data that relates to intervention.
For example, a researcher must know who are the appropriate subjects, what kinds
of treatment or intervention strategies may be considered efficacious, and, in order
to further knowledge in the field, must have a plausible theoretical idea about why
a particular intervention is appropriate for a given group of individuals.

In accordance with this overall plan, in 1962 we examined intensively a group of
207 Danish children at high risk for schizophrenia (they have schizophrenic mothers). We also examined 104 control subjects. We followed this group until 1967
when 20 of them evidenced a variety of psychiatric breakdowns. In good agreement with the general theory guiding this research (Mednick, 1962), an autonomic
nervous system variable (fast skin-conductance recovery rate) proved to be the best
discriminator of the breakdown subjects from their carefully chosen high-risk and
low-risk controls (Mednick & Schulsinger, 1973). Some time later, after psychiatric diagnoses had been given to each subject (H. Schulsinger, 1976), ANS
variables were also shown to predict to schizophrenia (Mednick et al., 1978),
especially for the male schizophrenics.

RATIONALE FOR THE MAURITIUS PROJECT

The ANS variables (particularly ANS recovery) proved to be the premorbid variable that best distinguished the 20 HR individuals who suffered breakdowns. In
accordance with our overall plan the next step involved examining "a normal
population with our tests [in order to] detect those individuals who are potential

schizophrenics and then explore the possibility of interventions (Mednick, 1960, p. 69).

We were planning this project for Copenhagen when we were offered the opportunity and initial financial support from the World Health Organization (WHO) to conduct the research in Mauritius. A visit to Mauritius indicated that local vaccination records would enable us to identify a birth cohort that had survived to age 3. All the 3-year-olds in two communities (Quatre Bornes and Vacoas) gave us a study population of about 1,800 children. We combined forces with Professor Peter Venables of York University and with Dr. A. C. Raman, a Mauritian, English-trained psychiatrist. We established a laboratory in Quatre Bornes; and as a result of the energetic efforts of Brian Bell, an English psycho-physiologist who managed the project, the 1,800 children were psychophysi-ologically assessed in the year beginning August, 1972. In addition to obtaining the psychophysiological assessment, we observed and coded play behavior and examined cognitive development of the 1,800 children. This aspect of the project was directed by Brian Sutton-Smith. Turan Itil and George Ulett taped electroen-cephalograms (EEGs) for a part of the population. A family interview, a medical examination, and perinatal information were also recorded.

In contrast to the work in Copenhagen where selection of the children at high risk was made on the basis of known parental characteristics, the Mauritian high-risk subjects were identified on the basis of psychophysiological data. This was because physiological data (in the Copenhagen Project) appeared to be the best predictors of later breakdown, and because physiological variables were more likely to show cross-cultural robustness. The research also represented the first attempt at fairly large scale screening of a population by psychophysiological tech-niques with the aim of early detection of high-risk children. But of equal impor-tance, the project sought to define a prevention program in which the identified risk children would be helped to learn adequate social functioning under low-threat conditions.

In undertaking this work we were aware that there were many potential pitfalls involved in the assumption that autonomic deviance in childhood (assessed by peripheral measures) would predict adult mental illness, especially when our ex-pectations were based on preliminary results on adolescents in Copenhagen, and we were now moving into a very different culture, with different races and climatic conditions. A longitudinal study of a psychophysiologically assessed, large, un-selected population of children in Mauritius was deemed of sufficient importance in its own right to justify the project, however. In any case, were we to wait for evidence adequate enough to forestall criticism (Garmezy & Streitman, 1974), we should certainly not survive to attempt the work at all.

This report will concern itself only with data related to the skin-conductance measures. The physiological records for the Mauritian 3-year-olds were scored by hand in Mauritius, then coded and sent to Venables in England for analysis; 1,796 usable records were obtained. Distributions of the skin-conductance measures were plotted. Children with deviant skin-conductance characteristics such as those displayed by the Copenhagen breakdown group were identified. Smaller groups with other deviance of special interest such as electrodermal nonresponders and controls with average skin-conductance functioning were also identified. A total of 200 such children from the population of 1,796 were identified. One hundred were placed in two specially established nursery schools; the remaining 100 were selected as matched controls and permitted to remain in the community (community controls).

Beyond the design of the nursery schools, no specific intervention program was attempted. The nursery schools had several distinctive features, however, which should be mentioned:

1. The 100 children were almost completely from poor families. The children were bussed to and from school; the hours were 9:00 a.m. to 3:00 p.m. The nursery-school children were given a hot, protein-rich lunch. The community controls consumed only minimal amounts of protein, their diet consisting almost completely of rice and vegetables.
2. Because of the selection procedures, the nursery schools had a very high density of autonomically sensitive children (about 50%).
3. The directors and teachers were very highly motivated and well trained and had a remarkable esprit de corps.

It should be stated that at no time was anyone in Mauritius informed about the autonomic status of the children.

Why nursery schools?

It may be of value to present the thinking that directed us to choosing nursery schools as a vehicle for intervention. We considered a number of possibilities before making our choice. The earliest possible intervention may occur before conception in the form of genetic counseling. In view of relatively low rates of schizophrenia among children with one schizophrenic parent, it would only be two-parent families that might be appropriate for such intervention. However, in view of the fact that two-thirds of the children of schizophrenic women are born before the schizophrenic woman is diagnosed, this procedure is of doubtful utility (S. A. Mednick, Mura, Schulsinger, & Mednick, 1971).

Those who consider improving the conditions of pregnancies and deliveries involving schizophrenic parents, must also face the fact that they will only be able to identify one-third of cases at the time of pregnancy. This would seem a worthwhile goal except for the fact that this one-third, born to women already schizophrenic, tend to have relatively problem-free pregnancies and deliveries (S. A. Mednick et al., 1971). Perinatal intervention may be extremely effective, but identification of risk will have to be made by some means other than the diagnostic status of the prospective parent.

The neonatal period suggests itself as a time when society and the investigator have access to the child and the parent. Further, some longitudinal research has suggested that neonatal status *has* predictive value for adolescent behavior (B.

Mednick, 1977). This period, then, has potential for early detection and, conceivably, intervention. It should be mentioned, however, that society's contact with the neonate (in the maternity hospital) is rather brief.

In terms of early intervention, nursery schools have much to recommend them. Nursery schools are in growing demand in Western society as more women enter the work force. Children spend from 4 to 8 hours a day at nursery schools being observed by teachers who are potential raters. This also gives the investigator ample opportunity to observe *and* intervene. The advantages of using nursery schools for intervention research are spelled out in detail in S. A. Mednick and Witkin-Lanoil (1977) and Mednick and Garfinkel (1975).

Results of nursery-school experience

The autonomically deviant (High-Risk) and normal (Low-Risk) groups were first admitted to the nursery schools in 1973. They continued until 1976, when they all entered the primary school system. The community controls (matched for age, sex, race, and *autonomic* characteristics) remained undisturbed by us during this period except for some psychophysiological retesting in a laboratory in one of the nursery schools.

Just before the 100 community control and 100 nursery-school children began primary school in December, 1976, they were invited in for a behavioral assessment session in order to compare them and estimate the effect of the nursery school. We will report the results of this behavioral observation shortly. It should be noted that these children have been systematically observed at regular intervals throughout the course of the project. The analysis of this larger data set of observations will be reported at a future time and will provide the basis for a more comprehensive evaluation of the effectiveness of the nursery school. The data of the behavior observation session offer certain advantages in terms of the controls instituted.

In order to bias the testing as little as possible, the play-observation session did not take place at either of the nursery schools, but at a third building. All the children were dressed in new, identical uniforms. Trained observers who had not previously met the children provided standardized ratings of their behavior, using an adaptation of a system devised by Bell, Weller, and Waldrop (1971). New toys were provided for the play period. In other words, attempts were made to reduce the possibility of the identification of the nursery children by the observers or any advantage of the nursery children in familiarity with the setting, play materials, or observers.

The children were brought to the observation setting in buses in groups of four, one child from each of the two nursery schools and one child from each of the communities. (Thus none of the children knew each other.) The four children were brought together in a playroom; during the play period each child was observed for a period of 8 minutes. Aspects of their behavior were counted or timed. We shall report on the timed behavior, which consisted of:

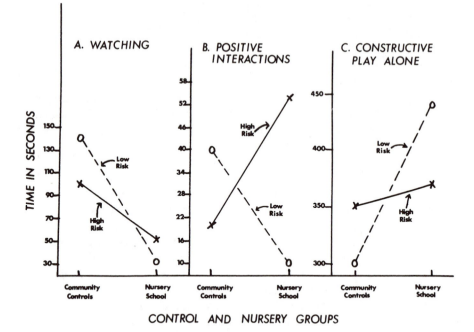

Figure 1. Time spent in watching, in positive interactions, and in constructive play alone for High-Risk and Low-Risk groups.

Watching: The observer timed periods when the child was inactive and watching others.
Positive interaction: The observer timed periods when the child talked or played cooperatively with the other children.
Constructive play alone: The observer timed the total number of seconds the child played constructively with toys by himself.

Because the total observation time for each child was 8 minutes, the periods spent in the three activities were not mutually independent.

Figure 1 compares the High-Risk and Low-Risk groups that had experienced the nursery schools with the psychophysiologically matched community controls who had not attended the nursery schools. Note that both the High- and Low-Risk groups decrease substantially their inactive watching after having attended the nursery schools. The Low-Risk (community) children are relatively high in positive interactions and watching. After the nursery experience, they reduce both of these activities to the benefit of indulging in constructive play. The High-Risk (community) children tend not to engage in positive interactions, but are high in constructive play. It is gratifying that the greatest effect of the nursery-school experience for the High-Risk children is their increase in positive interactions of a social nature (this at the expense of time spent in isolated, inactive watching).

We offer the following interpretations of these results:

1. The psychophysiological selection criteria are correlated with specific characteristic behaviors before the influence of the nursery school.
2. The nursery-school experience affects the social and play behavior of the children.
3. The nursery school affects behavior in the children differentially as a function of the psychophysiological characteristics used in selection.

What is most encouraging is the fact that the greatest change for the High-Risk group is an increase in positive social interactions. This increase is seen in an observation situation in which they are thrown in with peers and adult observers who are unknown to them. In terms of the interventive goals of this project, these results are not disappointing.

FURTHER DATA COLLECTION: THE 11-YEAR FOLLOW-UP

Since this assessment was completed in 1976, we have collected information on the entire cohort's progress through the school system by means of teacher questionnaires. At the present time we are bringing the cohort in for an intensive assessment. The assessment is being conducted in the setting of an education camp, which will provide an environmental studies course during term time and part of the holidays. Each child is attending the camp for 1 week. The provision of teachers and teaching facilities has been made by the Mauritian Institute of Education. Prior to their attendance, a social worker is obtaining parents' ratings of children's behavior and reports on parental attitudes and home environment. The camp ratings are being made of characteristics such as aggressiveness, hyperactivity, withdrawal, schizoid tendencies, and sociability/social competence. Psychophysiological measures include bilateral skin-conductance and heart-rate orienting responses to stimuli presented from a standard auditory tape. Event-related cortical potentials elicited by visual stimuli will enable measures of input processing to be made. Additionally, smooth-pursuit eye tracking is being assessed. All these measures have been shown to be predictive of, or related to, schizophrenic breakdown.

IMPLICATIONS

Nursery school

One important message which the Mauritius Project suggests regards the feasibility of conducting experimental–manipulative intervention research in the field of schizophrenia. The practical success of the project in relation to psychopathology will depend, in part, on the correctness of our assumption that a fast recovering ANS is partially predisposing to mental illness, particularly schizophrenia. If the number of psychiatric disabililities among the ANS–High-Risk community controls is not substantially elevated over the population risk, we cannot hope to show a positive prevention effect of the intensive nursery-school experience on later psychiatric diagnosis. But in any case, it will be possible to compare the level of psychological adjustment in the nursery-school and community-control samples. Other outcomes can also be examined.

Birth cohort study

The assessment of the 1,800 children at 3 years of age and the ensuing follow-up data have prepared the stage for a unique longitudinal study. It is rare in birth-cohort studies that physiological characteristics are available on a relatively large population at such a young age. It will be fascinating to observe the long-term life-history correlates of the skin-conductance, heart-rate, and EEG data in the context of the psychological, cognitive examination, and the medical and sociofamilial information. This portion of the investigation was conceived as a multipurpose study. It will be possible to investigate the early antecedents of interactions with more proximal experiences in the development of psychopathology, delinquency and criminality, alcholism and other substance abuse, and so forth on the one side and positive life outcomes on the other. As the lives of our children unfold and resolve into young adult life we anticipate the exciting task of discovering in what ways the child is father to the man.

Delinquency study

As mentioned in the introduction, the children are entering adolescence. Some will begin to evidence delinquent behavior. In order to prepare for the prospective study of these outcomes we are planning interviews with the cohort children and their families. This part of the project is directed by Katherine Van Dusen.

The delinquency study is guided by control theory as expressed by Travis Hirschi (1969). Biological, psychological, social, and ecological levels of controls are being assessed for each member of the cohort in order to determine how they individually and in interaction relate to subsequent development of delinquency.

PART II

The UCLA Family Project: 1964–1982

The Danish project exploited a well-documented actuarial feature of schizophrenic disorders, namely, that the biological offspring of schizophrenic parents have unusually high risk for the disorder themselves. Beginning just 2 years later, the UCLA Family Project approached the problem in an entirely different way by exploiting a complementary rationale: Although the overwhelming majority of schizophrenics do *not* have schizophrenic parents, many of them are reared in families with disturbances in patterns of communication and relationship among their members. Clinical observations along these lines have a long and established tradition in clinical psychology and social psychiatry, owing much to the teaching of Harry Stack Sullivan and Adolph Meyer. However, the more immediate impetus for the UCLA approach was a decade of experimental research in the 1950s by Eliot Rodnick, in collaboration with Norman Garmezy at Duke University.

Tracing the fascinating history of that collaboration from its beginning in the 1930s, when both men were young apprentices of David Shakow at the Worcester State Hospital in Massachusetts, could fill a book all by itself. Ironically, the research at Duke focused mainly on perceptual and reaction time experiments with hospitalized schizophrenics, in the classical tradition of experimental psychology to which Shakow's career was dedicated. In the course of their experiments, the young collaborators observed that the laboratory performance of schizophrenics deteriorated sharply in response to implied censure by parental figures. Consequently, much of the subsequent research at Duke was directed toward exploring the implications of disturbances in the dynamics of family relations for understanding eventual schizophrenic disorders in the offspring.

The horses were already out of the barn before they were corralled for study at Duke. On moving west to UCLA in 1961, Rodnick was determined to study the problem of schizophrenic development prospectively. (Garmezy did likewise on moving to Minnesota.) A new alliance was forged with Michael Goldstein, and the UCLA Family Project was launched in 1964. It remains the only project in the Risk Research Consortium that does not base the evaluation of risk on schizophrenic parentage, although there are many points of convergence in approach with several of the other teams. Part II presents two reports that summarize the methods and findings of this project.

79

5 Parental communication style, affect, and role as precursors of offspring schizophrenia-spectrum disorders

ELIOT H. RODNICK, MICHAEL J. GOLDSTEIN,
JULIA M. LEWIS, AND JERI A. DOANE

The UCLA Family Project was designed to provide evidence concerning behavioral and familial precursors of schizophrenia and related disorders sometimes termed the *extended schizophrenia spectrum*. Unlike other high-risk projects, which have defined risk for schizophrenia on the basis of parental psychopathology, this project has utilized a series of risk indicators that became more developed and refined as the study proceeded. The sample for the study was a series of 65 intact families containing a disturbed but nonpsychotic adolescent for whom help was sought from the UCLA Psychology Clinic. Disturbed adolescents were hypothesized as a class to be at higher-than-average risk for schizophrenia because of their failure to master the developmental tasks of the teenage years and also because other follow-up studies of comparable populations (Robins, 1966; Nameche, Waring, & Ricks, 1964) have supported their greater risk for schizophrenia.

In the initial stages of this project, and prior to the availability of follow-up data, we attempted to define subgroups of disturbed adolescents within the sample who were at greater risk than their peers. The sample of disturbed adolescents was divided into four groups based on certain key features of their behavioral difficulties. These four groups were (1) aggressive antisocial, (2) active family conflict, (3) passive negative, and (4) withdrawn and socially isolated. Criteria for defining each of these four groups are contained in Goldstein, Judd, Rodnick, Alkire, and Gould (1968). Two of the groups were hypothesized to be at greater risk for schizophrenia-spectrum disorders; Groups 2 and 4, the latter by virtue of their resemblance to the adolescent history of the poor premorbid schizophrenic and the former's resemblance to Arieti's description of the preschizophrenic *stormy* personality. In the early stages of this project we attempted to relate various measures of parental attributes and aspects of intrafamilial behavior to the form of the adolescent's behavioral disturbance. Findings at this stage revealed some interesting concurrent relationships between intrafamilial behavior and the form of the adolescent's behavioral disturbance (Goldstein et al., 1968; Alkire, Goldstein, Rodnick, & Judd, 1971; McPherson, 1970; and Goldstein, Rodnick, Judd, & Gould, 1970).

Another approach contributing to the definition of risk for schizophrenia involved parental attributes. Using leads provided by Wynne and Singer in their studies of communication deviance in parents of schizophrenics, we broadened

81

our use of the Thematic Apperception Test (TAT) to tap signs of communication disorder in parents of these disturbed adolescents. James E. Jones (1977) developed a coding system for communication deviance (CD), and applied it to data from the Wynne-Singer NIMH sample to determine factor profiles that discriminated parents of schizophrenics from parents of other psychopathological groups. He then applied these profile criteria to the verbatim parental TATs of our sample of disturbed adolescents and generated three groups: high, intermediate, and low risk for offspring schizophrenia based on the quantity and quality of CD behavior observed in these parental projective test data. Note that Jones' three groups are not based upon actual interactional data but on individual transactions between a parent and a tester. Thus, the CD data can serve as marker variables of intrafamilial behaviors but not as direct reflections of them. The importance of the distinction between marker variables and actual observed interactions will become clearer in this chapter.

RELATIONSHIP BETWEEN RISK INDICATORS

How does the risk derived from the adolescent's behavior problem group relate to that based upon parental CD? At first, when the sample was largely male (Jones, Rodnick, Goldstein, McPherson, & West, 1977), they seemed very close as only Group 2 and 4 adolescents had high CD parents; however, this relationship was not a perfect one as some adolescents from these two groups had parents with low or intermediate CD as well. As the sample was expanded (and more females were included), the relationship seemed to weaken and was no longer a statistically significant one, except when the sample was divided by sex, where the male subsample still revealed the original association between high CD and Group 2 and 4 type adolescent behavioral difficulties. In the females, the association broke down because there were some Group 1 cases (aggressive antisocial teenagers) with high CD parents, where no such relationship was noted in the males. Aggressive antisocial behavior in a female adolescent with its emphasis on sexual acting-out, reflects quite a different process than that observed in males. Group 1 females may turn out to be a more heterogeneous group than is the case for the acting-out males.

AFFECTIVE COMPONENTS OF INTRAFAMILIAL BEHAVIOR

As the project progressed, and more families in our sample were studied intensively, we were impressed by the wide variability in affective messages emanating from parent to child. The literature on families containing schizophrenic offspring frequently mentioned disturbed affective messages, whether described as the ambivalent affective messages of the double-bind hypothesis or the more consistently aversive messages noted by Lidz and his colleagues (1965). Interest in parental affective messages was enhanced by the publication of the work of Vaughn and Leff (1976a), who, although focusing upon familial factors related to the course of schizophrenia, identified some particularly aversive parental affective attitudes toward offspring that they grouped under the rubric of *expressed emotion* (EE). The key elements of high expressed emotion are criticism, overinvolvement, and hostility directed at the identified patient.

Doane, while a postdoctoral trainee on our project, was working on the problem of coding key affective attitudes in the transcripts of the directly observed interaction among family members obtained during the confrontation session. This session, the fourth in a series of six weekly contacts with families studied, involved several moderately stressful family discussions of idiosyncratically developed emotional problems within each family. These discussions were carried out in dyads with the adolescent and each parent separately as well as in a triadic situation involving both parents and the adolescent. In later stages of the project, control siblings of the same age were also included, where available, which added a tetradic interaction to the design. There are too few cases in the sample to include a comparative analysis at this time. In subsequent samples of hospitalized adolescents, the expanded procedure was used uniformly, and in subsequent reports we will deal with changes in family behavior as a function of the different contexts. This provides a comparison of the adolescent's behavior as he/she interacts with more complex segments of the family system.

In these discussions, all family members were asked to indicate how they felt about the problem and to attempt some resolution in a 5–7 minute period. While reading these transcripts, Doane was struck by the marked variability in affective messages observed in the verbatim transcripts. She identified some key affective messages that resembled a number of the components of the Vaughn–Leff construct as they might be revealed interactionally. This was done despite her unfamiliarity with the Vaughn–Leff research at the time. Her measure of affective style (AS) is composed of statements of personal criticism, guilt induction, and intrusiveness directed at the adolescent in the directly observed interaction. The Doane Affective Style Index was then introduced as a third risk indicator.

FOLLOW-UP PROCEDURE

Any high-risk study requires follow-up of the population into the risk period for schizophrenia. At the present time, we have only followed our teenage sample for 5 years so that their average age at the time of follow-up was 21.5, which is barely into the risk period for adult schizophrenia. A longer-term 15-year follow-up is currently in progress. Nevertheless, there is a wide variety of outcomes, ranging from definite schizophrenia to relatively normal adjustment, to warrant some preliminary tests of our risk indicators.

Before we present these data, a word about the follow-up procedure is in order. Of the 65 offspring, 52 were seen for a face-to-face detailed psychiatric interview and received a battery of psychological tests. All of these interviews were recorded on audiotape and listened to blindly by two psychologists who independently made diagnoses using the Research Diagnostic Criteria (Spitzer, Endicott, & Robins, 1975), as well as the criteria for the Borderline Syndrome of Gunderson (1977). Reliability of these assessments was extremely good. For purposes of data analysis,

Table 1. *Problem group versus outcome*

Outcome	Problem group ($N = 52$)[a]			
	I	II	III	IV
1–4	8	10	10	7
5	3	2	0	4
6–7	2	3	1	2

Outcome	Males ($N = 28$)[b]				Females ($N = 24$)[c]			
	I	II	III	IV	I	II	III	IV
1–4	4	4	6	2	4	6	4	5
5	1	1	0	3	2	1	0	1
6–7	1	3	1	2	1	0	0	0

[a]$\chi^2 = 5.47$; $p < .49$.
[b]$\chi^2 = 7.77$; $p < .26$.
[c]$\chi^2 = 4.44$; $p < .62$.

the cases were ordered on a 7-point scale originally devised by Wender, Rosenthal, and Kety (1968) for their adoption studies, in which Categories 1–4 are considered nonschizophrenic spectrum disorders (1 = normal; 2 = normal with mild neurotic traits; 3 = neurotic; 4 = mild to moderate character disorders) and in which Categories 5–7 are considered the extended schizophrenia-spectrum (5 = severe character disorders and probable borderline cases; 6 = probable schizophrenic and definite borderline cases; and 7 = definite schizophrenia). Within that spectrum we made a distinction between Category 5, the so-called soft spectrum and Category 6–7 the hard spectrum in which definite signs of schizophrenia or borderline syndrome are noted.

RELATIONSHIP BETWEEN RISK INDICATORS AND EARLY ADULT OUTCOME ASSESSMENT

Adolescent behavior problem. Table 1 presents the relationship between the fourfold problem grouping and the frequency of spectrum and nonspectrum cases. The relationship is not significant. However, as noted earlier for the CD problem group relationship, the relationship for males is somewhat sharper than that for females. For males, mainly Groups 2 and 4 show subsequent hard-spectrum outcomes. Table 1 also indicates that all but one of the hard-spectrum outcomes are found in the male subsample. It should be noted that although the overall chi square is not significant, there is an essential absence of Group 3 adolescents (passive–negative) in the schizophrenia-spectrum outcome group. Adolescents

Table 2. *Communication deviance versus outcome[a,b]*

Outcome	Level of communication deviance		
	Low	Intermediate	High
1–4	9	11	6[c]
5	0	1	5
6–7	0	0	8[c]

[a]$N = 40$; 12 cases with outcomes did not have verbatim TAT records required for CD analysis.
[b]$\chi^2 = 20.23$; $p < .0004$.
[c]Sibling diagnosed as definite schizophrenic. Target adolescent received Level 4 diagnosis of character disorder.

manifesting this pattern show a particularly low risk for subsequent schizophrenia or related disorders.

Parental communication deviance. The relationship between level of parental CD and spectrum versus nonspectrum outcomes is presented in Table 2. Here we see a highly significant relationship in which only high CD parents have offspring who subsequently develop schizophrenia-spectrum outcomes. If we consider the most serious outcome in the family and consider that two siblings who manifested definite schiziphrenia represent the outcome for a parental unit, the relationship between CD and schizophrenia-spectrum disorders 5 years later is even more significant.

Despite the positive results, one can see in Table 2 that although low or intermediate CD is almost always associated with nonspectrum outcomes, there is a wide variety of outcomes in high CD family units.

AFFECTIVE STYLE AS A PREDICTOR

A similar analysis was done with Doane's AS profile categorized into three groups, Benign, Intermediate (negative affective messages associated with at least one positive support statement), and Negative (instances of personal criticism, guilt-induction, or excessive intrusiveness without a strongly positive support statement). Table 3 presents the relationship between this categorization and outcome diagnosis. These data resemble the CD–outcome relationships as benign AS profiles in the triadic interaction are strongly associated with relatively good early adult outcomes. Similarly, the schizophrenia-spectrum outcomes occur in families where parents express negative or intermediate AS statements toward the adolescent. As with the CD data, negative AS profiles are not uniquely associated with subsequent schizophrenia-spectrum disorders as a number of more favorable outcomes occur in this group.

Table 3. *Affective Style profile versus outcome*[a,b]

| | Affective Style profile | | |
Outcome	Benign	Intermediate	Negative
1–4	23	5	7
5	2	4	4
6–7	0	1	6

[a]$N = 52$.
[b]$\chi^2 = 17.9$; $p < .005$.

Table 4. *Communication Deviance and Affective Style versus outcome*[a]

Outcome	Low or Intermediate CD and Benign AS	Low or Intermediate CD and Intermediate or Poor AS	High CD and Benign AS	High CD and Intermediate or Poor AS
1–4	9	10	7[b]	0
5	0	2	1	4
6–7	0	0	0	7[b]

[a]$N = 40$.
[b]Sibling diagnosed definite schizophrenia. However, unlike CD, AS is measured between parent and a specific offspring, diagnosis for sibling was ignored, and that of target adolescent used in this analysis.

COMMUNICATION DEVIANCE AND AFFECTIVE STYLE AS CONJOINT PREDICTORS

As our research evolved, we developed a working model that communication deviance and affective style may represent orthogonal parameters of the intrafamilial environment which combine to raise the likelihood of subsequent schizophrenia. First, we examined the relationship between CD and AS and found, indeed, that they were not related (Cramers V = .12, not significant). We then were secure in combining data from the two measures as a conjoint predictor of outcome. Next, we compressed our groups into four categories as seen in Table 4 and found this combination to predict outcome rather precisely. Schizophrenia-spectrum disorders, particularly those termed hard spectrum (6 and 7 on the Wender et al. Scale) only arise in families where parents manifested both high CD and negative AS. Negative AS or CD alone did not predict these severe outcomes. A more detailed presentation of the relationship between these two predictors and specific diagnostic outcome categories is contained in Doane, West, Goldstein, Rodnick, and Jones (1981).

Naturally, these results must be interpreted with extreme caution as we are barely into the risk period for schizophrenia. High CD cases without the negative AS may break down later on, and the AS factor may operate much as its analog in the Vaughn–Leff research, EE, as a predictor of course from adolescence to early adulthood rather than a determinant of ultimate outcome.

These data were examined in a different fashion using multiple regression techniques in which CD and AS were predictors and the Wender Scale diagnosis was the criterion. The latter was divided in two ways, as a 3-category (1–4, 5, 6–7) and 2-category (1–4, 5–7) grouping. The multiple r for the two predictors was .75 for the former and .74 for the latter. When a step-wise regression approach was used, CD was the first to enter with a beta weight of .50 and AS second with a beta weight of .28; each contributed at a statistically significant level to the prediction of outcome.

INTERACTIONAL CORRELATES OF COMMUNICATION DEVIANCE

The measure of communication deviance clearly serves as an effective marker of parental attributes associated with subsequent schizophrenia-spectrum disorders in offspring. However, unlike the AS Index, which is derived from directly observed interaction between parent and teenager, CD is based upon transactions between a parent and a tester during the administration of a projective test, the TAT. But, what does this index reveal about actual ongoing family interaction? Researchers from our group previously reported on some correlates of CD (Goldstein et al., 1978) which revealed that in the triadic interactions, high CD parents manifested significantly more nonacknowledging behavior than parents classified as intermediate or low, particularly when responding to the offspring. Also, Lieber (1977) found that high CD parents, when observed in a structured discussion of videotapes of their own triadic interaction, were less likely than other parents to use task-focusing comments when the discussion drifted away from the requested structure. Both of these studies support the idea that high CD parents, when actively involved in a three-way emotionally charged discussion with their disturbed teenager, have difficulty maintaining an effective focus of discussion.

A recent study by Lewis (1979) pursued this issue in more detail as she examined aspects of role structure, communication drift, and nonverbal behavior in these triadic family discussions. Her role-structure estimates were based on speaking patterns of *who* talks and *who* is the recipient of others' remarks. Using a profile approach, she characterized families as (1) father-central, (2) mother-central, (3) dual parental focus, and (4) mixed. Father- and mother-central are self-explanatory as each contains a single parent who is the primary speaker and recipient of the other two family members' remarks. Dual parental focus characterizes a triadic interaction in which both parents are equally active and direct the majority of their comments to the teenager. In the mixed pattern either the parents speak only to one another, or one parent talks to the child, who, in turn, addresses another parent, who in turn addresses another speaker, a ronde if you will. Lewis predicted, based on research in families containing a schizophrenic offspring, that

Table 5. *Parental-role structure versus communication deviance*[a,b]

| Level of communication deviance[b] | Parental-role structure | | | |
	Father central	Mother central	Dual parental focus	Mixed patterns
Low	10	2	0	0
Intermediate	5	2	0	8
High	5	8	6	1

[a] $N = 47$; 47 of 65 cases had both CD ratings and ratable interaction transcripts.
[b] $\chi^2 = 30.96$; $p < .0001$.

the father-central pattern would be less common in the high CD family units. Her results are presented in Table 5. Here we see that her prediction is indeed confirmed although the rates for high and intermediate CD groups are the same. In addition, we see that other patterns are noted in high CD family units, particularly mother central and dual parental focus, which are rarely noted in intermediate or low CD family units. Obviously, there is more heterogeneity in the role-structure patterns of high CD than the other two CD groups, but father-central occurs much less frequently than in low CD families. The discrepancy between high and low CD families is particularly noteworthy for the mother-central and dual parental focus family structures.

The heterogeneity in the high CD groups may explain why previous attempts to compare families containing schizophrenic offspring with other groups on similar measures may have produced a "now you see it, now you don't" pattern of results. These have all looked for a single pattern, such as maternal or paternal dominance, when, in fact, Lewis' data suggest strongly that there may be a number of distorted role patterns in preschizophrenic families that are lost when simple averages are used to contrast groups.

Lewis went one step further in attempting to account for the heterogeneity in role patterns. She hypothesized that they may reflect different types or patterns of CD in the parents. The criteria developed by J. E. Jones (1977) for the high CD classification utilized the multifactorial nature of the index. Jones found that when a single parent scored high (T score > 60) on Factor 2 (misperceptions) or 6 (major closure problems) the probability of offspring schizophrenia was high. Therefore, he classified a parental unit as high CD if either parent manifested a high score on Factor 2 or 6 independent of the other parent's score. For the remaining CD factors, Jones found that T scores greater than 60 were required from *both* parents for offspring schizophrenia risk to be high. Therefore, another group of parents in the UCLA sample were classified as high CD only when *both* parents manifested T scores above 60.

Lewis next grouped the high CD parents on the basis of the different criteria

Table 6. *Parental communication-deviance Inclusion Criteria and role-structure pattern*[a]

	Role structure		
CD Factor pattern	Father central	Dual parental focus	Mother central
Father high (2, 6) *or* both parents (2, 6)	4	1	2
Both parents high (1, 3, 4, or 5)	0	4	2
Mother only high (2, 6)	1	1	5

[a]$N = 20$.

suggested by Jones for entry into the high CD group (e.g., single or dual parent requirement). As shown in Table 6, there is a close correspondence between these criteria and role-structure pattern. Where father was high CD on the basis of the Factor 2, 6 pattern (regardless of mother's pattern), we see the father central structural pattern; where mother was classified as high *CD* on the basis of the Factor 2, 6 pattern, we see a mother central pattern; and where *both* parents manifested high CD on the remaining factors, the dual parental focus pattern is noted. Thus, not only was Lewis able to demonstrate parallelism between CD criteria and role structure, but she found that it is the parent or parents who actually have the high CD deficit that are central in the triadic family discussion. This means that such parents are actively involved in family relationships and may, in fact, dominate the family environment. Were this not the case, a theoretical embarrassment would exist. If the high CD parent was relatively inactive or ignored, then we would have to explain the mechanism by which the CD Index translates into pathological family relationships. The high activity level of the parent or parental unit manifesting the high CD projective test pattern suggests that high CD parent(s) are very significant in setting the form and probably the intensity of family discussions.

In order to understand better what type of tone is set within these parental structures, Lewis investigated the two other dimensions of communication drift and nonverbal affect display. Communication drift was measured with regard to two factors, adherence to the topic and expression of feelings. Failure to adhere to the topic was indexed by one of two patterns, drift away from the assigned problem for discussion or rigid adherence to the topic as defined that precluded meaningful discussion. For sharing feelings, two parallel deviations were excessive outpouring of feelings or rigid suppression of all feelings. High CD families ($p < .04$) generally avoided sharing feelings with each other and they were more likely to show distorted communication of the assigned topic, but surprisingly the tendency was

Table 7. *Nonverbal behaviors versus communication deviance*[a,b]

Level of communication deviance	Nonverbal behavior		
	Nonavoidant and relaxed	Nonavoidant and rigid	Avoidant and rigid
Low	8	0	2
Intermediate	2	6	1
High	2	4	9

[a]$N = 34$; only 34 families had CD ratings and usable videotapes for rating facial expression and body position.
[b]$\chi^2 = 20.12; p < .0005$.

toward the rigid, adherence to the topic rather than the drifting, disorganized style. However, the relationship between CD and communication drift was not as sharp as was noted for the previously mentioned role-structure measures.

Where notable rigidity and avoidance of feelings were both observed, it was most common in father-central family units. This was an important difference between father-central families in the high and low CD groups. In the low CD groups, high father activity was associated with clear communication and affect sharing. In the high CD group, the same role structure was associated with rigid adherence to the topic and avoidance of affect sharing. Thus, in the high CD families of this subgroup, paternal activity blocks rather than facilitates family communication. Simply categorizing families as father- or mother-central, as has been done in prior family research, would lose this qualitative difference and lead to the erroneous conclusion that schizophrenic and nonschizophrenic families were similar.

The third correlate of CD explored by Lewis was nonverbal aspects of parental behavior noted during the triadic discussion. The components were: eye contact, facial expression, and voice tone. Voice tone did not relate to the other nonverbal measures but did relate strongly ($p < .01$) to Doane's Affective Style Index, which was derived from content analysis of verbal transcripts only. The eye contact and facial expression measures were combined into profile groupings as follows: (1) avoidant eye contact, rigid facial expression; (2) nonavoidant eye contact; rigid facial expression; and (3) nonavoidant eye contact; relaxed facial expression. In Table 7, we can see that high CD is associated with parental avoidance of eye contact with the adolescent and an unchanging facial expression, whereas the other CD groups show less avoidance behavior and emotional rigidity.

In summary, high CD on a projective test is associated with unusual parental-role structures, a skewed communication style, and a rigid, avoidant nonverbal style directed toward the disturbed adolescent. It is not closely associated with our measures of affective style, either in terms of content or voice tone, both of which are closely associated with each other. Furthermore, the interpersonal correlates of CD

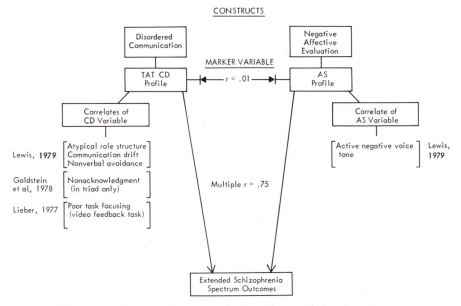

Figure 1. Parental factors predictive of extended schizophrenia-spectrum disorders.

do not relate closely to interpersonal measures of affective attitude directed at the target adolescent, suggesting that affect and communication are independent dimensions of family life.

EVOLUTION OF A MODEL OF PARENTAL FACTORS
ASSOCIATED WITH SCHIZOPHRENIC-SPECTRUM
DISORDERS IN OFFSPRING

Figure 1 presents the matrix of relationships among the variables discussed so far. We can see that two broad constructs, CD and AS, are necessary to predict offspring diagnostic status at the time of the 5-year follow-up. Communication deviance, as measured by an individual projective test administered to the parents clearly indexes more than its name would imply and reveals family units generally lacking in effective paternal participation that are poorly organized to deal with emotional material and show signs of marked interpersonal tension between parent and teenager. The affect measures, which are most parsimoniously thought of as measures of an affective evaluation of the teenager expressed in words and tone of voice, appear orthogonal or at least oblique to the interpersonal correlates of the CD Index. Furthermore, they are a necessary ingredient for accounting for the variation in early adult outcomes. Poorly organized and tense family structures lacking negative evaluative attitudes (criticism, guilt induction, or intrusiveness) do not contain early onset, definite or probable schizophrenia, or borderline personality disorders. Of course, as indicated earlier, we are barely into the risk period for schizophrenia in our sample and it is difficult to evaluate the contribution of negative affective evaluation to the course of psychiatric disorder from adolescence through adulthood. It may function as Vaughn and Leff (1976a) suggest for their measure of expressed emotion, as an accelerator of a likely relapsing course, so that it is a necessary condition for early deterioration in the period between mid-adolescence and the early twenties. Thus, we might expect that later onset cases will come from high CD home environments in which affective evaluation of the teenager was less harsh.

On the other hand, should our cohort of severe outcomes remain localized primarily among the high CD-negative AS subjects, then it would suggest that certain patterns of family disorganization or distortion must be accompanied by negative affective attitudes directed at a specific offspring in order for schizophrenia-spectrum disorders to appear subsequently. Interestingly, this reemphasis upon affective evaluative factors, such as personal criticism, brings this research full circle to the earlier experimental studies of Garmezy and Rodnick (1959) who emphasized the significant role of these evaluative messages in producing behavioral disorganization in adult schizophrenics while performing relatively simple laboratory tasks.

6 Measurement strategies in family interaction research: a profile approach

JERI A. DOANE AND JULIA M. LEWIS

In the past two decades family factors in schizophrenia and related disorders have been studied extensively. Two methodological strategies are often employed in these studies: (1) Obtain a sample of family behavior from one experimental context and then assume it reflects an enduring characteristic of the family; and/or (2) use some single measure of a construct in an attempt to describe or capture adequately a complex dimension of family functioning.

The purpose of this chapter is to report a methodological strategy that we have found useful in our analyses of interactional behavior observed in high-risk families. Very briefly, our approach involves assigning subjects or families to groups that reflect a profile of characteristics of family behavior derived from two or more criterion measures. These measures may be obtained from multiple contexts; or alternatively, they may reflect independently assessed component parts of some dimension of family functioning. We hope to demonstrate that using a configural method of grouping families or cases allows significant increments in prediction of outcome in a sample of families at risk for producing schizophrenia in the offspring.

The construct, which we will use to illustrate this methodological approach, is that of the affective tone or quality of the family environment. Recent research by Vaughn and Leff (1976a), building upon the work of Brown, Birley, and Wing (1972), has shown that this dimension of family functioning plays an important role in the course of schizophrenia. These investigators found that patients returning to environments rated high on expressed emotion (high-EE) had a greater likelihood of relapse than patients returning to low-EE environments. Expressed emotion is a construct reflecting negative attitudes directed toward the patient, including criticism, hostility, and overinvolvement.

Two recent reports from the UCLA Family Project have suggested that measures similar to EE have relevance for studying families of adolescents thought to be at greater-than-average risk for subsequent development of schizophrenia and related disorders (Doane et al., 1981; Lewis, 1979). Some of the data from these two reports will be presented here to illustrate the advantage of using a configural approach to data analysis.

93

The UCLA Family Project is a longitudinal, prospectively designed study that attempts to determine whether unique intrafamilial relationships exist in family units where offspring subsequently develop disorders in the extended schizophrenia spectrum (Wender, Rosenthal, & Kety, 1968). The 52 families examined in this report were studied initially when they sought help for a disturbed, but nonpsychotic teenager. They were then followed up 5 years later through the early period of risk for schizophrenia and related disorders. Further detailed description of the sample can be found in Chapter 5, this volume.

DIRECT INTERACTION PROCEDURES

Included in the initial 6-week assessment battery were direct interaction tasks, involving various combinations of family members in a discussion. In this report, data from two of these 7–10 minute situations are used – a dyadic discussion between the adolescent and each of his parents, and a triadic discussion in which both parents participate with the adolescent. The structure of the task was a modification of the revealed differences technique developed by Strodbeck (1954), in which we presented the dyad or triad with problems for discussion that had previously been identified as idiosyncratically relevant to each family. This was done in order to maximize the likelihood of obtaining an emotionally charged sample of interaction.

AFFECTIVE STYLE MEASURES

The Affective Style (AS) coding system is described in the Rodnick et al. chapter in this volume and further elaborated in Doane et al. (1981). Very briefly, the coding system identifies certain criterion negative remarks from typed transcripts: (1) overly harsh or personal criticism, (2) guilt inducement, or (3) excessive intrusiveness. The codes are thought to reflect interpersonal analogs of some of the components of the EE construct.

Each parent was assigned to one of the following two profile groups based on whether or not the parent used any of the key negative codes in a specific interaction, such as a dyadic or triadic discussion:

> *Benign*: The parent does not use any of the criterion negative codes.
> *Negative*: The parent uses at least one of the criterion negative codes.

VOICE TONE MEASURE

The affective quality of the parents' tone of voice (VT) as they spoke to the adolescent in the triadic discussion was coded independently by Lewis (1979). A total of 33 of the 52 families whose videotapes were of sufficient technical quality to permit adequate scoring were used. Parental speech in the interaction was unitized, and each unit was coded for voice tone quality. Families were then categorized into one of four groups reflecting the predominant VT quality used by the parent who had the greatest amount of interaction with the adolescent during the triadic discussion:

> *Positive*: VT reflects warmth, interest, regard, support, concern, etc.
> *Neutral*: VT is neither positive nor negative.
> *Passive Negative*: VT sounds negative *without* sounding actively upset, hostile, or challenging. VT may include defensiveness, whining, or lecturing.
> *Active Negative*: VT is forcefully negative (e.g., anger, hostility, frustration, antagonism).

It is important to remember that Voice Tone was coded by raters who were blind to the AS status of the family and who were participating in a different study, independent of the AS project. Further detailed description of the VT codes is presented in Lewis (1979).

FIVE-YEAR FOLLOW-UP ASSESSMENT

Five years after the initial contact, the families were reassessed to determine the psychiatric status of the index adolescents, then young adults between 20 and 23 years of age. For a more complete description of these procedures, see Doane et al. (1981). Very briefly, on the basis of psychological tests and an intensive clinical interview, clinicians blind to any information about the family made a psychiatric diagnosis for each young adult using the RDC Criteria developed by Spitzer, Endicott, and Robins (1975) and the Borderline Evaluation Schedule, developed by Gunderson (1977). On the basis of these diagnoses, each case was then assigned to one of the seven levels of the diagnostic scale originally used by Wender et al. (1968). These levels are discussed in further detail in Chapter 5 by Rodnick et al., this volume. For a complete diagnostic breakdown of all 52 cases, see Doane et al. (1981).

RESULTS

Single-setting versus cross-situational measures as predictors of outcome

We first examined the mothers' and fathers' AS profiles from a single setting separately to determine their respective contributions to prediction of subsequent offspring outcome. A significant number of both false positive and false negative errors in prediction occurred when separate parent AS scores from either the dyadic or triadic situations were used.

We next developed cross-situational profile groups for mothers and fathers based on their AS behavior across both the dyadic and triadic situations. Thus three groups were formed: (1) parents who had a Benign AS in both settings; (2) those who had a Negative AS in both settings; and (3) those who had a Benign AS

Table 1. *Parental cross-situational AS profiles as predictors of offspring diagnosis*[a]

Parental AS profile from dyad to triad	Nonspectrum (1–4)	Extended schizophrenia spectrum	
		Soft spectrum (5)	Hard spectrum (6–7)
Mothers			
Benign in both dyad and triad	23	0	1
Benign in one setting; Negative in the other	10	4	4
Negative in both dyad and triad	2	6	2
Fathers			
Benign in both dyad and triad	26	1	0
Benign in one setting; Negative in the other	7	7	5
Negative in both dyad and triad	2	2	2

Note: The degree of relationship was determined by a 2 × 3 chi-square test, collapsing the Wender 5–7 categories: for mothers – $\chi^2 = 20.18$, $df = 2$, $p < .001$; for fathers –
[a]$N = 52$. $\chi^2 = 21.88$, $df = 2$, $p < .001$.

in one setting, but were Negative in the other. Table 1 illustrates the relationship of maternal and paternal AS to outcome when these configural profiles were used as predictors. Consistently Benign mothers and fathers have offspring with good outcomes, whereas parents who are consistently Negative are more likely to have offspring with poor outcomes. The relationship of the inconsistent parents (mothers or fathers who are Benign in one setting, but Negative in the other) to outcome appears random, however. See rows 2 and 5 in Table 1.

The next step in our analysis was to determine whether combining *both* parents' cross-situational AS behavior improved prediction. Thus we next built higher-order profiles that combined the information from *both* parents across *both* situations. We were now able to categorize families on the basis of the cross-situational behavior of both parents together as a system, rather than predicting from either parent's behavior in isolation.

In Table 2, maternal and paternal cross-situational AS profiles were combined, and families were divided into five groups depending on whether one or both parents were consistent across settings in the quality of AS expressed. As shown in Table 2, prediction of outcome is improved and the information gained from

Table 2. *Maternal and paternal cross-situational AS profiles as a combined predictor of offspring outcome[a]*

Parental dyadic/triadic Affective Style profile pattern	Nonspectrum (1–4)	Extended schizophrenia spectrum	
		Soft end (5)	Hard end (6–7)
Bilateral Benign Both parents consistently benign across settings	19	0	0
Unilateral Benign One parent consistently Benign; other is Inconsistent across settings	11	1	1
Bilateral Inconsistent Both parents are Inconsistent across settings	3	3	3
Unilateral Negative One parent consistently Negative; other is Inconsistent across settings	2	4	2
Bilateral Negative Both parents are consistently Negative	0	2	1

Note: The degree of relationship was determined by a 2 × 3 chi-square test, collapsing the Wender Scale Categories 5–7; the Bilateral and Unilateral Benign AS groups, and the Bilateral and Unilateral Poor groups: $\chi^2 = 27.2$, $df = 2$, $p < .001$.
[a]$N = 52$.

including both parents' data in the profile allows one to obtain a clearer clinical picture of various families' system dynamics with respect to the expression of AS. Families with at least one parent who is consistently Benign both when alone with the child and when the other parent is present produce offspring with good outcomes (see rows 1 and 2, Table 2). Conversely, the presence of a consistently negative parent is associated with a poor outcome (see rows 4 and 5 in Table 2). We can also see that this method of grouping families illuminates further the relationship of parents with an inconsistent AS pattern to offspring outcome. It will be recalled from Table 1 that mothers or fathers who were inconsistent in their AS behavior across settings were as likely to have a nonspectrum as a spectrum offspring. We can see from Table 2 that just one inconsistent parent in a parental pair has little impact on a consistently benign or consistently negative spouse (see rows 2 and 4, Table 2). However, when *both* parents are inconsistent in the way

Table 3. *Affective Style content profile in the triadic interaction as a predictor of outcome*[a]

		Extended schizophrenia spectrum	
		Soft	Hard
	Nonspectrum	spectrum	spectrum
Affective Style profile	(1–4)	(5)	(6–7)
Benign	12	0	0
Negative	9	5	7

Note: The degree of relationship was determined by a 2×2 chi-square test, collapsing the Wender 5–7 categories: $\chi^2 = 8.45$, $p < .01$.
[a]$N = 33$.

they relate to the child, a spectrum outcome occurs in six of the nine cases (see row 3, Table 2).

Unidimensional versus multidimensional measures as predictors of outcome

In this section we will present a related but slightly different measurement strategy. Again, the emphasis is on building higher-order profiles tu form configural groupings in order to improve prediction as well as provide more clinical information about our families. The two measures which will be combined here are obtained from a single experimental situation but are independently assessed component parts of the affective dimension of family functioning. These measures are AS, which assesses the affective nature of verbal content, and Voice Tone (VT) which reflects how the parents *sound* as they deliver verbal messages to their child.

In order to illustrate the benefits of this type of approach, we will first present the association between each measure and outcome when they are *not* combined. Table 3 lists two groups of AS profiles from the triadic interaction for the 33 families for which both AS and VT could be rated. For this analysis, each family was assigned a familial AS profile that was based upon whether at least one parent used at least one negative AS code (Negative group). As seen in Table 3, although familial AS profile in the triadic situation is a statistically significant predictor of outcome, several false positive errors occur. That is, although all of the 12 extended schizophrenia-spectrum cases had parents with a Negative AS profile, there were nine cases with nonspectrum diagnoses with parents who also had a Negative profile.

The VT profiles were dichotomized by contrasting the Positive, Neutral, and Passive Negative groups with the Active Negative group. The assumption here was that the Active Negative voice tone was qualitatively more harmful by virtue of its mobilized, more aggressive affective impact. In Table 4, it can be seen that the

Table 4. *Voice tone as a predictor of outcome in the triadic interaction*[a]

		Extended schizophrenia spectrum	
Voice Tone profile	Nonspectrum (1–4)	Soft spectrum (5)	Hard spectrum (6–7)
Benign	18	2	2
Active negative	3	3	5

Note: The degree of relationship was determined by a 2 × 2 chi-square test, collapsing the Wender 5–7 categories: $\chi^2 = 7.22$, $p < .01$.
[a]$N = 33$.

Table 5. *Affective-style content profile and voice tone as combined predictors of outcome*[a]

		Extended schizophrenia spectrum	
Affective Style and Voice Tone profiles	Nonspectrum (1–4)	Soft spectrum (5)	Hard spectrum (6–7)
Benign VT and Benign AS	10	0	0
Negative VT and Benign AS	2	0	0
Benign VT and Negative AS	8	2	2
Negative VT and Negative AS	1	3	5

Note: The degree of relationship was determined by a 2 × 3 chi-square test, collapsing the Wender 5–7 categories and the Negative VT and Benign AS and Benign VT and Negative AS categories: $\chi^2 = 16.82$, $p < .001$.
[a]$N = 33$.

association between VT and outcome is also significant. Again, however, several errors in prediction occur. Although there were fewer false positive errors, more false negative errors occur. That is, 18 of the 21 nonspectrum cases are correctly identified, but 4 of the 12 schizophrenia-spectrum cases came from families exhibiting Benign voice tones during the experimental interaction.

The next step involved combining the AS and the VT profiles into higher-order configural groupings. These groups are thus a composite of the parents' affective attitude toward the child, reflecting both the affective quality of the verbal content and the emotional tone conveyed in the delivery of the words. In Table 5 it can be seen that combining component parts of this construct results in better prediction of outcome and, again, in a richer overall clinical picture of the data. Without exception, families who are *not* affectively negative in either what they say or how they say it, produce offspring with benign outcomes. Conversely, in families where parents say harshly negative things and deliver them in a hostile, angry, or challenging tone of voice, the result is almost always a schizophrenia-spectrum outcome (eight of nine cases). In those cases in which there is inconsistency across affective channels (rows 2 and 3, Table 5), the relationship to outcome is less dramatic. It appears as though an absence of negative affect in one affective channel may mitigate the harmful effect of the negative affect expressed through the other channel. In 10 of 14 cases in which the AS and the VT are inconsistent, the offspring show nonspectrum disorders (see rows 2 and 3, Table 5).

COMMENT

The purpose of this chapter has been to illustrate a methodological strategy for studying family characteristics that we have found useful in our study of families at risk for schizophrenia. This methodological strategy has been employed in two ways. In the first approach, a single variable was used to predict offspring outcome. Maximum prediction was achieved when the variable was measured in multiple settings (dyadic and triadic interactions) and when the behavior of both members of the parental subsystem was combined. More specifically, when the single index of affective style was used as a predictor, increasing increments in prediction were achieved when each parent's AS behavior was assessed across situations (see Table 1), and when *both* parents' cross-situational behavior was combined to form higher order groupings of parental subsystems (see Table 2). The best prediction occurred when both parents' AS behavior *across situations* was used to form profile groups. One can conclude from Table 2 that offspring of families in which at least one parent displays a consistently Benign affective style uniformly have a relatively good outcome as young adults (19 of 19 cases). Conversely, for offspring of families where at least one parent is consistently Negative in AS, the reverse is true. These cases are more likely to develop schizophrenia-spectrum disorders (9 of 11 cases). Families in which both parents are inconsistent across situations in their affective style of relating to the child are also more likely to produce offspring who develop spectrum outcomes (6 of 9 cases).

In a second illustration of the methodology, two different indices of family affect were examined in a single experimental context. Here, we used two independently measured component parts of affect – verbal content and voice tone – to predict outcome. Again, maximum predictive value was achieved when *both* indices were combined to form family profiles. In this example, the profiles reflected the parental behavior on both of the measures of affect. Thus, when the affective attitudes reflected in both voice tone and verbal content were taken into account, a significant improvement in prediction of offspring outcome occurred. To recapitulate briefly, when parents say relatively innocuous things in a relatively benign tone of voice, the offspring show nonspectrum diagnoses at follow-up. Conversely, when both voice tone and verbal content are overly harsh or critical, a poor outcome is more likely. Finally, when the affective quality between VT and content (AS) was inconsistent the results suggest that negativity expressed through one affective channel may be somewhat attenuated by a more benign attitude shown in the other channel (e.g., a Negative Benign voice tone). In 10 of 14 cases in which the parents conveyed inconsistent affective messages via content and voice tone, the offspring had nonspectrum outcomes. These results (shown in Table 5) corroborate Vaughn and Leff's position that tone of voice is a crucial component of the Expressed Emotion construct.

Obviously, the results used to illustrate the value of these methodological strategies also have theoretical relevance for the relationship of familial affective tone and subsequent schizophrenia-spectrum disorder. We also recognize the obvious limitations of the findings, such as a small sample size and lack of cross-validation. Further elaboration of the theoretical implications and limitations of the results presented in Tables 1–5 are discussed elsewhere (Doane et al., 1981; Lewis, 1979; and Rodnick et al., this volume). The purpose of this presentation has been to illustrate a specific methodological approach to data analysis, and space does not permit lengthy interpretation of the substantive nature of the findings.

Limitations of multidimensional profile strategies

Although we have found that this methodological approach has been useful in our own work, there are disadvantages inherent in this type of strategy which should be noted. First, when scores are combined from two or more separate measures, the measures must often be split into dichotomous groupings so that a manageable number of higher-order profile groups result. In the process, some information is invariably lost. For example, in the AS profiles in Table 2, we don't know what type of negative AS (criticism, guilt, intrusiveness) was expressed in a particular family. In a second example, dichotomizing the VT measure into Benign versus Negative limits our knowledge of a parent labeled *Benign* to only the fact that the parent's VT is *not* Active Negative. Although this type of information loss does occur with this approach, the information which is gained by adding measures (such as adding AS to VT) may result in a richer overall clinical picture of the family system characteristics, as well as improve prediction.

A second disadvantage is that profile scores may not be as stable or reliable as the individual measures used to form the profile. However, the results suggest the value of profiles for increasing predictive power may make using them with caution worth the risk.

Another disadvantage of this approach is that statistical procedures such as analysis of variance, which many investigators consider more powerful, are no longer an option when the data are grouped qualitatively. For example, the four AS and VT profiles presented in Table 5 are clearly not interval or even ordinal-level data. Thus, nonparametric statistical techniques such as chi-square tests must be used to test research hypotheses. This being the case, however, it is noteworthy to point out that a clear advantage of using statistical procedures such as chi square is that it permits one to examine families on a case-by-case basis, and to make predictions about risk for poor offspring outcome based on the individual family's marker attributes.

PART III

The St. Louis Risk Research Project: 1966–1982

When the St. Louis Risk Research Project began its pioneering efforts in 1966, the advantages and disadvantages of selecting certain samples of subjects and research methods versus other samples and methods were by no means worked out. Quite appropriately, this group deliberately took a more exploratory approach than most other studies that started a few years later. This exploratory stance was especially apparent in the diversity of subjects studied: The parents could have any type of functional psychosis, or be in tubercular and normal comparison groups; both male and female offspring were included; there was a black and white racial mix; and all socioeconomic groups were represented. Unstructured clinical and anthropological-style home visits were included along with experimental procedures that have dominated more recent risk studies, in St. Louis and elsewhere.

In the Progress Report from St. Louis, many of the vicissitudes of this richly multifaceted program are sketched out. However, for those readers who began following the risk-research field only recently, it also will be rewarding to consult directly the publications of this program stemming from the first phase in 1967–1972. These reports provided many suggestions that were invaluable in helping other investigators to plan their studies.

Later, in the second phase (1975–1979) of this program, the St. Louis group modified and added to their procedures by drawing upon the interim experience of other risk researchers. Thus, this Progress Report illustrates very well the constructive interchange among investigators that has been facilitated by the Risk Research Consortium.

The other two chapters in this part provide examples, by no means exhaustive, of the complex interrelationships of variables that are currently under examination by the St. Louis team.

7 St. Louis Risk Research Project: comprehensive progress report of experimental studies

JULIEN WORLAND, CYNTHIA L. JANES,
E. JAMES ANTHONY, MANON McGINNIS, AND
LORETTA CASS

The objective of this review of the experimental aspects of one of the earlier risk research projects is to acquaint the reader with the development over a 13 year period of the ongoing, prospective study of children at risk carried out in St. Louis under the direction of E. J. Anthony. We will attempt to point out the increase that our study has made in our knowledge of the particular families that we have studied, while pointing out how our thinking has changed about the importance of assessing different aspects of children's functioning.

THE BEGINNING

The proposed investigation is concerned with the psychological and social effects on children of growing up in an environment that includes contact with a parent requiring [hospitalization] for a psychotic illness. These effects will be compared and contrasted with those occurring in children whose parents have been admitted to a hospital for a physical illness. Two sets of studies are contemplated: (1) *a clinical evaluation* of the impact of the psychotic system of ideas and affects on the child and his immediate environment at the different stages of his development; and (2) *an experimental investigation* (cognitive, perceptual, communicative and psychophysical) of possible factors [conducive] to vulnerability to the psychotic influence.

With this preamble, the initial proposal, "The Influence of Parental Psychosis on the Development of the Child," was submitted to NIMH in 1966. Importantly, the initial project had a focus quite different from the one it has taken over the years.

Specifically, the initial project sought to study the children of "psychotics," with no specific interest in differentiating between children of schizophrenics and children of manic-depressives. This global beginning has enabled the St. Louis Project, which included both children of manic-depressives and children of schizophrenics from the beginning, to have an important control group for the kind of psychosis exhibited by the parents. Interestingly, also, there was no intent in the

This research was funded by NIMH Grants MH-24819 and MH-12043 to E. J. Anthony, M. D., principal investigator, and Grant MH-50124 to Drs. Anthony and Worland.

105

initial proposal to have a group of children of normal controls because "the additional expenditure of time and money would not be justifiable at this stage of the exploratory study." The inclusion of a large group of normal controls, despite this initial humility, was an important addition as the project developed.

The initial investigators felt that the type of disturbance by close contact and communication with a psychotic parent was, from a phenomenological point of view, a condition sui generis not hitherto described in the literature, although hinted at in earlier work on *folie à deux* (Anthony, 1969a, 1969c). The intent then was to describe in these children their response to being parented by a psychotic parent, and to do this by comparing and contrasting them with children who were being parented by a physically ill parent (Anthony, 1970a).

The hypotheses (Anthony, 1968b) for the initial study involved a comparison of children of psychotic parents with children of control parents in terms of their clinical disturbance, intrapsychic symptoms, peer-group relationships, "precursor" symptoms, intelligence, and "organic" features. With a goal of nearly 3 hours of testing for each child (psychiatric evaluation, 1 hour of psychological evaluation, and 1 hour with a psychophysiologist) plus a similar expenditure of time for the child's parents, an enormous amount of data was to be generated, allowing the testing of more than 28 general and then an additional 28 specific hypotheses related to the emergence of disturbance.

The theoretical concept underlying the initial proposal was that because "the evidence at present available suggests that the association between mental illness in the parent and mental illness in the child is not attributable in any large part to genetic factors," the high rate of psychiatric disturbance in the children of psychotic parents and the adverse effects manifested in the family as a whole is supportive of an environmental influence (Anthony, 1969b, 1970b). Thus the detailed study of the child, the family environment, and the presence of precursor symptoms were all goals of the initial project.

Reading this proposal, much of the impetus appears to have derived from the then new procedure of discharging mentally ill patients after short hospitalizations (Anthony, 1970b; Anthony & Rizzo, 1971), leading many to suspect that the ongoing relationship of the developing child with a psychotic parent would increase the child's vulnerability to later breakdown. The writers of the initial proposal saw failure in differentiation, both differentiation between the child and the psychotic parent as well as differentiation of the child from the environment in general, as important results of parental psychosis and precursors of individual psychosis.

THE PHASE I ASSESSMENT

The sample

Instead of a well-defined sample of children, the St. Louis Risk Project has a set of samples within samples drawn from a population of available offspring. Our index

Table 1. *Hospitalization characteristics of psychotic parents*

	Diagnosis		
	Schizophrenic	Manic-depressive	t^a
Ill parents			
N	30	18	
Admissions before testing			
M	2.87	3.11	.21
SD	2.02	2.65	
Range	1–9	1–9	
Admissions, lifetime to 1979			
M	4.50	4.61	.12
SD	3.18	3.15	
Range	1–15	1–12	
Days hospitalized before testing			
M	497.13	138.44	1.55[b]
SD	787.54	181.85	
Range	9–2462	14–810	
Days hospitalized, lifetime to 1979			
M	600.20	181.50	1.37[b]
SD	844.49	205.37	
Range	9–3560	33–936	

[a]df = 46; no tested differences are significant.
[b]t-test done on log-transformed scores.

parents were 30 hospitalized schizophrenics and 18 hospitalized manic-depressives who met the following criteria:

1. Married;
2. Marital family continuous and intact except for the patient's period of hospitalization;
3. Hospital diagnosis of psychosis, without findings of such contaminating factors as serious physical disability or organic brain syndrome; and
4. At least one child between 6 and 12 years of age.

These parents were located through psychiatric hospitals, and each patient had a review of his or her case record and an interview with a project social worker before being admitted to the study. Table 1 shows their hospitalization history up to the time of first testing and again up to 1979.

The comparison group consisted of 19 parents with a disabling, chronic physical health problem that had required hospitalization. This illness was usually tuberculosis. These parents met similar criteria to those noted previously except that

Table 2. *Demographic characteristics of population*

Variable	CSZ	CMD	CPI	CN	Total
			Group[b]		
Children					
N	100	60	78	130	368
Sex					
Male	50	28	34	67	179
Female	50	32	44	63	189
Race					
Black	35	21	46	48	150
White	65	39	32	82	218
Age (months)					
M	113.95	122.98	109.00	110.71	113.18
Families					
N	30	18	19	38	105
Sex of ill parent					
Father	13	7	9	—	29
Mother	17	11	10	—	38
SES, M[a]	47.92	39.33	54.89	35.03	42.96

[a]Hollingshead: Class I, 11–17; II, 18–27; III, 28–43; IV, 44–60; V, 61–77.
[b]CSZ = parental schizophrenia; CMD = parental manic-depressive illness; CPI = parental physical illness; CN = normal parents.

they had to have no history or evidence of serious psychiatric disorder, nor could their spouses have any such psychiatric disorder.

A normal control group was also used. The parents in this group had no history of either a disabling physical health problem or of any psychiatric illness requiring treatment, but otherwise met the same criteria.

Unlike several of the other risk research projects, both male and female offspring of both black and white parents of varying social classes were included in the sample (Anthony, 1968a, 1971). The total population of available offspring is represented in Table 2 and Figure 1, although it should be noted that for any individual assessment battery or test, the number of tested children or parents was less than the number shown.

Diagnoses of the ill parents. At the time the St. Louis Risk Research Project began, the refinement of psychiatric diagnoses was not as highly developed as it is now. Each parent received a DSM-II project diagnosis after a 90-minute interview, usually with Anthony, and after he had reviewed the hospital chart and talked with the patient's spouse and children.

We have calculated diagnostic reliability on these diagnoses in various ways. In one approach (Worland, Lander, & Hesselbrock, 1979) we compared Anthony's diagnoses with those of the hospital, not strictly proper since they were not com-

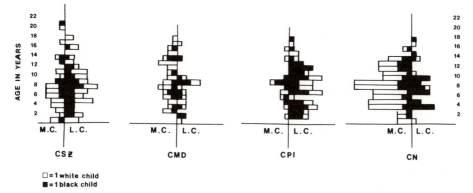

Figure 1. Population distribution of offspring by age, race, and class at Phase I.

pletely independent. This comparison yielded a kappa (J. A. Cohen, 1960) of .79, with total agreements for cases of manic-depressive patients, but for 5 of the 30 project-diagnosed schizophrenics the hospital diagnosis was manic-depressive illness.

Recently, with the advent of DSM-III (American Psychiatric Association, 1980) we have attempted to blindly rediagnose our sample, using the available original hospital admission and discharge notes, with names and hospital diagnoses deleted. This procedure has revised our sample composition and has forced us to delete some of the original cases from the sample in recent reports (e.g., Worland, Weeks, Weiner, & Schechtman, 1982). Unfortunately, this means that the earlier work reported in this chapter does include offspring from some cases that would no longer be considered psychotic.

The assessment battery

Between the proposing, the funding, and the beginning of assessment, an extensive research battery was gradually devised that, in some ways, carried out the plans of the initial proposal, but took some new directions as well. Shaping these initial decisions, in addition to E. J. Anthony, were Loretta K. Cass, Manon McGinnis, Norman L. Corah, and John A. Stern. A heavy clinical influence can be read in the selection of the initial research instruments. Loretta Cass, for example, was the chief psychologist in a child guidance clinic also associated with the Department of Child Psychiatry at Washington University, where the project has been carried out. The use of a child guidance clinic model in the assessment of the children is obvious in the kinds of instruments that were selected.

In what has been termed by Norman Garmezy the "day in the life" approach to assessing the effects of psychosis, the battery eventually settled on represented an enormous effort, not only in terms of the professional time involved, but also in terms of the time required from the project families. Even considering the relatively deflated currency of the day, subjects participated for the modest remuneration of $25 per family.

Psychological assessment

Here the child guidance clinic influence is apparent. Each child and each parent was seen individually to receive a "full" psychological evaluation. The tests used were the Wechsler Preschool and Primary Scale of Intelligence (WPPSI; Wechsler, 1967) or the Wechsler Intelligence Scale for Children (WISC; Wechsler, 1949), the Beery–Buktenica Developmental Form Sequence (Beery, 1967) which is a test of visual–motor coordination, the Rorschach Inkblot Test, the Thematic Apperception Test (TAT; Murray, 1943), and human figure drawings (DAP; D. Harris, 1963).

Intelligence. The 10 subscale scores including Digit Span but excluding Mazes were calculated and recorded, plus Verbal IQ, Performance IQ, Full-Scale IQ, the range of subtests (highest subtest score minus lowest), and the difference between Verbal and Performance scores.

Beery. This test of visual–motor coordination was scored according to the manual instructions (Beery, 1967). The age norms were used to compute a developmental quotient, which was the score used for the analyses we performed on the Beery.

Rorschach. The 10-card Rorschach was administered, and the examiner's handwritten protocol was typed and then scored by one of our four project psychologists (Loretta Cass, Lois Franklin, Larry Bass, and Ruth Rosenthal). They were kept blind to all information about the child except for age and sex. Each response was scored for its Integration Level according to W. C. Becker's (1956) adaptation of Friedman's (1952) system. Scores were given on six scales from global, unarticulated, or inaccurate form level, to highly articulated, well-differentiated, and accurate form level. Each scale was then summed to produce six Integration Level scores (the number of responses scored as representing each category). Scoring a response within one category excluded scoring the same response in another category. Each response was also scored for location, determinant, accuracy, and content, as described in Ames, Learned, Metraux, & Walker (1957) and in Beck, Beck, Levitt, and Molish (1961). Accuracy scores were determined by Beck et al., with recourse to Hertz (1961) when Beck did not list a particular response.

TAT. Cards 1, 2, 3BM, 6BM, 7BM, 7GF, 8BM, 10, and 16 were used. The handwritten protocols were typed and scored by Patty Evans and Linda Teal. These research assistants were blind to each child's identifying information. Each story was scored for time span according to Wohlford's (1966) adaption of the Epley and Ricks (1963) system. No distinction was made between cognitive and empirical time span, as the larger score for either category was given. This yielded one retrospective, one prospective, and one total time span score for each card. The three scores were individually summed across cards to give each child three total scores. Each TAT was also scored for affect (positive, negative, both, neither), coping (constructive, destructive, evasive, or no problem), and interaction (positive, negative, both, none).

Interrater and intrarater reliability (*r*) on coping ranged from .490 to .960, and averaged .654 on nine separate tests of 126 rescored protocols. Reliability for time span ranged from .640 to .970 and averaged .879, evaluated from 23 tests on 363 rescored protocols.

Figure drawings. The child was asked to draw a picture of a person and then asked to draw a picture of a person of the opposite sex. For each drawing the child was asked the person's sex, age, occupation, three wishes, and three best and three worst characteristics. Drawings were scored according to Harris's (1963) revision and extension of Goodenough's (1926) method, and age-normed standard scores were assigned to each drawing. Each child was scored on each drawing for the total extra items included (above those expected at age level), and the total omissions (items not included in a drawing but expected at age level).

Clinical ratings. From the complete protocols, psychologists made a series of ratings of psychopathology (Cass, Franklin, & Bass, 1973; Franklin, Worland, Cass, Bass, & Anthony, 1978).

The *clinical disturbance ratings* were psychologists' evaluations of 12 personality processes made from each child's responses on intelligence (WPPSI or WISC), visual–motor (Beery), and projective tests (Rorschach and TAT), plus a sum of these 12 ratings, and finally a global rating of disturbance based on each person's protocol taken altogether.

The selection of the 12 variables was accomplished through repeated interprofessional discussion and experimentation. They were chosen because of their demonstrated importance in psychodynamic personality theory and because they are evidenced in characteristics of test responses. The 12 variables are: logicality of thinking, reality testing, concreteness, anxiety, object relations, identity, superego, emotionality, aggressivity, conflict and defenses, coping, and pathology of content. Characteristics of the test responses used in the rating of the variables included both actual content and formal scores. The intelligence and visual–motor tests and Rorschachs were scored first and these scores, as well as the typescripts of all the tests, were given to the raters with only age and sex of the subject indicated.

Each of the 12 variables was rated on a 5-point scale from 1 (not pathological) to 5 (incapacitating pathology) using a manual developed for the project (Cass, 1973). For each variable, each point on the scale was described in terms of score values or kind of content from the various tests. For example, the description for a rating of 3 (moderate) on reality testing is: "moderate departure from stimulus accuracy: Rorschach 10–20% below norm for age; in TAT, one or two misperceptions in stimuli details; a few (two or three) instances of inaccurate elaborations on WISC or WAIS." The 3 rating was made if most (over half) of these conditions were met.

The *global rating of disturbance* is a more clinical and informal judgment of the overall disturbance seen in all the test protocols taken together without requiring equal weight for the variables. For example, a set of protocols filled with primitive and/or aggressive content might earn a global rating of 4 or 5 even though the test scores for reality testing, concreteness, and coping were not in the pathological range. The global rating was made without considering the sum of ratings of the 12 variables described, which was an additional score, referred to as the total pathology score.

Interrater reliability among three of the psychologists was determined for the individual ratings and for the total pathology score. Interrater agreement on 831 individual ratings from 63 protocols was assessed by J. A. Cohen's (1960) kappa statistic. Kappa was used because it takes into account agreements based on chance. It, therefore, produces coefficients somewhat more conservative than those found using Spearman's or Pearson's correlations on the same data. Pearson's r was used to determine the reliability of the total pathology score.

For the three pairs of raters, on the individual ratings, κ averaged .61, .68, and .57; the overall average κ on all protocols was .61. The reliability coefficients (r) of the total pathology score for the three pairs of raters were .94, .84, and .97.

Cognitive assessment

The experimental investigation included many research tasks designed to assess the degree of each child's differentiation and egocentricity (Anthony, 1975a). The construct of *differentiation* was based on Werner's (1957) concept that development "proceeds from a state of relative globality and lack of differentiation to a state of increasing differentiation, articulation, and hierarchical integration" (p. 126). We used several cognitive tasks to measure various aspects of psychological differentiation. First was a measure drawn from the Rorschach of a person's ability to analyze and structure ambiguous visual stimuli, discussed earlier in the section on Rorschach Integration Levels. Second, we used the Children's Embedded Figures Test (Karp & Konstadt, 1963) which taps the ability to disembed figures from background. Finally, the ability to be analytical in intellectual activities was measured by three tests, the Block Design, Picture Completion, and Object Assembly subtests of the intellectual evaluation.

Differentiation was studied using the Rod and Frame Tests, an apparatus so unwieldy that few data were ever collected. We also attempted a measure of "psychophysiological differentiation" which will be discussed later.

A further cognitive battery assessed *egocentricity*, a Piagetian concept that refers to the ability of a person to "decenter" and see the world from points of view other than his or her own, versus a unitary perception of the world that lacks even the knowledge that others have different views of experience. Our measures of this construct were the Three Mountains Test (Piaget & Inhelder, 1956), in which a child is presented with three papier-mâché mountains of three colors and a photographer doll. The child is given photographs of the mountains taken from different points of view and, without moving, is asked where the photographer was when the photos were shot. Our second index of egocentrism was the Broken Bridge Test (Piaget, 1932), a measure of notions of causality, imminent justice, and moral reasoning. *Impulsivity* was assessed using the Draw-A-Line and Draw-A-Circle tests.

Altogether, these cognitive measures were used to help identify the undifferentiated disturbances in children at risk, which would comprise prepsychotics, pseudopsychotics, and egocentric children. The psychological properties of the undifferentiated group would include an ego weakness; lack of self-regard; misinterpretation of the external world; dominance by primitive feelings; the determination of thinking by the circumscribed, the accidental, and the magical; the perception of meaning in insignificant, irrelevant material; and an opposite of active, wish-fulfilling fantasy.

Psychosocial evaluation

The psychosocial evaluation, under the direction of Manon McGinnis, included a home visit by Ms. McGinnis, John Lescow, and assistants, who then used the Behrens–Goldfarb Scale and the Witkin Schedule of Differentiation to assess such dimensions of family life as mutual support, alignments, home atmosphere, and sharing of parents. Also used were the now famous living-in experiments. It should finally be stated that these living-in episodes were done with only a handful of families for a total of 1 or 2 days. The data abstracted from these visits were never more than anecdotal and, despite frequently expressed hopes from other risk researchers, the outcome from them never quantified (Anthony, 1975c).

Psychophysiological assessment

Lastly, each child was asked to submit to a psychophysiological investigation. Thanks to the popularity, at that time, of *2001: A Space Odyssey* and the space program, many children were convinced that by allowing the application of sticky electrode paste and electrodes they could recapture the pleasures of John Glenn's soaring into outer space.

At first only offspring between 6 and 12 years of age were tested, but after 1969 the psychophysiological testing was expanded to all the available offspring and their parents as well. Altogether, 206 offspring and 33 parents received this evaluation (Janes et al., 1978).

The procedure has been described previously (Janes, Worland, & Stern, 1971, 1976; Janes et al., 1978) and will be reviewed briefly here. The child was seated in a comfortable chair, and transducers were applied for the bilateral recording of *skin potential* (SP) and *vasomotor activity*. For recording of SP, Beckman biopotential electrodes filled with Beckman electrode paste were attached to the abraded inactive site (the volar surface of the forearm, one-fifth the distance from elbow to wrist), and to the active site (thenar eminence of the palm). A hair-dryer blower was positioned about 15 cm above the child's wrist, and when activated the fan would blow air onto the back of the wrist.

The stimulus series consisted of 10 habituation trials of 20 seconds cool air, 20 conditioning trials (20 seconds cool air, the CS, followed immediately by 10 seconds warm air, the US), and 5 extinction trials (20 seconds cool air). Intertrial intervals varied between 25 and 35 seconds.

The measures abstracted were:

1. Responses to stimulus onset and offset.
    a. HOR (habituation trial orienting response). Response to stimulus onset dur-
        ing habituation trials.
    b. HTOR (habituation trial terminal orienting response). Response to stimulus
        termination during habituation trials.
    c. COR (conditioning trial orienting response). Response to cool air onset
        during conditioning trials.
    d. UR (unconditional response). Response to onset of warm air.
    e. CTOR (conditioning trial terminal orienting response). Response to offset of
        warm air.
2. Anticipatory responses.
    a. HAR (habituation trial anticipatory response). Any SP activity occurring
        within the 5-second period prior to stimulus termination.
    b. CAR (conditioning trial anticipatory response). Any SP activity occurring
        within the 5-second period prior to warm air onset.
3. Between-trial responses.
    a. HITR (habituation trial intertrial responses). SPRs between trials within the
        habituation phase.
    b. CITR (conditioning trial intertrial responses). SPRs between trials within the
        conditioning phase.
4. Derived measures. Three additional scores were computed for each subject based
    on the response categories.
    a. Habituation – Number of habituation trials to three successive nonresponse
        (no HOR) trials on the right hand.
    b. Differentiation – Number of trials on which HORs were greater in ampli-
        tude on the stimulated (right) hand than on the nonstimulated (left) hand,
        divided by number of trials with response, times 100. Thus with 5 trials on
        which HORs were larger in the right hand, and responses in at least one
        hand on 10 trials, the differentiation score would be 50. It was hypothesized
        that response amplitude would be greater on the stimulated side.
    c. Conditioning – The degree of SP conditioning was determined by substract-
        ing the percentage of trials on which HARs occurred from the percentage of
        trials on which SIRs (second interval response) occurred. A positive SP
        conditioning score indicated proportionately greater frequency of anticipato-
        ry responses during conditioning trials than during habituation trials, and was
        taken as evidence for conditioning.
5. Movement artifacts. These were scored as the number of times during the series
    of trials the vasomotor channel was interrupted by a sharp deflection of at least .5
    cm amplitude. This was scored separately for habituation and conditioning
    phases.

FINDINGS FROM THE INITIAL ASSESSMENT

Psychiatric vulnerability

In a study carried out by Lander, Anthony, Cass, Franklin, and Bass (1978) the
ratings of psychiatric vulnerability given to each child after the psychiatric evaluation were studied in an effort to determine whether the specific measures of

vulnerability were in any way associated with increased psychological disturbance. The measures of vulnerability included the following eight items that made up the Vulnerability Rating Scale:

1. Identification with the ill parent;
2. Credulity about parental delusions;
3. Influence of parental illness;
4. Undue submissiveness;
5. Undue suggestibility;
6. Involvement with the ill parent (Three Wishes Test);
7. Involvement with the ill parent (Three Houses Test); and
8. Involvement with the ill parent (Three Dreams Test).

Items 1, 2, and 3 were rated on the basis of interview information from both the well parent and the children. *Undue submissiveness* was measured by the child's willingness to perform certain unusual acts without prior explanation, such as putting a finger in the nostril or lying down on the floor. The child's response to suggestions about body sway, eye closure, and fist closure determined his or her rating on *undue suggestibility*. There were three tests of involvement. The Three Houses Test assessed the child's expressed desire to live with the ill parent; the others tapped the child's inclusion of the ill parent in his or her wishes and dreams. Subjects received 1 point for each factor rated present; possible scores ranged from 0 to 8. Two groups of subjects were then drawn from the total number, one group at the highest end of the vulnerability scale ($N = 19$) and one at the lowest end ($N = 21$).

The dependent variables for this evaluation were the ratings that psychologists had made based on their psychological testing. These ratings were made completely independently of the ratings of vulnerability that the psychiatrists had given to each child. Since these ratings were described in great detail earlier, they will not be explained at any length here.

When Lander evaluated her data, it resulted that the children rated in the highest vulnerability group showed more disturbance than the children in the low vulnerability group in all of the predicted areas of psychological functioning as well as in several others. Thirty-seven percent of the high vulnerables were rated as showing serious or incapacitating disturbance, whereas only 9% of the low vulnerable subjects were placed in this category.

Lander interpreted the results as indicating that the impact of parental psychopathology was measurably greater for those children who were designated as "high vulnerables." These were the children who were the most involved and identified with the ill parent and showed personality traits of suggestibility and submissiveness. They were readily identified by means of the rating scale administered by the psychiatric interview.

Clinical psychological evaluation

Psychological differentiation. Since differentiation was the major concept underlying the original grant proposal, we will present first a doctoral dissertation that tested the hypothesis that offspring of psychiatrically disturbed parents would exhibit poorer differentiation than the offspring of nonpsychiatrically disturbed parents (Franklin, 1977). The tests that Franklin used to evaluate this were the Block Designs, Picture Completion, and Object Assembly subtests from the Wechsler Intelligence Test for Children; the Children's Embedded Figures Test (CEFT), the genetic level from the Rorschach (Lerner, 1975), and the Sophistication of Body Concept Scale (SOBC). Franklin drew her sample from the St. Louis Project, using children between 6 and 11 years of age. She considered the CEFT measure (Karp & Konstadt, 1963) a measure of perceptual–cognitive differentiation in children 6 to 12 years of age. In the test, it was the child's task to locate and outline on request a simple figure (a tent or a house) that had been hidden in a larger, more complex picture. The child's accuracy score was the total number of correct locations on the 25 items that made up the test. Only correct first attempts at tracing the hidden figures were counted in the accuracy score.

The Rorschach measures that Franklin used were ratings made from typed transcripts of each subject's response according to the rating scale developed by Witkin et al. (1962). This system identifies 10 measures of the structuring of Rorschach percepts: (1) definiteness of percept; (2) passive acceptance versus active dealing with specific blot characteristics; (3) stability of percepts; (4) handling of alternatives; (5) ability to respond differentially to changing stimulation; (6) confusion in elaborating percepts; (7) special aspects of verbalization; (8) handling of the whole/space response (Ws); (9) interest in card coverage; and (10) general impression of competence and adequacy of resources in dealing with the task. Using a manual with specific instructions, the raters made assessments on 5-point scales from least to most structured, and the final score used in Franklin's study was the sum of the ratings for the 10 listed cues.

The Sophistication of Body Concept Scale provided a measure of the degree of articulation of body concept, as an indicator of the extent of progress toward psychological differentiation. This scale, consisting of a series of ratings covering three categories of drawing characteristics, was applied to the graphic features of the human figure drawings produced by each subject. The final score was a global rating ranging along a 5-point scale from the most sophisticated to the most primitive drawing. This procedure was taken from Witkin et al. (1962).

Franklin analyzed the data using an analysis of covariance, to control for significant intergroup socioeconomic status effects (Hollingshead, 1968). No significant main effect for parental diagnosis was found for any of the three WISC subtests, $2.81 > F > .01$, or for any other WISC subtests; nor for the CEFT, $F(1, 41) = 1.48$; nor for the SOBC, $F(1, 41) = .69$; nor for the Rorschach scoring, $F(1, 41) = .99$. Each of the three latter measures, however, yielded significant age effects, as would be expected.

Franklin concluded that the results did not support the assumption that parental psychosis resulted in any differences in the level of cognitive and perceptual differentiation in children 6 through 11 years of age, as measured by the test that she used in her study. No other risk research projects have looked specifically at differentiation as a measure of a child's response to parental psychosis, but some other projects that have assessed the intelligence of offspring of schizophrenics have yielded results that indicate that these offspring have lower IQ than normals (e.g., Mednick & Schulsinger, 1968). Franklin did not find this in the St. Louis Project, nor did Worland and Hesselbrock (1980) when they evaluated the entire sample, which is discussed below.

Egocentrism. The first results of the St. Louis study that addressed the question of egocentrism were provided by Bruno J. Anthony at the 1974 Meeting of the International Association of Child Psychiatry and Allied Disciplines (B. Anthony, 1978b). As a measure of Piagetian egocentrism, Anthony chose the Affect Discrimination Test (ADT) from the battery. In the ADT, a child was asked to "feel like" somebody in a photograph. These photographic stimuli were chosen from 43 facial shots of professional actors asked to produce nine different emotions: "happy," "sad," "surprised," "angry," "pleased," "disgusted," "afraid," "suspicious," and "worried." This test had been previously developed and normed by Gerry Clack in his doctoral dissertation at Washington University (Clack, 1970). In the actual experiment, the child was given the nine photographs in an array, and then was presented with a specific situation. For example, the child was given a situation such as "This person is sad because his best friend is sick," or "This person is angry because someone has wrecked his new car." The child was asked to select the photograph that best represented the feeling that a person might have in that situation.

Anthony's hypothesis that there would be a developmental trend in the ADT within the 6- to 12-year period was clearly born out. Eleven-year-olds were much more able to select the appropriate photograph than were 6-year-olds. In addition, children who performed poorly on the Affect Discrimination Test also were rated as more disturbed by clinical psychologists in the psychological battery; and the top quartile of children, as judged from school ratings of adjustment, were significantly more differentiated by their ADT scores than were the bottom quartile, $t = 2.30$, $p < .025$. If these children's disorders (judged from clinical rating and school behavior) could be traced in part to delays in affective role taking, causing them to be egocentric in their interpersonal interactions, Anthony speculated that the ADT seemed to illuminate this egocentric, nonemphatic attitude.

When Anthony evaluated the ADT by the parental diagnosis, the effect was not significant, and children of psychotic parents were not found to be more egocentric than the offspring of normal parents. However, when these analyses were broken down cross-sectionally into groups corresponding to the youngest, middle, and oldest children in the sample, they produced a pattern indicating that there was initially a large influence of parental health on the ADT scores of children, and that this influence abated as time passed. The younger children of psychotic parents did significantly worse on the ADT than did the children of two healthy parents. At the younger age, this factor accounted for the greatest proportion of the variance, a greater proportion than either race, social class, or sex. In the older children (9 years old and up), parental health became less of a factor in ADT performance, and no significant differences appeared between the oldest groups.

However, within the experimental group, the children of manic-depressives scored no differently than did controls and dramatically split from the children of schizophrenics, performing significantly higher in the oldest age group. Children in homes dominated by a schizophrenic parent scored far lower in the early years and were at a disadvantage throughout the age range.

How to interpret these results has been questioned recently by Rosanne Edenhart-Pepe, a psychology graduate student at Washington University, currently working in our project. Her interpretation of B. Anthony's data is that the offspring of schizophrenic parents scored lower on the ADT than the offspring in the other group, not because of a delayed decentering process, but because they responded more impulsively, did not consider the alternatives, and failed to completely search the visual array before making their conclusions. Thus, we have a finding in search of an interpretation: whether this task really represents a failure in the Piagetian sense of a developmental process, or whether impulsivity, poor visual searching, and carelessness are the underlying operating mechanisms. Edenhart-Pepe is currently beginning a doctoral dissertation on eye movements in offspring of schizophrenic parents to test her hypothesis.

Intelligence

There have been many reports on the intellectual level of children of schizophrenic parents. As noted above, Mednick and Schulsinger (1968) reported that children of Danish schizophrenic mothers scored significantly lower than control children on the Arithmetic and Coding subtests of the WISC; and Landau et al. (1972) reported some equivocal findings when they compared Israeli children of psychotic parents with a control group of slightly higher socioeconomic status. Other investigators have reported that the intelligence of children of schizophrenic parents is not significantly lower than that of children of normal parents (Cohler et al., 1977; Rieder, Broman, & Rosenthal, 1977; Rutter, 1966), and is not significantly lower than the childhood IQs of their schizophrenic parents (Lane, Albee, & Doll, 1970).

In addition, there has been little published data on the tested intelligence of the offspring of parents with affective disorder, although Cohler et al. (1977) presented data on the intellectual functioning of this group. Cohler reported that the children of mothers showing manic-depressive or depressive psychosis had IQ scores that averaged 12 points less than the scores of either children of schizophrenic or of well mothers. Cohler's group was quite small, and because we had data on a relatively large number of the offspring of manic-depressive parents, as well as on the offspring of parents with schizophrenia, we decided to take a look at our data in this way. Our purpose was to attempt to replicate in a sample of older children the finding of Cohler et al. (1977) that young children of psychotic depressed mothers had significantly lower IQ scores than the children of normals or the children of schizophrenics. Furthermore, we were attempting to determine whether this could also be demonstrated in the children of psychotic depressed fathers. Another goal was to determine the degree of correlation in the IQ scores between children and parents of these various groups.

When we performed our analysis by parental diagnosis, we found that there were no significant effects for Verbal IQ, Performance IQ, or for Full-Scale IQ, although highly significant race effects were found for all tested contrasts. When we evaluated the intelligence of children in the schizophrenic, manic-depressive, and physically ill parent groups, having added the sex of the ill parent as an additional independent variable, we found that children of ill mothers had lower scores than children of ill fathers on Performance IQ, $F(1, 148) = 5.23, p < .025$; and on Full Scale IQ, $F(1, 148) = 4.76, p < .05$. We could find no parental diagnosis-by-sex of the ill parent interaction effects, but there was a significant race-by-sex of the ill parent interaction effect on PIQ. Children of black, ill mothers had a mean PIQ of 91.66. Means for other subgroups were 99.16 for children of black, ill fathers; 108.52 for those of white, ill fathers; and 110.27 for white, ill mothers. There was no similar interaction effect for FSIQ.

We also attempted to look at the correlation between parents' and children's IQ scores. As we had expected, we found lower child–parent correlations in families with a schizophrenic parent than in families with a manic-depressive parent, a physically ill parent, or two well parents. However, all child–parent correlations were significant and child–schizophrenic parent correlations for VIQ and FSIQ were slightly higher than the corresponding child–nonschizophrenic parent correlations.

In families with an index manic-depressive parent, the child–index parent correlation for VIQ, PIQ, and FSIQ were almost equivalent to the child–nonindex parent correlation. A detailed look at this data is available in Worland and Hesselbrock (1980) where we also present some data on the IQs of offspring and the parent–child IQ correlations broken down by the parental diagnostic subtype.

Psychological disturbance. A great deal of effort in the St. Louis Project was spent in deriving measures of psychological disturbance from the psychological protocols, including not only the projective material but using the intelligence assessment and visual motor assessment as well. These ratings were the *clinical disturbance ratings*, which we analyzed together with the other clinical psychological variables (Worland, Lander, & Hesselbrock, 1979).

The task for this portion of the data analysis was complicated by the presence of 89 measures that were drawn from the test battery. These included 16 scores from the intellectual assessment, 1 score from the Beery–Buktenica Developmental Form Sequence, 31 scores from the Rorschach, 16 scores from the TAT, 10 scores from the DAP, plus the 14 clinical disturbance ratings and their sum. To handle this mass of data without performing 89 separate, one-way F tests, thereby amplifying our Type 1 error, we reduced the battery through a principal axis factor analysis. Using a Varimax solution we were able to produce eight orthogonal factors that accounted for 51.8% of the total common variance in the original pool of variables. We selected only factors that had eigenvalues greater than 2.5, and each factor accounted for 3% or more of the total common variance. Using a factor loading of greater than or equal to .30, we were able to isolate eight factors that represented 73 variables from the clinical psychological assessment, with only 6 variables having loadings on more than one factor.

The eight factors that were abstracted were "Intelligence," "Psychopathology," "Rorschach Productivity," "Complex TAT," "Primitive Rorschach Content," "Rorschach M," "Aggressive TAT," and "Good DAP." After we had abstracted these eight factors, we then computed factor scores for each child in our study. We then analyzed separately these eight factor scores for effects due to parental diagnosis, and the age, race, and sex of the child.

When these factor scores were analyzed, we found a significant main effect for the diagnosis of parents on the factor labeled "Psychopathology," F (3, 239) = 4.09. This factor represented the clinical disturbance ratings. The children of manic-depressive parents and the children of schizophrenics had higher scores (more psychopathology) than the children of physically ill or normal parents. This effect was also significant for the factor Primitive Rorschach Content, F (3, 239) = 3.68, with the children of schizophrenics having the highest scores and the children of manic-depressives the lowest. Aggressive TAT also produced a significant main effect for the diagnosis of the parents, F (3, 226) = 7.09, with the children of manic-depressives having the highest scores and children of schizophrenics having the lowest.

When we visually inspected the distribution of scores on the Psychopathology factor, we found that more children of schizophrenics and children of manic-depressives had above average (not extreme) scores on this factor, and the children of physically ill parents had no high scores at all. At the highest level of this factor, the children of manic-depressives, children of schizophrenics, and children of normal parents were equally represented.

On the other two factors, however, group differences were the result of extreme scores by the children of schizophrenics or the children of manic-depressives. For example, on the TAT Aggression factor, only the children of manic-depressives were significantly represented with high scores, whereas only children of schizophrenics had high scores on the Primitive Rorschach Content factor.

We interpreted these results as indicating support for previous findings that there was greater disturbance in children of schizophrenics than children of normals (Fowler, Tsuang, & Cadoret, 1977; Heston, 1966; Rosenthal, Wender, Kety, Welner, & Schulsinger, 1971; Rosenthal, Wender, Kety, Schulsinger, Welner, & Rieder, 1975; Rutter, 1966; Schulsinger, 1976). However, the overlap in scores on the Psychopathology factor demonstrated that there was not a critical cutoff that would differentiate these groups, nor was there any evidence that parental schizophrenia had effects that were any different from parental manic-depressive illness in terms of their association with a child's clinical disturbance as rated by psychologists from test data.

Another question that this investigation attempted to answer was whether the test behavior of children at risk would be similar to the test behavior of disturbed adults. Evidence that children at risk demonstrated difficulties similar to those of adult psychotics was found for the children of schizophrenics in their high scores on the Primitive Rorschach Content factor. The pattern of Primitive Rorschach Content by children of schizophrenics (anatomy, blood, fire, food, sex, and stain) mirrors the content found in the Rorschach of adult schizophrenics (Draguns, Haley, & Philips, 1967), although none of these children of schizophrenics was hospitalized for schizophrenia at the time of the testing. We felt that this supported the hypothesis that early indicators of vulnerability in children at risk could be found as emerging difficulties in areas continuous with deficiences observed in adult schizophrenics (Erlenmeyer-Kimling, 1972a). The children of manic-depressives differed from the children of schizophrenics on this variable, making the relationships specific to children of schizophrenics. This group difference was contributed to by 7% of the children of schizophrenics with scores higher than 99% of the offspring in the other three groups.

Mednick and Schulsinger (1968) had hypothesized that children of schizophrenics might develop a thought disorder that consisted of a set of conditioned avoidance responses that become operantly strengthened as threatening situations were successively avoided. In our evaluation, using projective techniques, we found that the children of schizophrenics certainly avoided aggressive content and themes in their stories to the TAT. In the Aggression Content factor, we found that the children of schizophrenics had the lowest scores of the three groups studied, with the children of manic-depressives having the highest scores, and children of normals and children of physically ill parents falling in between. We interpreted this result to indicate that the children of schizophrenics were avoiding producing aggressive content in their TAT stories as a result of a generalized conditioned avoidance response. Since the children of manic-depressives had the opposite tendency on the TAT, it appeared that parental schizophrenia specifically, rather than parental psychosis, might be related to the pattern of avoidance of conflict in offspring.

More on Rorschach signs of disturbance. A variable that has been abstracted from the Rorschach and that relates to the diagnosis of adult schizophrenia is H. Friedman's (1952) Developmental Level (DL) score, based on Werner's (1948) developmental theory, and adapted by Becker (1956). The DL score is an index of the maturity of visual perception and analysis, and ranges from global, unarticulated perceptions (at the least mature), to articulated, integrated, and accurate perceptions (at the most mature).

Friedman, for example, considers responses that are based solely on chromatic or achromatic aspects of the inkblots as being examples of the most unarticulated or amorphous type. "Black paint" is an example of this kind of response. On the other hand, responses in which a blot is perceptually articulated and then reintegrated into a well-differentiated and unified whole are the most mature type. Since reviews of the use of the DL score (Goldfried, Stricker, & Weinert, 1971; Lerner, 1975) supported that the DL score was a valid indicator of cognitive and perceptual levels of functioning, with lower scores in schizophrenic than in normal populations, and since it appeared to be related to indices of prognosis for psychotic patients (Becker, 1956), as well as to schizophrenics' level of social competence (Lerner, 1968), we decided to determine whether the children of schizophrenics might be lower in their DL score than were the children of normal, manic-depressive, and physically ill parents. A full report of this investigation is available in Worland (1979).

We analyzed the DL score, treating race, sex, and parental diagnosis as the independent variables, and covarying out socioeconomic status, age, and Full-Scale IQ. The analysis yielded a significant main effect for parental diagnosis, F (3, 241) = 3.98, $p < .01$. The main effects for sex and race were not significant; and none of the interaction effects was significant.

Using the Newman Keuls procedure, planned comparisons indicated that the children of schizophrenics had significantly lower DL scores than the children of manic-depressives, $p < .05$; than the children of physically ill parents, $p < .01$; and lower than the children of normals, $p < .05$. The differences between the other groups were not significant.

More on TAT pathology. Peter Shabad, a graduate student at Washington University, did a retrospective analysis of the TATs that were collected on children during the first phase of our project in an effort to differentiate the TATs of the children who subsequently suffered breakdowns from those who had apparently healthy development in adolescence (Shabad, Worland, Lander, & Dietrich, 1979). He did this by carefully reading all the protocols and attempting to isolate those factors that differentiated the two sets of TATs.

To make his task a little bit more difficult, he divided our sample into four groups: children whom Anthony had rated as disturbed in childhood and who had subsequently had breakdowns, children Anthony rated as disturbed who had had subsequently healthy histories, children rated healthy by Anthony who had had subsequently healthy adjustment, and a group of normal children. The breakdowns mentioned here were transient mood disturbances in adolescence that in all cases but one necessitated in-patient psychiatric treatment. They were not psychotic episodes.

By rereading the TATs, Shabad was able to isolate six characteristics that were associated with functioning in the children 6 to 10 years later. The characteristics included a lack of individual initiative, a denial of the mother–child relationship, a denial of negative outcomes, and a lack of autonomy. The TAT characteristics that he isolated were independent of the level of adjustment at the time the TATs were administered; were not related to the child's IQ, socioeconomic status, race, or other family characteristics; and were only moderately, negatively correlated with story length.

The most dramatic finding was on card 7GF, a picture of an older woman reading with a young girl holding a doll. The children who were disturbed in childhood and who had breakdowns later in life did not perceive the woman as the girl's mother in their stories as frequently as the children who were sick in childhood and had apparently healthy development. However, the children at risk who had apparently healthy later development, although they did perceive the woman as the child's mother, perceived her as a malevolent, punishing, and hostile person. A further finding on this card was that only the children who had disturbed later adjustment made any mention of the theme of the little girl's or baby's "growing up big" or "getting married." The impression was of a precipitious jump to adulthood.

Shabad interpreted these results as suggesting that the disturbed offspring at risk either with disturbed or unremarkable later adjustment told TAT stories that suggested they were having major problems in their relationships with their mothers. When disturbed offspring at risk dealt with these maternal problems through massive denial, this pattern was associated with subsequent breakdowns. However, when the disturbed offspring at risk dealt with their maternal difficulties by perceiving her as a negative and punitive figure, it was associated with apparently healthier development. More information on this study is available in the Shabad et al. (1979) report, where it is pointed out that a prospective study of these TAT signs would be essential before asserting that they are predictive of breakdown.

Psychosocial investigation

The study of the family background of the developing child developed a little beyond the original proposal and added a crucial dimension to our understanding of the psychotic influence. We used the term *unroofing* in this context from the story by a French novelist of a demon who unroofed houses to find out exactly what was going on in the families underneath.

The unroofing was done in several ways: by living-in with certain families (Anthony, 1973a), by home visiting (Anthony, 1972), and by seeing the family in the research center (Anthony, 1973b). The naturalistic observations were supplemented by structured interviewing, what we called *focal* interviewing, and by rating the family interaction and child-rearing procedures on the Behrens–Goldfarb and Witkin scales.

The living-in procedure was supervised by the anthropologist Jules Henry, before his death. The observer recorded the day's events with the family in verbatim fashion. The protocols revealed a number of striking dynamic findings. Life in such families oscillated between poles of rationality and irrationality, realism and unrealism. The experience was also radically different in households with an involving psychosis as contrasted with a noninvolving psychosis. The contagion of the environment was demonstrated by the fact that the observer found the family less crazy, as a rule, at the end than at the beginning of her visit, so that a kind of psychotic acculturation appears to take place. The protocols revealed, among many other things, a high percentage of negative interactions between family members, a low expectation of pleasure and satisfaction, an overt or covert tendency to "drive the other person crazy," a lack of reconciling power on the part of the adults, and an inability to cope with mounting tensions, an exhibitionistic and voyeuristic reaction on the part of the children, and an acceptance of deviant behavior without comment or criticism. The scapegoat effect, involving a particular child, could also be easily discerned.

As might be expected, depending on the premorbid history of the family, families varied with regard to their resilience to the impact of psychosis (Anthony, 1975b, 1976). Some families seemed to do better than before the crisis, some developed a transient maladaptation, whereas others gradually disintegrated and deteriorated. The family members, especially the children, were deeply affected by the change in the personality and behavior of the psychotic parent and responded with confusion to the loss of continuity in the previously loved and normal parent (Anthony, 1973b). Small epidemics of disturbance among the family members took place in conjunction with the onset of psychosis and, as one child put it, "when Mother becomes sick, we all become sick" (Anthony, 1974a).

The technique of focal interviewing entailed an interview in depth that focused on the response to psychosis and the way that it affects the life, thoughts, and feelings of the person interviewed. The technique provided a vivid picture of the development of psychosis within a family and the very different ways in which the different members reacted to it. It also demonstrated that the response to delusional ideas was closely bound up with the emotional relationship to the deluded one, so that acceptance or rejection of the delusion was related to acceptance and rejection of the delusional parent or acceptance and rejection by the delusional parent.

The two full-time team members of the psychosocial unit (McGinnis and Lescow) had difficult tasks to perform requiring tact, consideration, understanding, and persistence in the face of suspiciousness and hostility or apathy and disinterest. They visited hospitals and schools to find research subjects and to establish a research alliance strong enough to withstand the intensity of the investigative process. The work was time-consuming because of the necessity to keep in constant communication with a large number of hospitals and because home visiting covered wide areas of a large city. The research demands made upon the subjects were heavy, and it was necessary at the beginning to assess the capacity of the families to carry through with the program. The second task involved carrying out intensive psychosocial studies of the family and supervising the clinical care of children designated vulnerable as a result of investigation. Our project social workers have been called upon also by project families for crisis intervention and for ongoing psychological support (Anthony & McGinnis, 1978).

Because of the differences in ability to communicate verbally, class differences, and cultural expectations, it was difficult to use the Witkin Schedule of Differentiation for all families. Like most schemes devised to permit quantification of psychosocial data, the direction is pointed to a middle-class, white, liberal way of life. We, therefore, had to devise variables that would take class and cultural factors into consideration. With these provisos in mind, the mother's child-rearing practices can be related without prejudice to her capacity to permit her children to differentiate and individuate.

The two lowest social class groups (IV and V according to the Hollingshead–Redlich classification) tend to be restricted, inarticulate, and inhibited with regard to sexual and aggressive feelings. They avoid stepping out of geographic, intellectual, and emotional areas in which they feel safe and comfortable. There was some evidence to suggest that the psychotic mother, in particular, was low on empathy, communicative skills, the capacity to invest herself in the child, and in constancy of affection and her givingness.

The indicators in the Witkin Scale were found to have a certain value although his categories are not always pertinent for getting at the factor of differentiation in our socially stratified sample.

The Behrens–Goldfarb Scale, on the other hand, proved both usable and useful for quantifying the home visit impressions. They are detailed and somewhat tedious, but with continued use their value became increasingly apparent. Unlike the Witkin Scale, the categories are devised to cut across class lines.

On inspection of our data, we came across the finding that the psychotic families scored consistently lower than control families on the categories of verbal interaction, parent–child interaction, sibling interaction, and the interaction of the family as a group. Behrens and Goldfarb found that when the child and not the parent was psychotic, it was the intergenerational interaction that suffered most.

The Behrens–Goldfarb data showed a consistently lower overall score in all categories of the scale for the psychotic families as compared with the comparison and control families. There was more scatter in the scores of the physically ill than in the psychotic or normal families. The four categories that differentiated most significantly between the groups were mutual support, alignments, home atmosphere, and sharing of parents. There was a definite lack of support between family members in the psychotic households. The members tended to act as isolated individuals who got caught up in alignments with the well or sick parent. The attempt to deny the fact of illness created an unpleasant atmosphere. The sibling rivalry was often intense, possibly because one of the parents abdicated his or her parental role and became a grown-up child with childish needs. When the sick member was out of the home, the family as a whole appeared less suspicious and more open and responsive.

The incestuous element in the parent–child relationship was much more evident in the psychotic homes, the well parent turning to the children of the opposite sex to fulfill the emotional needs denied by the sick parent. As a result of the disturbed and unsatisfactory marital relationship, the children not only became objects of gratification but were aware of their increased value in this respect and may have traded on it.

In general, we had the feeling that nothing in these families ever gets defined or brought to a closure. The members learn to live with ambiguity and vacillation. To what extent this tendency is transmitted from family to family, we shall only be able to learn from a three-generational assessment. So far, we have had no families with a grandparent living in the home, but retrospective reports from the parents indicated that the curious atmosphere generated was known to them in their childhood. We are, at present, collecting a small sample of families who are willing to let us investigate the grandparents.

Comments on home visits. The Behrens–Goldfarb Scale provided us with structured and unified ways of viewing the manifold behavior and communication of the family system. It concerned itself with the observable and audible aspects of family life, and from its findings one can derive a sense of family style. The class factor became very obvious in rating families. The observers had to work harder in the quiet, uncommunicative, lower-class families. The use of two observers, although enhancing the reliability of the observations, often had the effect of polarizing the family, especially in psychotic households. The observers were often caught up in the strong alignments that characterize the family group with a psychotic member. The tension engendered by the visit was related mostly to the nervousness round the tabooed subject of psychosis. The symbolic death of the "crazy one" had to be kept away from public scrutiny at all costs.

Home visiting with psychotic parents was exasperating. The times were never right, appointments were often broken, no directions were given, doorbells were frequently out of order, family members were often missing, and the most careful planning often went awry at the last minute. In addition, no matter what explanations were offered, the families were deeply suspicious about the purpose of the visit and had difficulty in being friendly or positive. In the middle-class psychotic families, the visit was often overorganized by the family, so that the visitors were ferried through the home and through the family with very little spontaneous contact. Sometimes entertainments (by the children) were put on for the benefit of the visitors. In the lower-class psychotic homes, disorganization was rampant, and confusion was everywhere evident. The families also tended to be unnaturally quiet and passive, as if they were waiting for the visitors to make the first move. The children of the psychotic families tended to two extremes: either they were attention seeking, demanding or aggressive, or frozen, isolated, and unrelating.

Family functioning

The family's role as the primary socializing agent makes the family environment a natural place to look for origins of mental disorder. As reviewed by Jacobs (1975) researchers have proposed a number of family climate-related explanations of mental illness, especially schizophrenia, including double-bind communications, marital schism and skew, pseudomutuality, emotional divorce, and the schizophrenogenic mother. Research into expressed affect in families that have produced a schizophrenic member is mixed, but, in general, more negative affect has been found in families with a disturbed member, almost always a child.

Two instruments assessing family environment have been used in the St. Louis High-Risk Project. The first, used in all phases of the study, is the Bene–Anthony Family Relations Test (FRT). Children and parents, tested individually, drop cards describing family members into a series of postal boxes representing each member of the family. Statements vary on three dimensions: positive–negative, incoming–outgoing, and mild–strong. Samples are: "This person in the family sometimes gets too angry" (outgoing, negative, mild), and "This person in the family hits me a lot" (incoming, negative, strong).

Stiffman (1976) compared FRT family *incongruity* scores of schizophrenic, manic-depressive, and normal parents. These scores were derived discrepancies between the child's perception of positive or negative statements coming from a parent (incoming), and the parent's assignment of the statements to the child (outgoing). The major finding was that only in normal families did children perceive more positive feelings being directed from parents than parents actually awarded the children. This positively skewed perception of parental affect was not perceived by children of manic-depressive or of schizophrenic parents.

Janes, Hudson, Hesselbrock, and Anthony (1975) and Janes (1975) reported that fathers and children in manic-depressive families were more involved affectively with one another than were children and fathers in normal or schizophrenic families. Parents in schizophrenic families showed evidence of reduced involvement with their children. Quantity and quality of intrafamily involvement as measured by the FRT did not differ among families in which one parent was diagnosed as manic-depressive, in which one parent was physically ill, and in control families. Differences in involvement patterns were noted when one parent was schizophrenic. When the father was schizophrenic his involvement with the mother was greater than that of control fathers. When the mother was schizophrenic her involvement with the father was greater than that of control mothers. These differences were in total number of statements placed in spouse's box, that is, *quantity* of involvement; no differences in *quality* of involvement were demonstrated. Schizophrenics' responses to spouse did *not* differ from those of control in degree of positivity, in direction (incoming or outgoing), or in potency (mild or strong). See also Janes (1976).

Finn (1975) used the FRT to focus on sibling relations in families with a psychotic parent. He reported that although children of normal parents do not differ from children of psychotics in number of statements attributed to themselves or to their parents, they are more involved with their siblings than are children of psychotics, and this involvement is primarily negative. An independent assessment of sibling rivalry, the Three Houses Test, substantiated the notion that sibling rivalry was more frequently found in psychiatrically normal families as compared with psychotic ones. Further analysis showed that this rivalry was related to children's perceptions that siblings received too much attention and protection.

Psychophysiology

Although the type of abnormality reported appears to depend on medication, stimulus intensity, signal significance, hand from which electrodermal activity is recorded, and behavioral activity level, studies almost uniformly agree that schizophrenics' electrodermal activity differs from that of normal subjects. Does aberrant electrodermal activity precede behavioral manifestations of schizophrenia? Mednick and Schulsinger (1968) have published the only report to date directly relevant to this question. They reported that electrodermal activity of adolescents who subsequently (in the next 4 years) "manifested severely abnormal behavior" (p. 278) was significantly different from those who did not. Breakdown children had higher levels of responding, shorter response onset latency, and faster response recovery.

If abnormal electrodermal activity precedes the onset of schizophrenia and if a higher proportion of children of schizophrenics than children of normals become schizophrenic (and they do), then the proportion of children with abnormal electrodermal activity should be higher among offspring of schizophrenics than among offspring of normal parents. Three studies (Mednick & Schulsinger, 1968; Van

Dyke, Rosenthal, & Rassmussen, 1974; and Klein & Salzman, 1977) have reported at least some evidence that offspring of schizophrenics are more responsive electrodermally than are offspring of normals in some experimental situations, although there are a number of unreconciled differences in the findings. In our population, however, children of schizophrenic and of manic-depressive parents were not more or less responsive than children of normal and of physically ill parents. Complete results can be found in Janes, Hesselbrock, and Stern (1978).

A comparison of the results from our study with those from previous reports is constrained by sample and procedural differences. For example, the present study examined skin potential, whereas those of Mednick and Schulsinger (1968), Van Dyke et al. (1974), and Klein and Salzman (1977) used skin conductance. A review of these differences points out the problems with generalizing from the findings of any single study on psychophysiology. Mednick and Schulsinger, as well as Klein and Salzman, reported response amplitude, whereas the present report examined frequency, and Van Dyke et al. considered both measures. The auditory stimulus in previous studies was more intense than the present study's thermal stimulus. Ages were 10 to 18 in the Mednick and Schulsinger study, 21 to 55 in the Van Dyke et al. study, 10 in the Klein and Salzman study, and 6 to 18 in our study. Only children of chronic schizophrenic mothers were used in the Mednick and Schulsinger study. Ill parents were process schizophrenics in the Van Dyke et al. study and included both mothers and fathers. Klein and Salzman's ill parents were schizophrenic and schizoaffective mothers. The sample in the present study included offspring of schizoaffective, reactive, and chronic schizophrenic mothers and fathers. Families were intact in the present study and in Klein and Salzman's, whereas many of Mednick's subjects were from broken homes. Van Dyke et al.'s subjects were adoptees.

An additional finding from the St. Louis study was that movement artifact, a reflection of impatience or agitation or lack of impulse control, occupied a greater proportion of the psychophysiological records of children of psychotics than of the other childrens' records. This was attributable largely to greater activity of children of manic-depressives. The notion that this measure was a reflection of degree of maturation is strongly supported by its highly significant negative relationship with age (Janes et al., 1978).

Mednick and Schulsinger (1968) introduced evidence for a relationship between psychopathology and the configuration of the terminal portion of the electrodermal response. They reported that among children of schizophrenic mothers, those that eventually broke down psychiatrically had steeper slopes during the termination portion of a skin conductance response than did children who did not break down. Reasoning that steep skin *conductance* response termination was analogous to a biphasic response shape in a skin *potential* response (i.e., both positive and negative deflections in a single response), we compared psychological ratings for biphasic and uniphasic responders. We hypothesized that biphasic responders would be rated as more disturbed than uniphasic responders. For this analysis, children who gave a fair number of electrodermal (skin potential) responses (above the median) during the psychophysiological study were classified either as uniphasic or as biphasic responders on the basis of the characteristic shape of their skin potential responses. Both uniphasic and biphasic responders were found in all groups based on parental diagnosis. It was found that, independent of parental diagnosis, biphasic children were rated by psychologists as more pathological than uniphasic children, based on their psychological testing responses, mentioned elsewhere in this report. Details are found in Janes and Stern (1976). These results were interpreted within a framework provided by Edelberg's (1970) work on the information content of the electrodermal recovery limb. The biphasic response mode may reflect deficient information processing resulting from malfunctioning of the brain's gating-out mechanism. It was hypothesized that this, coupled with other genetically and environmentally determined factors, could lead to serious psychological pathology, and perhaps, in some cases, to schizophrenia (Janes & Stern, 1976).

Consistent with the overall thrust of the project as originally designed, the psychophysiological study was designed around the concept of differentiation. Psychophysiological differentiation was defined as the degree to which children responded on the stimulated side of the body, as opposed to bilaterally. The stimulus was a warm puff of air from a hair dryer applied to the right wrist. As discussed earlier in this report, less differentiated children were expected to be concentrated in families with a psychotic parent. Like other kinds of differentiation, psychophysiological differentiation was viewed as a developmental phenomenon, with younger children expected to give more global, whole-body responses to a given stimulus, whereas older children's responses were expected to be restricted to the right side of the body (stimulated side). Other variables of interest in the psychophysiological study were speed of habituation, degree of autonomic conditioning, and amount of movement artifact.

Evidence of differentiation was rare and did not occur more frequently among children with a psychotic parent when compared to those with psychiatrically normal and physically ill parents (Janes, 1974). Furthermore, if a more "advanced" type of responding, differentiation should have occurred more frequently among older children than younger children. This did not happen. Further examination of the stimulus situation led us to conclude that psychophysiological responses reflected activity contingent upon the sound of the hair dryer, which generated the puff of air, as well as contingent upon the puff of air itself. Although the puff of air was presented to the right wrist only, the sound of the hair dryer turning on (and off) was available to both ears. We must conclude that the differentiation hypothesis was not tested.

With respect to responsiveness, black children were more responsive than white children in vasomotor activity, whereas white children responded more frequently than black children in the electrodermal mode (Janes et al., 1976). Younger children were more responsive than older children.

Research clinic

In 1967, Anthony received funds from NIMH to pilot a system of corrective interventions in the research population that was under investigation (Anthony, 1977). This project funded a "preventive substation," or "research clinic," to evaluate the efficacy of a wide variety of systematically applied preventive measures in diminishing the testable vulnerability of children with psychotic parents. For each child seen in the clinic, a risk profile was constructed to establish the child's total risk on a series of seven ratings. These included: family history of illness, pregnancy and birth complications, constitution, development, physical health, environment, and specific traumata. Although Anthony considered this measure a very crude expression of a complex reaction tendency, it had the advantage of furnishing a numerical assessment as well as a more analytic approach to a very global concept.

The following four kinds of intervention programs were employed. These differed over several dimensions: short versus long; specific versus nonspecific; technically complex requiring the use of professionals versus technically simple; and costly versus inexpensive (Anthony, 1974b; 1977).

1. *Compensatory measures.* These were various nonspecific interventions aimed at building up ego resources, strengthening self-confidence, and bringing the child into contact with benevolent figures. The opportunities offered including individual tutoring, camp experiences, Big Brothers and recreational and creative opportunities outside the psychotic family. These activities were mostly carried out by nonprofessionals.

2. *Classical measures.* Individual and group psychotherapy were undertaken under supervision by full-time residents in child psychiatry. *Classical* interventions refer to the traditional therapeutic techniques with individual or groups of children employed at child guidance agencies throughout the country and based on psychodynamic conceptualizations, interpersonal transactions, and the therapist–child relationship. With younger children this takes the form of play therapy, and with older ones, verbal interchanges that aim at clarifying the anxious concerns of the patients. The novelty in this approach is the application of a mode of therapeutic intervention customarily used for emotionally disordered children to a preventive intervention that anticipates the development of potential disorder. In keeping with traditional psychotherapy, the disturbed parents were also seen in counseling with a child-centered focus.

3. *Cathartic measures.* These interventions were conducted either individually with each member of the family or with the family as a whole. In both styles, a focal interview encouraged each member of the family to report his or her individual experience of the family psychosis as it developed and enveloped the person and influenced his or her life, both inside and outside the family. A whole range of affects, such as fear, shame, guilt, anger, hatred, and compassion were abreacted.

4. *Corrective measures.* The rationale behind the corrective intervention stemmed from direct experiences with the children. The attempt here was to counter the increased suggestibility, submissiveness, and involvement in the psychotic illness with specific exercises to work against the tendency.

The evaluation of this extensive procedure, without benefit of control group, was carried out by readministering portions of the research battery to the children involved in the various different kinds of interventions. With this methodological caveat in mind, some tentative conclusions were drawn. It seemed that external behavior was a little more sensitive to change than internal behavior, or else that there might have been a lag in internal changes. There was some indication that the amount of intervention might have had quite a powerful effect on the vulnerability scores. It seemed to Anthony that the amount of interest that the research clinic took in a particular family seemed to exert a special influence of it's own, irrespective of the type of intervention. The classical interventions, which were the most massive ones, yielded the best results, and the cathartic ones, which seemed very efficacious on short term evaluation, did not appear to have much effect on the vulnerability scores. There appeared to be some relationship between the degree of change in the vulnerability score of the child and the degree of change in the vulnerability scores for the entire family. One additional difficulty with the methodology of the intervention program was the difficulty of obtaining comparable intervention and nonintervention groups. It seemed as if the volunteers for the intervention were not only highly motivated but also change-susceptible individuals who, more or less, picked themselves in a desire for change.

SUMMARY OF MAJOR FINDINGS FROM THE FIRST
ASSESSMENT

Our major findings about the children of psychotic parents after our first 5 years of evaluation were that our psychological testing yielded support for previous findings that children of psychotic parents, indeed, have greater clinical disturbance than children of normal parents, and that the assessed level of disturbance was not due to, or complicated by, the interactions of socioeconomic class status, race, or the age of children. Psychological disturbance was greater in those children most identified with their ill parent and those most suggestible. Psychophysiologically, we found that, at least in children with a high rate of exosomatic responding, children with biphasic responses were more likely to be rated disturbed by psychologists than were children with uniphasic responses, and this finding appeared to be independent of parental psychosis.

Unlike previous reports on the intelligence of children of psychotic parents, the children of psychotic parents in the St. Louis sample did not have lower intelligence than control children. A further finding was that the children of psychotic parents, particularly the children of schizophrenics, had more problems in the area of cognitive decentering in the Piagetian sense than did control children or the children of manic-depressive parents, and that this measure of egocentricity was related to the children's actual behavioral functioning, at least in those children where we had a school measure of their behavior.

Strengths and weaknesses of the initial battery

The major focus of the initial study had been to describe clinically the children of psychotic parents. For this reason, the initial battery was clinically (and psychiatrically) oriented toward pathology. Only a small number of the children had had school behavioral measures, and parents had not been asked to comment on the behavioral development of their offspring. Thus, except in those cases where we were lucky enough to have the school assessments, we had no external criterion for the children's actual mode of behavior. We had emphasized an "inside" view of the child, and had deemphasized an "outside" behavioral description of the child. At the end of the first assessment, we became aware of the number of behavioral indices of later disturbance being suggested in other projects, and feeling these were sorely needed in the St. Louis Project, we added many of these measures to our second assessment battery.

An additional problem with the extensive clinical assessment done in the first battery was that it was enormously expensive, requiring the aid of well-trained clinical psychologists and psychiatrists. The clinical ratings, for example, done in a skillful manner by child clinicians who between them had decades of clinical experience, were time-consuming and prohibitively costly. An additional problem was that by having clinicians assess children's test behavior to make ratings, we felt we perhaps had placed a potentially biasing screen between the children and our view of them; and we hoped to remove this screen partially in our reassessment.

THE SECOND ASSESSMENT OF THE SAMPLE (1975–1979)

After an interim grant between 1972 and 1975, during which much of the preparation for the analysis of the Phase I data was completed, the St. Louis Project applied for funding to recontact the sample and reassess the offspring at risk, the offspring of physically ill parents, and the offspring of controls. This phase of the project, under the direction of Cynthia Janes, emphasized the importance of external, behavioral criteria, and as a result, the more purely clinical assessments decreased in their importance. Funding was secured, and this assessment was carried out between 1975 and 1978. Continuing evaluation of the Phase I data was a parallel aim during this period.

Recontacting the research sample

Our first goal was to recontact and revaluate all the offspring and parents seen originally between 1967 and 1972. Contact and at least partial testing was accomplished on 73% of the original sample, with greater attrition in schizophrenic and physically ill families (66 and 68% retested, respectively) than in the manic-depressive and control families (76 and 81% retested). These data are in Table 3. It will be noted that although our overall reassessment rate of 73% is quite respectable, we were less successful in reassessing families of schizophrenics and physically ill parents than the families of manic-depressive and normal parents, a difference we felt was due to a social class effect, since our higher social class subjects were in the latter two groups. Also we were somewhat more successful at attracting mothers for reassessments than fathers. Another hardly surprising finding was that we were able to get more data when we assessed families at home or at school than when we asked them to come to the Research Center for testing.

Table 3. *General rates of reassessment during Phase II, partial reassessments included*

Group	Fathers		Mothers		Offspring		All subjects	
	(*N*)	(%)	(*N*)	(%)	(*N*)	(%)	(*N*)	(%)
Schizophrenic	29	41	29	66	94	73	152	66
Manic-depressive	17	65	17	82	56	77	90	76
Physically ill	19	53	19	58	73	75	111	68
Normal control	38	76	28	82	121	82	197	81
Total	103	60	103	73	344	77	550	73

Note: N = all subjects who made up the original sample; % = percentage of subjects in category who have had any reassessment.

The revaluation of the research sample

We selected a triannual assessment scheme for the 1975–1978 reassessment. Each offspring was scheduled for testing during the month of his or her 7th, 10th, 13th, 16th, 19th, 22nd, or 25th birthday. Because the entire project period lasted 4 years, this allowed us to see each child once and have some time left over to pick up stragglers. The advantages of this system were that it allowed us to have larger *N*s per cell at each age gate, that we were assessing children at the same ages as the Rochester High-Risk Project, and that since families were tested in a jumbled order our testers could be blind to their parents' diagnostic status. The major disadvantage was that the repeated recontact as various children reached time to be tested was an annoyance, especially for the larger families (Fig. 2).

Phase II represented a very exacting research schedule, especially as the task of collecting data and analyzing it within the ongoing longitudinal design was constantly punctuated by recurrent and urgent crises on the part of certain families that lived in a state of insistent emergency and used the Child Development Research Center as their first port of call. Despite the pressure of our work, this was encouraged – not only because it helped to dissipate mounting stresses that led up to psychotic breaks and hospitalizations, but also because it tied the subjects effectively to the ongoing research. This kept the refusal and dropout rates within workable proportions.

By the end of 1978, the family structure with which we began the research in 1967 had altered because time, psychosis, and the usual life stresses had taken their expected toll (Table 4). All the above factors brought about radical changes in the family structure so that the impact of psychosis no longer affected the children directly within the household. But although away from home and even out of the city, there was a curious and strongly ambivalent tie that persisted, making the parents' psychosis still the crucial event in the lives of the children, so much so that some of the children's first breakdowns have coincided with the rehospitalization of their ill parent.

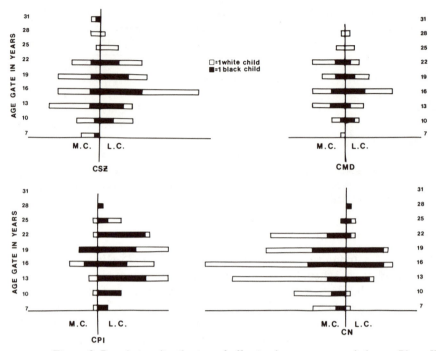

Figure 2. Population distribution of offspring by age, race, and class at Phase II.

In one somewhat unusual case, the parent had a psychotic relapse on the day of her father's death and the husband had predicted this: What he did not predict was that at the same time one of their children would be hospitalized for her first breakdown.

One effect of the physical emancipation was that the children seemed more able to talk about the parents' psychosis with more clinical detachment and objectivity and to show less gross involvement in it. They no longer felt as overwhelmed, but they were exasperated and ashamed. In fact, frequently they recommended separation or divorce as a relief for the nonpsychotic parent.

There was also no doubt that the psychosis with which we started the research no longer seemed to be the same psychosis. During the years, it altered almost kaleidoscopically. Time and the aging process continued their influence, but repeated electroshock treatments, the prolonged use of medication, protracted periods of unemployment and, in a number of cases, religious conversions (especially to such churches as Jehovah's Witness, Pentecostals, Scientology, the Charismatic Movement, etc.) appeared to have restructured and reshaped these psychotic profiles. The children reported that the parent seemed less frightening, less peculiar, and mellowing.

This was not, however, always the case, because we also watched a manic patient over a period of 10 years change from a moderately disturbing psychosis to

Table 4. *Incidence of stressful events in families during 1976–1978*

	Deaths	Murders	Suicides and attempts	Separation and divorce	Hospitalizations	Unplanned moves	Unemployed
Vulnerable – breakdowns (N = 6)	3	0	2	3	17	7	6
Vulnerable – no breakdown, but microepisodes (N = 9)	6	2	5	3	21	12	19
Vulnerable – no breakdown, no microepisodes (N = 4)	1	0	1	3	5	5	1
Total vulnerable group (N = 19)	10	2	8	9	43	24	26
Matched controls (N = 22)	1	0	0	2	1	1	1

a disastrous one causing upheaval throughout the family. Her husband had died, the children had all left home, any religiousness that had been a comfort to her became a religious mania.

The Phase II assessment battery (Table 5)

Psychiatric assessment. The psychiatric aim of Phase II was to make a detailed clinical analysis of those children who are considered most likely to suffer a breakdown in adolescence, in order to obtain as clear a picture as possible of the nature, intensity and course of the breakdowns before, during, and after the event.

Psychological assessment. The psychological battery used in the second assessment of the children attempted to repeat certain aspects of the initial assessment, so that longitudinal linkages could be made; but we also attempted to expand the battery to include areas not previously covered. Since the median age of the offspring for the second assessment was greater than 16 years, we were able to add the Minnesota Multiphasic Personality Inventory (MMPI; Hathaway & McKinley, 1942) to our battery. We also attempted to design the battery for children at the different ages of assessment in a way that would maximize our data with a minimum of effort. For example, we decreased the Rorschach from 10 cards to 5, and the TAT from 11 cards to 5. The test battery for the revaluation, then, included the following items:

1. The Wechsler Intelligence Scale for Children – Revised (WISC-R; Wechsler, 1974), or the Wechsler Adult Intelligence Scale (WAIS; Wechsler, 1955).
2. The Rorschach (I, II, IV, VII, IX). Our effort in selecting a subset of cards was to have a balance between chromatic and achromatic cards and between "broken" and "unbroken" cards in Becker's sense.
3. The Thematic Apperception Test (1, 2, 3BM, 7GF, 8BM).
4. The Continuous Word Association Test (CWAT). This was administered to about 40 children. Despite the use of a word association test during Phase I (Kahana, Stern, & Clack, 1969; Kahana & Sterneck, 1969), when we were unable to establish accurate interjudge reliability for any of the scoring systems that appeared useful to us, we dropped the test.
5. The Wide Range Achievement Test (WRAT; Jastak, Bijou, & Jastak, 1965). This test enabled us to get a quick estimate of each child's academic achievement in the areas of word recognition, mathematics, and spelling.
6. The Beery–Buktenica Developmental Form Sequence. This is a test of visual–motor coordination and is sensitive both to organicity and schizophrenia.
7. The Minnesota Multiphasic Personality Inventory (MMPI; Hathaway & McKinley, 1942). This test was given to children 16 years old and older.

The WAIS was given in its full form to subjects 19 years old and older, but those subjects 22 years old and older had a WAIS short form (Vocabulary and Block Design).

Table 5. *Test battery for Phase II (1975–1978)*

	Level		
	Life patterns	Life competence	Inner life
Moos Family Environment Scale	**	**	*
Bene–Anthony Family Relations Test	*	**	***
General Information Questionnaire (GIQ)	***	**	*
Rochester Adaptive Behavior Inventory	***	***	
School assessment	**	***	
Psychiatric interview	*	**	***
Intellectual assessment		***	
Beery–Buktenica Developmental Form Sequence		***	
Speech sample		***	
Wide Range Achievement Test (WRAT)		***	
Thematic Apperception Test (TAT; 1, 2, 3BM, 7GF, 8BM)			***
Rorschach (I, II, IV, VII, IX)			***

* = light emphasis.   ** = moderate emphasis.   *** = strong emphasis.

Behavioral functioning. In an effort to collect a broad-spectrum representation of each child's behavioral competence, the St. Louis Project expanded its assessment to include aspects of daily living, an objectively scored test for family environment, teachers' reports, and most importantly, an extensive self-report (Janes, Hesselbrock, Meyers, & Penniman, 1979). These items are described in detail.

The General Information Questionnaire. This instrument was developed by the project staff, led by Janes with the help of Darcy Gilpin Myers and Janet Penniman, as a means of obtaining specific information regarding the life patterns of our subject population, parents as well as offspring. It was a self-administered questionnaire that required approximately 2 hours to complete. It was administered at the home with each family member filling out a form. The questions on the forms varied with the age and marital status of each respondent, but the areas of functioning were the same for all. These areas were: job and/or school, family relationships, friendship patterns, leisure-time activities, participation in community affairs, health, and religious life. The majority of questions were multiple choice. The questions were a composite of items from the life events–stress literature, structured interviews used within the Washington University Department of Psychiatry, and items related to theoretical and empirical factors relevant to the development of psychosis.

Moos Family Environment Scale. A second instrument for evaluating family environment is Moos's Family Environment Scale (FES; Moos, 1974), a 90-item true–false test in which each family member indicates his or her perception of family attitudes and attributes. The subscales can be roughly grouped into three types: those involving perceptions of interpersonal relationships within the family, those dealing with directions of personal growth emphasized in the family, and those concerned with perceptions of the organizational structure of the family. Comparing high-school age offspring of schizophrenic and normal parents, children of schizophrenic parents rated their families significantly lower on 2 of the 10 subscales: Intellectual–Cultural Orientation and Active–Recreational Orientation. Overall, the results seemed to indicate that the teenager in the family with a schizophrenic parent is more likely to view his or her home environment as one in which family members generally stay at home and, perhaps somewhat reluctantly, stick together (Janes, 1976).

The Bene–Anthony Family Relations Test. This is a standardized test administered to all family members (Bene & Anthony, 1957). It evaluates each family member's feelings toward the other family members, and each family member's perception of the other family members' feelings toward him or her. We had used this test in the first battery and repeated it in the second.

Rochester Adaptive Behavior Inventory. This is a structured interview developed by Fred Jones and other risk researchers at the University of Rochester (Jones, 1977). Each mother was interviewed about each child. The interview covers such areas of the child's behavior as school behavior and achievement, friendship and peer interactions, family interactions, bizarre and unusual behavior, and sexual behavior. It also asks the parent to make predictions about the child's later competence. The total interview took a minimum of 90 minutes.

School achievement. Subjects who were in grade school or high school during the time of our Phase II evaluation were evaluated by means of two instruments each, filled out by as many teachers (up to four) as the child had. The first instrument was the Pupil Rating Form developed by Watt at the University of Massachusetts, which was being used at three risk research centers. It taps behavior observable to teachers and empirically demonstrated to relate to the development of schizophrenia. The second instrument, depending on the child's age, was either the Devereux Elementary School Behavior Rating Scale (Spivack & Swift, 1967) or the Hahnemann High School Bahavior Rating Scale (Spivack & Swift, 1972), comparable forms. These are well standardized and are widely in use.

Speech sample. Each parent was asked to make a 5-minute extemporaneous evaluation of each child. The parent was asked to evaluate how the child was growing up, what kind of person the child was becoming, what were the child's strengths and weaknesses, and what in the parent's behavior had either a good or a bad influence on the child's development. These speeches were audiotaped and transcribed.

Cross-sectional Phase II analyses

At the time of this writing, few analyses have yet been carried out on the data collected at Phase II. Although much of these data is ready for analysis at this time, the major effort of the project staff has been to complete the final preparation of the complete data file. However, a few studies have been carried out and will be reported here.

Family climate. In a master's thesis from St. Louis University, Saul Hopper (1976) studied two groups of families using the Moos Family Environment Scale (FES) and the Marlowe–Crowne Social Desirability Scale in order to explore the clinical usefulness of the FES and to investigate the differences in family climate between disturbed and normal families. The experimental group was composed of 12 families in which a parent had been diagnosed as either schizophrenic or manic-depressive; this group comprised 46 individuals. The control group, matched for race and social class, consisted of 16 normal families having 66 individuals.

Not only did Hopper investigate differences in scores between groups, but he computed a Family Incongruence Score, a measure of variance within families. He found that, as a group, the experimental subjects tended to have greater variance within their families than controls on most comparisons. Especially on the Moos scale labeled Cohesion, he found support for Anthony's (1972) description of family climate in families of psychotic parents and for earlier work by McGinnis and Sumer (1978). Since the experimental group was assumed to contain both families with an involving psychosis and a noninvolving psychosis, it was reasonable to surmise that low scores and high scores on the Cohesion factor would characterize the responding of the experimental group as a whole. This was indeed the case, whereas families in the comparison group had scores on this factor that were more normally distributed.

In addition, Hopper found differential effects of social desirability tendencies on FES subscales, a different pattern for the two groups. He also found a number of differences on mean FES subscale scores in a variety of group comparisons in-volved family means, parents' scores, children's scores, and the congruence of scores within the families. In conclusion, Hopper suggested that the FES was a clinically useful instrument, and the results presented strong evidence for its validity. However, his study suggested the need for further research on the effects of social desirability in order to make proper interpretations of the FES scores as well as the need for further research to establish the clinical sensitivity of the scale.

Two measures of communication deviance. Susan R. Randich conducted a study in cooperation with Esther Csapo, an undergraduate student from Washington University, comparing two measures of communication deviance that had been collected in our study (Csapo, 1977). Since both the Rorschach and the TAT had been used in previous evaluations at other risk research settings to measure communication deviance, we decided to take a look at the congruence between these two measures. The only subjects in our sample during the Phase II evaluation who received both the Rorschach and the TAT assessment were children; and since we assumed that communication deviance might increase with age, we concentrated on a group of 16- to 25-year-olds who had received both of these assessments. We understood that it might have been more desirable to study communication de-viance in adults, but adults were being given only the TAT communication deviance measure, so they were ruled out. The sample consisted of 30 individuals. The TATs were scored by two project psychologists (Worland and Lander), and we had achieved an interscorer reliability of r (47) = .97. Our differences had been resolved by discussion. Randich and Csapo used the Singer (1973) scoring manual and established interrator reliability on 15 nonsample pilot Rorschachs of r (15) = .76.

Following this, a system of scoring was devised such that several nonsample protocols could be periodically scored and reconciled by both scorers during the scoring of the actual sample, in order to maintain high reliability while minimally affecting the scoring of the sample protocols. Mutual drift, which might have led to spuriously high reliability despite low validity, would be minimized. A Spearman correlation was calculated on the total communication deviance scores. The Spearman coefficient of r_s (30) = .133, failed to show statistical significance; and, in fact, this correlation suggested that no relationship existed between the Rorschach and the TAT measures under examination.

One possible interpretation of these findings was that there was more communication deviance on the Rorschach, which is presumed to be a more anxiety-provoking test, and that since communication deviance might increase as a function of anxiety, high scorers on the Rorschach might have been low scorers on the TAT. If this were indeed the case, it would be expected that individuals with high communication deviance on the TAT would also score high on the Rorschach, although the reverse would not necessarily be true. However, an investigation of the distribution of scores indicated that this was not the case.

Their conclusion is that these two measures of communication deviance may assess different aspects of a single underlying communication problem, and that using the two together might yield a more predictive reliability in terms of their effect on childhood disturbance than the use of either one alone.

Psychophysiological methodology. One of the main issues to be explored during the Phase III grant period was bilateral differences in skin conductance level (SCL) and responding (SCR) and skin potential level (SPL) and responding (SPR) as functions of parental and child psychopathology. To validly make left- and right-hand comparisons of these EDA measures it was necessary to rule out variance attributable to extraneous factors. To do this it was essential that we place electrodes where recording was more reliable and that we precisely equate left- and right-hand recording sites. It was also essential that we choose electrolytes for SC and SP that would most validly reflect EDA. Janes has carried out this series of studies with the help of Wendy Katz; they investigated electrode placements for skin conductance, skin potential, and electrolyte effects. Their search for optimal electrode placements led to the discovery that there were regular, but complex, differences in EDA as a function of placement. The phalanges, thenar, and hypothenar eminences of the palmar surface were explored in a series of studies. It was found that reliable and stable skin-conductance recordings could be obtained from placements on the hypothenar eminence below the crease beneath the meeting of the metacarpus and phalanges. The search for good skin potential placements was more difficult and was complicated by significant electrolyte effects (summarized later), but standardization of placement within the thenar eminences was found crucial for reliable skin-potential recordings. The system arrived upon is simple and, therefore, placements are highly replicable.

The importance of the electrolyte chosen for either SC or SP recording has been brought to the attention of psychophysiologists by a number of investigators, but has not yet been fully appreciated. Electrolytes have been shown to differ in the degree to which they hydrate the skin and consequently affect amplitude, frequency, and shape of the EDR. They evaluated electrolytes for both skin conductance and skin potential. Unibase was found to be the electrolyte of choice, mainly because of its resistance over time to hydration effects.

Regarding skin potential, the search for a suitable electrolyte has been much more difficult. One of the most commonly used electrolytes, Beckman paste, was found to eliminate the electrically positive component of responses over time. This is undoubtedly due to its high salt concentration that contributes to skin hydration.

Longitudinal findings

Prediction of competence. In a doctoral dissertation from the University of Texas at Austin, Gail Overbey (1979) carried out a study using data from the St. Louis project, on the prediction of competence in children at risk.

The academic and social competence of children at high risk for the later development of mental illness was investigated using the psychological test measures and teacher ratings obtained during the 1967–1971 assessment period in elementary school and in 1975–1978 in high school. Four issues were addressed: (1) the power of such measures to differentiate between groups of children at risk; (2) the relationship between psychological test battery measures of competence and teacher ratings of competence; (3) the stability of these measures from early elementary school to high school; and (4) the combination of measures given during early elementary school that can best predict competent performance during high school.

The sample was drawn from the larger project and consisted of 30 children with one schizophrenic parent, 18 children with one physically ill parent, 17 children with one manic-depressive parent, and 40 control children whose parents had no physical or mental illness.

Subjects were evaluated during early elementary school and again at age 16. The following measures were obtained as potential components of competence: Verbal, Performance, and Full-Scale IQ, Rorschach Genetic Level score, and assessments of Positive Affect, Positive Interaction, and Constructive Coping taken from the Thematic Apperception Test. In addition, during both phases of the study teacher ratings of academic and social skills were obtained to provide an external indication of a subject's level of Academic Competence, Social Competence, and Total Competence.

With respect to the variables which differentiate groups at risk, results indicated that children of psychotic parents could not be distinguished from controls on any of the measures given during early elementary school. By age 16, however, the children of manic-depressive parents were significantly lower in teacher-rated Social Competence and Total Competence than controls. Children of schizophrenic parents were not significantly different from controls at either phase of the study.

In examining the relationship between psychological test measures and teacher ratings, a consistent positive relationship was obtained between IQ and teacher ratings. Furthermore, the TAT assessment of Constructive Coping was moderately correlated with Academic Competence in early elementary school but not at age 16. Rorschach Genetic Level was not associated with teacher-rated competence at either phase of the study.

Results further indicated that IQ and teacher ratings of competence remained fairly stable over the long time period. However, Rorschach and TAT measures of competence did not remain stable.

Finally, with demographic variables such as age, socioeconomic status, and race held constant, the single best predictor of Academic Competence in high school was the teacher rating of Academic Competence in elementary school. Teacher-rated Total Competence in elementary school was the best predictor of both Social Competence and Total Competence at age 16.

Prediction of psychiatric treatment. In a doctoral dissertation at St. Louis University, Harold Altman (1980) investigated the concepts of Lidz's theory of schism and skew and attempted to determine their utility in predicting later psychiatric treatment in children of psychotic parents. The schism and skew measures used in his study were drawn from the Bene–Anthony Family Relations Test that were taken between 1967 and 1971, and these have been used to predict psychiatric treatment up to December, 1978. Through a very complicated process of weighting, the Bene–Anthony items and evaluating whole families to determine family patterns, Altman succeeded in producing a schism score and a skew score for each family, and these were used, together with measures of demographic and intelligence factors and a measure of personal psychopathology and teachers' ratings, to jointly and separately predict later psychiatric treatment. Psychiatric treatment included any counseling, out-patient psychotherapy, or in-patient treatment; and this measure was operationalized by giving a score of from 0 to 3 for each child's experience with psychiatric treatment. The three individual predictors of psychiatric treatment together accounted for 19% of the total variance in offspring treatment. Each of the predictors alone added significantly to the proportion of variance contributed by the two other measures, $p < .05$. The variance contributed by the skew factor was 3%. However families with as few as one out of three indicators of skew were three times as likely to have a child receive psychiatric treatment as were those families with no evidence of skew. Schism was not a significant predictor. The best single predictor of later psychiatric treatment was the diagnostic status of the parents, which alone accounted for 12% of the variance in psychiatric treatment.

Table 6. *Summary of Phase III Assessments of Offspring*

Assessment	Age cohorts							Notes	*N*
	7	10	13	16	19	22	≥25		
Diagnostic psychiatric assessments					19	22	≥25	$+$ A − a	267
								B − b	53
Clinical psychiatric assessments	7	10	13	16	19	22	≥25	B − a	53
School ratings	7	10	13	16				C − a	45
Parent ratings of offspring (RABI, speech sample)	7	10	13	16				C − a	43
Psychophysiological measures[a]									
Questionnaires									
MMPI				16				$+$ A − a	66
								C − a	177
General Information Questionnaire (GIQ)	7	10	13	16	19	22	≥25	A − b	267
Moos Family Environment Scale			13					A − a	21
Personal Reaction Inventory			13					A − a	21
Psychological battery WISC-R or WAIS, Rorschach, TAT, WRAT	7	10	13	16	19	22	≥25	C − a	80

Note: A = all offspring (estimated *N* = 267); B = Vulnerable Risk offspring (*N* = 53); C = offspring not previously assessed; a = one assessment; and b = yearly assessment.
[a]Funded by MH30682, Cynthia Janes, P.I.

PHASE III EVALUATION (1979–1982)

In December, 1979, the St. Louis Project received requested funding for a diagnostic follow-up of our research sample. In this phase, under the direction of Anthony and Worland, co-principal investigators, we are primarily interested in making a reliable psychiatric diagnosis for each of our project children. Thus, our major interest has switched from predictor measures to a criterion measure, although the diagnoses made between 1979 and 1983 will not be assumed to be our final outcome measure, as the modal age of the research sample in 1979 was only about 20 years old.

The entire assessment package for this third phase of our evaluation includes other evaluations than the diagnostic assessments. We continue to evaluate offspring during the month of their birthday every 3 years from 7 or 10 years on up. In general, our assessments are divided into those given to subjects up to 16 years of age and those given to offspring 16 years of age and over. The details of our Phase III assessment procedure are included in Table 6. The major responsibility for this assessment is under the direction of Janet Penniman.

Diagnostic psychiatric assessment

Determining reliable diagnoses for each of our risk offspring and of a representative sample of offspring at low risk to use as a comparison is our major current concern. To accomplish this we will use the Diagnostic Interview Schedule (DIS), which has several distinct advantages.

The DIS is a structured interview that enables nonphysician examiners to decide whether criteria have been met at any time in the individual's lifetime for each of the diagnoses for which a set of operational diagnostic criteria have been outlined by Feighner, Robins, Guze, Woodruff, Winokur, and Munoz (1972), as well as the Research Diagnostic criteria of Spitzer, Endicott, and Robins (1977), and the DSM-III (American Psychiatric Association, 1980) criteria. The interview has a number of important features: (1) each question is to be read by the examiner exactly as written; (2) probes to clarify respondents' answers are specified; (3) positive answers to questions serve as the criteria for diagnosis, without requiring judgment by the interviewer as to whether some underlying concept has or has not been described; (4) mental status items are included and methods of ascertaining them completely spelled out, so that they can be evaluated by lay interviewers; (5) diagnostic scoring is done by computer; and (6) age of onset is provided for each diagnosis.

Another important aspect of the interview is that no arbitrary hierarchical ranking of diagnoses is imposed. Thus, subjects can qualify for a diagnosis of both schizophrenia and depression. Diagnoses can be made by computer or scored by the interviewer. Because of the possibility of clerical error, we will have the diagnosis done by computer.

The DIS is given to each offspring in the project at least once during the triannual assessment period. In addition, yearly assessments will be given to all offspring who meet any of the following criteria and are thus considered to be in the Vulnerable Risk (HRHV) subgroup:

> Previously considered a "breakdown" case;
> Rated as high-risk/high-vulnerable during the initial Phase I assessment;
> Major impairment in life functioning either observed by General Information Questionnaire (see below) or by social worker or by any other project staff.

Thus the HRHV subgroup will be under more diagnostic scrutiny in order that we can define the stages of development of psychosis or, on the other hand, the healing process that leads them away from pathology and toward competence.

Clinical psychiatric assessment

Anthony proposed that each HRHV subgroup be scheduled to see a project psychiatrist during the course of Phase III. The assessment will allow the psychiatrist to use Bellack's *Manual for Rating Ego Functioning from a Clinical Interview* (Bellack, Hurvich, & Gediman, 1973).

This was most congenial to Anthony's frame of reference, and it also seemed to him that the items in the Ego-Function Scale were highly relevant to the detection of latent, incipient, developing, or developed psychosis. There were two further positives for the use of Bellack's scales: It had already been extensively used for schizophrenic subjects, and it could be applied to a battery of psychological tests.

Each of the functions (reality testing, judgment, sense of reality, regulation of drives, object relations, thought processes, adaptive regression, defensive functions, stimulus barrier, autonomous and synthetic functions, and mastery/competence) has a series of test questions related to it, some of which we anticipated would be especially valuable in Phase III of the research. The interview is not difficult to carry out and provides the profile for each child on the ordinal scales as well as overall ratings on a 13-point scale.

Academic ratings

The academic ratings collected during Phase II provided the project with a thorough assessment of the performance and behavior of offspring in school. Our goal will be to obtain at least one rating during Phase III for each offspring for whom we were unable to obtain at least one during Phase II. This will include all offspring 18 or under who are still in school, whether living within the St. Louis metropolitan area or now living elsewhere.

Psychophysiological measures

Reduction of funding level accompanied the grant awarded for 1976–1979. As a result, separate funding was sought and obtained for the psychophysiological phase of the project. With the generous aid of the William T. Grant Foundation, we were able to purchase a Beckman R-611 polygraph.

The design of the new study was dictated primarily by current work being done on electrodermal activity (EDA) of schizophrenics, as well as a less well-developed literature dealing with EDA and depression. Issues of current greatest interest are (1) Are schizophrenics hyperresponsive, hyporesponsive, both, or neither? (2) Are there left–right responsiveness differences related to psychopathology? (3) Does the recovery limb of the EDR of schizophrenics differ from that of normals? Does it seem to have anything to do with psychopathology? (4) What is the significance of fast and slow ED recovery? Does it have anything to do with stimulus significance?

We devised the following experimental design to address these issues: Every trial consists of presentation of a simple tone to one ear or the other. Between-trial intervals will be random lengths (8–15 seconds). The subject is told to release a foot pedal when a tone comes to either the left or right ear if and only if the previously heard tone was heard in the right ear. Thus each stimulus presentation will contain two pieces of information – (1) *Execute*: The subject should release the foot pedal now if this is a press trial; and (2) *Alert*: Whether or not the subject should press the foot pedal on the next trial.

Because each trial contains both execute and alert information, activation level will not be confounded with one of these types of information and should remain constant from tone to tone. This design allows for testing the main effects of alerting and executing as well as interactions between the two.

One of our primary goals is to identify differences in EDA as a function of parental and child psychopathology. We hypothesized (Janes & Stern, 1976) that some kinds of less healthy individuals may attach inappropriate signal significance to stimuli. Within the present paradigm we therefore expect to see smaller executing and alerting effects for these less healthy people than for more healthy individuals. If healthy individuals show a higher degree of differential responding (as measured by amplitude, frequency, and configuration) this parameter has potential as a laboratory-based indicator of mental status.

Questionnaires

A continuing major emphasis is being given to the General Information Questionnaire, our main source of routine data about the daily life of our sample. This is administered yearly to each offspring during Phase III to assess the *quality* of their lives, their degree of *participation* in activities, *friendship* patterns, *health,* and to determine the degree of perceived change in life events (Holmes & Rahe, 1967). Changes in life events are not only important in the increase they cause in illness susceptibility (Holmes & Masuda, 1973), but perceived change in events has also been linked to depression (Schless, Schwartz, Goetz, & Mendels, 1974). This questionnaire will be administered in the homes of offspring.

The Minnesota Multiphasic Personality Inventory (MMPI) was administered to all offspring 16 or older in Phase II, leaving approximately 66 offspring who will pass the 16-year-age gate during Phase III. Each of these offspring will complete the MMPI at that time, as will all offspring not assessed during Phase II for reasons other than age. Again, the MMPI will be completed by the offspring at home and will be picked up (and monitored if necessary) by a project worker. Similarly, the Moos Family Environment Scale, the Personal Reaction Inventory, Marital History, and Absences will be administered to all subjects who either pass the appropriate age gates for these assessments or were not tested in Phase II.

Psychological assessment

The psychological assessment during Phase II consisted of a wide range of clinical instruments including the WISC-R or WAIS, Rorschach, TAT, and WRAT. No additions to this battery are being considered for Phase III, and only those offspring that were not assessed during Phase II will be tested during Phase III. This Phase III assessment group will include hopefully about 150 offspring who were not tested during the previous period either because we were unable to motivate them to come into the center or because they now live outside the St. Louis area.

Triannual assessment schedule

We will continue in Phase III the use of the triannual system of scheduling reassessments. Offspring are scheduled during the months they celebrate their 13th, 16th, 19th, 22nd, etc., birthdays. The advantages of this procedure are:

1. A greater number of offspring at each age gate can be assured than by random testing or by testing on a family-by-family basis.

2. The age gates were selected to dovetail with those used by other risk research centers.

3. Randomized assessment across risk groups decreases the biases of assessors who might otherwise become aware of which risk groups were under scrutiny during different periods of the project.

Summary

The battery of assessments for Phase III is summarized in Table 6. The table lists assessments, the age cohorts of offspring who receive each, plus notes on the groups and assessment schedules specific to each type of testing.

8   Cognitive evaluation of children at risk: IQ, differentiation, and egocentricity

JULIEN WORLAND, ROSANNE EDENHART-PEPE,
DAVID G. WEEKS, AND PAULA M. KONEN

In a previous report (Worland & Hesselbrock, 1980) we reported that the IQs of the children of psychotic parents in the St. Louis Risk Research Project were not lower than those of children of physically ill or of normal parents. Our findings agreed with previous reports on the IQ scores of the children of schizophrenics (Cohler, Grunebaum, Weiss, Gamer, & Gallant, 1977; Rieder, Broman, & Rosenthal, 1977; Rutter, 1966) but not with those of Mednick and Schulsinger (1968) or Landau, Harth, Othnay, and Sharfhertz (1972); and our findings disagreed with the findings of previous reports on the IQ scores of children of psychotic depressed parents (Cohler et al., 1977).

The purpose of the present report was to present follow-up IQ data on the same sample of offspring in the St. Louis Project. In addition we have analyzed the findings from a group of other cognitive tasks and attempted to determine whether these tasks would yield differences between the offspring of psychotic and nonpsychotic parents. These cognitive tasks were measures of psychological differentiation and egocentrism.

DIFFERENTIATION

The concept of psychological *differentiation* is derived from an organismic view of developmental psychology and is stated specifically in the writings of Heinz Werner. The foundation of Werner's theory is the *orthogenetic* principle of development, which states that "wherever development occurs, it proceeds from a state of relative globality and lack of differentiation to a state of increasing differentiation, articulation, and hierarchic integration" (Werner, 1957, p. 126).

In Witkin's operationalization of Werner's assertions, he supports a dichotomization in differentiation of psychological functioning into two broad categories: (1) the degree of analysis and structuring of the world; and (2) the degree of analysis and structuring of the self (Witkin et al., 1962).

This research was funded by NIMH Grant MH-24819 and MH-12043, to E. J. Anthony, M.D., principal investigator, and Grant MH-50124 to Drs. Anthony and Worland. The authors would like to thank the staff of the Child Development Research Center, especially Harriet Lander and Susan Randich for psychological testing and Janice Hensiek for helping with preparation of the manuscript.

148

The first category concerns the manner in which "objects," that is, those things external to the self, are analyzed as separate elements from their context and structured into wholes. The tasks related to this category measure a variety of abilities, among which are the ability to dis-embed figure from background, the ability to exercise analytical problem solving in intellectual activities, and the ability to make fine discriminations among multiple alternatives or along a stimulus dimension, among others.

Witkin maintained that the "structuring tendencies" underlying both of these categories are manifestations of "an underlying process of development toward greater psychological complexity" (Witkin et al., 1962, p. 16). This assertion is repeatedly supported by evidence showing that differentiation, in the form of field independence, appears to increase with increasing age, until the age of about 17 years. In addition, longitudinal evidence indicates that individuals typically maintain their relative position on the field dependence–independence continuum with increasing age. This latter finding lends support to Witkin's notion that differentiation is also a dimension within which individuals display stylelike modes of perceiving that endure across situations and over time. Thus, differentiation is conceived not only as "an underlying process of development" but also within any given age as a dimension of cognitive style.

EGOCENTRISM

We defined *egocentrism* in accord with Piaget's definition: a state of thought and perception in which the individual sees the world through his or her own point of view without knowledge of the existence of other viewpoints, nor the knowledge that he or she is a prisoner of his or her own perspective.

As individuals become less egocentric, their ability to differentiate self from other, or subject from object, increases. In this way, Piaget's and Witkin's notions are quite similar. Both theorists subscribe to the belief that development is a gradual process composed of progressively structured interactions between the individual and the environment for the purpose of constructing a representation of experience and knowledge of the self and the world. However, unlike Piaget, Witkin postulated that various aspects of the child's relationship to the parent either fostered or inhibited differentiation. Many of the characteristics cited by Witkin, although not confirmed using their empirical method, concerned the degree to which a mother's concern for and sensitivity toward her child's needs promoted her/his autonomy, assertiveness, and sense of separate identity. Development in each of these areas would have the effect of enabling the child to perceive the self and the environment more objectively, to infer cause and predict outcome more accurately, and to choose selectively values and attitudes to be internalized.

HYPOTHESES ABOUT DIFFERENTIATION AND EGOCENTRISM

It was our belief that children raised by a psychotic parent would be subjected to a relatively disorganized, inconsistent environment that lacked the elements necessary to promote adequate development. One would, therefore, expect these children to be markedly less differentiated than children of similar age who had the advantage of healthy parent models and an environment that fostered psychological growth. Second, it was expected that the disordered, illogical thinking of a psychotic parent would prevent adequate social interaction and would, therefore, predispose children to maintain their egocentric mode of thought beyond its normal tenure.

Our specific hypotheses about differentiation and egocentrism were that, in both these areas, children of psychotic parents would show more disturbance than children of normals.

Previous work in the St. Louis Risk Research Project by Bruno Anthony (1978) had yielded some support for the presence of impoverished performance on the Affect Discrimination Test, interpretable as a test of empathy, in young children of schizophrenics compared with young children in a comparison group.

In terms of longitudinal predictions for *egocentrism,* there is considerable evidence to support the assertion that children with emotional disturbance, when compared with control groups of normal children, perform in a more egocentric fashion on a variety of Piagetian tasks (Anthony, 1966; Cowan, 1966; Goldschmidt, 1967; Lerner, Bie, & Lehrer, 1972; Neale, 1966; Pimm, 1972). We predicted, therefore, that those offspring at risk who have had psychiatric treatment would show retrospectively greater evidence of earlier egocentrism than offspring with no psychiatric treatment.

As to *differentiation,* our hypothesis is tempered somewhat because Witkin (Witkin et al., 1962; Witkin, 1965) has emphasized that pathology is equiprobable at either the very differentiated or the very undifferentiated ends of that continuum within any specific age sample. What will vary, he says, is the sophistication of the defenses and, therefore, the kind of disturbance manifested. It was our belief, however, given our age sample and the measure of disturbance we used, that only the more outstanding affect and cognitive disturbances will be apparent, and these affect disturbances will be associated with a relatively undifferentiated earlier level of functioning. Thus, we predicted that offspring at risk who have signs of emotional disturbance would have been less differentiated than children without such indicators, as determined by a retrospective study of their earlier tests.

METHOD

Subjects

The index parents were 13 male and 17 female schizophrenics, 7 male and 11 female manic-depressives, 9 male and 10 female physically ill parents, and 38 control couples. These parents represented 105 intact families with 339 offspring of whom 94 were children of a schizophrenic parent (CSZ), 53 were children of a manic-depressive parent (CMD), 73 were children of a physically ill parent (CPI), and 119 were children of two parents with no hospitalizations for psychiatric or prolonged physical illness (CN). Children ranged in age from 6 to 20 years when tested. When possible the data presented are from testings of all offspring between the stated ages. Demographic features of the children and families are summarized in Table 2 of the St. Louis Project's Progress Report.

Families with a psychotic parent were asked to volunteer to participate in this study during or just after the hospitalization of the ill parent. Families with a physically ill parent were asked to participate during or just after one parent's hospitalization for a chronic or acute physical health reason, usually tuberculosis. Parents with any psychiatric history were excluded from participation in this group. Normal families were recruited through their children who attended schools located near the site of the project. Families with positive psychiatric histories or prolonged physical illness were excluded from the normal group. Each family was paid $25 for participation.

A DSM-II diagnosis of each psychiatrically ill parent was made by a project psychiatrist after interviews with the patient, the patient's spouse and children, and after a review of the hospital chart. There was diagnostic agreement between the project psychiatrist and the hospital diagnosis (i.e., schizophrenia vs. manic-depressive illness) in 43 of 48 cases ($\kappa = .79$; J. A. Cohen, 1960). There was total agreement for the diagnosis of manic-depressive parents. In 5 of 30 schizophrenic parents, the hospital diagnosis was manic-depressive illness. These five subjects were considered schizophrenic for these analyses.

Characteristics of the psychiatrically ill parents are presented in Table 1 of the progress report. The number of hospitalizations and number of days parents were hospitalized were determined from admission and discharge notes obtained from hospitals. Schizophrenic and manic-depressive parents were compared in terms of the number of admissions each had had before testing and again for all admissions up to 1978 (on the average 6 years since testing). No differences were found. Because of high variance in the number of days hospitalized, group differences were examined on log-transformed data. No differences were found between schizophrenic and manic-depressive parents in terms of total days hospitalized either before testing or during their lifetimes.

Diagnostic subtypes of the schizophrenic parents were paranoid (11), schizoaffective (11), catatonic (3), chronic undifferentiated (1), acute reaction (1), hebephrenic (1), and unknown (2). In parents with manic-depressive illness, there were 10 with only depressive episodes (who will be referred to as unipolars) and 8 with manic or with both manic and depressive episodes (referred to as bipolars). There were no reliability checks available for these subtype diagnoses.

Testing

The intelligence tests were administered between 1967 and 1972 and again between 1975 and 1978. The tests used were the Wechsler Preschool and Primary Scale of Intelligence (WPPSI; Wechsler, 1967) and the Wechsler Intelligence Scale for Children (WISC; Wechsler, 1949) at the first assessment and the Wechsler Intelligence Scale for Children–Revised (WISC-R; Wechsler, 1974) and the Wechsler Adult Intelligence Scale (WAIS; Wechsler, 1955) at the second assessment, according to the age of the child.

Tests of differentiation and egocentricity were administered between 1967 and 1972. The Children's Embedded Figures Test (CEFT; Karp & Konstadt, 1963) was used as our measure of differentiation. On this test a child is required to search through increasingly complex pictures in order to locate a previously designated figure (tent or house). The data analyzed were the numbers of correctly located figures.

The Three Mountains Test (TMT; Piaget & Inhelder, 1956) was the test we selected for a measure of egocentricity. This test is presented on a 5 cm × 5 cm board that contains three clearly distinguishable papier-mâché mountains. The child is asked (1) to identify a photograph that matches the view that two toy photographers would have in each of four positions; (2) to select a picture and then place the photographer in the appropriate position; and finally (3) using a smaller set of model mountains, to reconstruct the view seen by the photographer in each of four positions. The data analyzed were the number of correct responses in all three conditions combined.

RESULTS

Group differences in tests of intelligence

Sample and design of the analyses. The main analysis reported here is based on the two testings of 137 individuals, once between 1967–1972 (Phase I) and once between 1975–1978 (Phase II). Of these individuals, 35 were the offspring of one schizophrenic parent, 23 were the offspring of one manic-depressive parent, 22 were the offspring of one physically ill parent, and 57 were the offspring of two control parents. Actually, 176 children received both Phase I and Phase II testing. However, children less than 72 months old at Phase I were dropped from cross-sectional analyses because apparently only brighter young children were tested. Young children who exhibited distracted, inattentive behavior during the earlier testing were not required to complete the test battery, resulting in a biased sample. No attempts to test children less than 72 months of age were made during the Phase II testing period. Data from all 176 children were used for the predictive analyses reported below.

In addition, data were available from the assessments of 134 children tested only during Phase I of this project, and other data were available from an additional 96 children who were tested only during Phase II of the project.

Because of significant SES correlations with our intelligence measures, and because there were significant group differences in SES, this variable and age were covaried out of all the analyses.

The main analysis presented here is a repeated measures analysis of covariance for those subjects tested at both Phase I and Phase II. We have used the data available for those subjects tested only at Phase I or at Phase II to determine the representativeness of those subjects who were tested twice, and have used age at Phase I and age at Phase II as covariates. Persistent race effects for all analyses are not reported.

Table 1. *Means and standard deviations for IQ measures at Phase I and Phase II by group*

Group	Verbal IQ		Performance IQ		Full-Scale IQ	
	I	II	I	II	I	II
CSZ	106.41	94.69	107.91	95.80	107.04	96.59
	(12.12)	(9.27)	(12.05)	(9.25)	(11.56)	(9.10)
CMD	102.72	92.23	106.76	93.73	104.30	94.21
	(16.16)	(13.29)	(16.47)	(13.92)	(16.93)	(14.62)
CPI	108.11	97.52	108.58	97.48	108.22	98.35
	(14.16)	(14.62)	(15.79)	(13.90)	(15.34)	(13.67)
CN	112.12	105.65	113.37	105.25	113.12	105.88
	(12.24)	(15.12)	(12.11)	(14.61)	(11.97)	(13.27)

Note: CSZ = children of schizophrenic parents; CMD = children of psychiatric controls; CPI = children of physical illness controls; CN = children of normal controls.

In order to determine whether those subjects tested *both* at Phase I and Phase II were representative of *all* the available subjects tested, one preliminary analysis contrasted the subjects who were tested only at Phase I with those tested at both Phase I and Phase II. A second preliminary analysis contrasted those tested only at Phase II with those tested both at Phase I and Phase II. When these subjects were contrasted, there were no significant differences between these groups for Verbal IQ, Performance IQ, or for Full-Scale IQ. Consequently, we concluded that those offspring who were tested twice were a representative sample of the available pool of subjects.

Findings. The repeated measures analysis of covariance for Verbal IQ yielded a significant group effect, $F(3, 127) = 3.64$, $p < .02$; a moderate but nonsignificant time effect, $F(1, 128) = 3.38$, $p < .07$; and a significant time-by-race interaction effect, $F(1, 128) = 4.24$, $p < .05$. Children of schizophrenics and children of manic-depressive parents did not differ significantly from one another but both had significantly ($p < .05$) lower VIQ scores than the offspring of normals. The time effect was due to marginally lower VIQ scores at Phase II than at Phase I. The significant time-by-race interaction effect was due to a 11.19 point drop for blacks from Phase I to Phase II versus a 7.40 point drop for whites.

For Performance IQ there were no significant effects, other than the race effect. However, for Full-Scale IQ there was a significant group effect, $F(3, 126) = 2.67$, $p < .05$. Again children of control parents had higher FSIQ scores than children of schizophrenics ($p < .05$) or children of manic-depressive parents ($p < .01$). The other main effects and their interactions were not significant for FSIQ.

The data for the repeated measures analyses are presented in Table 1, where it can be seen that offspring in all four groups had slightly lower IQ scores at the second testing than at the first testing.

In our earlier report (Worland & Hesselbrock, 1980) we had discovered that children of ill mothers, despite the mothers' diagnoses, had lower IQ scores than children of ill fathers. However, when we tested those offspring at Phase II, we did not find a significant sex of ill parent effect for VIQ, F (1, 127) < 1; for PIQ, F (1, 127) = 2.44, p > .10; or for FSIQ, F (1, 127) < 1; although children of ill mothers still had PIQ and FSIQ scores 2 or 3 points lower than children of ill fathers.

Longitudinal prediction of phase II IQ

Design of analysis. In an effort to develop a predictive model of Phase II intelligence, we have used 94 variables that included 13 original variables: race, sex, sex of ill parent, age, father's IQ, mother's IQ, socioeconomic status (SES) at Phase I, IQ at Phase I, age at Phase II, SES at Phase II, and three variables representing diagnostic status. The three diagnostic variables were parental schizophrenia (CSZ), parental manic-depressive illness (CMD), and parental physical illness (CPI). Another 75 variables were created to represent all possible two-way interactions among the 13 original variables. In addition, six three-way interaction variables of a piori interest were calculated: sex-by-sex of ill parent by each of: -CSZ, -PI, -MD, -father's IQ, and -mother's IQ; and SES at Phase I-by-SES at Phase II-by-sex of ill parent.

In order to reduce the number of variables to a manageable size, only those two-way interaction variables that correlated significantly (p < .005) with IQ at Phase II were retained. This left a pool of 41 variables, the 13 original variables, 22 two-way interactions, and the 6 three-way interactions.

The 41 variables defined above were used as potential predictors of IQ at Phase II in a stepwise multiple regression analysis. For purposes of this analysis only 176 subjects with complete data on all variables were used. Five predictors were selected which contributed a significant (α = .05) proportion of variance over and above previously entered predictors.

Findings. The predictors in order of their entry into the equation are listed in Table 2. Not surprisingly, IQ at Phase I is the best predictor of IQ at Phase II, accounting for most of the predictable variance. That father's IQ is a significant predictor after the child's IQ implies that father's IQ continued to exert an influence on the IQ of the child during the testing interval. It should be noted that mother's Phase I IQ is somewhat more highly correlated with IQ at Phase II than is father's Phase I IQ (.67 vs. .62). But being more highly correlated with the child's IQ at Phase I also, mother's IQ would add less over this first predictor. In addition, what mother's IQ does not share with her child's IQ, it does share with father's IQ; thus mother's IQ does not become a predictor later on.

The third predictor, the CSZ-by-IQ at Phase I interaction, is negatively related to the criterion (note the sign of β in Table 2). However, the raw correlation between this variable and IQ at Phase II is positive (.24). This phenomenon is best understood by considering the stability of IQ within diagnostic group. The cor-

Table 2. *Prediction of IQ at Phase II*

Variable	Cumulative R^2	R^2 Added	β
IQ at Phase I	.679	.679	.759
Father's IQ	.710	.031	.225
CSZ by IQ at Phase I	.744	.034	−.214
Race by age	.754	.009	.106
MD by sex by sex of ill parent	.760	.007	−.082

relations between IQ at Phase I and Phase II are .59 for the schizophrenic group, .87 for the physically ill group, .87 for the manic-depressive group, and .83 for the control group. There is a positive relation between IQ at Phase I and Phase II in the schizophrenic group, which accounts for the positive raw correlation between the interaction variable and IQ at Phase II. However, the temporal stability of IQ is much higher in the other three groups. Thus when combining all four groups, IQ at Phase I will carry more weight for the schizophrenic group. Consider the child of a schizophrenic with a high IQ at Phase I. By the modest correlation (.59) for this group, we would predict only a moderately high IQ for Phase II. But the heavy weight on Phase I IQ in the prediction equation (for all groups) would inflate the prediction of the Phase II IQ for this child. The negative weight on the interaction variable brings the prediction down to a more conservative level.

The last two predictors each add less than 1% of variance. It may be well not to take them too seriously until and unless they are found to be predictors in an independent replication. Briefly, we can note the nature of these effects, if they are reliable. The race-by-age effect is such that the difference in Phase II IQ between black and white children is slightly less for older than for younger children. The sex-by-sex of ill parent-by-MD interaction indicates that children the same sex as the manic-depressive parent fare less well (in terms of decrease in IQ) than their opposite-sex siblings. (This effect also holds for children of schizophrenics, but not quite as strongly.)

Tests of differentiation and egocentricity

Sample and design of analyses. Our initial task was to investigate the hypothesis that individuals raised by a psychotic parent and presumably in a more pathogenic environment would be less differentiated and more egocentric than individuals raised in a more normal environment. We felt it appropriate to examine this hypothesis within our entire available sample, which comprised 40 CSZ, 28 CMD, 35 CPI, and 67 CN. We treated parental diagnosis as one independent variable and age (blocked into three levels: 6–7, 8–9, 10–11 years) as a second. We treated SES and age as covariates.

Findings. The analysis yielded highly significant effects for age on the CEFT, F (2, 159) = 38.98, $p < .0005$, and the TMT, F (2, 156) = 29.53, $p < .0005$. However we did not find any significant differences between offspring of parents in the different diagnostic groups on either the CEFT, F (3, 159) = .25 or on the TMT, F (3, 156) = .63.

We then attempted to improve the focus of our investigation by using smaller groups based on a more homogeneous parental psychopathology grouping to contrast with the controls. Using hospital admission notes for the parents' index admission, we formed two discrete groups: children of a psychotic parent with Schneiderian first-rank symptoms (Taylor, 1972), and children of schizophrenic parents without Schneiderian symptoms. Interrater reliability for the Schneiderian diagnosis (made by Loretta Cass and Judith Schechtman) was $\kappa = .74$. To children of parents in these two groups we added children of nonpsychotic parents to form the three levels of the independent variable for the following series of one-way ANCOVAs, which treated SES and age as covariates.

The dependent measures for these analyses were scores for the TMT, CEFT, and a score called *differentiation.* This later score was created in order to approximate closely Witkin's concept of differentiation, since we did not have available exactly the same items that Witkin had used. We extracted this score from test scores residualized for SES and age from the CEFT; the Affect Discrimination Test (B. Anthony, 1978a; Clack, 1970); WISC Block Design, Picture Completion, Object Assembly; Rorschach Genetic Level (P. M. Lerner, 1975); and TAT Coping (Worland, Lander, & Hesselbrock, 1979).

The reasons for choosing these variables were established from the Witkin et al. (1962) derivation of their differentiation variable. WISC Block Design, Picture Completion, and Object Assembly are all highly correlated with an Analytic–Global Field Approach factor that Witkin extracted from various tests measuring field dependence–independence. The CEFT is the children's form of Witkin's Embedded Figures Test, one of the three measures comprising the same factor. Witkin showed that the ability to make multiple discriminations along a continuum was related to his concept of differentiation. The Affect Discrimination Test (Clack, 1970) taps the child's ability to make multiple discriminations between photographs of various facial expressions, and thus was included in our Differentiation score. The ability to impose structure on a relatively disorganized field has been shown to relate to differentiation, and for this reason the Rorschach Genetic Level (P. M. Lerner, 1975) was included. TAT Coping scores were used in an attempt to measure the directedness with which instrumental activity is applied to ambiguous situations, similar to Witkin's TAT *directedness of activity* concept. All of these variables were combined, using weights obtained when they were subjected to a principal components analysis that yielded a one-factor solution.

Results from these three one-way ANCOVAs showed no significant differences between children of a psychotic parent with Schneiderian symptoms, children of a schizophrenic parent without Schneiderian symptoms, and children of controls on the CEFT, $F (2, 101) = .64$, the TMT, $F (2, 101) = 2.28$, or on the Differentiation factor, $F (2, 92) = 1.82$.

Longitudinal analyses. We further hypothesized that children who had developed emotional disturbance requiring psychotherapy would have been, as children, significantly more egocentric and less differentiated than children without such subsequent disturbance. To test this assertion, we assigned each subject a score of 0 if they had never received any psychiatric treatment or counseling, 1 if they had received outpatient psychotherapy, 2 if they had had a psychiatric hospitalization, or 3 if they had received both in-patient and out-patient psychiatric treatment (Altman, 1980). Our anticipated significant negative correlation between this index of treatment and the measures of differentiation and egocentricity was not realized. The correlations ranged from .002 to .02, and given our N of 187, none of them reached significance.

DISCUSSION

The conclusion that children of schizophrenic and manic-depressive parents have lower IQ scores than children of physically ill or control parents finds some support in these analyses. However, a later analysis of these data with additional subjects and deleting offspring of parents who did not meet DSM-III (American Psychiatric Association, 1980) criteria for psychotic diagnoses failed to substantiate the finding that children of psychotic parents have lower scores on IQ tests than children of nonpsychotic parents. However, the sex of the psychotic parent is an important mediating variable (Worland, Weeks, Weiner, & Schechtman, 1982). When we had tested such children at an average age of 9 years (between 1967–1972), we did not find any significant effect for parental diagnosis. However, in the current investigation we did find such an effect when we tested a sample at an average age of 16 years, 59% of whom had been tested before but 41% of whom were siblings of previously tested individuals. The major contribution to this finding was not from the new siblings' scores but from the scores of those children tested twice.

In view of the difference in age between the earlier tested and the recently tested groups, it is tempting to say that the effect of parental psychosis on measures of intelligence only appears after the passage of years. However, Cohler, Grunebaum, Weiss, Gamer, and Gallant (1977) found lower IQ scores in the offspring of psychotic depressed mothers at less than 6 years of age.

Another possibility is that, with a 50% attrition of cases from Phase I to Phase II, the parental diagnostic subtypes could have been represented with different frequencies at the Phase II testing when compared with the Phase I testing. The breakdown, however, indicated that this was not the case, with approximately 45% of the children of schizophrenics coming from a paranoid parent, 34% from a schizoaffective parent, 13% from a catatonic parent, and about 8% unknown, at both the Phase I and Phase II assessment. Similarly, the percentage of offspring coming from unipolar as opposed to bipolar depressed parents was approximately equal at both assessment periods, with the ratio about two offspring of unipolar to three offspring of bipolars.

It should be mentioned in connection with the observed lower IQ scores in children of schizophrenic and manic-depressive parents that two other risk projects are finding that offspring of schizophrenic patients have lower IQs than the offspring of matched controls. Watt, Grubb, and Erlenmeyer-Kimling (Chapter 13, this volume) found lower IQ in the offspring of one schizophrenic parent compared with the offspring of parents selected to control for socioeconomic status. Their findings – as well as those of Weintraub and Neale (Chapter 17, this volume) plus those reported by Mednick and Schulsinger (1968) and those reported in the present chapter – provide evidence that parental schizophrenia is associated with slightly diminished offspring IQ.

The data presented on the prediction of intelligence are consistent with the issues raised above. The IQ of children of schizophrenics is lower at Phase II than would be estimated on the basis of the relationship between the Phase I and Phase II scores of the offspring of nonschizophrenic parents. Why this is not also true for the offspring of manic-depressive parents is not clear. In any case it appears that, with increasing age, the offspring of schizophrenics being followed in St. Louis are losing ground in IQ when compared with our other groups.

One possible explanation of their lower than expected IQ scores is that there might be a subgroup within the children of schizophrenics who are substantially lower in IQ at Phase II than would be expected, thus reducing the mean of the entire group. This would be supported by the lower Phase I/Phase II correlation coefficient for children of schizophrenics than for other children, but a scatterplot of the Phase I and Phase II IQ scores shows no such discernible pattern. The group mean for Phase II IQ in those children of schizophrenics tested twice is lower than anticipated, and there is more shifting of ordinal position within that group than within the other groups.

As with Phase I IQ, significant differences between diagnostic groups were not obtained for our other cognitive measures that were taken at the same time. Thus we found no support for the initial hypothesis that children of a psychotic parent are less differentiated and more spatially egocentric than children of controls (between 6 and 11 years of age). Moreover, within the offspring of psychotic parents, severity of parental disturbance, indexed by Schneiderian first-rank symptoms, did not appear to influence the children's degree of egocentrism or differentiation. With respect to egocentrism, this finding is contrary to that of Struass, Harder, and Chandler (1979) who reported significant differences in spatial egocentrism scores between groups formed on the basis of this parental dimension. Differences between the sampling procedures and measures used might account for this discrepancy, however.

Our method of determining the presence of Schneiderian symptoms was based on material contained in the sometimes vague and incomplete hospital admission notes. The Schneiderian determination of Strauss et al. appears to have been based on more concrete information. Our measure of egocentrism was one used by Piaget and it correlated highly with age ($r = .48$) and Full-Scale IQ ($r = .49$).

The measure used by Strauss et al. was derived from Flavell et al. (1968), and when used by Strauss et al. correlated neither with age nor IQ, although Flavell had reported a significant relationship between his measure and both grade level and IQ. Such relationships would be expected of a measure of egocentricity, since it is a developmental phenomenon. Our conclusion is that Strauss et al. had available a better measure of Schneiderian symptoms, but that their measure of egocentrism seems problematic.

Although it has been shown that children with emotional disturbance are, concomitantly, more egocentric than nondisturbed controls (Neale, 1966; Simeonsson, 1973), to our knowledge no one has demonstrated whether there are cognitive antecedents to such disturbance. We investigated the possibility that children manifesting various degrees of emotional disturbance would show, retrospectively, a prior high degree of egocentrism and less differentiation than children without such disturbance. Our results indicated that emotional disturbance manifested up to 10 years later could not be predicted by earlier levels of egocentricity or differentiation.

Our conclusion concerning these results has been forestalled until such time as we have completed the analysis of our entire battery of cognitive tests. To date, we believe that our inability to locate significant differences in egocentricity and differentiation between children of our diagnostic groups is a product of at least two causes. First, egocentricity and differentiation are global concepts, operationalized by tests that tap a variety of subskills, such as resistance to distraction, persistence, and figure–ground reversal. Had we chosen tests that measured very specific skills, we might have improved the likelihood of discovering group differences. Second, differentiation and egocentricity both develop at greatly different rates from one child to another, implying that normal and deviant groups of young children will have overlapping distributions of scores, especially on global tests like the ones we used.

In conclusion, the following points merit consideration: (1) Compared with preadolescent children of nonpsychotics, in the St. Louis sample, preadolescents of psychotic prarents are not noticeably impaired in either cognitive or intellectual development; (2) In adolescence, children of one psychotic parent have lower IQ scores than children of nonpsychotic parents; (3) Children of a schizophrenic parent seem most vulnerable to loss in IQ over the passage of time; and (4) Compared with children who have apparently healthy development, psychiatrically treated children had not been more egocentric or less differentiated earlier in childhood.

Our conclusions on the IQ score analyses should be considered tentative until we have completed these analyses on our full retested sample.

9 Interrelationships among possible predictors of schizophrenia

CYNTHIA L. JANES, JULIEN WORLAND,
DAVID G. WEEKS, AND PAULA M. KONEN

A consistent finding in retrospective studies of childhood antecedents to schizophrenia is that the school behavior of preschizophrenics, particularly as reflected in teachers' ratings, differs from that of children who do not eventually become schizophrenic (Watt, 1972, 1978; Watt & Lubensky, 1976). Especially in the area of social competence, preschizophrenics have been rated lower than children who do not develop schizophrenia (Roff, Knight, & Wertheim, 1976; Watt, 1978).

In addition to reduced competence in school, factors that may increase a child's risk for developing schizophrenia in adulthood include parental schizophrenia, low intelligence, and electrodermal hyperactivity (Kety, Rosenthal, Wender, and Schulsinger, 1971; Lane & Albee, 1964; Mednick & Schulsinger, 1968).

Previous reports from the St. Louis Risk Research Project and others have provided equivocal evidence of interrelationships among these factors. For example, Worland et al. (1982) reported that the IQs of children of schizophrenic mothers are lower than those of children of non-ill parents. Janes, Hesselbrock, and Stern (1978) found no relationship between parental schizophrenia and childhood electrodermal activity, although others have reported a weak relationship (Prentky, Salzman, & Klein, 1981; Van Dyke, Rosenthal, & Rasmussen, 1974; Salzman & Klein, 1978).

If parental schizophrenia, low intelligence, electrodermal hyperactivity, and incompetence in school are risk factors for schizophrenia, it is reasonable to hypothesize that psychiatric diagnosis of parents, intelligence, and electrodermal activity in children are associated with subsequent school behavior. Competence in school may be useful not only as a predictor of schizophrenia, but also as a significant intermediate outcome, measurable before the onset of schizophrenia. The purpose of the parent study was to determine to what extent factors identified in previous research as related to schizophrenia are associated with each other. This study focuses on the degree to which risk factors assessed prior to adolescence (parental schizophrenia, low intelligence, and electrodermal hyperactivity) are associated with school competence of adolescents.

160

METHOD

Subjects

Subjects were all the offspring of schizophrenics ($N = 25$) and offspring of non-ill parents ($N = 50$) for whom we had complete data in childhood electrodermal activity and Full-Scale WISC IQ, and teacher-rated classroom behavior in adolescence. Diagnostic details for parents may be found in the St. Louis Progress Report (Chapter 7, this volume). Demographic information is presented in Table 1.

This sample did not differ from subjects with partial data nor did the offspring of schizophrenics differ from offspring of non-ill parents on sex, age at childhood testing, or age at adolescent testing. They did differ from one another with respect to race, χ^2 (1) = 4.15, $p < .05$, and SES, χ^2 (1) = 15.98, $p < .001$, with more offspring of schizophrenics black and from lower social classes than offspring of non-ill parents.

Electrodermal activity

The electrodermal data used in these analyses were six measures, each one the primary marker variable of each of six factors obtained in a previously reported factor analytic study (Janes, Hesselbrock, & Stern, 1978). These included five factors of electrodermal activity and an index of movement (subjects had been instructed not to move). We recorded skin-potential activity from left and right hands during a habituation series of 10 puffs of cool air to the dorsal side of the right wrist, and a conditioning series of 20 puffs of cool air paired with warm air. Procedural details are given in our Progress Report (Chapter 7, this volume).

Movement index

The movement index was a measure of the child's inability to keep fingers still during the 45-minute psychophysiological procedure. It was derived from finger movement artifact on the psychophysiological record. A high score indicated that finger movement occurred during a large portion of the record. Each child was instructed to keep fingers still.

Teachers' ratings

Two behavior assessment forms were completed by junior high school and high school teachers. The Pupil Rating Form (PRF; Watt, Grubb, & Erlenmeyer-Kimling, Chapter 13, this volume), developed specifically for evaluating behaviors relevant to the development of schizophrenia, is a 28-item Likert-Scale rating sheet on which teachers indicate the degree to which a child's behavior fits a given descriptor. For analysis, these 28 descriptors were grouped into four factors, labeled Scholastic Motivation, Extraversion, Harmony, and Emotional Stability.

Table 1. *Demographic features of the sample*

Offspring of	N	Race		Sex		SES		Childhood assessment (age)		Adolescent assessment (age)	
		Black	White	Male	Female	Lower	Middle	Mean	SD	Mean	SD
Schizophrenics	25	12	13	14	11	13	12	8.2	1.8	16.5	2.4
Nonschizophrenics	50	11	39	33	17	4	46	7.8	1.7	15.2	2.0

The Hahnemann High School Behavior Rating Scale (HHSB; Spivack & Swift, 1971) contains 45 phrases describing specific behaviors at school. The 45 items comprise 13 scales, which were further reduced to two scales for the purpose of the present study. These are labeled Personal and Social Competence, and Academic Competence. The first included the following HHSB factors: rapport with teacher, general anxiety, quiet–withdrawn, dogmatic–inflexible, verbal negativism, and disturbance–restless. Academic competence included reasoning ability, originality, verbal interaction, anxious producer, poor work habits, lacks intellectual independence, and expressed inability. As adolescents, all offspring had several teachers. Up to four teachers for each child completed the PRF and HHSB. To ensure teachers' familiarity with students, it was required that each teacher have the student for at least 4 hours per week in a major subject. The average number of teachers' assessments per offspring was 3.7.

RESULTS

Simple correlations

We computed correlations between childhood demographic and psychophysiological variables and teacher-rated adolescent behavioral factors from the PRF and HHSB. These correlations are presented in Table 2. The positive correlations for sex indicate that as compared with boys, girls were seen as more academically inclined, and more personally and socially competent. Neither race nor socioeconomic status correlated significantly with teachers' ratings. With respect to parental psychiatric status, children with a schizophrenic parent scored lower on Personal and Social Competence, Scholastic Motivation, and Emotional Stability than children of nonpatients. The WISC IQ was associated with Academic Competence and Scholastic Motivation.

With regard to psychophysiological factors, nontrivial correlations were found for electrodermal nonspecific responding (i.e., electrodermal activity other than that occurring in response to stimuli presented) and the movement index. Electrodermal nonspecific responding was significantly associated with Emotional Stability. The movement index was significantly associated with Academic Competence, Personal and Social Competence, Scholastic Motivation, and Emotional Stability. Relatively high levels of electrodermal nonspecific responding and hyperactivity were associated with lower scores on Emotional Stability, Academic Competence, Personal and Social Competence, and Scholastic Motivation.

Partial correlations

Could associations between parental schizophrenia and teachers' ratings of adolescents be accounted for by IQ or psychophysiological responding? The presence of significant correlation of intelligence and psychophysiological activity with teachers' ratings raised that possibility. Consequently, we performed a series of partial correlations between parental diagnosis and school factors in which either

Table 2. *Childhood variables versus teacher ratings of adolescents: simple correlations (Pearson r)*

	HHSB			PRF		
Childhood variables	Academic Competence	Personal and Social Competence	Scholastic Motivation	Emotional Stability	Harmony	Extraversion
Sex	.23*	.20*	.25*	.01	.26*	.03
Race	-.05	.01	-.09	-.03	.04	.09
Socioeconomic status	-.04	.05	-.04	-.04	.07	-.05
Parental diagnosis	.10	.19*	.20*	.29**	.10	.02
WISC FSIQ	.31**	.17	.26*	.15	.11	.12
Electrodermal nonspecific responding	-.08	-.17	-.18	-.20*	-.19	.00
Movement index	-.21*	-.23*	-.19*	-.29**	.02	.02

*p < .05. **p < .01.

WISC IQ, electrodermal nonspecific responding, or the movement index was held constant.

The significant association between parental diagnosis and the teachers' rating of Scholastic Motivation, to which IQ was also significantly related, failed to remain significant when IQ was held constant, r (73) = .09. A similar control for nonspecific responding did not eliminate the significant relationship between parental schizophrenia and Emotional Stability, r (73) = .24, p < .05.

As can be seen in Table 2, the movement index was significantly associated with the same three school factors correlating with parental diagnosis. What happened to the latter relationships when the movement index was partialed out? Interestingly, with the movement index held constant, the correlation between parental diagnosis and Personal and Social Competence became nonsignificant, r (73) = .16, as did that with Scholastic Motivation, r (73) = .18; whereas the correlation of parental diagnosis with offspring Emotional Stability remained significant, r (73) = .22, p < .05.

Could IQ data or psychophysiological responding increase our ability to predict teachers' ratings of adolescents over and above the prediction we could make from parental diagnosis alone? This question was approached by partialing out parental diagnosis in cases in which we had found that both parental diagnosis and either IQ, nonspecific responding, or the movement index were significantly related to a given school-behavior factor. If the association of IQ, nonspecific responding, or movement with the teachers' ratings remained significant when parental diagnosis was partialed out, this would imply that the additional variable improved our ability to predict the teachers' ratings over and above our prediction from parental diagnosis alone. When we used this procedure, we found that the relationships that remained significant were those between IQ and Scholastic Motivation, r (73) = .19, p < .05; nonspecific responding and Emotional Stability, r (73) = −.20, p < .05; the movement index and Emotional Stability, r (73) = −.26, p < .01; and between the movement index and Personal/Social Competence, r (73) = −.21, p < .05. However, the correlation of the movement index and Scholastic Motivation with parental diagnosis partialed out was nonsignificant, r (73) = −.17.

DISCUSSION

We found some evidence for an association between parental psychiatric status and both teacher-rating instruments. Personal and Social Competence from the HHSB, and Scholastic Motivation and Emotional Stability from the PRF all were significantly related to parental psychiatric status. Adolescent offspring of schizophrenics tended to score lower than offspring of normals on these factors. These associations replicate retrospective reports of preschizophrenics' teacher-rated classroom behavior (Watt, 1972, 1978; Watt & Lubensky, 1976), as well as previous reports of teacher-rated behavior in offspring of schizophrenics (Weintraub, Neale, & Liebert, 1975), in which children at risk for schizophrenia were viewed by teachers as lacking emotional maturity and stability.

Each of the three factors associated with parental psychiatric status was also associated with the psychophysiological movement index. In addition, Scholastic Motivation was associated with WISC IQ, a not unexpected finding, whereas Emotional Stability was related to electrodermal nonspecific responding. Further analysis of these relationships by means of partial correlations showed that psychophysiological variables and IQ sometimes accounted for, and may have mediated the relationships between, parental diagnosis and teacher-rated behavior. Parental psychiatric status did not add significantly to associations of the movement index or IQ with HHSB Personal and Social Competence and PRF Scholastic Motivation. For Emotional Stability, however, a significant additional contribution was made by parental diagnosis over and above associations with the movement index and electrodermal nonspecific responding. Thus, knowledge of parental psychiatric status aided a prediction of Emotional Stability scores from psychophysiological data alone.

Conversely, we found also that the movement index and electrodermal nonspecific responding increased our ability to predict Emotional Stability scores beyond our predictions from parental psychiatric status alone. Furthermore, predictions on the basis of parental diagnosis were improved by considering IQ in predicting Scholastic Motivation scores and by the movement index in predicting Personal and Social Competence scores.

It is not yet possible to make statements about the correspondence of these teacher-rated traits and adulthood schizophrenia, since this population is just now approaching the age of maximum risk. The most reasonable implication, based upon previous research and the present results, is that parental schizophrenia, low IQ, and extraneous activity both electrodermally and in hand movement, are probably all related to the likelihood of eventually becoming schizophrenic.

PART IV

The New York High-Risk Project: 1971—1982

By 1971 the high-risk method was generally accepted as a viable approach to research in schizophrenia, and the National Institute of Mental Health placed a priority on it for research funding. Almost simultaneously, the projects in New York, Minneapolis, and Stony Brook were initiated, and the following year the URCAFS project began in Rochester.

The director of the New York High-Risk Project, Nikki Erlenmeyer-Kimling, is a behavior geneticist who worked with Franz Kallmann at the New York State Psychiatric Institute. At its inception the project replicated some features of the Danish project, but with more explicit focus on studying attention and information processing and interactions between genetic and environmental factors in the etiology of schizophrenia. As it developed Erlenmeyer-Kimling broadened the scope of the study, enlisting consultative collaborations with Clarice Kestenbaum for clinical psychiatric examinations, Herbert Vaughan for psychophysiological measurements, Norman Watt for behavioral evaluations at school, and Irving Gottesman for Minnesota Multiphasic Personality Inventory (MMPI) assessments.

The vast population of the New York area yielded large samples for research, even including a unique sample of "dual mated" children at risk, that is, offspring with two schizophrenic biological parents. Part IV comprises five chapters from this project, starting with a comprehensive progress summary, followed by more focused reports of the psychophysiological studies, attentional studies, analyses of school behavior, and clinical assessments of research subjects with early psychological difficulties as adolescents.

10 *The New York High-Risk Project*

L. ERLENMEYER-KIMLING, YVONNE MARCUSE,
BARBARA CORNBLATT, DAVID FRIEDMAN,
JOHN D. RAINER, AND JACQUES RUTSCHMANN

THEORETICAL ORIENTATION

The several high-risk studies of schizophrenia represented at the San Juan plenary conference share certain common goals, including the hope that it will be possible to identify characteristics that typify the premorbid status of individuals who will later become schizophrenic. The models of schizophrenia that guide the various studies are not all the same, however, and expectations about factors that will turn out to be important differ, as do expectations about the variables that can most profitably be pursued in high-risk research.

The New York High-Risk Project differs from most of the other studies in its strong genetic orientation. The underlying theoretical model is based on four assumptions:

1. Except for nongenetic phenocopies, schizophrenia occurs in persons with a genetic predisposition in interaction with probably nonspecific environmental stresses;
2. Genetic predisposition is expressed in dysfunctions that antedate the appearance of the schizophrenic disorder by many years;
3. Such dysfunctions appear first in biological and behavioral processes that occur relatively early in the pathway stemming from a genetic defect(s); and
4. Therefore, these latter dysfunctions precede psychosocial and clinical deviances.

More specifically, it is assumed that the genetic error(s) is reflected in neurotransmitter disturbances, possibly in the dopamine system. The latter, in turn, are hypothesized to be translated into a neurointegrative defect (Fish, 1957; Meehl, 1962, 1972b) which is expressed phenotypically in neuromotor signs, psychophysiological deviations, and attentional and information processing disorders.

This research is supported, in part, by Grants MH19560, MH30921, and MH28648 from the National Institute of Mental Health, by a grant from the W. T. Grant Foundation, and by the Department of Mental Hygiene of the State of New York. We wish to thank our collaborators, Drs. Hector Bird, Joseph Fleiss, Irving Gottesman, Clarice Kestenbaum, Elizabeth Koppitz, Dolores Kreisman, Herbert G. Vaughan, Jr., and Bernard Tursky for their contributions to various parts of the research cited in this chapter. We thank Anne Moscato, Thomas Chin, Joseph Gallichio, Ulla Hilldoff, Ruth Meyerson, Barbara Maminski, Rochelle Schwartz, and Noreen Dodge for help in preparing the manuscript.

The cumulative genetic data collected on twins and other relatives of schizo-phrenic probands (see reviews in Erlenmeyer-Kimling, 1978; Gottesman and Shields, 1976) have not been capable of distinguishing between a polygenic-threshold model (see Edwards, 1960; Gottesman & Shields, 1972, 1976) and a single-major-locus model with multiple thresholds (see Matthysse & Kidd, 1976; Reich, Cloniger, & Guze, 1975), each of which appears to give an equally good fit to existing data and to have the possibility of accounting for spectrum conditions or variable expressivity. Fortunately, the distinction may not be crucial for the attempt to identify early indicators of vulnerability. High-risk researchers must be alert to another possible complication, however – namely, that schizophrenia is genetically heterogeneous (Erlenmeyer-Kimling, 1968; Erlenmeyer-Kimling & Paradowski, 1966; Hamburg, 1967; Kidd & Matthysse, 1978). Although a final common neu-robiological pathway is likely to be implicated in most cases, genetic heterogeneity raises the possibility of different types of interactions with environmental factors and different levels of severity of expression. Experimental work in genetics and behavior genetics offers numerous examples of differential responsivities of differ-ent genotypes to the same environmental conditions leading to the same phe-notypic outcomes (see Erlenmeyer-Kimling, 1972b; Ginsburg, 1967).

The fact that most schizophrenics do not have a schizophrenic parent is com-patible with either a polygenic or a single major-locus threshold model of schizo-phrenia. (Genetic heterogeneity may be represented by two or more independent single major genes and is thus included under expectations for a single major-locus.) There is no reason to assume that schizophrenic individuals with un-affected parents differ genetically or biologically from schizophrenics with affected parents. Thus, unlike the situation for environmental variables, it may be possible to generalize from the children of schizophrenic parents about certain types of psychobiological variables that are thought to be relatively close to the site of gene action and that have already been shown to be deviant in schizophrenic patients.

A point of view about environmental factors

Many of the high-risk studies focus on hypotheses concerned with the possible etiological role of specific environmental variables. Although one of the early goals of the New York project was to chronicle environmental events in high-risk and comparison children, and although such data have been collected, we have come to question the meaningfulness of environmental data collected on samples such as ours and those of many of our colleagues. For one thing, although environmental factors are undoubtedly important in the development of schizophrenia, they are – we believe – not necessarily, nor even likely to be, specific. Although numerous attempts have been made to identify environmental events that are common to all persons who have become schizophrenic, no such event has been found. Samples of psychiatric patients do not show patterns of life-history events that are specifi-cally distinguishable from the life-history patterns exhibited by matched normal control subjects (Morrison, Hudgens, & Barcha, 1968; Gottesman & Shields, 1972), and even precipitating events of a *non*specific nature are lacking in the histories of many schizophrenic patients (Birley & Brown, 1970). Thus, it appears likely that, for most schizophrenics, the environmental contribution to the development of the disorder consists of cumulative, nonspecific stresses that are equally often experienced by other members of the population – who have different genotypes – without resulting in schizophrenia.

The second reason for questioning the meaningfulness of environmental data in a study such as ours is that we examine children of schizophrenic parents, as do most of the other high-risk studies. Living with a severely disturbed parent, or being separated from one's parent at an early age because of the parent's illness, certainly introduces environmental variables that may have detrimental effects on the high-risk child. But, although such variables may look promising for inclusion in a causal model of schizophrenia, they may be misleading. High-risk researchers must face the fact that only 10 to 15% of persons who become schizophrenic have an overtly schizophrenic parent. The home backgrounds of the majority of preschizophrenics can, therefore, be expected to differ in a multitude of important ways from the home backgrounds of those preschizophrenics who happen to have a schizophrenic parent. Extrapolation from studies of the latter in assuming causal connections between environmental factors and schizophrenia is, therefore, tricky at best.

For these reasons, our chief interest in environmental variables is to identify *positive* aspects of the environment that might help to buffer a genetically predisposed high-risk child from psychopathological development. The difficulty will lie in distinguishing such children – that is, genetically predisposed children who do not become schizophrenic because of buffering – from children who do not become schizophrenic because they do not have the gene or genes that are implicated in the pathogenesis of schizophrenia. Thus, there are two classes of *invulnerable* individuals that need to be sharply distinguished and that have very different implications for our understanding of the ingredients that make up the brew of invulnerability. Our hope is that, if it is possible to identify psychobiological precursors in the children who eventually become ill, it will also be possible to flag a group of false positives, who showed the same early characteristics but remained free of schizophrenia, and then to examine the environmental histories of these subjects for possible positive features. Our expectation is that, whereas the environmental histories of children who later develop schizophrenia and other high-risk children who both fail to show the early precursors and fail to have a schizophrenic disorder might not differ greatly, the histories of the false positives might include a greater number of buffering factors.

Selection of variables. A basic assumption in the formulation of the New York High-Risk Project, as well as of most other high-risk studies, is that it will indeed be possible to detect deviant characteristics early in life in genetically predisposed individuals. Such characteristics are presumably ones that are seen as disturbances in schizophrenic patients. The array of dysfunctions that have been reported to characterize at least some schizophrenic patients is, however, extremely wide, so that the choice of variables to be emphasized in studies of high-risk subjects

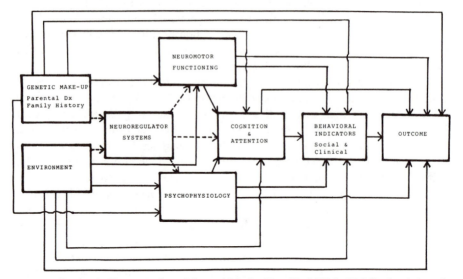

Figure 1. Theoretical model on which the New York High-Risk Project is based.

becomes difficult. Our selection of variables to be examined in the New York High-Risk Project was guided by the assumptions outlined in a preceding section. A diagram of an underlying schematic model based on these assumptions is presented in Figure 1. It should be noted that the model is conceptually similar to, but perhaps more testable than, one developed by Meehl (1972b). Since the beginning of the study – when our earliest thinking about a model stemmed from our interest (Erlenmeyer-Kimling, 1968) in hypotheses suggesting that genetically vulnerable individuals have difficulty in attending to and processing stimuli normally either because they are unable to maintain normal filtering of incoming stimuli (Erlenmeyer-Kimling, 1968; McGhie & Chapman, 1961; Kornetsky & Mirsky, 1966) or because they are unable to disengage attention from a stimulus after having attended to it (Matthysse, 1974) – a number of lines of evidence have emerged that lend support to such a model. Data are now available from the New York High-Risk Project to apply to the schematic model at all levels except those of neurotransmitter activity, and it is expected that the pertinent data will be collected on the latter area.

Implications for intervention. Although it is sometimes assumed that conditions with a genetic basis cannot be prevented through intervention, this is a misconception (Erlenmeyer-Kimling, 1977). Our program, which assumes gene–environment interaction as its basic premise, is directed toward the early identification of specific deficits that precede the schizophrenic illness because we postulate that, once such deficits are pinpointed, it will be possible to develop specific intervention strategies that can be applied to vulnerable (genetically predisposed) individuals in an effort to prevent a schizophrenic disorder from becoming manifest. Although many types of global intervention may improve the quality of life for pre-schizophrenic individuals, most are unlikely to have a significant impact on the prevention of mental disorder. On the other hand, specific interventions aimed at specific deficits that characterize persons at high risk for the disorder may meet the goal of prevention. It is reasonable to assume that intervention will be more effective if it is aimed at deficits that occur relatively early in the pathway between the genetic defect and eventual psychopathological behavior than at deficits that probably occur much later. (For example, in phenylketonuria, a genetic metabolic disorder that results in mental retardation if not treated, intervention is aimed at the immediate consequence of the enzyme deficiency – that is, at the prevention of the overaccumulation of phenylalanine – rather than at the later consequence, mental retardation.) Although the optimal interventions might be those operating at the biochemical level, the application of such interventions to high-risk individuals is currently not feasible or practical. Attentional and information-processing deficits, however, appear to be one level of dysfunction that intervention efforts might attack. These deficits are found in many schizophrenic patients, as noted earlier, and our own work indicates that they appear in a subgroup of high-risk subjects and are associated with the development of clinical deviance. Attentional and information-processing deficits are probably closer to primary defects caused by the genetic error than are many other types of deficits (e.g., social) that can be examined in high-risk subjects, and, at the same time, they are potentially modifiable with behavioral techniques.

DESCRIPTION OF THE NEW YORK HIGH-RISK PROJECT

The New York High-Risk Project was initiated in 1971 and called for the longitudinal study of a large number of variables in high-risk and comparison children from the greater New York metropolitan area.

A first sample (Sample A) of subjects has been followed continuously since its recruitment in 1971–1972. Sample A consists of 205 children who were between the ages of 7 and 12. (Three more children with a schizophrenic mother and manic-depressive father were excluded from the tallies and the analyses.) As shown in Table 1, Sample A includes 80 subjects at high-risk for schizophrenia (the HR group), consisting of 44 children of schizophrenic mothers, 23 children of schizophrenic fathers, and 13 children at exceptionally high risk by virtue of having two schizophrenic parents; 125 subjects at low risk for schizophrenia, consisting of 100 (the NC group) whose parents had never been hospitalized or treated for a psychiatric disorder at the time of intake into the study and 25 (the PC group) with one or two parents who had psychiatric disorders not related to schizophrenia – in all but one case an affective disorder. It is important to note that rediagnosis of Sample A using Research Diagnostic Criteria (Spitzer et al., 1977) is under way and that the numbers of subjects in the HR and PC groups may change.

Collection of a second sample (Sample B) has recently been completed. Sample B affords a test of the replicability of findings derived from the study of Sample A as well as a means of testing hypotheses that may be suggested by data generated

Table 1. *Samples in the New York High-Risk study*

Group	Sample A		Sample B	
	Study children	Siblings	Study children	Siblings
High-Risk (HR)	80	53	45	34
Psychiatric Comparison (PC)	25	20	40	19
Normal Comparison (NC)	100	49	65	33
Total	205	122	150	86

on Sample A. As in Sample A, Sample B children were between the age of 7 and 12 years at intake. Sample B includes 45 HR children (25 with a schizophrenic mother, 12 with a schizophrenic father, and 8 with two schizophrenic parents), 40 PC children – all of whom have a parent with an affective disorder – and 65 NC children (see Table 1). Sample B was diagnosed using Research Diagnostic Criteria (RDC) from the beginning of intake.

Subjects who were in the target-age range at the time of intake are designated the *study children* to distinguish them from their younger (below age 7) and older (above age 12) siblings who have been studied less intensively. Developmental data and follow-up histories, but no laboratory data, have been collected on the 122 siblings in Sample A and the 86 siblings in Sample B (see Table 1).

Recruitment of the samples

In both samples, the children of mentally ill parents were ascertained though the admission of a parent to one of several state psychiatric facilities in the New York metropolitan area. Consecutive admissions at these facilities were screened to identify patients who were white, English-speaking, still married to the biological parent of a child (or children) in the target-age range and who had at least one 7–12-year-old child. The intact-marriage criterion was waived if both parents were schizophrenic. (An effort was made to obtain families with two or more target-aged children, so that sibling comparisons might be made in analyses of gene–environment interaction.) Patients with diagnoses of chronic alcoholism, drug addiction, brain trauma, or psychoses of toxic origin were excluded.

As an initial diagnostic evaluation, records of patients who passed the screening criteria were reviewed independently by two psychiatrists in our group after all references to hospital diagnoses and medications had been removed from the records. Each of the reviewers assigned a diagnosis based on the record materials, completed a symptom checklist, and scored the 100-point Global Assessment Scale (Endicott et al., 1976) assessing the severity of functional impairment. Only those cases in which there was full diagnostic agreement were retained for the study. In Sample B, in addition, the RDC were used in the initial diagnostic evaluation.

A further diagnostic evaluation is being obtained on parents in Sample A using the Schedule for Affective Disorders and Schizophrenia – Lifetime Version (SADS-L, Spitzer & Endicott, 1979). Additional evaluations on parents in both samples will take into account all of the accumulated material on each patient, including the Minnesota Multiphasic Personality Inventory (MMPI) which is administered during a home visit.

In Sample A, the Normal Comparison (NC) group was obtained with the cooperation of two large school systems that agreed to send our letter, asking for participants, to families that met the screening criteria described above (i.e., white, English-speaking, intact family, one or more 7–12-year-old children). The obvious disadvantage was that the NC group was a volunteer group. For Sample B, the latter problem was avoided by enlisting a population-sampling firm to conduct a survey for the purpose of obtaining demographic information on a large number of families, which then formed a pool from which matches for the Sample B high-risk subjects could be drawn. Matching was based on the family's socioeconomic level and the age and sex of the children. In both samples, families were excluded from the NC group if either parent was found to have had psychiatric treatment.

Study design and procedures

The plan of study calls for reexamination of the study children every 2 to 3 years. Sample A has now been examined on three separate occasions, and plans have been developed for a fourth round of examinations for this sample as well as a second round for Sample B. Each round of examinations consists of a home visit to the family and a visit to our laboratory by the study children. Between rounds of testing, contact is maintained with the families by telephone at 3- to 6-month intervals. In addition, teachers' evaluations and school record data are obtained on the study children once they reach junior high school age in a separate substudy (reported in Chapter 12 of this volume).

The initial home visit includes a 2- to 3-hour structured interview conducted with the well parent (or the more functionally intact of two schizophrenic parents or a randomly chosen parent in the NC group). The interview covers the family histories of each parent and complete developmental histories on each child in the family, including older and younger siblings of the study children. Each parent also receives a clinical interview and the MMPI. At the same time, a second interviewer obtains a shorter interview with the other parent regarding his or her perceptions of the children and also conducts an interview with each study child separately. The Bender–Gestalt and Human Figure Drawing tests are administered to the study children.

Subsequent home visits include interviews with the parents, focusing on changes in the family situation and developmental changes in all of the children and treatment received or needed by the children. The study children are administered a life-events questionnaire, an adaptation of the Physical Anhedonia Scale (Chapman, Chapman, & Raulin, 1976), and, if aged 14 or older, the MMPI. Data on social support networks will also be collected in future rounds of testing.

Following the home visit, the study children are tested in the laboratory. (The order of home and laboratory visits was reversed for budgetary reasons in the third round for Sample A.) Table 2 lists the principal measures that have been administered in the laboratory during the various rounds of testing.

Interim assessment of current clinical status

Although the ultimate assessment of clinical outcomes in the High-Risk group cannot be made until all of the subjects have passed through, or, at least, are well into, the schizophrenia risk period, interim assessments of the current clinical status of the subjects can be made. Several systems of assessment are being used or developed.

One means of evaluating current clinical status that has been used is a semistructured 30-minute psychiatric interview (developed for the New York High-Risk Project by Clarice Kestenbaum and Hector Bird) that is videotaped and subsequently rated for clinical deviance and symptomatology on the Mental Health Assessment Form (Kestenbaum & Bird, 1978) by three child psychiatrists who are blind with respect to a given subject's parental group. The interview is now being expanded to permit assessment in greater depth of each subject's clinical status in subsequent rounds of testing. In addition, the parent interview is being expanded to incorporate a number of areas of behavior from the Achenbach Scale (1977), questions from the Columbia-Psychiatric Interview for Children and Adolescents pertaining to schizophrenia, depression, and mania, as well as questions on behavioral assets. Subjects who are flagged as showing psychopathology in the expanded psychiatric interview or in the parent interview will be administered a standardized interview (e.g., the SADS or Kiddie-SADS). The psychiatric interview has thus far yielded (1) a Global Assessment Scale (GAS) rating of degree of psychopathology similar to that obtained on the parents from the clinical interview conducted in the home; and (2) a profile of symptoms. The expanded psychiatric interview, coupled with the expanded parent interview, will yield a diagnostic statement in addition to the GAS rating and symptom profile.

A second kind of assessment is being made to determine each subject's clinical status at the time of entry into the study. As described in Erlenmeyer-Kimling, Kestenbaum, Bird, and Hilldoff (Chapter 14, this volume), Kestenbaum and Bird are conducting a review (blind with respect to parental group) of data collected on each subject during the first round of testing to arrive at a predictive statement as well as a GAS rating of the child's status at that time. The first round data being reviewed include statements about the child from the parent interview, the interview conducted with the child, psychological test data (WISC, Bender–Gestalt and Human Figure Drawing), and data from the neurological exam and Lincoln–Oseretsky test of motor impairment.

Another type of assessment of current clinical status has been employed based on follow-up data obtained in the telephone contacts at 3-month intervals and in other contacts with the families. Behavioral disturbances are measured according to a 5-point Behavioral Global Adjustment Scale (BGAS) which is described in Cornblatt and Erlenmeyer-Kimling (Chapter 12, this volume). The ratings take

Table 2. *Laboratory procedures administered to date*

Procedure	Sample A (round):			Sample B
	1	2	3	(round 1)
Anthropometric measures and photographs	X	X	X	X
Attentional–cognitive measures				
Wechsler Intelligence scales	X		X	X
CPT (Carousel presented card version)	X	X		
ATS (Attention span)	X			
CPT1 (Computerized vigilance task)		X	X	X
CPT2 (Computerized discrimination task)		X	X	X
IOT (Information overload test)			X	X
STM–Lag (Short term memory lag test)			X	
VADS (Visual aural design test)				X
Neurological, motoric, and laterality				
Neurological examination	X			X
Lincoln–Oseretsky Test of Motor Impairment	X			X
Purdue Pegboard				X
Dichotic Listening Test			X	X
Psychophysiology				
Conditioning paradigm, GSR	X			
Resting EEG		X		
Auditory event-related potentials				
to repetitive stimulation		X		
to task-relevant stimulation			X	X
Visual evoked potentials to CPT 1 and CPT 2			X	X
Auditory thresholds (absolute and aversion)		X	X	X
heart rate and skin conductance		X	X	X
Magnitude estimation and psychophysical judgments		X		
Stimulus level intensity gradients		X		
Clinical and social measures				
Structured videotaped interview	X			
Videotaped psychiatric interview		X	X	X
Friendship and intimacy interview			X	X

into account family relationships and the child's general development, peer relationships, and functioning in school (or work if the subject has left school). Inter-rater reliability among three raters for 50 subjects selected at random from Sample A was .94. Raters were blind with respect to subjects' parental groups.

The 5-point BGAS can be further collapsed into three categories for purposes of data analyses. These are (1) major impairment of functioning in more than one area (scale points 1 and 2); (2) moderate difficulty in functioning in some areas (scale point 3); and (3) good functioning in family, school and peer relations (scale points 4 and 5). Scale point 1 is reserved for subjects who have been hospitalized for psychiatric problems and scale point 2 for those who have been in treatment for serious problems or warrant treatment (see Erlenmeyer-Kimling et al., Chapter 14, this volume). Results of the BGAS ratings are discussed in Cornblatt and Erlenmeyer-Kimling (Chapter 12, this volume) where a highly significant overlap between deviant (scale points 1 and 2) BGAS ratings, and deviant performance on attentional measures in the first round of testing is described.

SUMMARY OF SELECTED RESULTS TO DATE

As was indicated in Table 2, a large number of measures have been administered to the subjects in both samples of this longitudinal project. In this report, we will focus on three major domains of variables: attentional measures, neuromotor measures, and a limited set of the psychophysiological measures. Data reported in Cornblatt and Erlenmeyer-Kimling (Chapter 12, this volume) or in Friedman et al., (Chapter 11, this volume) will not be repeated in detail here. Analyses of genetic data emerging from the project will be reported at a future date.

Attentional measures

Sample A, rounds 1 and 3. As described in Cornblatt and Erlenmeyer-Kimling (Chapter 12, this volume), attentional measures have been employed in all testing rounds on Sample A and in the first round of testing on Sample B. The data suggest that an important attentional dysfunction appears at relatively early ages in high-risk children, or at least in a subgroup of high-risk children.

Two attentional measures were administered to Sample A during the first round of testing and three were administered during the third round of testing. (The second round of testing is of less interest because different versions of the CPT were administered to each half of the sample.) Measures in rounds 1 and 3 were as follows:

First round
1. A version of the Continuous Performance Test (CPT), a test of sustained visual attention in which the subject is required to respond to the second of two identical stimuli; distraction and no distraction conditions were given.
2. An Attention Span task (ATS) that requires immediate recall of auditory stimuli consisting of a three- or five-letter series presented at a fast or a slow rate; distraction and no distraction conditions were given.

Third round
1. A computerized version of a vigilance task, in which the subject was required to respond to a given stimulus.
2. A computerized version of the CPT given in Round 1, in which the subject was required to respond to the second of two identical stimuli.
3. An Information Overload Test (IOT) that requires the subject to point to target stimuli in the absence and presence of different types of background distraction.

4. A Short-Term Memory Lag Test (STM-Lag) that requires the subject to state whether a stimulus word or trigram has already been presented in the list of stimuli or is "new."

As noted in Cornblatt and Erlenmeyer-Kimling (Chapter 12, this volume) and elsewhere (Erlenmeyer-Kimling & Cornblatt, 1978, 1980; Rutschmann et al., 1977), the HR group performed significantly more poorly than the comparison subjects on the CPT in Round 1. Although the computerized versions of the CPT in the third round of testing showed age ceiling effects that prevented significant group differences from emerging, a consistent *trend* was apparent for the computerized CPT which was similar to that observed for the CPT version in Round 1: viz., HR subjects tended to show worse performance on several of the response indices than did the comparison subjects. There was no indication that *response bias* (i.e., signal detection theory indices log Lx or B'H) discriminated between groups on either version of the CPT in Round 3 or on the Round 1 CPT. Thus, the lower performance of the HR subjects on these tests of sustained attention appears to be attributable to a decreased capacity for discrimination and not to group differences in test-taking attitudes or motivation.

Group differences were also found on the ATS in Round 1, with HR subjects doing significantly worse on the five-letter trials at the fast rate of presentation than the NC subjects (see Cornblatt & Erlenmeyer-Kimling, Chapter 12, this volume; Erlenmeyer-Kimling & Cornblatt, 1978, 1980). In the third round of testing, the STM-Lag Test was substituted for the ATS. Data analyses on the STM-Lag have recently been completed (Rutschmann et al., 1980). Although no group differences are to be found on the condition using words as stimuli, several important differences emerge on the condition using trigrams as stimuli. The data on the trigram condition demonstrate a decreased memory strength (as assessed by signal detection theory indices, d' and P(I) – where d' is a parametric sensitivity or discriminability index and P(I) is the nonparametric sensitivity index) for the HR group and suggest that, under the most delayed interval between initial presentation of the trigram and second presentation (at which time the subject should recognize the trigram as not new), performance does not improve with age in the HR group but does so in the NC group. As noted in Cornblatt and Erlenmeyer-Kimling (Chapter 12, this volume), HR subjects in the first round of testing were deficient in the recall of longer stimulus sequences in the ATS. Thus, the same capacity limitation appears to be revealed in different but related tasks across age and appears to be consistent with an assumption of longitudinal continuity of an attentional dysfunction.

The IOT administered in the third round of testing is considered to be a measure of distractibility and of ability to process information overload. Cornblatt and Erlenmeyer-Kimling (Chapter 12, this volume) have reported that the IOT showed no differences between the HR and NC subjects in the task requiring the subject to point to target stimuli in the absence of distraction but that a significant decrement in the performance of the HR subjects was seen in the distraction conditions. Moreover, in the condition which required the subject to attend to the background story as well as carrying out the main pointing task, the HR subjects did less well than the NC subjects on the secondary task (answering questions about the background story) as well as on the target task. Thus, the IOT appears to show deficits in HR subjects with respect to both simple distraction effects and capacity to process information overload. The findings with respect to distraction reinforce those obtained on the CPT in the first round of testing. The deficit in processing capacity on the IOT further suggests that HR subjects may not only be less efficient in screening out irrelevant and distracting stimuli, but that they may also be less able to shift attention between competing sources.

Comparisons of signal detection index, d': Sample A, Rounds 1 and 3. The results on the CPT and ATS from Round 1 and the computerized CPT, the STM-Lag Test and the IOT from Round 3 clearly support the interpretation that the Sample A HR subjects showed attentional difficulties when they were first tested between the ages of 7 and 12 years and continue to show such difficulties in adolescence. The main strategy of the New York High-Risk Project, however, is concerned not so much with group differences, but with the attempt to identify subgroups of outliers on the measures under study and to examine the relationship between performance deviance on the various measures and clinical deviance. Thus, for example, Cornblatt and Erlenmeyer-Kimling (Chapter 12, this volume) have presented analyses demonstrating that performance deviance on the CPT and ATS in Round 1 shows significant overlap with poor BGAS ratings in 1978 and 1979; and Erlenmeyer-Kimling et al. (Chapter 14, this volume) have shown the same results when the data are limited to the 15 clinically deviant HR subjects versus all other HR subjects.

Comparison of HR subgroups with respect to the signal detection index, d', is of particular interest as d' can be viewed as a standardized measure of sensitivity which is computable for several of the attentional measures. In Figure 2, d' values are presented for the CPT from Round 1, the computerized CPT from Round 3 and the STM-Lag from Round 3 for the clinically deviant subgroup of HR subjects (see Erlenmeyer-Kimling et al., Chapter 14, this volume), the remainder of the HR subjects, the PC and the NC groups. As can be seen, the clinically deviant subgroup of HR subjects has a much smaller d' – indicating lower sensitivity or capacity to discriminate – on each of the three measures (one from Round 1 and two from Round 3) in comparison with the remainder of the HR group, which is not currently showing clinical deviance. The nondeviant HR subjects are not different from the NC group. The PC group actually has the highest (best) mean d' on the two measures from the third round of testing, but this may be a function of relatively small sample size.

Sample B replication. In Cornblatt and Erlenmeyer-Kimling (Chapter 12, this volume), we have pointed out that data on the attentional performance of subjects in Sample B support the importance that we place on the findings from Sample A. Sample B was administered the computerized vigilance task, the computerized CPT and the IOT that were administered in Round 3 of Sample A, and the Visual–Aural Digit Span (VADS) developed by Koppitz (1973). The VADS was

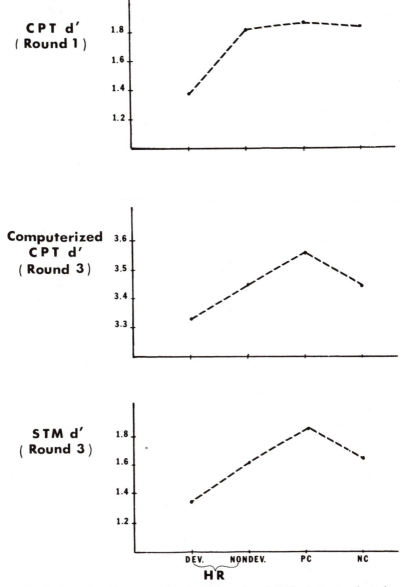

Figure 2. The d' on three attentional measures for clinically deviant and nonde-
viant HR subjects and comparison subjects in PC and NC groups in Sample A.
Measures are the CPT from Round 1 and the computerized CPT and STM-
Lag from Round 3.

used to substitute for the ATS, which had been administered to Sample A in Round 1, and extended immediate recall to the visual as well as the auditory modality.

Compared to the NC and PC subjects in Sample B, the HR subjects showed: (1) significantly poorer performance on the computerized CPT, with lower d's; (2) a trend toward poorer performance on the IOT similar to that seen in the third round of testing of Sample A (the IOT was introduced after a large proportion of the Sample B subjects had been tested, so the number of subjects on whom data are available is small); and (3) significantly fewer digits recalled on all but the easiest of the four subtests of the VADS.

Thus, data from the independently ascertained Sample B appear to replicate closely the attentional data obtained on Sample A at the same ages of testing (ages 7–12 years) as well as the Sample A data obtained at older ages.

Psychophysiological functioning

Electrodermal measures, Sample A, Round 1. In the first round testing of Sample A, an attempt was made to replicate the psychophysiological procedures used by Mednick and Schulsinger (1968) in the study of children of schizophrenic mothers in Denmark. In the Mednick and Schulsinger study, electrodermal responses were recorded to a 54-dB tone which was initially neutral (the conditioned stimulus, or CS) and a 96-dB noxious noise (the unconditioned stimulus, or UCS). Following an orienting session consisting of eight 1000-Hz and eight 500-Hz tones presented in random order, a *conditioning* session was started. The conditioning session consisted of 12 pairings of the CS+ tone with the 96-dB UCS, six presentations of the CS+ alone, and six presentations of a CS− tone. (In our laboratory, one of two stimulus tapes was randomly assigned to the subjects: Tape A used the 1000-Hz tone as the CS+, which was paired with the UCS during conditioning, and the 500-Hz tone as a CS−, which was never paired with the UCS; Tape B reversed the frequencies of the CS+ and CS− tones.) An extinction session, consisting of two CS− and six unpaired CS+ trials, was followed by reconditioning (2 CS+ pairings with UCS) and generalization, in which two unpaired CS+ trials and two generalization tones (1967 and 1311-Hz for the 1000-Hz CS+ and 320 and 250-Hz for the 500-Hz CS+) were presented.

A comparison of Mednick and Schulsinger's and our electrodermal results is presented in Table 3.

Although the pattern of short latency, increased amplitude, fast recovery, and lack of habituation was first reported for Mednick and Schulsinger's high-risk subjects as a group, it was subsequently reported to characterize only those high-risk subjects who were considered, by the time of the 1968 evaluation, to have become sick. The best discriminator among the Sick and Well subgroups of the High-Risk group and the Normal control group was considered to be recovery.

Although our Sample A high-risk subjects as a group failed to show the pattern described by Mednick and Schulsinger – and although the only statistically signif-

Table 3. *Electrodermal results*

Mednick and Schulsinger	Our Sample A
High-risk subjects had shorter response *latencies* to the UCS	High-risk subjects had longer response *latencies* to the UCS
High-risk subjects had *greater amplitude* of response than controls	High-risk subjects had the *same amplitude* of responses as controls
High-risk subjects had *shorter recovery* times than controls	High-risk subjects had *longer recovery* times than controls
High-risk subjects *failed* to *habituate* to UCS over the course of testing but controls habituated	All subjects habituated to UCS over the course of testing

icant differences between high-risk and control subjects was found for latency of response, in the opposite direction from that reported by Mednick and Schulsinger – some additional analyses with respect to recovery have been carried out to allow further comparisons between our subjects and the Danish ones. The mean recovery rates (i.e., mean time to half-recovery) of each group are as follows:

HR[a]	6.17 sec	($N = 54$)
PC	7.56 sec	($N = 20$)
NC	6.46 sec	($N = 87$)

[a]One schizophrenic parent only.

As may be seen, the children of schizophrenic mothers or fathers showed very slightly faster mean recovery than the children in the NC group but this difference was not significant. When recovery data are examined for the children of schizophrenic mothers separately from the data on children of schizophrenic fathers, a nonsignificant trend in the direction of Mednick and Schulsinger's findings for the children of schizophrenic mothers does come to the fore. In our sample, children of schizophrenic mothers ($N = 35$) had a mean recovery of 5.13 sec compared to 6.46 sec for the NC group and 8.08 sec for the children of schizophrenic fathers. The difference between the children of schizophrenic mothers and the NC group is not significant, and, in view of the fact that the schizophrenia risk is the same for children of affected mothers as for children of affected fathers, it is puzzling to find such a large difference between these subgroups if recovery is, in fact, predictive of genetic risk for schizophrenia.

Mednick (1978) has reported more recently that the entire difference between his risk groups on all of the autonomic nervous system variables is due to children in the High-Risk group from nonintact families. [In the New York High-Risk Project, all of the families were intact at the time of intake into the study in the sense that the parents had not divorced or separated (although many did so not

long after entry into the study). However, as the case vignette presented in Erlenmeyer-Kimling et al. (Chapter 14, this volume) shows, "intactness" of the family
does not necessarily mean that each high-risk child remained continuously in the
family home with both parents present.] One interpretation of the intactness
variable is that it is associated with severity of the illness of the affected parent.
Thus, it might be expected that children reared in a nonintact family in Mednick's
sample tend to be those with severely disturbed mothers, whereas those from
intact families tend to have less severely ill mothers. (If that is not the case, the
reported association between autonomic nervous system variables and the intactness variable has no interpretation under any genetic model.)

In our study, it is not possible to compare subjects on the intactness of the
family, but the scores assigned to the schizophrenic mothers on the Global Assessment Scale (GAS) can be examined in relation to their children's recovery data.
The GAS, as noted earlier, yields a rating of severity of functional impairment on a
100-point scale ranging from superior functioning (100) to extreme deterioration
(0). Correlation of the schizophrenic mothers' GAS scores with the recovery data
obtained on their children yields a correlation coefficient of $-.23$, indicating that
the children with the *least* severely ill mothers (high GAS scores) tended to have
faster recovery than children of more severely ill mothers. Thus, in our intact
families, there is no indication that recovery is associated with severity of mother's
illness in a way that would be expected if recovery is relevant to the prediction of
risk for schizophrenia.

In Erlenmeyer-Kimling et al. (Chapter 14, this volume) we have reported recovery data on the 23 subjects who are now showing clinical deviance (8 hospitalized
and 15 in psychiatric treatment). As noted there, the five hospitalized high-risk
subjects have a mean recovery of 6.65 sec – slower than for the HR group as a
whole or for the NC group as a whole. The 10 high-risk subjects in treatment have
a mean recovery of 5.72 sec, which is the fastest of any subgroup (see Table 4,
Chapter 14, this volume), although it is not significantly different from the HR or
NC groups as a whole. Two of the subjects in treatment have a schizophrenic
father, and two have two schizophrenic parents. When their recovery times are
subtracted, the mean for the in-treatment children of schizophrenic mothers is
7.80 sec. Thus, in our data it is difficult to conclude that recovery of the electrodermal response in those offspring of schizophrenic mothers who are going to
become clinically deviant is in any way different from recovery time of other
subjects.

Cortical event-related potentials. The psychophysiology battery adopted for Sample
A subsequent to the first round of testing and for Sample B includes measures that
have been selected principally on the basis of prior demonstration of deviant
findings in patients with schizophrenic illness. The specific procedures have been
designed to maximize the possibilities for quantitative analysis of behaviorally
significant indices of specific central processes that have been postulated to be
deviant in schizophrenics. Particular attention has been paid to mechanisms of
selective attention and to dynamic storage mechanisms.

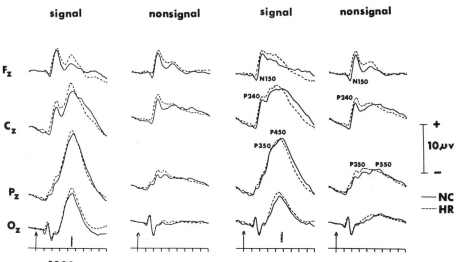

Figure 3. Grand mean ERP from Sample A, third round, recorded in response to the CPT and vigilance procedures. Arrows mark stimulus onset and vertical bars mark mean reaction time. [Reprinted by permission from E. Calloway & D. Lehmann, *Human Evoked Potentials: Applications and Problems,* 1979. New York: Plenum Press.]

Detailed descriptions of several of the psychophysiological procedures and preliminary results have been reported elsewhere (D. Friedman, Vaughn, & Erlenmeyer-Kimling, 1978; Friedman et al., 1979a, 1979b) and in Friedman et al. (Chapter 11, this volume).

Cortical event-related potentials (ERPs) were recorded in the third round of testing of Sample A (N = 30 HR and 30 NC) and Sample B (N = 15 HR and 18 NC) during the administration of the computerized vigilance task (CPT1) and the computerized version of the CPT (CPT2), as well as during several other procedures (Friedman et al., 1978; Friedman et al., 1979a, 1979b). Pass, Klorman, Salzman, Klein, & Kaskey (1977), using a version of the CPT, found, as others have for auditory stimuli, that adult schizophrenics produced less P300 amplitide (a positive peak 300 msec after stimulation) than normal controls to signal stimuli. In our samples, a pattern of mean differences between high-risk and normal comparison subjects was found to be remarkably consistent for the two samples.

Figure 3 presents the grand mean visual ERP for the computerized CPT (CPT2) and the computerized vigilance task (CPT1) for Sample A, third round, and Figure 4 presents the resultant factor structures. These derived waveforms are statistical representations of peaks in the original waveforms. A high factor loading indicates a high correlation between the factor and amplitude of the cortical potential at a particular point in time. Each factor can, therefore, be associated

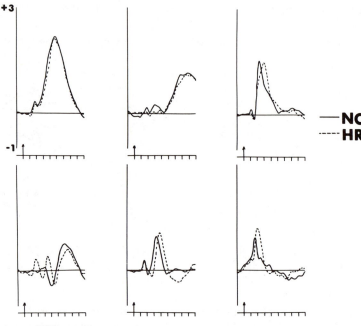

Figure 4. Rotated factor loadings from the CPT and vigilance procedures for Sample A, third round. The Principal Components Analysis was performed across ERP elicited by the stimuli from both tasks. Arrows mark stimulus onset. Factors referred to in the text are indicated by number. [Reprinted by permission from E. Calloway & D. Lehmann, *Human Evoked Potentials: Applications and Problems*, 1979. New York: Plenum Press.]

with amplitude peaks in the original waveforms that are active in different time regions. Thus, Factor 1, which peaks at 450 msec is associated with P450 in the original waveforms; Factor 2, which cannot be associated with a specific peak, and is reaching its peak at a point in time when P450 is decreasing, appears to represent resolution of this late positive activity. Factor 3 peaks between 240 and 300 msec and is identified with P240. Factor 4 peaks at 600 msec and is associated with P550. Factor 5 is highly correlated with time points at 300 to 350 msec and is identified with P350, and Factor 6 peaks at 150 to 200 msec and is associated with N150 (a negative peak 150 msec after stimulation). The amplitude of each peak in a given subject's cortical waveform can then be estimated using the factor score obtained for each of the six factors.

Significant differences or trends toward significance were evident in the same components for both samples: the HR children produced less initial negativity (N150), less P350 amplitude, greater frontal P240-P250, and greater frontal P450–P500 amplitude than their NC counterparts.

Outliers from Sample A, third round, were identified on the basis of their pattern of factor scores. Of the subjects chosen on this basis, 10 HR and 2 NC children had extreme scores on four or more factors. Among these subjects, four, all of whom were high-risk subjects, showed a consistent pattern of factor scores: Their ERPs were characterized by low initial negativity, large amplitude P240 components, and large amplitude frontal P450 waves to signal stimuli and low amplitude P450 components to nonsignal stimuli. Inspection of these outliers' grand mean ERP revealed abnormally small between-task differences in cognitive- and attention-related components. When the outliers were subtracted from the grand mean for the HR group, the residual mean was very similar to the NC mean. Thus, the most consistent ERP findings relating to the CPT and vigilance tasks are in components reflecting cognitive and attention-related processes. Less initial negativity may indicate poor attentional processes in these HR children, as in- creases in this component's amplitude have been related to attentional level. The absence of between-task differences in the cognitive-related components might reflect deficient information processing or a difference in the way these HR children (as opposed to the remainder of the sample) analyze the relevant informa- tion from the two tasks. Thus, the ERP data are consistent with the findings on the attentional measures for both samples.

Neuromotor functions. Several types of measures have been administered in an effort to assess neuromotor functioning. A modified Lincoln–Oseretsky Test of Motor Impairment and a pediatric neurology examination were given in the first round of testing to both samples. The neurological examination given to Sample A was revised and improved for Sample B to focus more heavily on soft neurological signs. As reported previously (Erlenmeyer-Kimling, 1975), the Lincoln–Oseretsky Test discriminated significantly between the HR and NC groups in Sample A; this finding was replicated in Sample B, with the NC group performing better than the HR group in both samples.

Significant group differences were not found on the neurological examination in Sample A, although a trend was noted suggesting that HR males under 11 years old displayed somewhat greater neurological impairment than same-aged NC males. This trend, which was relatively weak in Sample A, was consistent with data reported by Marcus (1974) on a high-risk sample in Israel. On the improved version of the neurological examination given to Sample B, however, a number of significant differences emerged on items related to right–left orientation, gait and position, and eye movement ($p < .05$), as well as on scales measuring fine-motor movement ($p < .001$) and overall neurological abnormality ($p < .01$) (Marcuse & Cornblatt, in press). Directional trends for all main effects in Sample B were consistent with the trends noted in Sample A, in showing poorer neuromotor functioning in HR subjects, males, and children under 11 years of age, thus supporting Marcus's (1974) findings and those of other investigators who have noted fine-motor impairment in high-risk children (Fish, 1975; Rieder & Nichols, 1979).

A preliminary attempt has been made to compare deviance on other measures (for Sample A only because there are as yet no follow-up data on Sample B). Nine (out of 50, or 18%) of the HR subjects who were under 11 years of age in Sample

A had scores on the neurological summary scale and/or the motor scale of the examination that were beyond the score cutting off the poorest 5% of the NC group (four subjects) of the same age on each scale. Seven of the nine HR subjects so identified had BGAS (1979) scores between 1 (impaired) and 3 (moderate difficulty in functioning) and two of the NC subjects had BGAS scores of 3. As noted in Erlenmeyer-Kimling et al. (Chapter 14, this volume) the HR subjects who have been hospitalized or are in treatment tend to have relatively poor neurological summary scores.

Other fields of data

The three areas of data discussed here in some detail represent an important part of the New York High-Risk Project, but other types of data are being collected and analyzed as well. The first report on the teachers' evaluations of Sample A subjects is presented in Watt et al. (Chapter 13, this volume) and indicates that HR subjects tend to be seen less positively than the NC subjects by their teachers. Data on friendship patterns and degree of intimacy and confiding in the friendship relationship are being analyzed by our collaborator, Dolores Kreisman. In addition to being used as a part of the child psychiatrists' (Kestenbaum and Bird) clinical assignment of the subject, the data from the parent interview will be combined into several empirical scales regarding a subject's functioning in a Ph.D. dissertation that Michael Glish is undertaking. Life-events data and the physical anhedonia scale remain to be examined on Sample A subjects (and to be administered to Sample B in the second round of testing). These additional fields of data on high-risk and comparison subjects will provide a broader picture of their functioning as whole people.

DISCUSSION

At this stage of the longitudinal study, it appears that we have been able to identify subgroups of HR children who exhibit attentional dysfunctions at early ages, early neuromotor disturbances, and evoked-response patterns that differ from those of the comparison subjects or the remainder of the HR group. The subjects who are now showing clinical deviance in adolescence overlap significantly with the subjects who had early attentional dysfunctions; they also tend to have relatively poor neuromotor performance. We hope to pursue these promising leads further and to determine whether there is evidence supporting the tentative and simplistic model outlined in Figure 1.

Whether a significant number of the subjects belonging to any of the deviant subgroups identified thus far will later become schizophrenic can be seen only after further follow-up. In view of the fact that we expect schizophrenia to be genetically heterogeneous, we would not be surprised to find more than one subgroup, with differing response characteristics emerging from the overall High-Risk group. Thus, there may be more than one set of characteristics that will be found to predict to schizophrenia. Moreover, our subgroups may contain some false positives who will not become schizophrenic. False positives may be very important for further scrutiny because they may be genetically predisposed individuals who are fortunate enough to have environmental buffering that enables them to avoid becoming ill. If so, such subjects might provide an important key to the understanding of environmental variables that help individuals with a schizophrenic genotype to avoid becoming ill.

The preliminary indication of a deficit in attention – both as measured directly and as reflected in the evoked-response components – in some young children who are at risk for schizophrenia is especially interesting in view of (1) the many reports of impaired attention in schizophrenic patients (Garmezy, 1977; Grinker & Holzman, 1973; Gunderson, Autry, Mosher, & Buchsbaum, 1974; Matthysse, 1977); (2) the strong suggestion of a correlation between attentional dysfunction and lowered MAO and DBH activity levels (Buchsbaum, Murphy, Coursey, Lake, & Ziegler, 1978); and (3) the reported reduction of MAO activity in schizophrenic patients (Wyatt, Potkin, & Murphy, 1979).

In our sample, the fact that attentional dysfunction is seen only in a subgroup of children of schizophrenic parents and that it does not cluster in siblings (Erlenmeyer-Kimling & Cornblatt, 1980) seems to rule out the possibility that this deficit is of strictly environmental origin as result of living with a schizophrenic parent. Thus, the current picture is compatible with the hypothesis that impairment in attention is an early indicator of vulnerability to schizophrenia – in at least some cases – and that it is possibly an early phenotypic sign of disturbed neurochemical functioning. A planned study on MAO and DBH activity levels in the high-risk and comparison subjects may help to establish this relationship further.

Our long-term goal is preventive intervention. Intervention is as yet premature because we do not yet know how to identify specific individuals for whom intervention is indicated, what problems really characterize such children, or what form intervention should take. If, however, we can learn to identify the truly vulnerable members of the High-Risk group and to understand what characteristics need to be modified in them, then we will be in a position to develop rationally based strategies for intervention.

11   Event-related potential (ERP) methodology in high-risk research

DAVID FRIEDMAN, L. ERLENMEYER-KIMLING, AND HERBERT G. VAUGHAN, JR.

The psychophysiological functioning of adult schizophrenics has received a great deal of attention over the past two decades (see reviews by Venables, 1977; Shagass, 1976; 1977; Buchsbaum, 1977; Roth, 1977; Zahn, 1977; 1979), but it is only relatively recently, with the advent of the high-risk longitudinal study, that the psychophysiological functioning of their offspring has come under close scrutiny. The few studies that do exist deal primarily with the autonomic nervous system (e.g., Zahn, 1977; Venables, 1977; 1978; Mednick & Schulsinger, 1968; Klein & Salzman, 1978; Erlenmeyer-Kimling et al., Chapter 14, this volume), as indices of autonomic functioning have been traditionally used to measure tonic levels of arousal and phasic-orienting responses. In the majority of these studies, the focus was on physiological responsivity with no behavioral responses concomitantly recorded.

Many investigators of the schizophrenias share the view that these disorders are manifestations of brain dysfunction. Thus, the study of the brain function of schizophrenics using the averaged evoked potential recorded from scalp electrodes has been an area of active research. In these investigations, the focus has been more psychophysiological, as both physiological and behavioral responses have been recorded simultaneously in an attempt to delineate the relationships between variables in the two domains. This is an exceptionally powerful methodology in the study of schizophrenia, as cognitive deficits and dysfunctional physiological responsivity have both been reported to characterize these disorders. This allows the investigator to determine under what circumstances psychological and physiological measures are coupled or uncoupled, and to what extent deficits in either domain are more severe in psychopathological states of consciousness. Few studies using this methodology with high-risk children have been carried out, and these will be reviewed below.

The authors would like to thank Mr. James Wilson, Jr. for data collection and Mr. Joseph Gallichio for his aid with data analysis, Mr. James Hollenberg and Ms. Henrietta Wolland for computer programming. This research was supported by Grant MH-19560 from the National Institute of Mental Health and by the New York State Department of Mental Hygiene.

THE EVENT-RELATED BRAIN POTENTIALS (ERP)

Stimuli in several modalities elicit a series of time-locked electrical components from the human brain that are recorded at the scalp as the evoked or event-related potential (ERP). The amplitudes and latencies of these components depend upon both physical and psychological conditions. Two types of ERP are recognized: *exogenous*, those that are greatly affected by stimulus parameters such as intensity and duration, and *endogenous*, those that are heavily influenced by the psychological context in which the eliciting stimulus is embedded. It is with this latter class of ERP that this paper will deal. The most well-known of the endogenous components is P300 (also known as the *late positive* component, or *association cortex* potential). The "P" refers to the fact that it is recorded as a positive voltage and the "300" refers to its latency in milliseconds after the onset of the stimulus. It is now known that the latency of this potential can vary over a wide range depending upon stimulus and task characteristics. In the years since the original report of this component (Sutton et al., 1965), P300 has been shown to be exquisitely sensitive to the cognitive structure of the task during which it is recorded. Recently, a longer latency waveform, labeled slow wave (SW), which overlaps with and extends beyond P300, has been shown to be sensitive to some of the same variables as P300 (e.g., N. Squires, Squires, & Hillyard, 1975; K. Squires, Donchin, Herning, & McCarthy, 1977).

ADULT SCHIZOPHRENIC WAVEFORMS

The most consistent ERP finding with adult schizophrenics is that components prior to 100 msec poststimulus are larger than normal, whereas those after 100 msec are attenuated and more variable relative to normal controls (for reviews see Shagass, 1976; Roth, 1977). This has led Shagass (1976) to postulate that, since the early, exogenous components are dependent upon the sensory parameters of the stimulus, the larger and less variable nature of these components in schizophrenics is indicative of an impairment of a central "filtering" mechanism. Thus, the reduction in amplitude of the longer-latency cognitive-related potentials may be the result of this deficient regulatory mechanism which is reflected in early ERP events. Investigations in this area have uniformly shown a reduction in the adult schizophrenic of P300 amplitude recorded during cognitive information-processing tasks (Roth & Cannon, 1972; Levit, Sutton, & Zubin, 1973; Pass et al., 1980; Roth, Pfefferbaum, Horvath, Berger, & Kopell, 1980; Timgit-Bertheier & Gerono, 1979).

ERP INVESTIGATIONS IN HIGH-RISK CHILDREN

Herman et al. (1977) reported that compared with normal controls ($N = 6$), high-risk children ($N = 6$) had larger amplitude and longer-latency components at 100 to 200 msec poststimulus to signal and nonsignal stimuli in a version of the Continuous Performance Test. As this report was based on an extremely small sample, general conclusions are difficult to draw.

Itil, Hus, Saletu, and Mednick (1974) and Saletu, Saletu, Marasa, Mednick, and Schulsinger (1975) reported finding no amplitude differences between high-risk ($N = 62$) and normal control children ($N = 62$), but that the high-risk children showed significantly shorter latencies of components after 100 msec poststimulus than their normal control counterparts. These latency differences, however, were significant at very modest levels ($p < .05$ for most), and were very small, on the order of 7 to 16 msec. In addition, a large number of statistical tests were made, detracting from the strength of the reported differences.

In the New York High-Risk Project, we (Friedman et al., 1979a) did not find faster latency auditory ERP in the high-risk children ($N = 20$) compared with the normal controls ($N = 20$), but did find a subgroup of high-risk children ($N = 5$) who had significantly longer latency ERP components compared with the remainder of the high-risk sample ($N = 15$) and the normal control group.

In a study with visual ERP, we (Friedman et al., 1979b) did not find large differences between high-risk and normal control groups using two versions of the Continuous Performance Test which differed in their processing complexity. However, a subgroup of children, all of whom were at risk for schizophrenia, showed abnormally small between-task differences in the late, cognitive-related ERP components. These results suggested that this subgroup of children may have differed from the remainder of the high-risk group and the normal control group in the way in which they analyzed the relevant information from the two tasks. These results reinforced our use of more cognitively oriented paradigms with high-risk children in order to obtain ERP correlates of information processing, deficits in which have been reported for high-risk samples (e.g., Asarnow et al., 1977; Cornblatt & Erlenmeyer-Kimling, Chapter 12, this volume; MacCrimmon et al., 1980; Rutschmann et al., 1977).

THE PRESENT STUDY

For the New York High-Risk Project (see overview by Erlenmeyer-Kimling et al., Chapter 14, this volume), we designed a paradigm in which we could record ERP and behavioral events simultaneously. The nature of the task ensured that we would record late positive components and slow wave, brain potentials known to reflect cognitive information processing. If the finding of reduced late positive component amplitude in adult schizophrenics is truly a manifestation of some biological and/or cognitive abnormality, and not simply a consequence of the schizophrenic disorder, then the child at genetic risk should exhibit the same tendency as the adult schizophrenic when compared to normal controls.

METHODS

Subject selection

For this preliminary analysis of the auditory ERP, data are included on the first 56 children (28 high-risk = HR; 28 normal controls = NC) from our initial cohort who came for the third round of testing (Sample A3) and on the first 30 children

(N = 13HR; 17NC) from our second cohort (Sample B1). Sample B1 serves as a replicate for Sample A.

Task procedures and stimuli

The task was designed to obtain ERP to relevant, irrelevant and background auditory events. During each block of trials, the children heard three kinds of events: a frequent tone pip (1000 Hz, 64 dB SPL), which occurred 66% of the time, a pitch change (PC), from the standard frequency (at 700 Hz, 64 dB SPL), and a stimulus omission or missing stimulus (MS); PC and MS each occurred 17% of the time. The stimuli were presented binaurally over headphones, with an interstimulus interval of 800 msec. Subjects were instructed to respond with a finger lift (which activated a reaction time key) to one of the infrequent events. The infrequent event that was relevant was alternated across four blocks of trials, for a total of 300 stimuli per block.

EEG recording procedures

EEG was recorded on a Beckman Type RM Dynograph with a time constant of 1 second and high-frequency cutoff at 30 Hz. Electrodes were placed at midline frontal (F_z), central (C_z), parietal (P_z), and occipital (O_z) scalp sites, with electro-oculogram (EOG) recorded from an electrode located above the right eye. All leads were referred to the right earlobe. Data acquisition and stimulus presentation were under the control of a PDP 11/10 computer, which digitized the physiological data at 4-msec intervals for a 100 msec pre- and a 700 msec poststimulus epoch and recorded it, along with reaction time, on digital tape for off-line analyses. Trials containing movement and/or eye artifact were removed from the analyses.

Data analyses

ERP components are known to overlap at the scalp. For example, two components with temporally adjacent peaks may summate with a peak latency intermediate to the two original components. This leads to error when attempting to estimate peak amplitude values by visual inspection since the measurement of one component may be contaminated by an unknown contribution from the amplitude of adjacent or overlapping components. Principal Components Analysis (PCA) has been used by ERP investigators to disentangle statistically these overlapping components (see, for example, Donchin & Heffley, 1978, for an explanation of PCA in an ERP context). Because P300 and slow wave are known to interact in this manner, PCA was used to obtain measures of these potentials uncontaminated by overlap.

PCA was used as an objective method of decomposing the ERP waveform, since this permits rigorous and objective definition of components, ruling out any subjective bias that might occur when hand scoring the data. The factors resulting from the PCA are statistical representations of "peaks" in the original waveforms. A high factor loading indicates a high correlation between the factor and the voltage of the scalp potential at a given point in time. Each factor can then be associated with voltage peaks that are active in different time regions in the original ERP waveforms. The amplitude of each of the peaks in a given subject's waveform can then be expressed using the factor score.

PCA of the averaged waveforms was performed with the BMDP Statistical Package (Dixon, 1975) using the time points as variables and the waveforms as cases. Because component amplitude might distinguish the groups, we wanted to maintain the original microvolt scale when performing the PCA. We, therefore, factored the cross products matrix, as there are no transformations performed on the data when obtaining it, thus retaining full amplitude information from each subject's original waveform. The PCA was performed separately on the PC and MS ERP. For each of these analyses, the number of cases entered was 2 (relevant/irrelevant), by 4 (F_z, C_z, P_z, and O_z scalp sites), by number of subjects, yielding 448 waveforms for Sample A3 (with 56 subjects) and 240 waveforms for Sample B1 (with 30 subjects). The number of time points, or "variables," was 66, with each point representing 12 msec of EEG.

RESULTS AND DISCUSSION

ERP waveforms

The grand mean ERPs averaged across subjects within each risk group and sample to the relevant and irrelevant infrequent events are depicted in Figure 1. As can be seen, the detection of a gap in stimulation, the *missing stimulus,* produces a large-amplitude potential referred to as the missing stimulus potential or MSP, comprised of a positive-going wave peaking at 400 msec, P400, and a subsequent slow wave. Stimulation with a change in pitch also produces a large amplitude potential, comprised of a positive wave peaking at 350 msec, P350, and a subsequent slow wave, but, unlike the MSP, this brain event is composed of earlier, stimulus-generated potentials, N100 and P200. The MSP is an *emitted* potential because its elicitation is not dependent upon the presence of a stimulus, whereas the ERP to the pitch change is known as an *evoked* potential, because it is dependent upon the presence of a stimulus. The late positivity-slow wave complex seen in each of these ERPs is endogenous and is thought to represent the same brain activity in both the MS and PC ERPs.

It is clear that the relevant events elicit larger-amplitude late positivity–slow wave complexes than the physically identical irrelevant events. Note also that mean reaction time (RT) occurs at about the same time that this late positivity reaches its peak. This finding is typical of many studies and has led to the conclusion that this potential indexes stimulus evaluation time. A striking feature of the comparison between HR and NC waveforms is the reduction in late positive component amplitude seen in the waveforms of the HR subjects in both samples and to both infrequent relevant events. This reduction does not appear to be due to differences in mean RT between groups, as mean RT and its associated variability are very similar in both groups within each sample. Slow wave is larger in the Sample B1 HR than NC subjects, a result not evident for Sample A3. As Sample

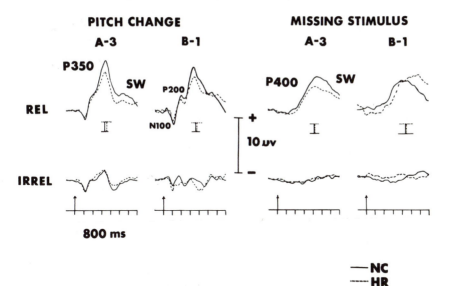

Figure 1. Grand mean ERPs averaged across subjects to the relevant and irrelevant events for each risk group and sample. Vertical bars mark mean reaction time, and horizontal bars indicate standard deviation associated with each reaction time mean. Arrows mark stimulus onset. Time lines every 100 msec. Data depicted were recorded from the parietal electrode (P_z). Rel = relevant; Irrel = irrelevant. SW = slow wave.

B1 subjects are younger than those of Sample A3, this discrepancy may be due to information processing strategies that differed for the younger HR subjects of Sample B1.

Statistical representation of the waveforms

The factor loadings after Varimax rotation to both infrequent events are shown in Figure 2. The two factors depicted for each event were the first two extracted from the PCA, accounting for at least 75% of the ERP variance. As can be seen, the factors are highly similar for each event and each sample. The shape and timing of the factors labelled P350, extracted from the PC ERP, peaking at 400 msec for B1 and 350 msec for A3, lead to their identification with P350 in the original waveforms, while the slower-onset, longer-latency factors are identified with slow wave in the original data. The shape and timing of the first factor depicted for the MS ERP (labeled P400), peaking at 400 msec for both samples, lead to its association with P400 in the original waveforms. The second, long-latency factor is identified with slow wave in the original waveforms.

The mean factor scores, corresponding to P350, P400, and slow wave components, averaged across groups within each sample, are displayed in Figure 3. The most striking aspect of these data is the reduction, in the HR subjects, of the amplitude of the factor scores associated with late positivity in both MSP and PC ERP. These are reliable findings as assessed by Group (HR vs. NC) by Relevance

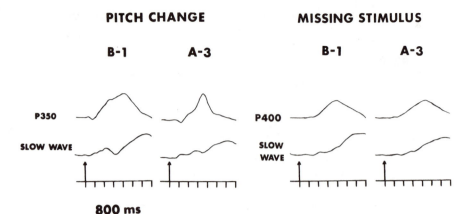

Figure 2. Factor loadings after Varimax rotation obtained from the cross products matrix. Principal Components Analysis was performed on the pitch change and missing stimulus ERP separately, pooling the ERP across HR and NC groups. Each late positivity (P350, P400)–slow wave complex accounted for better than 75% of the variance in both samples. Arrows mark stimulus onset; time lines every 100 msec.

(relevant vs. irrelevant) by Electrode (F_z, C_z, P_z, O_z scalp sites) repeated measures ANOVA.

SUMMARY AND CONCLUSIONS

The most consistent finding, replicated in two independent samples, is for P350 (PC) and P400 (MSP) amplitudes to be reduced in the HR children's ERP relative to NC children when the eliciting event is relevant. This reduction in late positive component amplitude is one of the most consistent findings with adult schizophrenics. Thus, late positive complex amplitude reduction may be one of the premorbid indicators for schizophrenia.

These findings are, of course, based on group mean differences. The next step is to determine which of the HR children display extreme amplitude reduction and to see if these subjects show consistent patterns of dysfunction in other psychophysiological, behavioral, and clinical measures, as these subjects may be the most vulnerable in the HR group.

Reduction of P300 and slow wave amplitudes can be caused by many different factors. Correlations between other variables in the test battery and ERP measures may aid in defining the particular problem areas these children demonstrate. It is only upon follow-up of those individuals displaying abnormal ERP patterns that we will be able to validate our psychophysiological measures against the crucial variable of clinical diagnosis. It is at that point that we should be able to detect ERP characteristics that are true premorbid indicators and those that are a consequence of mental dysfunction. Our data demonstrate the potential fruitfulness of the cognitive ERP components as premorbid indicators for schizophrenia.

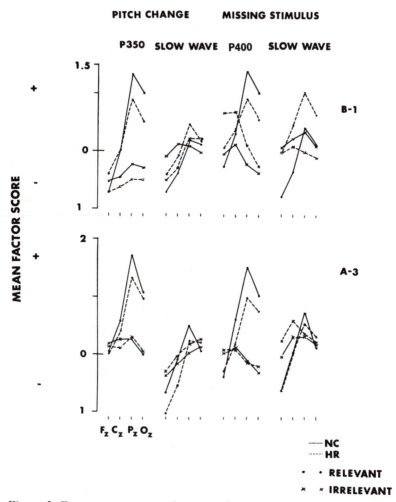

Figure 3. Factor scores averaged across subjects corresponding to the P350, P400, and slow wave factors depicted in Figure 2. Scores are plotted for relevant and irrelevant events for each risk group and sample at each of the four electrode sites (F_z, C_z, P_z, O_z).

12 Early attentional predictors of adolescent behavioral disturbances in children at risk for schizophrenia

BARBARA CORNBLATT AND
L. ERLENMEYER-KIMLING

Considerable evidence from both clinical and experimental research on schizophrenia indicates that schizophrenic adults cannot focus or maintain their attention as well as normal adults (e.g., Grinker & Holzman, 1973; Kornetsky & Mirsky, 1966; McGhie & Chapman, 1961). Recently, it has been recognized that such attentional deficits may be antecedents as well as prominent features of schizophrenia (e.g., Garmezy, 1977; Matthysse, 1977).

For this reason, a number of the investigations that prospectively study children who are considered to be at risk for eventual schizophrenia have included a variety of attentional measures in their test batteries. The five high-risk investigations that have most specifically studied attention in children of preschool and school age include:

1. The Massachusetts Intervention Project organized by Grunebaum and his associates (e.g., Cohler et al., 1977; Grunebaum, Weiss, Gallant, & Cohler, 1974; Grunebaum, Cohler, Kauffman, & Gallant, 1978; and Herman, Mirsky, Ricks, & Gallant, 1977);
2. The Waterloo-McMaster High-Risk Project being conducted in Canada by Asarnow, Steffy, and their collaborators (e.g., Asarnow et al., 1978; MacCrimmon, Cleghorn, Asarnow, & Steffy, 1980);
3. The Minnesota series of cross-sectional risk studies directed by Garmezy (e.g., Driscoll, 1979; Garmezy, 1973, 1978; Neuchterlein, 1979; Nuechterlein, Phipps-Yonas, Driscoll, & Garmezy, 1980 and Phipps-Yonas, 1979);
4. The Neale and Weintraub study underway at Stony Brook, New York (e.g., Harvey, Winters, Weintraub, & Neale, 1981, Oltmanns, Weintraub, Stone, & Neale, 1978; and Stone, Neale, & Weintraub, 1977);

This research was supported, in part, by Grant MH 19560 from the National Institute of Mental Health and by the Department of Mental Hygiene of the State of New York. Statistical and computing help was supported in part by NIMH Clinical Research Center Grant MH 30909-04.

We would like to thank Thomas Chin and Ryselle Cohen for their help in preparing the data and Henny Wolland and the Computer Center Staff for their contributions to the data analysis. The assistance of Yvonne Marcuse and Ulla Hilldoff in assigning the clinical ratings is most appreciated. Special thanks go to David Friedman and Jacques Rutschmann for their very helpful comments during the preparation of this chapter.

5. The New York Longitudinal High-Risk Project directed by Erlenmeyer-Kimling at New York State Psychiatric Institute (e.g., Erlenmeyer-Kimling & Cornblatt, 1978, 1980; Erlenmeyer-Kimling, Cornblatt, & Fleiss, 1979; and Rutschmann, Cornblatt, & Erlenmeyer-Kimling, 1977).

There is considerable diversity across these investigations in both the attentional processes being studied and the measures that are used. As a result, there are often inconsistencies in the specific preliminary results that have been reported. For example, the various versions of the Continuous Performance Test (CPT) that have been used to measure sustained attention in several of the projects have met with different degrees of success. When the procedure used is appropriate for the ages of the subjects being tested, the CPT has been found to discriminate effectively between high-risk and normal control children, as, for example, in Nuechterlein's study (1979) and in the findings of the New York High-Risk Project that will be discussed in the sections that follow. On the other hand, contradictory patterns of group differences have been found when the task is too easy to generate adequate individual differences (as in the double-digit version of the CPT used in the New York Project and as may also be the case in the results reported by Asarnow et al., 1978) or when other important design considerations are overlooked (such as the failure to control adequately for changes in the ages and composition of the samples being compared in the series of studies by Grunebaum and his associates).

However, despite such methodological problems, the results across studies generally support the expectation that early attentional deficits may be of considerable promise in predicting later psychopathology. This is demonstrated by the cognitive data obtained by the New York High-Risk Project in which attentional variables have been emphasized since the onset of the study in 1971.

METHOD

Subjects

The first sample – Sample A – has been tested on three occasions over an 8-year period. When initially tested in 1971–1972, Sample A consisted of 205 subjects between the ages of 7 and 12 years. Of these subjects, 80 were the children of schizophrenic parents (the High-Risk group), 25 were the children of parents with a psychiatric disturbance other than schizophrenia (the Psychiatric Control group), and 100 were the children of normal parents (the Normal Control group). Data obtained from the first round of testing and from the third round, which was completed in 1979, will be presented here.

The second sample – Sample B – was tested for the first time between 1977 and 1979 and recently completed a second round of testing (July, 1981). When initially tested, Sample B consisted of 150 subjects, also between the ages of 7 and 12 years, and included: 44 children in the High-Risk (HR) group, 40 in the Psychiatric Control (PC) group, and 66 Normal Control (NC) children. The Sample B first round attentional data will also be discussed in this chapter. (For more details about the two samples, see Erlenmeyer-Kimling et al., Chapter 10, this volume).

Procedures

The attentional measures administered to Samples A and B during their first rounds of testing and to Sample A during its third round are listed by round in Table 1. It is evident that changes have been made over the years of testing in the measures administered to each sample. In some cases, test substitutions in later rounds were made on the basis of information emerging from the first round of testing or because more difficult tasks were needed for older subjects. In other cases, design modifications were necessary to accommodate more sophisticated computer-controlled measurement procedures. It is important to note, however, that despite these changes continuity has been maintained throughout all testing rounds in the processes being tapped, with particular emphasis on three major areas of attentional processing: (1) sustained attention, (2) short-term memory/focused attention, and (3) distractibility.

Sustained attention has been measured in each testing round of the two samples by a version of the Continuous Performance Test (CPT) which measures a subject's ability to detect either a designated target stimulus (simple task) or the second of a stimulus pair (complex task) out of a quasi-random series of relevant and irrelevant stimuli. *Short-term memory/focused attention* was measured in the first round of testing of Sample A by the auditory Attention Span Task (ATS). In the first round of Sample B, the ATS was replaced by the Visual–Aural Digit Span (VADS) which extended the recall of information to include the visual mode as well as the auditory mode used in the ATS. In addition, short-term auditory recognition memory was also tested in a subgroup of older subjects (i.e., age 15 and above) during the third round of testing of Sample A. *Distractibility* was measured in Sample A during both the CPT and the ATS in the first round of testing and in the Information Overload Task (IOT) during the third round. No measures of distractibility were given to Sample B during its initial testing, although these have subsequently been included in later test rounds.

Each of the measures is described more fully below.

RESULTS

Sample A, Round 1

The major findings from the two attentional measures administered to Sample A during its first round of testing are summarized in Table 2. For all individual variables discussed in this chapter, significance of group differences was evaluated by means of multiple regression analysis controlling for age, sex, and age × sex in forced stepwise sequence. Significant group differences were found on many of the indices generated by these measures, with subjects in the High-Risk group performing more poorly than Normal Controls in all instances.

Table 1. *Attentional measures administered to Sample A, Round 1; Sample B, Round 1; and to Sample A, Round 3*

Measure	Task	Stimuli	Test description	Processes tapped
Sample A, Round 1 (1971–1972)				
CPT: Playing-Card Version	Keypress to identical card sequences	Slides of standard playing cards, including clubs and spades and numbers 2–10	Slides continually flashed on screen by carousel projector; alternating no-distraction and distraction conditions	Sustained attention Distractibility
Attention Span Task (ATS)	Immediate oral recall of target letters	Strings of 3 or 5 letters	Letters recited by tape-recorded female voice (target letters) or male voice (distractor letters); three conditions: No-distraction–Distraction–No-distraction. Trials counterbalanced for fast vs. slow presentation rates	Short-term memory Focused attention Speed of processing Distractibility
Sample B, Round 1 (1977–1979)				
CPT: Double-Digit Version				
(a) Simple Task	Fingerlift to designated target number (i.e., 08)	Double-digit numbers, ranging from 02 to 19	Digits computer generated and continually flashed on CRT monitor; visual evoked potentials recorded simultaneously with behavioral responses	Sustained attention
(b) Complex Task	Fingerlift to identical number sequences			
Visual–Aural Digit Span (VADS)	Immediate recall of digits (alternating oral and written recall)	Strings of digits, gradually increasing in length until error criterion reached	Digits presented by experimenter in alternating aural and visual modes	Short-term auditory and visual memory

(continued)

Table 1. (*cont.*)

Measure	Task	Stimuli	Test description	Processes tapped
Sample A, Round 3 (1977–1979)				
CPT: Double-Digit Version				
(a) Simple Task		—[a]	—[a]	Sustained attention
(b) Complex Task		—[a]	—[a]	Focused attention
Information Overload Task (IOT)	Point finger to one of four pictures	Names corresponding to pictures on test plates	Picture names continually recited by tape-recorded voice; picture test plates presented by experimenter. Three conditions: No-distraction–Distraction–Information Overload	Attentional flexibility and attentional shifts Distractibility
STM-Lag	Recognition of words/trigrams being new (first presentation) or old (second presentation)	Sequences of words and of consonant–vowel–consonant (CVC) trigrams	Stimuli continually recited by tape-recorded female voice; lag intervals for duplicated items vary (i.e., lags include 0, 3, 6, 12, 24, and 48 fillers intervening between first and second stimulus presentations)	Short-term auditory recognition memory

[a]Same as described for Sample B, Round 1.

Table 2. *Summary of statistical comparisons of HR and NC groups (Sample A, Round 1) on the attentional measures*

		p value
Playing Card CPT (complex task)		
Number of responses:		
Hits	HR group fewer corrects	.05
False alarms	HR group more errors	N.S.
Random commission errors	HR group more errors	.001
Signal detection indices:		
d' (sensitivity index)	HR group lower	.05
Log Lx (index of response bias)	HR group lower	N.S.
Distraction effect:	YES – Response decrement in D[a] compared to ND[b] trials in HR group	
Attention-span measures (ATS)		
Proportion of correct responses:		
ND fast five[c]	HR group lower proportion of corrects	.05
Rate index	HR group less improvement from slow to fast rate	N.S.
Proportion of incorrect responses[d]:		
ND fast five	HR group higher proportion of incorrects	.01
Rate index	HR group less improvement from slow to fast rate	.05
Distraction effect:	NO – apparent floor effect, D trials too difficult for all subjects tested	

[a]D = Distraction.
[b]ND = No-distraction.
[c]ND fast five = All no-distraction trials on which five letters were presented at the fast rate.
[d]Incorrect responses = commission errors only.

The version of the CPT given to Sample A during the first round of testing was a complex vigilance task tapping sustained attention and distractibility. The test consisted of slides of standard playing cards which were rapidly flashed in continous succession on a screen. The subject's task was to respond when two identical slides appeared in sequence. (For example, a six of spades following a six of spades). Correct responses to target pairs were called "hits." In an equal number of pairs the slides were matched in number but not in suit. (For example, a six of spades following a six of clubs). Responses to these pairs were considered systematic commission errors and were labeled "false alarms." The remaining stimuli were randomly organized "fillers." Responses to filler trials were called "random commission errors." Half of the trials were presented without distraction and half were presented in the presence of external auditory distraction – a tape-recorded female voice reciting numbers at varying speeds and levels of loudness.

The results of this version of the CPT have previously been reported in detail by Rutschmann et al. (1977) and by Erlenmeyer-Kimling and Cornblatt (1978). In summary, High-Risk subjects made significantly fewer correct responses (or hits) and significantly more random commission errors than did subjects in the Normal Control group. Furthermore, these performance decrements were enhanced in the presence of external auditory distraction. High-Risk subjects were also found to have significantly lower d's (the index of discriminability between signals and nonsignals) in a signal detection analysis, suggesting a generally lower sensitivity to critical stimuli in this group.

In the Attention Span (ATS), which measured both focused attention and distractibility, subjects were required to listen to and immediately recall sequences of three or five letters presented by a tape-recorded female voice at a fast (one letter per second) or slow (1 letter per 1.5 sec) rate. Half of the sequences were presented with distraction: letters recited by a male voice interspersed between the target letters in the female voice.

No differences were found between groups on the distraction trials, as these proved to be too difficult for all of the subjects. On the no-distraction five-letter trials presented at the faster rate, however, High-Risk subjects made significantly fewer correct responses and significantly more commission errors than did Normal Control subjects.

In addition to the group differences, a number of preliminary analyses combining attentional indices into composite performance measures have consistently identified a subgroup of particularly deviant performers within the high-risk group. For example, Erlenmeyer-Kimling and Cornblatt (1978) found that 19.1% of the High-Risk group compared to 4.4% of the Normal Controls scored extremely poorly on three or more indices out of a total possible of eight attentional indices (six from the CPT, two from the ATS). Furthermore, when two indices from the CPT, two from the ATS, and the raw score from the Digit Span Subtest of the Wechsler Intelligence Test for Children (WISC) were combined into linear discriminant function scores, Erlenmeyer-Kimling and Cornblatt (1980) found that 25% of the High-Risk children were classified as being deviant across measures compared to 5% of the Normal Control children.

These early findings were considered sufficiently encouraging to maintain our focus on the study of attention. Consequently, a number of attentional measures were pilot-tested during the second round of testing of Sample A, and the most appropriate of these measures were selected for the attentional batteries administered to Sample B during its first round of testing and to Sample A during its third. For budgetary reasons Sample A was divided into two subgroups during the second round of testing, with many of the attentional measures being administered to only one group of the other. Round 2 data are not presented here because only limited comparisons between subject groups could therefore be made.

Table 3. *Summary of statistical comparisons of HR and NC groups (Sample B, Round 1) on the attentional measures*

		p value
Double-Digit CPT (Complex Task)		
Number of responses		
Hits	HR group fewer corrects	.05
False alarms	HR group more errors	N.S.
Random commission errors	HR group more errors	N.S.
Signal detection indices		
d' (sensitivity index)	HR group lower	.05
Log Lx (index of response bias)	HR group lower	N.S.
Distraction effect	Not tested	
Visual Aural Digit Span (VADS)		
Number of digits correctly recalled		
Condition 1 – Aural stimulus/ oral response	HR group fewer digits correctly recalled	N.S.
Condition 2 – Visual stimulus/ oral response	HR group fewer digits correctly recalled	.05
Condition 3 – Aural stimulus/ written response	HR group fewer digits correctly recalled	.05
Condition 4 – Visual stimulus/ written response	HR group fewer digits correctly recalled	.01
Summary score – total across all four conditions	HR group fewer digits correctly recalled	.01
Distraction effect	Not tested	

Sample B, Round 1

The attentional data initially obtained from our second sample support the group differences found earlier for Sample A during its first round of testing. Two attentional tasks were administered to Sample B during the first round of testing. These were the Double-Digit version of the CPT, measuring sustained attention, and the Visual–Aural Digit Span or VADS, tapping short-term memory and focused attention. Findings from both of these measures are presented in Table 3.

The original playing card version of the CPT was revised for use in the subsequent testing rounds (i.e., for Sample B first round and Sample A third round). The Double-Digit version of the CPT was computerized and modified to allow measurement compatible with the recording of visual evoked potentials, which were obtained concurrently with the behavioral data. In the modified version double-digit numbers (ranging from 02 to 19) were flashed in a continuous series on a visual monitor. The overall measure was divided into two separate tasks: a simple vigilance paradigm, during which subjects responded whenever an 08 was presented; and a complex vigilance task – more comparable to the playing card version – during which subjects responded to the second of two identical stimuli in a row (for example, an 18 following an 18).

In general, the Double-Digit CPT turned out to be somewhat easier than the earlier playing card version, and the simple vigilance task was found not to discriminate between groups on any of the response measures. In fact, the simple task of the double digit CPT yielded no findings of interest in any age category for either Samples A or B. The results of this task will, therefore, not be discussed further and were not included in the tables presented. However, on the more complex task, High-Risk subjects made significantly fewer correct responses and had significantly lower signal detection d's than did their respective controls.

The VADS, developed by Elizabeth Koppitz, was administered to Sample B in place of the Attention Span which was given to Sample A. As mentioned, although the two tests are comparable, the VADS extends immediate recall to the visual as well as the auditory modality. Subjects were presented digit strings of increasing length in both the visual and aural modalities and were required to repeat the stimuli both orally and in written form. This yielded a total of four counterbalanced conditions and a summary score measuring total recall across all four conditions. High-Risk subjects recalled significantly fewer digits than the Normal Control subjects on all but the aurally presented–orally recalled condition, and had summary scores that were significantly lower than those of the Normal Control group.

The findings obtained from the complex task of the CPT and from the VADS are consistent with the earlier Sample A results and suggest that deficits in sustained and focused attention are generalizable across high-risk samples. The stability of such attentional impairments can also be examined with respect to the data collected during the third round of testing of Sample A, which was conducted approximately 6 years after the initial testing round.

Sample A, Round 3

The results of the attentional measures administered to Sample A in Round 3 are summarized in Table 4. The complex task of the revised CPT also proved to be too easy to yield individual differences in subjects between 13 and 18 years old (the age range of Sample A during the third round of testing), although there was a noticeable trend for the youngest subjects in the High-Risk group (i.e., those between 13 and 14) to perform more poorly than their same age Normal Controls. This ceiling effect, unfortunately, limits the conclusions that can be drawn about the continuity of deficits in sustained attention over time. However, more can be said about the stability of distractibility, in that the early CPT distraction findings were essentially reproduced by the Round 3 measure of distraction – the Information Overload Task, or IOT.

The IOT is considered to be a test of distractibility, attentional flexibility, and the ability to focus and shift attention between competing sources of information. The basic task required the subject to point to the one of four pictures on a test plate that matched a target word that was being recited on a tape recorder. Three background conditions were used. In the first condition, the pointing task was

Table 4. *Summary of statistical comparisons of HR and NC groups (Sample A, Round 3) on the attentional measures*

		p value
Double-Digit CPT (Complex Task)		
Number of responses		
Hits	HR group fewer corrects	N.S.
False alarms	Same for HR and NC groups	N.S.
Random commission errors	HR group more errors	N.S.
Signal detection indices		
d′ (sensitivity index)	HR group lower	N.S.
Log *Lx* (index of response bias)	NC group lower	N.S.
Distraction effect	Not tested	
Information Overload Task (IOT)		
Proportion of correct responses		
Quiet condition	Same for HR and NC groups	N.S.
Noise condition	HR group lower proportion of corrects	.05
Voice condition	HR group lower proportion of corrects	.01
Proportion of questions correctly answered	HR group lower proportion of correct responses	.001
Distraction effect	*YES* – HR group performed more poorly on all distraction conditions	

presented in the absence of background noise and served as a training condition during which baseline response levels were established. In the second condition, distraction consisted of very realistic sounds of a busy school cafeteria, which gradually increased in loudness. Distraction in the third condition consisted of a tape-recorded voice telling a simple story at the same time that the target words were being presented. Subjects were required to process rather than simply screen out this source of distraction, as they were told they would be asked questions about the story's content at the end of the pointing task. High-Risk subjects were found to perform the pointing task significantly more poorly than normal control subjects in both distraction conditions, and were also particularly deficient in answering questions about the background story.

A measure of short-term memory – The STM-Lag Test – was also included in the third round attentional battery. In this procedure, short-term memory for words and for consonant–vowel–consonant (CVC) trigrams was assessed by means of a continous recognition task. A continuous string of items (both words and CVCs) was presented, and the subject judged each item as to whether it was new or old. Because this test was considered to be quite difficult, it was only given to a subgroup of older Sample A subjects (i.e., those above 14) and cannot be directly compared to the other attentional measures. We will, therefore, only briefly summarize the results of this measure here (but see Rutschmann et al., 1980 and Erlenmeyer-Kimling et al., Chapter 10, this volume, for more details). With respect to short-term recognition memory for words, no differences were found between the High-Risk and Normal Control groups. For the trigrams, however, High-Risk subjects were found, in general, to have a lower overall memory strength than Normal Controls, and in particular, to be deficient in initial memory strength relative to Normal Control subjects. These findings are consistent with the Round 1 data indicating that High-Risk subjects have more difficulty than Normal Control subjects with the short-term recall of digits.

SUBGROUP OF DEVIANT PERFORMERS IN THE SAMPLE A HIGH-RISK GROUP

The consistent finding of a performance deficit in High-Risk subjects relative to normal controls across comparable measures of attention – both in two independent samples tested at the same ages, and in the same sample tested at two points in time approximately 6 years apart – supports the hypothesis that attentional dysfunctions are a characteristic of at least some children at risk for schizophrenia. However, detection of group differences is only a preliminary step in high-risk research. A more important goal, based on the expectation that only about 10 to 15% of the High-Risk group will ever actually manifest schizophrenia, is to identify a subgroup of particularly deviant performers within the High-Risk group.

One way of searching for outliers within the High-Risk group is to define deviance on any given measure with respect to the Normal Control group's performance levels. An analysis of this type has been done for Sample A based on data from Round 1 by selecting the score on a selected response index that identified the most poorly performing 5% of the Normal Control group and then considering all subjects performing below that cutoff score to be deviant. Next, a tally was made of the number of response indices on which each subject was deviant out of a total possible of 15 indices taken from the CPT, ATS, and the WISC. This deviance analysis differs from the two mentioned earlier in this chapter (i.e., Erlenmeyer-Kimling & Cornblatt, 1978 and 1980) in using a larger number of attentional indices. The current analysis is based on 15 attentional indices – 8 from the CPT, 5 from the ATS, and 2 from the Digit Span Subtest of the WISC. The two earlier analyses included fewer variables (i.e., 8 in the 1978 report and 5 in the 1980 report) because only indices yielding significant group differences were selected – and, in the case of the 1980 study, the number of indices was further reduced by randomly eliminating one index from any pair that intercorrelated significantly. In the current study, however, we decided to include all attentional indices that were considered to be relevant on theoretical grounds, whether or not they had generated significant differences between the High-Risk and Normal Control groups (on the suspicion that important variables might be lost in the deviance analysis by imposing the group differences requirement). Consequently, the current analysis contains all of the attentional indices used in the past but has added a number that were not previously included.

Table 5. *Behavioral–Global Adjustment Scale (B-GAS)*

Scale rating categories

(1) *Severely impaired functioning*
   Gross behavior disturbance requiring psychiatric hospitalization

(2) *Markedly impaired functioning*
   Unable to function in some but not all areas; behavior consistently deviant in at least one area, but not sufficiently severe to warrant hospitalization

(3) *Moderately impaired functioning*
   Moderate difficulty in functioning in two or more areas; difficult to judge whether will be within the normal range or develop into a real problem; minimal rating for therapy of any kind

(4) *Average functioning*
   Individual either consistently average in all three areas of functioning *or* experiences mild difficulties in one of the three but also excels in at least one of the remaining areas

(5) *Above average functioning*
   Above average individual; consistently appears somewhat above average in all three areas *or* must excel in at least one of the three and be, at minimum, average in the others.

Note: The three areas of functioning on which above ratings are based include: (a) family interrelationships and family's perception of subject's general emotional development; (b) peer interactions; and (c) school functioning (or functioning in a work situation if the subject no longer attends school).

High-risk subjects were found to be deviant on a significantly larger number of indices than were normal control subjects (M_{HR} = 1.93 vs. M_{NC} = .90, t = 3.80, $p < .001$). Further, a substantially greater proportion of the High-Risk group than the Normal Control group (25% compared to 5%) was found to perform deviantly on four or more of the selected attentional response indices, and 11% of the HR group were extremely deviant (i.e., on six or more measures) compared to only 3% of the NC group.

OVERLAP BETWEEN DEVIANCE IN ATTENTION AND IN
BEHAVIOR

Even more significant to the validation of early attentional dysfunctions as possible predictors of eventual schizophrenia, is the finding that the subgroup of High-Risk subjects who were identified as deviant on the Round 1 attentional indices has been found to show an increasing overlap with the subjects showing behavioral problems as they reach late adolescence.

Behavioral disturbances were measured according to a 5-point Behavioral–Global Adjustment Scale or B-GAS, which is summarized in Table 5. The

Table 6. *Behavioral–Global Adjustment Scale (B-GAS): Sample A Results*

	B-GAS 78			B-GAS 79		
Group[a]	N	M	SD	N	M	SD
HR	(72)	3.29	.99	(72)	3.14	1.01
NC	(84)	4.00	.68	(92)	3.81	.69
PC	(13)	3.54	.88	(18)	3.39	.85
F(HR vs. NC)		26.58			25.54	
p value		<.001			<.001	

[a]Neither age, sex, nor age $\times$ sex accounts for a significant proportion of the variance of B-GAS scores.

B-GAS ratings are based primarily on information obtained from the parents of the children during the routine follow-up telephone calls which have been made every 3 to 6 months since the onset of the project. The B-GAS scores represent our preliminary means of rating behavior; they will eventually be analyzed in conjunction with other clinical assessments currently being developed. Three major areas of functioning are taken into consideration in assigning the B-GAS ratings: (1) family relationships and the child's general development; (2) peer interactions; and (3) school functioning.

Ratings are scored in the direction of health, that is, the higher the score, the healthier the overall behavior is considered to be. The rating categories range from gross behavioral disturbance requiring hospitalization (a rating of 1) to above-average functioning in all three areas (a rating of 5). Interrater reliability on the B-GAS scores of 50 randomly selected cases was .94.

An entire set of ratings for Sample A was carried out in August of 1978. A complete updating of the Sample A scores was also made in August 1979. The results of both assessment periods are presented in Table 6. As can be seen, High-Risk subjects were considered to be a significantly more disturbed than Normal Control subjects on both occasions, although Psychiatric Controls did not differ from either of the other groups.

When the two sets of B-GAS scores are compared with each subject's deviance score on laboratory indices from the first round of testing discussed above, the High-Risk subgroup that is deviant on the laboratory measures is found to show an increasing overlap with the subjects who are exhibiting subsequent behavior problems. This is illustrated in Table 7. Both B-GAS 78 and B-GAS 79 ratings show a significant overlap with performance deviance on the early laboratory measures. Furthermore, the correlation between the two types of scores has increased as the behavioral ratings have been updated. This trend both suggests that Sample A subjects showing early deficits on laboratory measures are becoming increasingly deviant behaviorally as they get older – as might be expected – and supports the

Table 7. *Relationship between early laboratory performance and later behavior ratings: Sample A, HR group*

Deviance on A-1 lab measures	H (%)	M (%)	I (%)
1978 B-GAS scores[a]			
0–1	29	15	5
2–3	6	15	5
4+	7	9	9
1979 B-GAS scores[b]			
0–1	26	17	6
2–3	5	15	6
4+	3	10	12

Note: H = healthy functioning, including B-GAS scores of 4 and 5; M = moderately impaired behaviorally, including B-GAS score of 3; I = markedly to severely impaired, including B-GAS scores of 2 and 1.
[a]$r = -.30; p < .01$.
[b]$r = -.42; p < .001$.

hypothesis that attentional dysfunctions serve as early predictors of later psychopathology. Of course, final validation of attentional dysfunctions as specific predictors of schizophrenia awaits determination of the extent to which the early pathology, reflected by the B-GAS scores, relates to actual schizophrenia.

SUMMARY

Since the beginning of the New York High-Risk Report in 1971, a variety of attentional measures has been administered to two samples of children at high and low risk for schizophrenia. Despite the changes in testing procedures required as the samples get older and the addition of new measures when necessary, the emergence of attentional deficits in the children of schizophrenic parents relative to the normal control children has been remarkably consistent across samples and testing rounds. This is particularly evident in the areas of sustained attention, focused attention, and susceptibility to distraction in high-risk children.

Furthermore, when the early individual attentional measures are combined into an overall deviance score, a distinct subgroup of subjects can be identified within the High-Risk group. Subjects within this subgroup are not only impaired across a number of measures, but, in many cases, are also becoming increasingly disturbed behaviorally and socially as they reach their late teens.

Overall, our findings strongly suggest that attentional dysfunctions may be critical early markers of schizophrenia proneness.

13 Social, emotional, and intellectual behavior at school among children at high risk for schizophrenia

NORMAN F. WATT, TED W. GRUBB, AND
L. ERLENMEYER-KIMLING

Let us state at the outset a premise of this research program that is remarkably foreign to people outside the specialized field of longitudinal research in schizophrenia and remains controversial among investigators within that field (cf. Hanson, Gottesman, & Meehl, 1977); many, if not most, children destined to have adult schizophrenic disorders deviate from normal interpersonal, emotional, or intellectual behavior for a substantial length of time – often several years – before the onset of psychotic symptoms (Watt, Fryer, Lewine, & Prentky, 1979). It is awkward to regard the behavioral deviations as prodromal signs in the same sense that an aura foretells an impending epileptic seizure or a sudden loss of weight indicates the beginning of a severe depression. It seems more plausible to consider shyness, emotional volatility, abrasive interpersonal relations, or deficiencies in intellectual performance or motivation as outward manifestations of the epigenesis of human character than to construe them as incipient symptoms of psychosis.

This is not to deny that such deviant traits in childhood or adolescence may be functionally related – or even contribute causally – to future schizophrenic disorder. Obviously, the form and quality of one's character will reflect and may determine to some extent that person's prospects for adult mental health. The objective of this research is to find reliable associations between observable aspects of character development and adult mental health. If we find deficiencies of character or competence in the early lives of adult schizophrenics, then our goal would be to establish the causal relationships between the early features of development and the later features of breakdown and recovery. A complete explanation of that sort would have to include the mechanisms that mediate those relations, whether they

This chapter was previously published with the same title in the *Journal of Consulting and Clinical Psychology, 50, 171–181, 1982.*

The research is supported, in part, by Grants No. MH 19560, No. MH 30921, No. MH 28648, and No. MH 32667 from the National Institute of Mental Health, by a grant from the W. T. Grant Foundation, and by the Department of Mental Hygiene of the State of New York.

We wish to thank Philadelphia Cousins, Richard Lewine, and Michael Glish for their research assistance; Bob Engstrom, Dale Schellenger, and Chip Reichardt for expert computer consultation; and E. Faith Ivery, Debra Karas, and Linda Wilbanks for help in preparing the manuscript.

212

be biochemical or psychodynamic or neurophysiological in nature. All of us in the field of risk research are a long way from that level of explanation, but the capture of some salient longitudinal relationships may not be far out of our reach.

THE PROGRAMMATIC CONTEXT OF THIS INVESTIGATION

The New York Project is a prospective, longitudinal investigation of children of one schizophrenic parent, children of two schizophrenic parents, children of one parent with a different (predominantly depressive) psychiatric disorder, and children of normal parents. The long-term goals of the project are to analyze interactions between biological and environmental factors, to develop screening methods for early identification of vulnerable children, and to develop instruments for preventive intervention with children at risk for schizophrenia based on a more firm understanding of etiological factors and the premorbid state. Emphasis in the main project is placed on measures related to possible neurophysiological dysfunctions in the children, with some attention given to clinical psychiatric assessment of the entire family and to factors that differentiate vulnerable and resistant children within the High-Risk groups.

The Index parents were drawn from numerous psychiatric facilities in the New York metropolitan region. The diagnoses used were based on the clinical judgments of two psychiatrists prior to the development of the third edition of the *Diagnostic and Statistical Manual of Mental Disorders* (DSM-III, 1980). The psychiatrists reviewed the patients' hospital charts, from which diagnoses and information about medications had been removed. No case was included in the study without diagnostic agreement between the two psychiatrists, who reviewed the records independently and without consulting each other. The third round of assessments included SADS-L interviews of the patient parents, on the basis of which a few of the original diagnoses are being changed from schizophrenic to affective disorder. The net effect of these diagnostic reevaluations will be to reduce ultimately the size of the schizophrenic High-Risk sample and increase the size of the Psychiatric Control sample, with all diagnoses more closely aligned to the DSM-III classification system. When all of the diagnostic reevaluations have been completed, the data in the present report will be reanalyzed accordingly.

The present subsidiary project is designed to obtain objective assessments of social, emotional, and intellectual functioning in school to permit: (1) contemporary behavioral comparisons between the children at risk and their controls; (2) contemporary studies of correlations between school behavior and other (neurophysiological, demographic, and psychiatric) measures of the children and their parents from the main project; (3) theoretical predictions of vulnerability to future emotional breakdown, based on combinations of genetic and behavioral criteria; and (4) ultimately, retrospective description and post hoc theoretical analysis of the antecedents of schizophrenic (and other emotional) breakdowns.

When the subjects in the main project are studied initially, the families are intact and the children are 7 to 12 years of age. The school assessments begin when the children reach about 12 to 15 years old and are attending junior high school.

Ideally, a follow-up assessment takes place when the child reaches high school 2 or 3 years later. Our study has been criticized for not examining the children much earlier in their development, but this strategic decision was based on three practical considerations that we consider persuasive: (1) Our earlier retrospective studies of school records showed little discriminating predictive value in teachers' descriptions of the grade school behavior of preschizophrenics, in contrast to the sharp distinctions that emerged in junior and senior high school (Watt, 1978). (2) In most grade schools, pupils are taught all subjects by only one teacher, whereas in most junior high schools the pupils receive instruction from many teachers each year; earlier methodological studies (Shay, 1978) showed that median test–retest reliabilities for the 28 Pupil Rating Form scales increased with the number of pooled teacher ratings from .70 (one teacher) to .80 (two) to .84 (three) to .89 (four); similarly, median interjudge reliability coefficients for the 28 scales increased from .61 (two teachers) to .70 (three) to .76 (four), and median validity coefficients for seven scales, measured against the criterion of systematically recorded classroom observations, increased from .36 (one teacher) to .42 (two) to .48 (three) to .55 (four). Hence we had sound empirical reasons to prefer the psychometric leverage for our classroom measures that is first available in early adolescence. (3) The median age of onset for schizophrenic disorders is about 25, so that the average delay from our first school assessment to schizophrenic outcome can be estimated at roughly 10 years; starting school assessments at 6 or 8 years old would almost double the average time to schizophrenic outcome and delay commensurately any replication or intervention studies that might ensue.

This report analyzes the results of the first school assessments made for 114 subjects in Sample A, the first of two samples collected in the larger project, based on two of the three instruments for which data were obtained.

METHOD

Subjects

To date, school assessments have been completed for 120 (59%) of the children in Sample A. This includes 44 children of schizophrenic parents, 6 children of psychotic depressive parents, and 70 children of normal parents. School data were obtained for only 4 children of two schizophrenic parents, so for purposes of statistical analysis they are included among the 44 mentioned above. Because of their small number the six psychiatric control children are omitted from the analyses presented here. This report, therefore, focuses on the 44 children (25 boys, 19 girls) at high risk for schizophrenia and 70 normal control children (42 boys, 28 girls). Although subjects were not originally matched on age, the groups did not differ significantly in mean age, both averaging 15 years old at the time of the school assessment. Control families had higher socioeconomic status, which required statistical adjustment through analysis of covariance. There were no blacks in the study.

Measures

Four major-subject teachers were asked to rate each study child on the measures of classroom behavior after several months of acquaintance with the child. Referees were limited to major-subject teachers because they usually meet with their classes at least four times each week, so that they know their pupils well. They all teach academic subjects, which ensures a certain commonality of classroom experiences.

Pupil rating form (PRF). The PRF is an instrument extrapolated from a coding system developed by Watt, Stolorow, Lubensky, & McClelland (1970) for quantifying information in school records. The PRF consists of 28 behavioral and personality dimensions along which teachers are asked to rate each child by assigning a score from 1 through 5. The form requires approximately 15 minutes to complete. It is accompanied by a behavioral description of the end-points for each scale item to standardize, at least crudely, the meaning or definition of each scale. The PRF was factor analyzed in a study of 571 pupils (267 boys, 304 girls) from two junior high schools in Denver. The procedure adopted was the maximum likelihood confirmatory factor analytic technique developed by Jöreskog (1971) and Sorbom (1974). This yielded an extremely simple factor structure, identical for males and females, with four primary factors that we labeled: Scholastic Motivation (nine scales), Extraversion (eight scales), Harmony (seven scales), and Emotional Stability (four scales). Table 1 presents a summary of the factor structure of the PRF on which the present analysis was based. It is interesting to note that this factor analysis yielded four of the five clusters of scales that were originally planned in the study of school records on the basis of previous cross-cultural research by other investigators (Watt et al., 1970).

The reliability and validity of the PRF were studied intensively by Shay (1978). Pooling the ratings of three teachers (the average number available in the present study), he found test–retest reliabilities (with 1 month intervening) for the 28 scales ranged from .63 to .95 with a median of .84; all were significant at the .01 level or beyond. Ebel's (1951) intraclass correlation statistic showed that the average interjudge reliability of rating for all possible combinations of three teachers was not significant for one scale (independence) but ranged from .41 to .82 with a median at .70 for the other 27 scales; all were significant at the .01 level or beyond. The validity of three pooled teacher ratings was tested against the criterion of systematic classroom observations made by trained observers for 7 of the 28 scales, yielding coefficients that ranged from .26, which was not significant, to .69 with median of .48. Six of the seven validity coefficients were significant at the .001 level. The validity of 13 of the 28 scales altogether was assessed in multitrait–multimethod matrix analyses (Campbell & Fiske, 1959) against a variety of criteria, including systematic classroom observation, sociometric peer ratings, and self-report. The overall validity was judged excellent for eight of the scales, good for two, fair for one, and poor for two. Of greatest relevance for the present

Table 1. *Revised factor structure: pupil rating form*

Factor	Factor pattern loading[a]	
	Males	Females
Factor I: Scholastic Motivation (9)		
Achievement: achieving–underachieving	1.000	
Effort: motivated–unmotivated	.980	
Work habits: organized–disorganized	1.027	
Reliability: dependable–undependable	.732	
Attention: attentive–distractible	1.502	
Orderliness: orderly–careless	.951	
Maturity: mature–immature	.839	
Independence: independent–dependent	.525	
Confidence: confident–insecure	.662	
Factor II: Extraversion (8)		
Sociability: extraverted–introverted	1.000	
Loquaciousness: talkative–quiet	1.018	
Self-assertion: assertive–passive	.930	
Inhibition: inhibited–uninhibited	− .941	
Activity Level: high–low	.800	
Leadership: leader–follower	.685	
Group Participation: much–little	.720	
Presentation: exhibitionistic–modest	.912	.554
Factor III: Harmony (7)		
Disposition: pleasant–unpleasant	1.000	
Mood: cheerful–somber	.923	
Popularity: popular–unpopular	.797	
Cooperation: compliant–negativistic	1.223	
Adjustment: well adjusted–maladjusted	.716	1.286
Conduct: well behaved–misbehaved	.488	1.545
Consideration: considerate–egocentric	.597	1.273
Factor IV: Emotional Stability (4)		
Tension: calm–nervous	1.000	
Emotional Control: controlled–emotional	1.167	
Impulsivity: impulsive–deliberate	−1.216	
Aggression: aggressive–peaceful	− .514	

[a]If the scale's factor pattern loading is significantly different for males than females, both loadings are listed. Otherwise the single value represents the loading constrained to be equal for both groups.

study were Shay's multitrait–multimethod matrix analyses of the validity of the two primary PRF factors, Scholastic Motivation and Extraversion, which accounted for 49% and 26%, respectively, of the total variance. For these analyses each of the primary factors was represented by two scales and tested for validity against two independent criteria. The evidence for discriminant validity in both matrices was outstanding, and the convergent validity coefficients were .77 and .57 against systematic observation and .66 and .59 against sociometric peer ratings, all significant at the .001 level. With such exceptionally high validity coefficients, the reliability of measurement for the PRF factors must be quite satisfactory; in this case the test–retest reliabilities were .93 and .90 for Scholastic Motivation and .75 and .81 for Extraversion.

Hahnemann High School Behavior Rating Scale (HHSB). The HHSB was developed by Spivack and Swift (1972, 1977). It was designed to measure the behavior of junior and senior high school students that reflects their level of success in academic performance. Like the PRF, the HHSB requires teachers to rate their pupils along a number of behavioral dimensions on scales of 1 to 5 or 1 to 7 points. There are 45 items altogether, which are combined for scoring purposes into 13 Behavior Factors. The form requires 15 to 20 minutes to complete. The orientation of the HHSB differs from that of the PRF, in that the HHSB emphasizes behavior with specific relevance to academic achievement, whereas the PRF covers a broader spectrum of social and emotional behavior.

Procedure

Individual consent forms for the collection of school record data and teacher ratings were obtained from the study children and their parents. The principal at the junior high or high school attended by each child was initially contacted by a letter that explained briefly the request for information and included a copy of the consent forms. A follow-up phone call was made to arrange a date for the investigator to visit the school in order to procure the necessary information.

The principal, staff, and teachers were told that the child was part of a large developmental study and that they had been randomly selected in a phone survey, as the normal controls had been, in fact. In order to avoid stigmatizing the study children, school personnel were not informed of the psychiatric history of the child's parents nor of the true nature of the study. A predictable criticism is that many of the teachers may already have known about the parental illness and that this knowledge would cast a negative prejudice on their ratings. To ascertain what the teachers knew or suspected, we posed three open-ended questions about their impressions of each child: (a) What assets or advantages do you see that might favor healthy development in this child's adjustment? (b) What handicaps or disadvantages do you think might interfere with this child's health or adjustment? (c) Please describe in your own words this child's personality and behavior at school. These questions were phrased very cautiously so as not to draw attention directly to the parents or home situation, which we considered unethical, but to allow adequate opportunity for the teachers to express such concerns. Virtually all of the teachers (approximately 98% in this sample) answered the three questions, but their answers suggested concern about the home situation of only 6 of the 44 (14%) children of schizophrenic parents, which are summarized below:

1. (b) "His home situation makes it difficult for him to be 'around' other students after school or to really socialize with other boys and girls his age."
2. From one teacher: (a) "Despite apparent family problems, this young man seems able to adjust and is mature enough to handle the situation." (b) "Difficulties within his family have altered his life and forced him to become relatively independent." (c) "Sometimes interested in school, but other problems seemed to make school 'inconvenient.'" From another teacher: (a) "Stability of one good home environment." (b) "No community roots." (c) "Polite, intelligent, curious traits coupled with great concern over moving back and forth between two states."
3. (b) "Home environment, peers."
4. From one teacher: (a) "Perhaps a totally alien environment might help – away from home." (c) "She often missed concerts and musical events because of her home association." From another teacher: (a) "Going to school away from home."
5. (b) "Lives with relatives who sometimes impose conditions she doesn't accept."
6. From one teacher: (b) "Family background." From another teacher: (b) "She has grown up in an extremely unhealthy atmosphere." (c) "She is often distressed as a result of serious family problems."

From these remarks we conclude that general awareness of a problematic home situation (but possibly not of the psychiatric illness of a parent) influenced the teachers' evaluations for a small minority of the High-Risk subjects. Such "contamination" of judgment is not likely to distort the results for the sample as a whole to a substantial extent.

The research assistant met with each of the child's major-subject teachers to explain the rating scales and to ask their cooperation. All cooperating teachers were given copies of the forms which they completed in their free time and then mailed to the investigator in an envelope provided. Each teacher then received a five dollar honorarium check by mail. Most teachers agreed to make the evaluations and most delivered them as promised. The children in this study were rated by 3.15 teachers, on the average, which indicates a 79% response rate from teachers who agreed to participate. No child was rated by less than two or more than four teachers.

To compute the most stable item scores possible, all of the ratings available for each child were averaged. The PRF and HHSB factors consisted of the unweighted sum of all items comprising a particular factor.

Data analysis

Preliminary analyses were made to test for systematic sex differences or interactions of sex × risk classification. There were no significant sex differences nor interactions of sex by risk classification for any of the PRF factors. A significant sex difference (but no interaction) with risk classification was found for only one of the 28 PRF scales: orderliness. Girls were rated more orderly than boys: F (1,109) = 5.16, $p < .025$. Since this was the only sex difference on any of the dependent measures, the data for the two sexes were combined in all subsequent analyses.

The experimental sample was drawn from hospitalized populations, whereas the controls were obtained through random phone sampling of the communities in which the index patients resided. These sampling procedures led to an unfortunate systematic difference between the groups: Parental social class, as measured by the Two-Factor Index of Social Position (Hollingshead, 1957), was higher for the controls ($M = 55.73$, $SD = 27.11$) than for the high-risk group ($M = 84.21$, $SD = 27.13$): F (1, 112) = 8.48, $p < 005$. Social class correlated significantly with all of the dependent measures, so the social class discrepancy between the groups could inflate the group differences on the dependent measures to produce spurious "findings." For this reason, the results for the PRF and the HHSB were analyzed in one-way Multiple Analyses of Covariance (MANCOVA) with social class covaried out.

RATIONALE

It is extraordinarily complex to predict theoretically how children of schizophrenic parents will differ behaviorally from other children. Several premises require explication in order to understand our particular predictions. The first is that about 10% of the children of schizophrenic parents are destined to become schizophrenic as adults (Erlenmeyer-Kimling, 1977; Kety, 1978) and it has been estimated that as many as 40% more of them will develop adult psychological disorders of lesser severity (Mednick & McNeil, 1968). The risk for schizophrenia increases to approximately 40% in children with two schizophrenic parents (Erlenmeyer-Kimling, 1968). The second premise is that the preschizophrenics among the children at high risk are distinguishable behaviorally at school in at least a substantial minority of cases and possibly in a slight majority of them (Watt et al., 1979). Since we are using essentially the same empirical instrument as in our "follow-back" school records study, we, therefore, expect the preschizophrenics to replicate the behavioral deviations of the preschizophrenics in our earlier archival research. The third premise is neither as obvious nor as secure as the first two: Possibly with the notable exception of depressive disorders, many children destined for other functional psychiatric disturbances as adults deviate behaviorally at school in similar ways as preschizophrenics, but to lesser extremes (Watt et al., 1979).

It might be argued that these premises betray the crudeness of our theory and of our instruments for behavioral assessment; that the teachers' evaluations measure little more than global competence at school, and thus have very limited relevance for precise differentiation of premorbid behavior. If that criticism is accepted, our predictions condense to a single one with a corollary: Children of schizophrenics have lower than average competence at school, largely attributable to the most vulnerable children (among which preschizophrenics are the most emphatic cases). That modest rationale would be acceptable to us. However, by subdividing the high-risk sample on the basis of early indications of intermediate outcome (e.g., referral in adolescence for psychological treatment or psychiatric hospitalization) and by isolating the teacher evaluations for the children of two schizophrenic parents (who have the highest actuarial risk), it may be possible to tease from the school data whether useful differentiation of behavioral styles is possible with these methods, and encourage us to test more precise theoretical predictions, as follows.

Hypotheses

With the results of our follow-back research in mind (Watt et al., 1979), these predictions are listed in descending order of confidence or likelihood of confirmation:

1. Children (especially sons) of schizophrenic parents have less harmonious relations at school than normal children (PRF Factor III).
2. Children of schizophrenic parents are less stable emotionally than normal children (PRF Factor IV).
3. Children (especially daughters) of schizophrenic parents are less extraverted than normal children (PRF Factor II).
4. Children of schizophrenic parents have lower intelligence than normal children.
5. Children (especially sons) of schizophrenic parents are less motivated scholastically than normal children (PRF Factor I and HHSB factors).

RESULTS

Table 2 summarizes the results concerning the PRF factors, intelligence, and parental social class. The unadjusted means and standard deviations are listed in the two columns on the left of the table. The two middle columns present the same scores after covariance adjustment for the difference in parental social class. The column on the right presents the significant univariate tests of differences between the Index and Control groups. The F-tests in parentheses show the group contrasts after the covariance adjustment for the social class difference. The footnote indicates that the multiple analyses of variance for the PRF scores were significant both with and without the social class adjustment, which shows that the school behavior of the two groups differed reliably, even when the social class discrepancy was discounted.

A refinement of the PRF results is presented in Table 3, including the means, standard deviations, and statistical contrasts for each behavioral scale that yielded a significant group difference.

The multiple analysis of covariance for the Hahnemann High School Behavior (HHSB) rating scale results was significant: $F(13, 99) = 2.00$, $p < .05$. Table 4 presents the unadjusted means, standard deviations, and univariate statistical comparisons for the seven factors that significantly differentiated the risk group from the controls. The last three factors in the table were inversely coded, so the teacher ratings favored the control children in all seven domains of scholastic behavior.

Table 2. *Summary of the means, standard deviations, and statistical contrasts between high-risk group children and controls in Sample A of the New York Project – multiple teacher evaluations on the pupil rating form (PRF), intelligence, and parental social class (SES)*

| Variables | Raw scores | | Scores adjusted for social class (SES) | | Univariate contrasts (ANCOVA Fs in parentheses) |
	Index (N = 44)	Control (N = 70)	Index (N = 44)	Control (N = 70)	F
Factor 1. Scholastic Motivation					
M	3.04	3.74	3.14	3.64	31.04****
SD	.75	.71	.74	.67	(11.53****)
Factor 2. Extraversion					
M	2.91	3.21	2.95	3.18	4.02*
SD	.69	.62	.68	.61	(2.01)
Factor 3. Harmony					
M	3.40	4.00	3.52	3.94	24.32****
SD	.73	.59	.71	.57	(10.29***)
Factor 4. Emotional Stability					
M	3.31	3.76	3.37	3.71	11.99****
SD	.80	.61	.79	.59	(5.17**)
Composite PRF score					
M	3.13	3.65	3.21	3.60	29.80****
SD	.52	.51	.50	.49	(12.16****)
Intelligence					
M	103.34	118.43	104.87	117.66	44.07****
SD	11.45	12.09	11.20	11.90	(25.85****)
Parental Social Class					
M	84.21	55.73			8.48***
SD	27.31	27.11			

Note: The multivariate analysis of variance (MANOVA) for the four PRF factors was significant: $F_{(4, 109)} = 6.94$; $p < .001$. The multivariate analysis of covariance (MANCOVA) computed with parental social class covaried out was also significant: $F_{(4,108)} = 3.03$, $p < .025$. Scores on the PRF ranged from 1–5. High scores in the table indicate favorable ratings on the PRF, high intelligence, and *low* social class.
*$p < .05$.   **$p < .025$.   ***$p < .005$.   ****$p < .001$.

Harmony

As a group, the Index children clearly had less harmonious relations at school than the control children (Table 2). The teachers described the Index children as being significantly more unpleasant, unpopular, negativistic, and maladjusted (Table 3). It is also consistent with the PRF results that the teachers rated the Index children lower on rapport with the teacher in HHSB Factor IV and higher on class disturbance and restlessness in HHSB Factor 12 (Table 4). There were no important

Table 3. *Summary of the significant group differences on the individual scales of the pupil rating form*

Factor	SES[a]-adjusted means		F
	Index children ($N = 44$)	Control children ($N = 70$)	
Factor I: Scholastic Motivation (9)			
Achievement: achieving–underachieving	3.06	3.53	5.81**
Effort: motivated–unmotivated	3.23	3.56	
Work Habits: organized–disorganized	3.02	3.62	10.88****
Reliability: dependable–undependable	3.41	3.85	6.97**
Attention: attentive–distractible	3.29	3.60	4.07*
Orderliness: orderly–careless	3.15	3.60	11.97****
Maturity: mature–immature	3.32	3.69	9.02***
Independence: independent–dependent	3.49	3.65	4.13*
Confidence: confident–insecure	3.25	3.37	
Factor II: Extraversion (8)			
Sociability: extraverted–introverted	3.01	3.24	
Loquaciousness: talkative–quiet	3.03	3.16	
Self-assertion: assertive–passive	3.21	3.33	
Inhibition: inhibited–uninhibited	2.84	2.66	
Activity Level: high–low	3.20	3.22	
Leadership: leader–follower	2.85	3.01	
Group Participation: much–little	2.97	3.30	5.05*
Presentation: exhibitionistic–modest	2.48	2.53	
Factor III: Harmony (7)			
Disposition: pleasant–unpleasant	3.83	4.21	8.13***
Mood: cheerful–somber	3.32	3.56	
Popularity: popular–unpopular	3.26	3.54	11.70****
Cooperation: compliant–negativistic	3.56	3.92	6.19**
Adjustment: well adjusted–maladjusted	3.48	3.91	9.99***
Conduct: well behaved–misbehaved	3.94	4.18	
Consideration: considerate–egocentric	3.68	3.86	
Factor IV: Emotional Stability (4)			
Tension: calm–nervous	3.26	3.52	6.00**
Emotional Control: controlled–emotional	3.67	3.98	4.73*
Impulsivity: impulsive–deliberate	2.77	2.54	
Aggression: aggressive–peaceful	2.35	2.27	

[a]SES = parental social class.
*$p < .05$.   **$p < .02$.   ***$p < .005$.   ****$p < .001$.

Table 4. *Summary of unadjusted means, standard deviations, and statistical comparisons for significant results on the Hahnemann High School Behavior Rating Scale*

Factor	High-Risk children (N = 44)	Control children (N = 70)	Univariate analysis of covariance[a] $F_{1,\,111}$
1. Reasoning Ability			
M	14.97	18.64	6.34**
SD	3.85	4.66	
2. Originality			
M	8.55	10.94	7.32**
SD	3.23	3.10	
4. Rapport with Teachers			
M	10.59	12.16	7.23**
SD	2.57	2.59	
5. Anxious Producer			
M	5.62	7.26	9.87***
SD	1.51	1.95	
8. Poor Work Habits			
M	13.87	15.80	3.96*
SD	3.22	2.66	
9. Lacks Intellectual Independence			
M	19.28	22.24	10.05***
SD	3.73	3.11	
12. Disturbance–Restless			
M	16.88	18.78	4.21*
SD	4.69	2.46	

[a]The covariate was parental social class.
*$p < .05$.   **$p < .01$.   ***$p < .005$.

sex differences on this variable, though there were such differences in the follow-back study (preschizophrenic boys were much more disruptive).

Emotional stability

Index children were regarded as less stable emotionally than Control children (Table 2). There were significant group differences on two of the four scales comprising PRF Factor IV: Index children were rated more nervous and more emotional than Controls (Table 3). The results here replicate the follow-back findings despite the fact that two of the original Emotional Stability scales were shifted to the Scholastic Motivation factor (maturity and confidence) and two were shifted to the Harmony factor (mood and adjustment).

Extraversion

Factor II was the only PRF factor that did not retain its significant group difference after the covariance adjustment for social class (Table 2). Only one of the
eight scales on that factor showed a significant univariate group contrast: Index
children were judged to participate less in class than Control children.

Intelligence

The magnitude and significance of the IQ difference between the groups, even
after the social class adjustment, were considerably larger than we expected. The
mean difference exceeded one standard deviation. The very high average IQ of
our Controls (SES-adjusted $M = 118$) raises the question whether our sampling
procedures for the Controls may have introduced a bias for high intelligence
because all of the Controls were volunteers. This would be consistent with the
finding from another study in the larger project that there is no difference with
respect to IQ between High-Risk and Psychiatric Control groups, both of which
were recruited in the same way from New York area psychiatric facilities. Although
the average IQ of the Index children studied here (SES-adjusted $M = 105$) is
reasonably high in the normal range, there is no question that they are less
intelligent than this Normal Control group.

What happens if intelligence is covaried out of the statistical analyses in addition
to parental social class? That renders the multivariate tests for both instruments
insignificant. The only univariate contrast that remained significant after the double covariance adjustment was for PRF Factor III, Harmony: $F (1, 110) = 4.34, p
= .04$. Obviously, intelligence was a salient component of the children's adjust-
ment at school, as judged by their teachers. This is by now a familiar finding that
replicates many of our previous investigations. It leaves one important ambiguity
that cannot presently be resolved: whether the group differences in classroom
behavior are merely epiphenomena of a pathognomonic difference in intelligence
or may have some independent significance as precursors of psychiatric disorder.

Scholastic Motivation

The group difference for PRF Factor I, Scholastic Motivation, was even larger
than for Factor III, Harmony (Table 2). Seven of the nine Scholastic Motivation
scales showed significant group differences as well: Achievement, Work Habits,
Reliability, Attention, Orderliness, Maturity, and Independence (Table 3). This
finding is further reinforced by significant group differences on HHSB Factors I,
II, V, VIII, and IX: Reasoning Ability, Originality, Anxious Producer, Poor Work
Habits and Lacks Intellectual Independence. Clearly the Index children were less
motivated scholastically. However, as pointed earlier, this difference may reflect
primarily the group difference in intelligence.

DISCUSSION

Children at high risk for schizophrenia by virtue of having at least one schizophrenic parent do behave differently at school than other children. They present greater disharmony, less scholastic motivation, more emotional instability, and lower intelligence than controls. They are *not* significantly more introverted than other schoolchildren. It remains ambiguous whether the behavioral differences observed in the classroom have any significance as precursors of psychopathology that is independent of intelligence. There is further ambiguity because children of schizophrenic parents are an extremely heterogeneous group, especially as regards future outcome. That ambiguity should dissipate with passing time as their development and adult psychological adjustment unfold.

In the meantime we can approximate a glimpse of the future in two ways: (1) by breaking out the results for children of two schizophrenic parents, on the assumption that a substantially larger portion of them are destined to become schizophrenic themselves; and (2) by breaking out the results for those small subsamples that have already been treated psychiatrically or hospitalized since the school assessments were completed, on the assumption that such *intermediate outcomes* single out children with the highest likelihood of ultimate schizophrenic outcome. We can summarize our impressions of the behavioral profiles for four children with two schizophrenic parents, six high-risk children who have received treatment already, and three high-risk children who have been hospitalized.

The SES-adjusted scores for the four PRF factors, the PRF total and intelligence (as measured individually in the laboratory) were rank ordered from highest (indicating good adjustment) to lowest (indicating poor adjustment) for all 114 subjects. Precentile scores were then computed for each individual on each factor. Two of the four children with two schizophrenic parents fell in the bottom quartile for Scholastic Motivation, Harmony, Emotional Stability, Total PRF score, and Intelligence. A third of the four was rated at the 25th percentile for Emotional Stability. *None* of them was judged to belong in the bottom quartile for Extraversion. Indeed, two of the four were placed at or above the 90th percentile for Extraversion, and the lowest score on that factor was at the 37th percentile! Emphatically, children of two schizophrenic parents are *not* introverted at school, at least in this study.

Among the six treated children (which includes two with two schizophrenic parents), three were rated in the bottom quartile for Harmony and Emotional Stability. Those three and one more had total PRF scores in the bottom quartile for Scholastic Motivation. Three treated children were judged extreme on Introversion. Those three and one more had IQs at or below the 25th percentile.

Two of the three hospitalized subjects were rated in the bottom quartile on Harmony. One of those two was also in the lowest quartile on Scholastic Motivation, Emotional Stability, and Total PRF score. The other was also rated in the bottom quartile on Introversion and Intelligence.

By these criteria, one could infer that the most dependable markers for vulnerability to schizophrenia are Disharmony (unpleasant, unpopular, negativistic, and maladjusted), Emotional Instability (nervous, emotional), and low Intelligence. Low Scholastic Motivation has some discriminating value, but never by itself – always in combination with Disharmony or Emotional Instability. Introversion distinguished half of the treated children, but was a weak marker for hospitalization and had no relation to the highest actuarial risk for schizophrenia, namely having two schizophrenic parents. Introverted behavior may prove to relate to schizophrenic outcome most plausibly not as a *static typology* of childhood development, but as a *dynamic phase* in a process of withdrawal beginning with *protest*, followed by a stage of *despair* and ultimately giving way to *apathy* (Bowlby, 1973; Ricks, 1980). In this schema, preschizophrenics might be considered *not* as introverted types of children, but as coping individuals who react to stress with an understandable pattern of adaptations. The first two stages of reaction may be considered fairly reversible whereas the last, apathy, is far more stable and resistant to change. The protest and despair stages would still be considered as premorbid aspects of character development, because they may precede the onset of disintegrative psychotic symptoms by as many as 5 or 10 or even 20 years. This is an appealing rationale also because it is highly consistent with the remainder of our results: The children at risk for schizophrenia in our study certainly seem to be struggling and protesting and failing in their adjustment at school. If they have two schizophrenic parents or if they are destined for early hospitalization, their protest is strident, but withdrawal is not yet salient. An exception to this reasoning is that among those who will soon be treated as out-patients for psychological difficulties, an appreciable proportion already show some evidence of interpersonal retreat. Conceivably, theirs is a tactical or temporary retreat that will not transpose to the intransigent apathy typically associated with chronic schizophrenic disorder.

14 Assessment of the New York High-Risk Project subjects in Sample A who are now clinically deviant

L. ERLENMEYER-KIMLING,
CLARICE KESTENBAUM, HECTOR BIRD, AND
ULLA HILLDOFF

Subjects in the first sample (Sample A) of the New York High-Risk Project were first seen between the ages of 7 and 12 years in 1971–1972. The mean age of this sample is now 17.5 years, and most of the subjects have thus entered the schizophrenia risk period. Although we cannot expect to draw conclusions about final clinical outcome until this sample has passed through a much larger proportion of the risk years, it is of interest to examine the subjects who have already manifested some type of clinical deviance up to this point and to consider whether any of our early assessment measures could have led us to predict that these particular subjects would experience disturbances later on.

Of the 205 subjects in Sample A, 8 have been hospitalized for a psychiatric disorder and 15 are or have been in psychiatric treatment to date. (Three of the latter have not actually been treated but are experiencing severe problems for which treatment is indicated.) The problems exhibited by the subjects in the treatment group are diverse. Although it is clear that most of these subjects are functioning poorly, it is not clear whether two of the subjects (see THR3 and TPC2 in Table 2) should be classed with the others as showing significant psychopathology. These subjects are included for the present but may be removed from the clinically deviant group upon further follow-up.

For convenience in this report, hospitalized subjects with a schizophrenic parent are labeled HHR (hospitalized high-risk); hospitalized subjects whose parents have affective disorders are labeled HPC; hospitalized subjects with normal parents are labeled HNC; and treated subjects are labeled THR, TPC, and TNC, respectively.

As shown in Table 1, the eight hospitalized subjects include five with a schizo-

This research was supported, in part, by Grants MH 19560 and MH 30921 from the National Institute of Mental Health, by a grant from the W. T. Grant Foundation, and by the Department of Mental Hygiene of the State of New York.

We wish to thank Drs. Martha Trautman and Cyrus Ayromloui for their work in interviewing the subjects in the New York High-Risk Study and rating the videotaped interviews. We thank Drs. Barbara Cornblatt and Yvonne Marcuse, Ms. Ruth Meyerson, Rochelle Schwartz, and Barbara Maminski and Mr. Thomas Chin for preparing data and other materials for this report. We thank Mr. Jeff Adamo for carrying out diagnostic work on the parents and children using the RDC.

Table 1. *Subjects from Sample A hospitalized or in psychiatric treatment*

Group	Male	Female	Total	Group[a] label
Hospitalized				
Schizophrenic mother	1	3	4 ⎫	
Schizophrenic father	—	1	1 ⎬	HHR
Two affected parents	—	1	1 ⎫	
Depressed mother	—	1	1 ⎬	HPC
Normal parents	1	—	1	HNC
Total	2	6	8	
In treatment				
Schizophrenic mother	5	1	6 ⎫	
Schizophrenic father	1	1	2 ⎬	THR
Two schizophrenic parents	—	2	2 ⎭	
Depressed mother	2	2	4	TPC
Normal parents[b]	1	—	1	TNC
Total	9	6	15	

[a]Group labels assigned for this report.
[b]Does not include one (male) child dead of overdose.

phrenic mother or father, one child whose parents both have affective disorders, one child of a depressed mother, and one child of normal parents. Two of the hospitalized subjects (HHR3 and HHR4) with a schizophrenic mother are sisters, and they have a brother (THR5) in the treatment group; two of their older siblings, who were over the age of 12 at the start of the study and were therefore not included as study children, have also been hospitalized. Another hospitalized girl (HHR1) with a schizophrenic (or schizoaffective, mainly schizophrenic) mother has two brothers (THR1 and THR2) in the treatment group; the father in this family, although never hospitalized or treated for psychiatric disorder, appears to be a latent schizophrenic from his Minnesota Multiphasic Personality Inventory (MMPI) profile and clinical interview (I. I. Gottesman, personal communication). The hospitalized daughter (HHR5) of a schizophrenic father also has a brother (THR8) in the treatment group. The family history of the hospitalized subject (HNC1) with normal parents indicates some degree of psychopathology in the grandparents on both sides and possibly in a maternal aunt; the subject's father was hospitalized for "fatigue" while in the army.

The 15 subjects in treatment include eight offspring with a schizophrenic mother or father and two with two schizophrenic parents, four children with depressed mothers – constituting two brother–sister pairs – and one subject with normal parents. According to the RDC, the mother of THR1 and THR2 and the mother of THR6 are diagnosed schizoaffective, mainly schizophrenic. The mothers of

TPC1 and TPC2 are diagnosed by the RDC as schizoaffective, mainly affective. There is some history of psychopathology in the family of the subject with normal parents. (A male subject with normal parents who died of a drug overdose is not included with the psychiatrically disturbed group.)

In this chapter, we will briefly describe the problems for which the 23 subjects are being treated, the predictive statements made by two of us (CK and HB) – the child psychiatrists on the team – in blind assessments of materials collected on the children at their initial examination, and the standing of the children on several of the laboratory measures administered in 1971–1972 during the first round of testing.

PROBLEMS REQUIRING TREATMENT AND PREDICTIVE ASSESSMENTS BASED ON ROUND 1 TESTING

Table 2 lists the main problems shown by the subjects in the treatment groups and gives the diagnoses made according to the Research Diagnostic Criteria on the children in the hospitalized groups. The RDC were applied in a blind evaluation of case record and other materials on the hospitalized subjects. Predictive statements and Global Assessment Scale (GAS) scores made by CK and HB based on materials from the first round of testing are also given in Table 2.

The materials used in formulating the predictive assessments were: statements made by the parents about the children in the initial parent interview conducted in the subjects' homes, statements made by the children about themselves in the children's interview, a summary of psychological test data (WISC, Bender Gestalt, and Human Figure Drawing), comments by the pediatric neurologist, and total scores on the neurological exam and the Lincoln–Oseretsky Test of Motor Impairment. Assessments were made by CK and HB independently, and blindly with respect to parental group membership or with respect to the child's treatment status, on all of the hospitalized cases and an equal number of well-functioning children from all subject groups in Sample A. The same procedure was followed by CK for the subjects in psychiatric treatment. In addition to the predictive assessments, a Global Assessment Scale (Endicott et al., 1976) score was assigned to each child based on the same materials. The Global Assessment Scale (GAS) is a 100-point scale, ranging from superior functioning (100 points) to extreme deterioration (0 points). Table 2 lists the GAS scores assigned by CK who had an opportunity to rate each child.

As can be seen in Table 2, the predictive assessments of the two raters were in complete agreement for the hospitalized subjects and were correct in identifying seven of the eight subjects. Among eight currently well-functioning cases used to keep the raters blind, one child was predicted to be at risk by both raters, one was questioned as being at risk by both raters, and a third was predicted to be at risk by one rater (HB). Less accurate, but better than chance, predictions were made for the subjects who are now in psychiatric treatment. Mean GAS scores were: 43 for the hospitalized subjects, 56 for the THR subjects, 58 for the other treated

Table 2. Problems of the 23 clinically deviant subjects and predictive assessments and GAS scores made by child psychiatrists

Group	Case No.	Gender	Brief description of problem	Predictive assessment[a] CK	Predictive assessment[a] HB	GAS scores
HHR	(1)	F	RDC: Schizophrenia	Risk for Sz	At risk	40
	(2)	M	RDC: Atypical premorbid schizophrenia with organicity	At risk (already ill)	At risk	28
	(3)	F	RDC: Schizophrenia	Not at risk	Not at risk	65
	(4)	F	RDC: Schizophrenia	Risk for Sz	At risk	33
	(5)	F	RDC: Schizoaffective	Risk for Sz	At risk	35
HPC	(1)	F	RDC: Schizophrenia; clinical impression, Affective disorder	Risk for Aff	At risk	55
	(2)	F	RDC: Probable affective disorder	Risk for Aff	At risk	59
HNC	(1)	M	RDC: No diagnosis DSM-III: Paranoid with schizotypal features	Risk for Sz	At risk	32
THR	(1)	M	Loner; in room all day; won't leave house; refuses to talk	Not at risk	—	75
	(2)	M	Loner; watches TV all day; no friends; secretive; transvestite	Risk for Sz	—	49
	(3)	M	Varied problems; promiscuous homosexual; pederast (questionable whether he belongs in this group)	Not at risk	—	78
	(4)	M	Loner; no friends at all; withdrawn; nervous symptoms; up to age 8–9 years, rocking for hours; angry; suspicious; sleeps all day	Risk for Sz	—	42
	(5)	M	No friends; picked on and is scapegoated by others; fights a lot; poor school work	Risk for Sz	—	53

(6)	F	Paranoid, thought people talking about her behind her back, calling her a lesbian; isolated; sleeps all day; stayed in bed for a few months	Risk for Aff	—	49
(7)	F	Discipline problem from early years; frequently ran away; enuresis; history of dizzy spells	Dull normal making fair adjustment	—	70
(8)	M	Difficulties getting along with family, teachers, and peers; temperamental, fidgety all the time; tense and nervous	Risk for Aff with possible sociopathy	—	58
(9)	F	Highly disturbed behavior; killed pets; destroys own and others' belongings; used towels instead of toilet paper and hid them in closet; picks at skin; enuretic until age 15; steals money from family; threw knife at guardian; threatens to kill self or others	At great risk for Sz	—	38
(10)	F	Masturbates with animals; sexually molested a boy in 2nd–3rd grade; accident prone; withdrawn and depressed; isolated; feels others tell lies about her and blame her for things she didn't do; suicide attempt (gesture?); impulsivity	Behavior disorder	—	50

(continued)

Table 2. (*cont.*)

Group	Case No.	Gender	Brief description of problem	Predictive assessment[a]		GAS scores
				CK	HB	
TPC	(1)	F	Memory lapses; distant; stole money (questionable whether she belongs in this group)	Normal child	—	80
	(2)	M	Depressed, unhappy, tired; sleeping difficulties; lonely; picked on by others; easily frustrated; kissing other boys in 2nd–3rd grade	At risk for Sz	—	52
	(3)	M	Jail 3 times for stealing cars; shoplifting; gets drunk; uses drugs. *Prior:* bad temper; easily frustrated; fidgety, nervous; fights a lot; enuresis until 11.5 years; impulsivity	At risk for sociopathic problems	—	45
	(4)	F	No social life; depressed; unhappy; temperamental; ran away several times; school behavioral and academic problems; fights a lot; impulsivity	At risk for acting up, antisocial behavior	—	45
TNC	(1)	M	In therapy since 4th grade; frightened of everything; withdrawn from social interactions (but later improved); clumsy, uncoordinated; moody; easily frustrated; poor concentration	Some MBD indications with soft signs. At risk for possible depression	—	55

[a]Sz = schizophrenia; Aff = affective disorder.

232

subjects (TPC and TNC), and 62 for the well-functioning subjects. Thus, the data collected at the first round of testing provided a fairly good basis for making clinical predictions.

PERFORMANCE ON MEASURES FROM THE FIRST ROUND
OF TESTING

In the first round of testing in 1971–1972, Sample A was administered a battery of tests as shown in Table 2 of Chapter 10. Several of the tests are considered here where the standing of the 23 clinically deviant subjects on these measures can be compared with the performance of their main subject groups as a whole (i.e., the HR, NC, and PC groups).

WISC IQs. The mean Full-Scale IQ of the five HHR subjects is 11 points below the mean for the entire HR group (93 vs. 104). Whereas the HR group as a whole shows only a 2-point difference between Performance and Verbal IQ (105 vs. 103, respectively), the HHR subjects average 11 points difference favoring Performance IQ (99 vs. 88 for Verbal IQ); one subject (HHR2), however, does have a higher Verbal than Performance score. The THR subjects show no mean discrepancy at all between the Verbal and Performance scores, but this is due largely to one subject (THR6) with a Verbal IQ 28 points above her Performance IQ; without this subject, there would be a 13-point difference in favor of Performance IQ.

Each of the two HPC subjects has a Full-Scale IQ above the mean for the PC group as a whole (117 and 109 vs. 104), but the TPC subjects have a somewhat lower mean (100). The HPC subjects have higher Verbal than Performance scores (114 vs. 109, respectively), but the TPC subjects have a difference in the opposite direction (98 vs. 102). Thus, unlike the HHR and THR subgroups, the children from the PC group who are not showing clinical deviance do not appear to exhibit either a clear IQ decrement or a consistent direction of the difference between Performance and Verbal IQ.

The one HNC subject has a Full-Scale IQ of 123, a Performance IQ of 133, and a Verbal IQ of 109, in contrast to a mean of 116 for the entire NC group and a single point discrepancy between Performance and Verbal IQ. The TNC subject, however, is lower than the NC group as a whole, with a Full-Scale IQ of 109 and a 5-point difference favoring Verbal over Performance IQ (111 vs. 106).

Although the number of clinically deviant subjects is too small to permit any conclusions to be drawn regarding the possible role of IQ in relation to the development of early clinical problems, the data on the HHR and THR subjects are provocative. They suggest the hypothesis that subjects who are at high risk for schizophrenia *and* who have lower Full-Scale IQs may show clinical deviance at earlier ages than HR subjects with higher IQs – or, possibly, that fewer of the latter will develop serious clinical disorders even with further follow-up.

Bender–Gestalt Test. All of the HHR subjects performed relatively poorly on the Bender–Gestalt Test according to the Koppitz (1963) scoring system; the HHR subject with the best Bender score received a poorer score than 50% of all HR subjects and 80% of the NC subjects of his age. All but 3 of the 10 THR subjects received scores that were worse than at least 50% of the HR subjects as a whole and at least 80% of the NC-subjects of the same ages; the remaining 3 were outperformed by 20 to 25% of HR subjects and 30 to 45% of the NC subjects of the same age.

One of the HPC subjects also did poorly on the Bender, but the other was at top performance for PC subjects of her age. TPC subjects ranged in comparison to the PC group as a whole, from performances in the TPC group that were bettered by only 20% of the PC group to a TPC subject whose performance was bettered by 80% of the PC group. Both the HNC and the TNC subjects were among the worst performers in the NC group on the Bender-Gestalt Test.

Human Figure Drawing Test. The Human Figure Drawing Test did not discriminate consistently any of the subgroups of clinically deviant subjects from their main groups as a whole, either in terms of the number of Emotional Indicators flagged under the Koppitz (1968) scoring system, in terms of missing expectable items for their age groups (Koppitz, 1968), or in terms of total developmental score.

Neurological examination and Lincoln–Oseretsky Test of Motor Impairment. The clinically deviant subjects of all subgroups tended to have relatively poor total scores on the pediatric neurology examination or on the Lincoln–Oseretsky Test of Motor Impairment or on both. For example, subjects in the HHR group scored more poorly than 48% to 95% of the HR group as a whole on the neurological examination and more poorly than 10% to 90% of the entire HR group on the Lincoln–Oseretsky. All but one of the five HHR subjects had a score that was worse than the poorest performing 50% of the entire HR group on either or both measures. Results were similar for each of the other clinically deviant subgroups related to their own main groups with age taken into account. Nevertheless, it is important to note that individual members of the several subgroups performed very well on either the neurological examination or the Lincoln–Oseretsky Test of Motor Impairment and, in two cases (THR3 and TPC2), performance was excellent on both measures. As it happens, the latter two cases are the ones that are considered questionable for inclusion among the clinically deviant subjects.

Like the Bender-Gestalt Test, both the neurological examination and the Lincoln-Oseretsky Test of Motor Impairment appear to have some use, in conjunction with other data, in drawing predictions of psychopathological outcome. However, these three measures are evidently not related to parental diagnostic group or the type of psychopathology shown by the child.

Continuous Performance Test. The Continuous Performance Test administered in our laboratory on the first round of testing (Erlenmeyer-Kimling et al., Chapter 10; and Cornblatt & Erlenmeyer-Kimling, Chapter 12, this volume; Rutschmann et al., 1977) was a measure of sustained visual attention in which the subject was

Table 3. *Composite attentional score (number of response indices scored as deviant) for the HHR and THR subjects combined and the remainder of the HR group*

Number of response indices scored as deviant	HHR and THR (%)	Remainder of HR (%)
0–1	27	57
2–3	20	27
4+	53	16
Total	100	100

required to make a keypress to the second of two successive identical stimuli; on half of the blocks of trials, auditory distraction in the form of a tape-recorded voice was present. All of the HHR and the two HPC subjects – but not the HNC subject – had deviant scores and were below the cutoff score for the most poorly performing 5% of the NC group on two or more response indices. This was true also of 7 out of the 10 THR subjects and for the TNC subject, but not for any of the 4 TPC subjects.

Composite attentional indices (CPT and ATS). Another measure of attention administered to Sample A in the first round of testing was the Attention Span Task (ATS) in which the subject was required to repeat a series of letters (three or five letters) immediately after a tape-recorded voice had completed the series; distraction, in the form of a tape-recorded opposite-sex voice reciting digits, was inserted between the target letters on about half the trials. As noted in Cornblatt and Erlenmeyer-Kimling (Chapter 12, this volume), eight response indices were available from the CPT and the Attention Span. Deviance on any response index was defined as a score below the cutoff score that identified the most poorly performing 5% of the NC group. The number of response indices on which each subject was deviant by this criterion was tallied to provide a composite attentional score. Although HR subjects as a whole were found to be deviant on a significantly higher number of indices than were the NC subjects (see Cornblatt & Erlenmeyer-Kimling, Chapter 12, this volume), it is of particular interest that the HHR and THR subjects were among the worst performers on the composite score compared to the HR group as a whole. Table 3 shows the percentage of HHR and THR subjects by the number of deviant response indices compared with the remainder of the HR group.

The HNC subject was deviant on none of the response indices, but the TNC subject was deviant on four. (Data have not yet been scored on the PC group or its

Table 4. *Mean time to half-recovery of the electrodermal response*

Main subject group			Clinically deviant subgroup		
Group	N	Recovery time (sec)	Group	N	Recovery time (sec)
HR	54[a]	6.17[a]	HHR	5	6.65
			THR	10	5.72
PC	20	7.56	HPC	2	10.46
			TPC	4	7.09
NC	87	6.46	HNC	1	23.85
			TNC	1	11.16

[a]One schizophrenic parent only

HPC and TPC subgroups.) See Erlenmeyer-Kimling et al. (Chapter 10, this volume) for a discussion of the performance of the clinically deviant subjects on the signal detection index, d′, from three attentional measures.

Electrodermal response, half-time recovery. As reported in Erlenmeyer-Kimling et al. (chapter 10, this volume), electrodermal data were collected in the first round of testing of Sample A in a testing procedure similar to that used by Mednick and Schulsinger (1968) in their study of Danish children of schizophrenic mothers. In this procedure, electrodermal responses were recorded in relation to a raucous noise that was presented as an unconditioned stimulus to each of two tones, one of which was frequently paired with the raucous noise and was designated the conditioned stimulus (except that very little conditioning actually took place). The one significant difference that emerged in comparing the main subject groups in the New York high-risk study was a finding of longer response latencies in the children of schizophrenic parents – a result that was opposite to that reported by Mednick and Schulsinger. Recovery time (time to half-recovery) did not differ significantly among groups in the New York study. However, as Mednick and Schulsinger (1968) have reported that recovery time was significantly faster primarily in the high-risk subjects who became "sick," it is important to determine whether the clinically deviant subjects in the New York High-Risk Project show similarly fast recovery times even though the HR group as a whole does not.

Table 4 shows mean time to half-recovery for each of the main subject groups and for the clinically deviant subgroups. As can be seen, the HHR subjects have a somewhat larger (slower) mean recovery score than either the HR or the NC groups. The THR subjects, on the other hand, have a somewhat faster recovery time than HR subjects as a whole. Both of the HPC subjects have slower recovery than the PC group as a whole or than the TPC subgroups. The same is true of the HNC and the TNC subject compared to the NC main group. Thus, in the New York High-Risk Project, time to half-recovery of the electrodermal response in an experimental paradigm such as that used by Mednick and Schulsinger does not discriminate effectively between subjects who do and do not exhibit clinical deviance in adolescence in any of the subject groups. S. A. Mednick (1978) has noted that a major difference between the New York and Copenhagen projects in the selection of subjects is that the New York project excluded subjects from nonintact families whereas the Copenhagen project included a number of subjects from nonintact families. Mednick has indicated that this is the reason for the disparity between the two studies in their electrodermal findings. Although this may be so, it would suggest a lack of robustness in the relationship between risk for schizophrenia and the electrodermal pattern found in the Copenhagen project.

SUMMARY OF FINDINGS

In summary, the data on the subjects who have been hospitalized or in psychiatric treatment thus far suggest a pattern for the high-risk subjects in which lower IQ, a deficit in Verbal IQ, and relatively poor performance on the Bender-Gestalt Test, neurological examination, Lincoln–Oseretsky Test of Motor Impairment, and attentional indices at young ages (7 to 12 years) may be predictive of later psychopathological outcome. Although the first round of testing was conducted before the children had begun to show major signs of disorder, GAS scores based on a review of interview, psychological, and neuromotor data from that round were lower for the HR subjects who are currently clinically deviant than for other subjects in a blind (with respect to parent's diagnostic group or child's clinical subgroup) rating.

Subjects in the other clinically deviant subgroups are too few and the data too inconsistent to permit conclusions about possible patterns predictive of later psychopathological development in NC or PC subjects.

It must be kept in mind that the mean age of subjects in Sampe A is only 17.5 years. More subjects may develop serious enough disorders to require hospitalization or psychiatric treatment in the future, and it remains to be seen whether they will show the same pattern of early measures as has been observed in the HHR and THR subjects. Moreover, although the subjects who have already been hospitalized will clearly remain in an outcome group that could be labeled "sick," some of the subjects who are in treatment may outgrow their problems and move out of the sick group. Thus, it is premature to attempt to draw conclusions about the relationship of performance on the early measures and long-term psychiatric outcome of the subjects in our sample, although it is certainly possible to say that there is a strong relationship between performance on the early measures and the development of psychopathology in adolescence.

EPILOGUE

To illustrate the quality of illness and background of the HHR subjects, a case vignette follows.

Case HHR1

Daughter of a schizophrenic mother (schizoaffective, mainly schizophrenic by the RDC). Age 15 at first hospitalization. Subject's RCD diagnosis: schizophrenia, disorganized; subacute.

Family history. Schizophrenic mother has been hospitalized four times. Mother's twin sister is also schizophrenic, and mother's paternal aunt has been hospitalized 33 years. HHR1's father, deceased (diabetic coma), was described as suspicious and violently abusive toward wife and children. Although he was never hospitalized, his MMPI profile was interpreted as being consistent with latent schizophrenia or schizoaffective illness; his father was alcoholic. Two of HHR1's four siblings, all males, developed serious psychological difficulties and are currently considered at great risk for schizophrenic breakdown; both are included in the THR subgroup (THR1 and THR2, see Table 2). Home life was chaotic.

Round 1 findings. HHR1 was first studied at the age of 11.5 years. In the parent interview, she was reported to have been an overly active infant, whose development was early. At the time of the interview, she was described as moody and prone "since birth" to tantrums. In the interview with HHR1, when asked what she did with friends, she answered "walk around, make trouble, and annoy people." She described herself as getting angry and hitting people.

On the WISC, HHR1 obtained a Full-Scale IQ of 100, with a 16 point discrepancy between Performance and Verbal IQ (Verbal 92, Performance 108). The lowest score was Comprehension (2). The Koppitz Emotional Indicators on the Human Figure Drawing Test indicated timidity, impulsivity, and lack of organization. Her Bender Gestalt developmental score was at the 15th percentile of the HR group (i.e., 85% of HR subjects scored better than this subject). She scored relatively poorly on the neurological examination and on the Lincoln–Oseretsky Test of Motor Impairment. She was deviant on the CPT.

In the review of the first round findings, one rater (CK) observed: "This child is having difficulty controlling impulses and shows evidence of learning difficulties, specifically in language development. She may have increasing school and subsequent social difficulty as she gets older. She appears to be at risk for schizophrenia."

Developmental history. HHR1's early life was characterized by many separations and disruptions because of her mother's psychiatric hospitalizations. She was placed intermittently in institutions or foster care from age 6 to 12 and eventually was sent to live with a married half brother. At age 12 she became sexually involved with a 24-year-old alcoholic man. At age 14 she returned to live with her mother, continued to spend time with her alcoholic boyfriend, drinking beer and smoking marijuana. School work deteriorated. When HHR1's father died after a long illness (diabetes), she reportedly did not mourn his death. She became increasingly withdrawn, smiling and laughing inappropriately, neglectful of personal appearance. Following a fight with her boyfriend and her older brother, she threatened to kill her brother or herself, claiming she heard a voice telling her to kill her brother. She was hospitalized. During her hospitalization (interrupted for a month by her mother's removing her against doctors' advice) she was seen talking out loud and writing letters to her dead father; she was noted to have poor concentration, flight of ideas, concrete thinking, and visual and auditory hallucinations. On psychological tests she obtained a Full-Scale IQ of 85, Verbal 92 (same as at age 11.5) and Performance 81. She had a defective score in block design and much attentional fluctuation due to "preoccupation with inner turmoil."

HHR1 was discharged after 6 months to residential care but was unable to remain in the institution because of assaults on others, homo- and heterosexual preoccupations, and laxity in personal hygiene. She was eventually returned to residential care on maintenance phenothiazine medication.

Round 3 laboratory visit. HHR1 completed a second round of testing at age 13, before the manifestation of her illness and a third round at age 19 while she was still in residential care. She was maintained at that time on Mellaril (200 mg/day).

The laboratory staff noted that she demonstrated extremely poor social judgment, exhibited loosening of associations, and was concrete in her responses (e.g., "breakfast?, Oh, break—fast, I see!").

The Mental Health Assessment Form (see Erlenmeyer-Kimling et al., Chapter 10, this volume) was administered. She received low (poor) scores on items concerned with: constriction of affect, depressive affect, history of anger, depression, depressive equivalent, irritability, difficulty with parents and siblings, superficial relationships, dissatisfaction with behavior, presence of symptoms which interfered with function and drug abuse (alcohol, marijuana, and hashish). She was rated as having a GAS score of 32.5.

She described herself to the interviewer as always being fearful and shy. "I always knew there was something wrong with me." She said she was closer to her father than to any other human being. When asked about depression, she answered, "I am not too sure what depressed is."

Current status. HHR1 is currently in a group home, maintained on Mellaril, 100 mg b.i.d. She is obtaining a high school equivalency with the aid of a math tutor, does volunteer work in a hospital, and is taking driver's education training. She visits her mother at home each weekend, but is not yet able to live away from the structured setting.

PART V

The Stony Brook High-Risk Project: 1971–1982

The Stony Brook Project has developed into what might be termed a classic psychosocial study of children at risk for psychopathology. It began as a cross-sectional study of young school-aged children whose mother or father had a current schizophrenic or depressive psychosis. It combined (1) highly refined research diagnostic criteria for the clinical assessment of both parents; (2) laboratory measures of attention and cognitive functioning; (3) teacher and classmate peer assessments of social and academic functioning; and (4) parent and child ratings of family functioning. As the project moved into its current longitudinal phase, the investigators demonstrated their own considerable clinical, laboratory, and community experience by adapting their original measures to the now older high school samples. Most importantly, the Stony Brook Project now has the largest cohort of prospectively studied children at risk for psychopathology, with a considerable portion of its sample representing children at risk for affective disorders.

Still of great interest to this project are sets of dimensional variables that are viewed as important to the development of psychopathology. Their search for *precursors* of schizophrenia has focused on measures of cognitive slippage and attentional deficits. Relevant to the *environmental* dimension are family functioning variables, such as parenting characteristics and marital discord; this dimension considers "environment" as characterized by both stressful and protective factors. Finally, there is the dimension of *competence*, which is viewed as important because it allows them to develop a descriptive picture of the children.

The reader will find that as the result of the breadth of the measures chosen in the Stony Brook Project, there are numerous opportunities to compare their methodology and findings to those of most all the other risk projects in this volume.

241

15   *The Stony Brook High-Risk Project*

SHELDON WEINTRAUB AND JOHN M. NEALE

It is well established that children of schizophrenic parents are at high risk for the development of psychiatric maladjustment in adulthood, but relatively little is known about what they are like as children and how and why some of them start down a path leading to schizophrenia in adulthood. Thus the goals of the Stony Brook Project have been to: (1) obtain a detailed picture of the characteristics of children with a schizophrenic parent; (2) relate child characteristics to parental diagnosis and environmental variables in the home and school; (3) identify particularly vulnerable and invulnerable children; (4) assess the ways in which the child and family unit are affected by and cope with the stresses of psychiatric disorder and hospitalization; and (5) identify precursors specific to the development of schizophrenia.

The framework for the Stony Brook Project is derived from a diathesis–stress approach to schizophrenia, with a particular focus on the factors that might potentiate the diathesis. Because schizophrenics show such heterogeneity, in terms of symptoms, course, and outcome, we believe there is little justification to search for a single antecedent marker variable. It is more likely that there are multiple developmental pathways to schizophrenia, a position supported by our own data as well as by the follow-up and follow-back literature. Three strategies guided our selection of variables. First, drawing on current data and theory pertaining to schizophrenia, we selected variables that may reflect either the high-risk genotype or early signs of the disorder, and created downward extensions of these variables appropriate for school-aged children.

Our second strategy was to focus on the social and academic competence of the children gathered from parents, teachers, and peers and providing a broad-based descriptive picture of the high-risk child. The importance of competence to schizophrenia is indicated both by the schizophrenics' social incompetence, and by the fact that measures of competence prove to be the most powerful predictors of course and outcome for adult schizophrenics. Additionally, competence, as measured by teacher and peer ratings, is an effective predictor of later maladjustment.

Our third strategy attempts to characterize the environment of the high-risk

This research was supported by Grant MH 21145 from the National Institute of Mental Health and funds from the William T. Grant Foundation.

243

child. We are collecting the children's phenomenological ratings of the stressfulness of life events and of the child-rearing characteristics of their parents. We are trying to develop a picture of *environmental noxiousness* by examining marital discord, parenting practices, sibling relationships, family structure and dynamics, and behaviors directed toward the child by peers.

The first stage of the project was cross-sectional in design. Schizophrenic mothers and fathers were recruited into the project and administered a detailed diagnostic battery. Depressed and normal parents were selected and assessed as well. Evaluations of the spouse and home environment were conducted. Our cross-sectional sample now consists of 245 families, including 94 with a schizophrenic parent, 66 with a depressed parent, and 60 normal controls. Assessment of the children included an evaluation of their cognitive, social, and personal competence, and an attempt to identify precursor patterns, early signs, and variables hypothesized to be relevant to schizophrenia. In the first stage, 374 children were tested in our lab, including 147 with a schizophrenic parent, 93 with a depressed parent, and 134 normal controls. Outside the lab, 687 children were assessed in the schools, including 154 with a schizophrenic parent, 91 with a depressed parent, and 442 normal controls.

Although cross-sectional data allow important descriptive statements to be made about the adjustment and other characteristics of vulnerable children, the most important contribution of the high-risk method will come from studies in which these children are followed longitudinally. In a cross-sectional comparison, children in the High-Risk group might differ from controls on a variable which would in adulthood fail to differentiate those who break down from those who do not. It is only through a longitudinal study that one can examine the variables that are crucial for an adult schizophrenic outcome. Therefore, a better understanding of schizophrenia and the possible discovery of early signs of later maladjustment will come only through the longitudinal study of these children at risk, which constitutes the second stage of the project. One hundred ninety-seven families have participated in our follow-along evaluations, including 72 with a schizophrenic parent, 53 with an affectively ill parent, and 52 normal controls. The total number of project "casualties" (those who have moved plus those who refused to participate further) is 48, or 19.6%. We have lost 23.4% of our schizophrenics, 19.7% of our affectives, and 13.4% of our normal controls.

SELECTION, ASSESSMENT, AND DIAGNOSIS OF PARENTS

Two parent variables are being investigated: diagnosis (i.e., schizophrenic, depressed, normal) and sex (mother, father). Our primary focus is on schizophrenia, but by including depressed patients the effects of being reared by a parent with a psychiatric disorder may be controlled, while specific schizophrenic parent rearing patterns and genotype are allowed to vary. As Garmezy (1969, 1971) has noted, depressed parents constitute an excellent nonschizophrenic psychiatric control group because depression appears to be a distinct clinical entity, is not implicated as a precursor to schizophrenia (Heston, 1966), and is characterized by different patterns of premorbid social competence (Zigler & Phillips, 1960).

Children of both male and female psychiatric patients are studied to provide a more complete sample and to enable us to clarify the potential interaction effect of sex of patient with the sex of child on the child's adjustment (Gardner, 1967; Orvaschel, Mednick, Schulsinger, & Rock, 1979). Since marriage is an indicator of good premorbid status for male schizophrenics (Held & Cromwell, 1968), many of the schizophrenic fathers in our sample will be characterized by a good premorbid adjustment.

The selection process

All new psychiatric admissions with school-aged children at any of the four local inpatient mental health facilities were considered for selection. All inpatients hospitalized for reasons other than alcoholism, drug abuse, or central nervous system impairment were approached for selection into the study.

Two types of normal controls have been incorporated into the research design: classroom controls and family controls. For all school comparisons, each target child is compared with two classmates. One of these is a same-sex but otherwise randomly drawn child from the same classroom; the other is matched to the target child on sex, age, race, social class, and IQ. Matching was conducted to control for potential confounds, or *nuisance variables.* Social class, for example, might account for differences found between high- and low-risk children. On the other hand, matching involves the tacit assumption that the matching variables are merely peripheral correlates and unrelated to the development of schizophrenia. This assumption may not be warranted with variables such as social class and IQ. In addition, matching on one variable often produces systematic unmatching on another. For these reasons, it is important to select random controls (Meehl, 1970, 1971).

Sixty families of the matched and random-control children were recruited into the project. The cooperation rate was 75%. The same assessment battery administered to the patient and the spouse on their adjustment and the home environment was administered to the control parents, and their children received the same evaluation in the lab. Thus, there is a control group for the parents as well as the children. This evaluation also provides assurance that the control children have parents with no psychiatric history.

Diagnostic assessment

The reliability and validity of psychiatric diagnosis have been the *bête noir* of many a research project and are of paramount concern in a longitudinal study. The great effort and expense involved in the establishment of a high-risk sample and in data collection would be worthless in the absence of careful, adequate attention to the major independent variable, that is, the diagnosis of the patient–parent.

Therefore, we conducted a full and detailed assessment of every parent. The battery consisted of diagnostic and behavioral evaluations of current and past social functioning and psychiatric status, as well as hospital case record data. Information was collected with the following questionnaires and structured interview procedures: The Current and Past Psychopathology Scale (CAPPS; Spitzer & Endicott, 1968); Mini-Mult (Kincannon, 1968); and Mate Adjustment Form (MAF; Weintraub & Neale, 1978).

The CAPPS (Spitzer & Endicott, 1968) is a structured diagnostic interview and psychiatric history schedule, effective in measuring psychopathology and impairment in role functioning for both patients and nonpatients. The standardized interview schedule provides a natural progression of topics with predominantly open-ended questions to elicit information needed to rate a matching inventory of scales. On most of these, severity is rated from 1 (none) to 6 (extreme). These judgments are a weighted average for the time period under study and take into account both duration and severity.

Reliability and validity for the diagnostic section of the CAPPS are respectable (Spitzer, Endicott, Fleiss, & Cohen, 1970; Endicott & Spitzer, 1972). Interjudge reliability coefficients, as determined on a series of 46 newly admitted inpatients and as measured by the intraclass correlation coefficient, range from .57 to .99 with the median value being .89 for the symptom scales, and .66 to .98 for the role scales. Test–retest reliability coefficients, computed on 25 newly admitted psychiatric patients evaluated by different interviewers at different points in time (but within a week), range from a low of .30 for Speech Disorganization to a high of .85 for Depression–Anxiety, with the median value being .57.

The use of the CAPPS makes possible meaningful comparisons across other high-risk studies. This should facilitate the efforts of other investigators to replicate findings on truly similar groups of patients, rather than on an obviously heterogeneous and dissimilar group of patients who share little more than an arbitrary diagnosis of schizophrenia (Mosher & Gunderson, 1973). An instrument such as the CAPPS, however, requires that each interviewer be trained in its administration. Our research staff underwent an extensive training program in administering and scoring the CAPPS, which involved listening to training tapes, observing experienced clinicians interviewing, and consulting with the authors of the CAPPS and their staff. Weekly tape sessions were conducted to ensure a high degree of reliability in our ratings and consistency in interviewing procedures. Reliability checks, which were conducted frequently, have shown more than adequate values, typically in the .80s. For the last 10% of the patients admitted to the project, we replaced the CAPPS with the Schedule for Affective Disorders and Schizophrenia (SADS; Spitzer & Endicott, 1979), plus a few questions from the CAPPS which enabled us to complete it as well.

The *Mini-Mult* (Kincannon, 1968) was used as an aid to diagnosis and to provide additional descriptive information. The Minnesota Multiphasis Personality Inventory (MMPI) is an instrument of demonstrated reliability and validity and has been found effective in behavioral genetic studies of schizophrenics (Gottesman & Shields, 1966, 1972). In a critical afterword to Gottesman and Shields

(1972), Meehl warns: "There is little excuse for anyone subsequently to enter upon a costly and difficult study in human behavior genetics and fail to include the MMPI in his battery." Because of time constraints, the Mini-Mult was substituted for the full MMPI. Although efforts to demonstrate the effectiveness of the Mini-Mult have produced a mixed picture, most studies of psychiatric inpatients report scale and code-type correspondence between the Mini-Mult and the full MMPI that are comparable to MMPI test–retest reliability (Kincannon, 1968; Hartman & Robertson, 1972; Lacks, 1970; Ogilvie, Kotkin, & Stanley, 1976). Winters, Weintraub, and Neale (1979) found that Marks, Seeman, and Haller (1974) codetypes produced by the Mini-Mult were as effective as full MMPI codetypes in identifying schizophrenic and depressed patients. It also appears that considerable improvement in the ability of the Mini-Mult to estimate accurately MMPI scale scores and a profile's validity can be obtained by using information on the population of interest in converting from the raw Mini-Mult scores to estimated MMPI raw scores via a substitution equation (Faschingbauer, 1976).

The Mate Adjustment Form

The MAF (Weintraub & Neale, 1978) is a structured instrument devised to obtain in a reliable, objective way the spouse's ratings of (1) past adjustment; (2) current psychopathology; (3) functioning in the roles of worker, student, housekeeper, mate, and parent; (4) effect on the children; and (5) being a burden and source of stress to the family. This instrument is modeled after the CAPPS and incorporates many of the features of the Family Evaluation Scale (Spitzer, Gibbons, & Endicott, 1971). Administration of the interview is tape recorded, and we have found the interrater reliability to be comparable to that of the CAPPS. The MAF contains 15 scales that are similar to those provided by self-report on the CAPPS: (1) performance in the worker role; (2) performance in the housekeeper role; (3) performance in parent role; (4) social contacts outside of the family; (5) neglect of basic self-care; (6) sleep disturbances; (7) inactivity; (8) general anger toward others; (9) acting out behaviors and illegal behaviors; (10) anger specifically directed toward children; (11) paranoid behavior; (12) psychotic behavior; (13) neurotic behavior; (14) manic behavior; and (15) depressive behavior. Item to total correlations revealed that no item correlated more highly with another scale than with its own. The mean item–total correlations ranged from .52 to .82, the mean being .68. Coefficient alpha ranged from .15 to .88, the mean being .66. Because some scales have very few items, these internal consistency measures are somewhat lower than is generally desired in psychometric testing.

Diagnostic Rating Form

We developed a rating form based on all of the information available to us, including tape recordings of the interviews, computer diagnoses obtained from the CAPPS with DIAGNO II (Spitzer & Endicott, 1969), and ratings of overall severity on the Global Assessment Scale (GAS; Endicott et al., 1976). The first

Table 1. *Reliability of diagnostic ratings on a sample of 106 patients*

Symptoms	r
A. *Key admission*	
Tests for schizophrenia	
Thought disorder	.86
Poor insight	.85
Social isolation/avoidance	.60
Restricted affect	.36
Catatonia	.00
Delusions	.78
Hallucinations	.86
Auditory hallucinations	.78
Tests for mania	
Elevated mood	.84
Activity level	.92
Talkativeness	.88
Flight of ideas	.85
Inflated self-esteem	.90
Decreased need for sleep	.89
Distractibility	.89
Excessive involvement in activities with high potential for painful consequences	.71
Tests for depression	
Depressed mood	.86
Poor or increased appetite/weight loss or gain	.84
Sleep difficulty or too much sleep	.85
Loss of energy	.54
Loss of interest or pleasure	.75
Self-reproach/guilt	.66
Problems in thinking/concentration	.69
Suicidal thoughts or behavior	.80
Exclusion tests (OBS–drugs–alcohol)	
Disorientation–memory loss	.60
Alcohol	.97
Drugs	.60
B. *History*	
Schizophrenia tests	.86
Elevated mood	.66
Other manic symptoms	.88
Depressed mood	.93
Other depressive symptoms	.82
OBS–alcohol–drug	.83
C. *GAS*	.81

section is a set of eight criteria for schizophrenia: formal thought disorder, poor insight, social isolation/avoidance of others, restricted affect, obvious catatonia, delusions, auditory hallucinations, and other hallucinations. Section two is comprised of eight signs of mania: elevated or irritable mood, increased activity, more talkative, flight of ideas, inflated self-esteem, decreased need for sleep, distractibility, and excessive involvement in activities with high potential for painful consequences. Section three consists of nine signs of depression: dysphoric mood, poor/increased appetite/weight loss/gain, sleep difficulty/too much sleep, loss of energy, psychomotor retardation/agitation, loss of interest/pleasure, self-reproach/guilt, diminished ability to think/concentrate, suicidal thoughts/behavior. Section 4 includes items reflecting CNS impairment and alcohol or drug abuse. Reliability of the ratings, estimated by Pearson's r between two independent raters on a sample of 106 cases, was satisfactory for all but three infrequent symptoms (see Table 1).

Diagnostic assignments were independently determined by John Neale and Sheldon Weintraub using all available information. Using J. A. Cohen's (1960) kappa statistic, the reliability of diagnosis was .96 for DSM-II schizophrenia, .94 for DSM-III schizophrenia, .92 for unipolar depression, and .92 for bipolar illness. These reliabilities are higher than those reported typically because the sample was prescreened and only a small number of categories was used.

ASSESSMENT OF THE SPOUSE AND HOME ENVIRONMENT

As discussed earlier, high-risk research may play an important role in uncovering potentiators of the genetic diathesis. Two important factors here are the well spouse and the family environment. A complete assessment of the entire family unit is essential, for the psychiatric patient–parent is not the sole influence on the child. When one parent develops a psychosis, the quality of the adjustment of the spouse may exert a critical influence on the adjustment of the children (Rutter, 1966). In the high-risk area, this point has been well demonstrated by B. Mednick (1973). She reported that most of the offspring of schizophrenic mothers who had experienced an adult breakdown also had a deviant father.

To evaluate the characteristics of the patients' spouses, the same instruments and procedures as are used with the psychiatrically disordered parent have been administered to the spouse: (1) CAPPS, (2) Mini-Mult, and (3) MAF. This information, which is tape recorded, is collected during one of two home visits. Another home visit is made to describe the emotional climate of the home, to evaluate various sociopsychological influences on the children, and to administer measures of marital adjustment, family functioning, and parent–child relationships.

Marital adjustment

The parents were evaluated with a reliable, standardized questionnaire, the Marital Adjustment Test (MAT; Locke & Wallace, 1959; Coleman & Miller, 1975). Analysis of mean total MAT scores of patients revealed a significant main effect for diagnosis ($p < .001$). Newman–Keuls tests showed that controls were significantly higher in mean total MAT scores (more satisfied) than both schizophrenics and depressives ($p < .01$), and that schizophrenics were significantly higher than depressives ($p < .05$). Analyzing patient responses to the individual items, schizophrenics and depressives reported more disagreement with their spouses than did controls in demonstrations of affection, sex relations, and conventionality (i.e., deciding "right, good, or proper conduct"). Both groups were less likely than controls to settle disagreements by mutual give and take, to engage in outside interests together, to confide in their mates, and to marry the same partner if given another chance. In addition, both groups rated their marriages as significantly less "happy" than control marriages. Schizophrenics reported more disagreement with their spouses than did control couples on matters of recreation, selection of friends, and philosophy of life. Finally, depressives reported more disagreement with their spouses than did schizophrenics on selection of friends and sex relations, and rated their marriages as significantly less happy than schizophrenics.

Turning now to the spouse data, analysis of mean total MAT scores revealed a significant main effect for diagnosis ($p > .001$). Newman–Keuls tests showed that controls were significantly higher in mean total MAT scores than the spouses of schizophrenics ($p > .01$) and the spouses of depressives ($p < .01$). Analyzing spouse responses to the individual items, spouses of schizophrenics and depressives reported more disagreement with their partners than did controls in matters of recreation, demonstrations of affection, sex relations, conventionality, and ways of dealing with in-laws. Both groups were less likely than controls to engage in outside interests with their partners and to marry the same partner if given another chance. In addition, both groups rated their marriages as significantly less happy than control marriages. Spouses of schizophrenics reported more disagreement with their partners than did controls on philosophy of life. Spouses of depressives were less likely than controls to settle disagreements by mutual give and take, marry the same partner if given another chance, and confide in their mates. Finally, spouses of depressives reported being less likely than spouses of schizophrenics to marry the same person if given another chance.

Family functioning

This was assessed with the Family Evaluation Form (FEF; Weintraub & Neale, 1978). Any attempt to measure as broad a construct as family functioning must be limited in scope for obvious, practical reasons. Areas of inquiry for family functioning were developed through modifications of the St. Paul Scale of Family Functioning (Geismar & Ayres, 1960) and the Family Evaluation Scale (Spitzer, Gibbon, & Endicott, 1971). In addition, further questions evolved out of extensive, unstructured interviews that had been tape-recorded with the spouses of the first few families who entered the project. Administration of the FEF requires approximately 1 hour of interviewing, and is tape-recorded to permit continuous monitoring of reliability. Nine scales for the FEF were constructed through a combination of theoretical and empirical decision making using the method outlined by Jackson

(1970, 1971): (1) quality of household facilities; (2) problems with family finances; (3) family solidarity; (4) marital relationship; (5) relationship among the children; (6) family embarrassment due to the illness; (7) avoidance of family by others; (8) burden of the illness on the family; and (9) general burden of the illness on others. Results of one-way ANOVAs with the well spouse as informant indicate significant differences in ratings of family solidarity, children's relations, the marriage, household facilities, and financial problems. In each instance, the well spouses rated their family functioning as more disturbed than the controls. There were no significant differences between the two patient groups, although there was a trend for the spouses of schizophrenics to see a poorer relationship among their children than do spouses of depressives ($t = 1.81, p < .075$). The results of an assessment of family functioning from the perspective of the patient, using the shorter version of the FEF that is also administered to controls, revealed group differences on all of the scales. Patients evaluated their families as more disturbed than the controls, and the depressed patients made more negative evaluations than the schizophrenic patients.

Parenting characteristics

These were assessed with the Child's Report of Parental Behavior Inventory (CRPBI; E. Schaefer, 1965a). According to various clinical acounts, the child-rearing characteristics of psychiatric patients are marked by inconsistent patterns of reinforcement, emotional distance, communication deficits, irrationality, and bizarre behavior. The research literature, however, is surprisingly sparse and offers no coherent picture. The CRPBI assesses the child-rearing characteristics of parents from the perspective of their children, yielding three orthogonal factors describing dimensions of parental child-rearing behaviors: (I) Acceptance versus Rejection; (II) Psychological Control versus Psychological Autonomy; and (III) Lax Control versus Firm Control (E. Schaefer, 1965b). In the 56-item CRPBI (Burger & Armentrout, 1971), Factor I consists of the Acceptance and Child Centeredness scales, Factor II the Control Through Guilt and Instilling Persistent Anxiety scales, and Factor III the Discipline and Nonenforcement of Rules scales. The CRPBI factors have been found to have high test–retest reliability over a 5 week period, ranging from .79 to .95 (Margolies & Weintraub, 1977). We recently conducted an analysis of the CRPBI for our sample (Weintraub, Margolies, & Neale, 1980). Schizophrenic mothers were viewed as more accepting and child centered by their children than were normal mothers by their children. Child centeredness also characterized the depressed mothers. These two female patient groups differed in that the schizophrenic mothers were reported to be more lax in the discipline of their children. Schizophrenic fathers tended to be perceived more negatively than normal fathers; their children reported that they are somewhat unaccepting and uninvolved. Depressed fathers were not viewed by their children as reliably different from controls.

According to their children, husbands of schizophrenic women were very much involved in the making of rules and regulations, in the setting of limits, and in the enforcement of these rules and limits. They and the husbands of depressed wom-

Table 2. *Number of families in each group*

Sex of patient	Diagnostic status				
	Schizophrenic	Depressed	Control	Diagnostic[a] uncertainties	Other
Male	36	24			
			60	15	10
Female	58	42			
	94	66			

[a]This category contains 10 cases in which the confidence rating was too low to assign a diagnosis, and 5 cases in which different diagnoses were assigned by John Neale and Sheldon Weintraub.

en are similar to those described by Schaefer (1965b) as using "covert psychological methods of controlling the child's activities and behaviors that would not permit the child to develop as an individual apart from the parent" (p. 555). For the husbands of schizophrenics, this is accomplished primarily by instilling anxiety; for the husbands of depressives by control through guilt. There were no differences for the wives of patients and controls.

CHARACTERISTICS OF THE SAMPLE

As seen in Table 2, there are now 245 families in our project. Our critera for inclusion here are that there was a diagnostic evaluation of the patient, a home visit, and some data collected on the children. For reasons that we will shortly discuss, we do not have complete data on all members of these families. Six hundred eighty-seven children have been completely assessed in the schools, including 154 children with a schizophrenic parent and 91 children with a depressed parent. Three hundred seventy-four children have been tested in our lab, including 147 children with a schizophrenic parent, 93 children with a depressed parent, and 134 with a normal parent (see Tables 3 and 4).

Demographic characteristics of the sample are presented in Table 5, (excluding the 11 families that joined the project most recently). Schizophrenic patients had had more previous hospitalizations and more days in the hospital than the depressed patients, but there were no significant differences in demographic characteristics among groups. The scores on education and occupation require some current comment as they are drawn from the CAPPS. Education is rated on a 7-point scale ranging from professional degree to under 7 years of school. As can be seen from Table 5, all of our groups have mean scores close to 4, which denotes a high school graduate level. Occupational level is rated on an 8-point scale ranging from higher executive–professional to not working. Again all three groups have a mean close to 4, which is equivalent to the level of "clerical or sales worker, technician, or owner of a little business."

Table 3. *Child sample by age, sex, and parental diagnosis: school assessment*

	Grade	Schizophrenic	Depressed	Normal control
Boys	2–5	39	30	131
	6–9	31	16	80
Girls	2–5	51	23	140
	6–9	33	22	91
		154	91	442

Table 4. *Child sample by age, sex, and parental diagnosis: lab assessment*

	Age	Schizphrenic	Depressed	Normal control
Boys	6–10	34	31	29
	11–15	40	16	40
Girls	6–10	39	22	32
	11–15	34	24	33
		147	93	134

Table 5. *Demographic characteristics and psychiatric history of sample*

	Diagnostic status		
	Schizophrenic	Depressed	Control
Race			
Caucasion	82	61	56
Black	7	2	1
Puerto Rican	2	0	0
Other	3	3	3
Marital status			
Married	73	51	55
Separated	13	8	2
Divorced	6	5	3
Widowed	2	2	0
Average number of children	3.34	3.71	3.59
Education[a]	3.86	3.75	3.72
Occupational level[b]	3.92	3.63	3.80
Mean age of patient			
Male	34	34	35
Female	30	31	29
Previous psychiatric hospitalizations	2.30	1.49	
Previous days in hospital	139.6	86.7	

[a]Educational level scores range from 1 (professional degree) to 7 (under 7 years of school).
[b]Occupational level scores range from 1 (higher executive, major professional) to 7 (unskilled employee).

A comparison of the key admission characteristics may be found in Table 6. The schizophrenics were higher than the depressives in schizophrenic symptoms and were rated as more severely ill on the Global Assessment Scale (GAS). The depressives were significantly higher than the schizophrenics on depressed mood and other depressed features. Notice, however, that the schizophrenics were higher than the depressives in manic features, suggesting the presence of affective components in our sample of schizophrenics. For CAPPS Summary Scale Scores, schizophrenics scored higher on Reality testing, Social Disturbance ($p < .01$) and the depressives scored higher on Depression–Anxiety ($p < .01$). Eighty-six percent of the schizophrenics received a DIAGNO II computer diagnosis of schizophrenia, based solely on the CAPPS interview. An additional 12% were diagnosed as schizoid.

The Mini-Mult modal codes, using Marks et al.'s (1974) profile coding system, were as follows:

Male schizophrenics	8 – 4 – 2
Female schizophrenics	8 – 4 – 6
Male depressives	2 – 4 – 7
Female depressives	4 – 2 – 7

Patients with an 842 profile are described by Marks, Seeman, and Haller (1974) as distrustful, suspicious, and fearful or avoidant of emotional involvements and close personal relationships. Nearly 75% are diagnosed paranoid schizophrenic. The most frequent diagnosis of the 846 profile type is also paranoid schizophrenia. Patients with this profile are described by Marks, Seeman, and Haller, and by Gilberstadt and Dukes (1965) as having difficulty in concentration and showing disordered, unusual, and autistic thinking. Patients with a 247 or 427 profile are most frequently diagnosed as depressed, and described as anxious, worrisome, sad, and having low self-esteem.

Additional information on the characteristics of our sample may be gleaned from the spouse's perception of the patient's problems as obtained on the Mate Adjustment Form. Patients were described by their spouses as more deviant than controls on every scale at the $p < .001$ level. Schizophrenics are seen by their spouses as significantly more angry, paranoid, psychotic, and manic, whereas depressives are seen as being significantly more depressed. Furthermore, there are trends for schizophrenics to be rated as more angry with children and better in their work performance. This latter trend should be viewed with extreme caution, however, since the cell frequencies on the worker role scale are very small for the schizophrenics; many were unable to maintain employment and thus could not be rated along this dimension.

We also obtained the patients' perceptions of their well spouses. Two consistent patterns of results emerged. First, in all instances, spouses of controls are rated as being much less disturbed than spouses of patients with significant differences on worker role, housekeeper role, social contact, paranoia, neurosis, and depression. Second, in every instance, depressives' ratings of their spouses and families are more severe than schizophrenics' ratings. Neither pattern is readily explained.

Table 6. *Diagnostic ratings for key admission*

Variable	Group		t
	Schizophrenics	Depressives	
Σ Schizophrenia tests	6.80	2.67	7.62***
Though disorder			
Poor insight			
Social isolation/avoidance			
Restricted affect			
Catatonia			
Delusions			
Hallucinations			
Auditory hallucinations			
Elated Mood	1.02	.62	2.23*
Σ Other manic symptoms	2.39	1.04	3.31**
Activity level			
Talkativeness			
Flight of ideas			
Inflated self-esteem			
Decreased need for sleep			
Distractibility			
Excessive involvement in activities with high potential for painful consequences			
Depressed mood	1.55	2.84	−6.28***
Σ Other depressive symptoms	3.32	6.47	−5.23***
Poor or increased appetite/ weight loss or gain			
Sleep difficulty or too much sleep			
Loss of energy			
Loss of interest or pleasure			
Self-reproach/guilt			
Problem in thinking/ concentration			
Suicidal thoughts or behavior			
Organic/alcohol/drugs	.54	.75	−1.22
GAS[a]	27.38	33.98	−5.41***

*$p < .05$.   **$p < .01$.   ***$p < .001$.
[a]Global Assessment Scale. Lower scores indicate greater psychopathology.

Psychiatric patients may tend to marry people who are also somewhat disturbed (e.g., B. Mednick, 1973). Alternatively, the patients' psychopathology may produce biased ratings.

Sampling bias

An important issue in a study like ours is sampling bias. By collecting data on families that refuse participation or drop out, we may estimate the nature and extent of the bias. Refusal by the patient in the hospital before we conduct our evaluation is rare (only 10 cases), but even here we are able to analyze the patient's hospital records and compare them with those of the rest of the sample. On demographic characteristics such as age, religion, education, and occupation, there were no differences between patients who refused participation and those who consented. There was some evidence, however, suggesting that the refusers were both more severely disturbed and more paranoid than the consenters.

The second point at which we lose cooperation is when we approach the spouse for his/her participation and that of the family. Here we lost 25 families. Because for each of these families we have for the patient a CAPPS, Mini-Mult, and hospital record, we compared the patients in these families with those of the rest of our sample (see Table 7). Again we found no significant differences for the patient/parent in demographic characteristics, such as education and occupation, but additionally no differences appeared in severity, paranoid status, total time in psychiatric hospital, and number of previous hospitalizations. Whatever sampling bias might exist here would probably be found in spouse factors and family dynamics.

Although the nature and extent of the entire family's participation in our research project are fully detailed before consent is obtained, we permit families to remain in the project even though their participation might not be complete. That is, we have families in the project who choose not to participate in all aspects of our assessments. For instance, a patient's spouse may give consent to his/her family's participation, but personally refuse to be interviewed. Or another family might participate fully, except we are unable to obtain a school evaluation because the family lives in a school district that is not cooperating with us. This pattern of partial participation is quite vexing in our various analyses because they are characterized by varying Ns. On the other hand, this situation puts us in a unique position·to further analyze potential confounds because of dropouts, and, in our opinion, provides us with a more representative sample. We believe that if we selected only those families willing to participate in every aspect of our project, we would be left with a sample that is unrepresentative of families with a psychiatric patient/parent in general.

ASSESSMENT OF CHILDREN

In turning to our assessment of the children, we must first note that the offspring of schizophrenics are *not* grossly deviant as young children. The data available suggest that whereas high-risk children can be discriminated from others, the

Table 7. *Families that dropped out: patient characteristics*

Total N	25[a]
Male	8
Female	17
Diagnosis	
Schizophrenic	10
Depressed	5
Other or uncertain	10
Severity	3.96[b]
Marital status	
Married	18
Separated or divorced	6
Widowed	1
Occupational Level (mean)	4.06[c]
Educational Level (mean)	4.16[d]
Total time in psychiatric hospital	2.23[e]
Number of previous hospitalizations	2.18

[a]This number equals 14.4% of total patient sample; 16.1% of sample of schizophrenic and depressed patients.
[b]Severity ranges from 1 (least) to 6 (most).
[c]Occupational level ranges from 1 (higher executive or major professional) to 7 (unskilled employee).
[d]Educational level ranges from 1 (professional degree) to 7 (<7 years of school).
[e]2 = less than 6 months; 3 = less than 1 year.

differences are going to be subtle (see Garmezy, 1974a, 1974b, for a review). Our strategy for selecting variables followed from our general diathesis–stress view of schizophrenia. Within this context, the high-risk method can yield data reflecting the high-risk genotype, the earliest signs of the disorder, and potentiators of the diathesis. Thus, one of our strategies was to seek early indicators of symptomatic behavior, or the high-risk genotype, by using downward extensions of laboratory variables shown to be important by studies of adult schizophrenics. Our second strategy views the child's behavior as reflections of appropriate coping mechanisms, and focuses on the development of *general competence behaviors*. These behaviors have direct adaptational significance and are supported and rewarded by the environment. Our third strategy attempts to characterize the environment of the high-risk child. We are collecting the child's phenomenological ratings of the parents' child-rearing characteristics and the stressfulness of life events that have been experienced. We are also recoding data from both the home and school to provide a series of objective ratings of "environmental noxiousness." Here, we examine parenting, marital discord, sibling relationships, and behaviors directed toward the child by peers. We believe that these two sets of measurements will provide a comprehensive picture of the environments of our sample that can then be related to specific classes of behavior.

School assessment

The schools are a major source of data in our assessment of children. The school environment constitutes the most significant social and psychological arena a child encounters outside of the family, representative as it is of the competitive, work, and social demands of adulthood. A plan was worked out with the school superintendents so that the confidentiality of subjects and their families would be maintained. The reason for our choice of children is concealed from school personnel who have contact with them, and the names of the participating children are not identified to the teacher or the class members. As a further protection of the confidentiality of the children and their families, all children of the same sex as the target child are administered the same peer and teacher rating instruments.

In order to obtain a reliable, multifactorial assessment of the child from the perspective of his or her classmates, we developed two peer instruments: *The Pupil Evaluation Inventory* (Pekarik, Prinz, Liebert, Weintraub, & Neale, 1976) and *ASSESS: Adjustment Scales for Sociometric Evaluation of Secondary School Students* (Prinz, Swan, Liebert, Weintraub, & Neale, 1978). The format of each consists of an item by peer matrix in which the items appear as rows down the left side of the page and the names of the children in the class across the top of the page. The subject checks each child he or she believes to be described by a particular item. After rating the other children in the class, each child also completes a self-evaluation. The Pupil Evaluation Inventory (PEI) consists of 34 items, and factor analysis has revealed three major dimensions: (1) Aggressive–Disruptiveness; (2) Unhappiness–Withdrawal; and (3) Social Competence–Likeability. ASSESS consists of 45 items describing five factors: (1) Antisocial; (2) Interpersonal Competence; (3) Asocial; 4) Introversion–Extraversion; and (5) Self-Control. Both the PEI and ASSESS show high internal consistency, item to scale correlation, test–retest reliability, and interrater agreement between male and female raters.

Teacher ratings were also collected. For elementary school students, we use the *Devereux Elementary School Behavior Rating Scale* (Spivack & Swift, 1967). The scale consists of 47 items that define 11 factors: Classroom Disturbance, Impatience, Disrespect–Defiance, External Blame, Achievement Anxiety, External Reliance, Comprehension, Inattentive–Withdrawn, Irrelevant–Responsiveness, Creative Initiative, and Needs Closeness to Teacher. For junior and senior high school students, we administer the secondary School Behavior Rating Scale, which is an age-appropriate measure created from the DESB, and the Hahnemann High School Behavior Rating Scale (Swift & Spivack, 1969). It has 50 items and five clusters: (1) Academic Competence; (2) Social Competence; (3) Aggressive–Disruptive; (4) Anxiety–Withdrawal; and (5) Rapport with Teacher.

Assessment of the child in the home

Both parents evaluate the child's adjustment, using the Devereux Child Behavior Rating Scale (Spivack & Spotts, 1966). The scale consists of 97 items that define 17 behavior factors: Distractibility, Poor Self-Care, Pathological Use of Senses,

Emotional Detachment, Social Isolation, Poor Coordination and Body Tonus, Incontinence, Messiness and Sloppiness, Inadequate Need for Independence, Unresponsiveness to Stimulation, Proneness to Emotional Upset, Need for Adult Contact, Anxious–Fearful Ideation, "Impulse" Ideation, Inability to Delay, Social Aggression, and Unethical Behavior. Reliability of the scale, both in terms of interrater and test–retest agreement, is quite good.

Laboratory studies

In our laboratory assessment, two children are tested per day. The children are picked up at home at about 8:30 a.m., are taken out to lunch at midday, and returned home at about 3:30 p.m. A letter describing the results of our assessment is sent to the parents, and if any problem seems severe enough, an appropriate referral is made.

A primary focus of our studies is on information processing and attention. Several results from the high-risk studies suggest that these are indeed important areas (e.g., S. A. Mednick & Schulsinger, 1974; Erlenmeyer-Kimling & Cornblatt, 1978; Asarnow et al., 1978). Our laboratory battery includes measures of intellectual functioning, distractibility, maintenance of attention, referential thinking, and cognitive slippage. For a detailed presentation of these measures, see "Information Processing Deficits in Children at High Risk for Schizophrenia" (Neale, Winters, & Weintraub, Chapter 16, this volume).

Data analysis in the cross-sectional phase of a high-risk project presents a major problem. Because only a subset of the children of schizophrenic parents are expected to become deviant and/or have the schizophrenic genotype, traditional between-groups analyses of mean differences may be too insensitive. Imagine, for example, a sign that has a validity of .90 in predicting which of the offspring of schizophrenics will themselves become schizophrenic. Such a measure would identify only about 27 children in a sample of 200 children with a schizophrenic parent (.90 × 30), a subsample that may not be large enough to cause an overall mean difference between the offspring of schizophrenics and controls. Thus, it is important to move beyond an analysis of means and carefully examine distributions of scores. Such an analysis could reveal a group of outliers which was not large enough to produce an overall mean difference between groups.

Taking this argument one step further, it is also useful to search for deviance across a set of variables instead of a single one. The error associated with a single task makes defining deviance in this way undesirable. But we could be more confident about our designation of children as deviant if they showed a pattern of deviant responding across a set of tasks. The first question to be asked here is whether deviance can be found across tasks. In other words, is there a group of children who are deviant on several measures? Searching for such a group has several advantages. The subset of deviant children, for example, could provide a sample for testing hypotheses that would be too expensive to evaluate in the entire group. The same strategy, but in reverse, could also be used to identify a different, but perhaps equally important group. As Garmezy (1975b) and Anthony (1974a) have suggested, some children seem able to withstand and even overcome severe disadvantages. We know that about 50% of the children of schizophrenics will do well as adults. Can these "invulnerables" be identified in a high-risk project? Finding an invulnerable sample may allow us to examine environmental factors that, in some sense, innoculate these children against psychopathology. (The labels *vulnerable* and *invulnerable* are being used in the absence of outcome data but reflect our predictions about the two groups.) As a first step we decided to try to form two such groups using performance on cognitive tasks administered in our laboratory as deviance criteria. After forming the extreme groups, we attempted to validate them by examining data from their school behavior and some measures of the characteristics of their parents.

An initial analysis of these *outlier data* (Stone, Weintraub, & Neale, 1977) was limited to a sample of elementary and junior high school aged children, which included 139 target children with a schizophrenic parent and 57 control children with parents free of diagnosable psychopathology. Six measures were selected from our laboratory battery – Verbal IQ, Performance IQ, mean performance on the distraction trials of the distractibility task, mean search time for letters in quadrants 3 and 4 of the visual search task, mean performance on the free response trials of word communication, and number of superordinate responses on object sorting. First we had to define a cutoff for deviant performance. More than one-half of a standard deviation from the mean, in a specified direction, was selected. This somewhat liberal criterion was chosen to increase the chances of finding across-task consistency in deviance. This procedure varies from one used by Hanson, Gottesman, and Heston (1976), that of examining all possible outpoints in both positive and negative directions and selecting the cutpoint that was most discriminating for each measure. Because we specify whether the task is keyed negatively or positively, our procedure is less prone to Type I errors and avoids the interpretational difficulties when one simply scans data in every possible way looking for any result to maximize group differences.

Each of these six variables was first residualized using age, sex, Verbal and Performance IQ (except for the two IQ scores) and their interactions as variables in the regression equation. The variables were residualized so that we could perform subsequent analyses with a single group of children instead of being forced to work with subgroups formed by age, sex, and IQ. The resulting distributions of residualized scores were then standardized and with the adoption of the .5 *SD* cutpoint, subjects were classified as deviant or not on each measure. Next a distribution was formed, showing the percentage of the offspring of schizophrenics vs. controls who were deviant on 0, 1, 2, 3, etc. of the tasks. Chi-square values were computed at each point in an attempt to locate two maximal χ^2s to define the deviant and invulnerable groups. These two groups were then compared on our measures of school behavior and some parental characteristics. The school variables were the three factors (Aggression, Withdrawal, and Likeability) from the peer rated Pupil Evaluation Inventory, and four factors (Achievement Anxiety, Relatedness to Teacher, Social Compliant vs. Disruptive, and Cognitive Competence) from the Devereux Elementary School Behavior Rating Scale, an inventory completed by the child's teacher. The parent variables included several demographic variables, factor scores from the Current and Past Psychopathology Scale and the Mini-Mult scales.

To locate the highly vulnerable group, we looked for a maximal χ^2 with a higher percentage of subjects among the offspring of schizophrenics than of controls. The invulnerable group we defined by the maximal χ^2 with a higher percentage of controls than offspring of schizophrenics. Being deviant on four or more measures produced one of the maximal χ^2s, and this point became the criterion for our highly vulnerable group; 15% of schizophrenics and 0% of controls fell into the deviant group. Being deviant on one or fewer versus two or more measures produced the second maximal χ^2 and thus became our criterion for invulnerability; 31.7% of the offspring of schizophrenics and 57.9% of the controls fell into this group.

At this point we have answered one of our questions. Performance across laboratory tasks was rather consistent for some subjects, allowing us to identify groups of children who were either consistently deviant or consistently nondeviant. Then we attempted to validate these groups by comparing their school behavior. The deviant, vulnerable children were lower than the invulnerables in relatedness to teacher, cognitive competence and likeability, and higher in disruptiveness and withdrawal. The vulnerable group also departed substantially from the expected mean of a standardized distribution of scores ($Z = 0$) based on both control and schizophrenic families. This same tendency, although in weaker form, was present for the invulnerables. For example, they are over 1 *SD* from the mean, in the positive direction, on cognitive competence. These differences in school behavior are consistent with the results of follow-back studies which have found similar characteristics to be precursors of adult schizophrenia. These data, then, seem to provide strong validation for designating these two groups as vulnerable and invulnerable.

We were much less successful in validating our two groups based on parental characteristics. For this analysis we were careful not to count families twice. That is, even with multiple children in the same family classified as vulnerable or invulnerable, the family would only be entered once into this data set. Looking at demographic characteristics, the two groups of families with a schizophrenic parent did not differ in social class (education and occupation), race, parental age, number of children in the family, or marital status. From CAPPS data, the two groups did not differ on severity of psychopathology, total time of psychiatric hospitalization, or number of hospitalizations. Similarly, there were no differences on any of the CAPPS factors (Reality Testing, Social Disturbance, Anxiety–Depression, Impulse Control, Somatic Concern-Functioning, Disorganization, Obsessive-Guilt–Phobic, Elation–Grandiosity). There were also no significant differences on any of the Mini-Mult scales. Thus, we are forced to conclude that there are no obvious differences between the schizophrenic parents of vulnerable and invulnerable children in our sample. This null result may reflect the low level of variability within the schizophrenic group on these measures. Perhaps differences will be revealed in subsequent analyses of other familial variables. B. Mednick's data, for example, strongly implicate spouse characteristics as important in vulnerability. Marital adjustment would appear to be another likely candidate for further explorations. Fortunately, we have collected data on these variables and are now working on these analyses.

SUMMARY

Our findings indicate that the high-risk children are indeed vulnerable, evidencing patterns of social and cognitive incompetence. Children with a schizophrenic parent differed from children with normal parents on almost every variable we assessed, including aggressiveness, withdrawal, relatedness to teacher, distractibility, conceptual skills, and cognitive factors. They also differed from children with a depressed parent on certain of our variables, such as cognitive slippage, as indexed by object sorting performance. Children with a depressed parent, however, showed similar patterns of incompetence, even on supposedly schizophrenia-specific variables. The two chapters that follow provide more detailed information on these differences.

At this point in our research program, we are puzzled and intrigued by the similarities of the risk groups and have speculated about its causes. One possibility is that the high-risk children are responding in some reactive, temporary way to their parent's illness and hospitalization. As our own data indicate, a patient's problems, irrespective of diagnosis, can shake the equilibrium and stability of the entire family. A stable emotional climate, so important to a child's sense of security and conducive to growth and maturity, is often unavailable to the high-risk child. This possibility of temporary reactivity is unlikely given the considerable interval that obtained between parental hospitalization and child assessment, but will be tested more definitively with out follow-up data.

A second possibility is that our schizophrenic parent group, although reliably diagnosed, is overly heterogeneous. Indeed, our data indicate that patients who might be diagnosed as DSM-II schizoaffective frequent our schizophrenia group. A preliminary reanalysis of our data using narrow DSM-III criteria (Winters, Stone, Weintraub & Neale, 1980), however, does not yield substantially different results.

A third possibility is that the variables we measured are really not specific to schizophrenia. These variables were among the most salient in the psychological deficit and schizophrenia literature, but this literature characteristically reports only schizophrenic versus normal control differences. Recent evidence, however, suggests that many supposedly schizophrenic characteristics, including various cognitive, motor, and perceptual deficits, are found in adult depressed patients (W. R. Miller, 1975; Helmsley & Zawada, 1976).

A fourth possibility is that children with a depressed parent are themselves at especially high-risk and vulnerable to later psychopathology. Childhood vulnerability may, to some considerable extent, be unrelated to a parent's specific psychiatric diagnosis. Thus, we are very interested in expanding the focus of our project to include vulnerability to affective illness, as well as vulnerability to schizophrenia.

We should note, in closing, that many of the high-risk children and their families are adjusting quite satisfactorily and demonstrate impressive degrees of strength and resilience. We would like to learn more about the coping strategies and support systems required for the children Norman Garmezy and E. James Anthony have tagged "invulnerable," who are able to survive and even thrive where others break down.

16 Information processing deficits in children at high risk for schizophrenia

JOHN M. NEALE, KEN C. WINTERS, AND
SHELDON WEINTRAUB

The rationale for the Stony Brook Project's selection of cognitive and attentional variables is derived from a diathesis–stress approach to schizophrenia. Drawing on current data and theory pertaining to schizophrenia, we chose variables that are likely to reflect either the high-risk genotype or early signs of the disorder, and designed age-appropriate, downward extensions of these variables. This reflects an assumption of continuity between adult psychopathology and childhood behavior. Given the findings that schizophrenics generally perform more poorly than controls on measures related to attention (Venables, 1964), distractibility (J. S. Chapman & McGhie, 1962), cognitive slippage (Daut & Chapman, 1974), and intelligence (Lane & Albee, 1964), among others, it seems reasonable to expect that their offspring might show deficits on these measures as well. Several results from high-risk studies suggest that these are indeed important areas and that the assumption of continuity may be a valid one (e.g., S. A. Mednick & Schulsinger, 1974; Erlenmeyer-Kimling & Cornblatt, 1978; Asarnow, Steffy, MacCrimmon, & Cleghorn, 1977).

METHOD

The information processing tasks to be described below were administered in our lab to a total of 374 children, including 147 with a schizophrenic parent, 93 with a depressed parent, and 134 with normal control parents. For a description of the procedures used to select families and to diagnose the parents, see The Stony Brook High-Risk Project (Chapter 15, this volume). The description of the children by sex, age, and parent's diagnostic status is presented in Table 4 of that chapter.

We chose five measures to represent information processing: IQ (Verbal and Performance), object sorting, referential thinking, visual search (maintenance of attention), and distractibility.

This research was supported by Grant MH 21145 from the National Institute of Mental Health and funds from the William T. Grant Foundation.

Verbal and performance IQ

As school records began to be collected, we found that many children in our sample did not have an adequate intelligence estimate already in their file. Thus, we decided to include the WISC in our assessment battery. Due to time limitations, however, the full WISC could not be administered. Based on several studies of short forms of the WISC, we decided to use the most reliable tetrad of subtests: block design, picture arrangement, information and vocabulary.

Object sorting

This task was selected because it appeared to fulfill a number of criteria which are relevant to selecting variables in a high-risk study. First, responses on the task should follow developmental patterns that are meaningfully related to the individual's behavior in other situations and to overall adjustment. Second, the performance of adult schizophrenics must be significantly different from that of normals and other patient groups. Third, the type of response exhibited by schizophrenics should be found more frequently among their unaffected first degree relatives than in the general population. And finally, response characteristics on the task should show a familial pattern similar to that found for the clinical disorder. Sorting tasks, in which the subject is asked to either form or explain the rationale for a group of items, have tentatively been shown to meet all of these requirements, and may tap into the dimension of cognitive slippage.

Subjects' responses on sorting tasks have been classified in a wide variety of ways. Foremost has been the distinction between responses that specify clearly a particular common attribute of all the items selected (*superordinate* or *analytic* responses) and those which do not. Olver and Hornsby (1966) found that between the ages of 6 and 19 there is a progressive increase in children's use of superordinate classification. This same trend was observed by Kagan, Moss, and Sigel (1963) who also found that the type of sorting response made by both children and adults was remarkably consistent across a variety of perceptual and verbal tasks. Furthermore, this distinction in preferred mode of response was related to extra-laboratory behavior. Analytically inclined individuals were more ambitious and independent, more systematic in intellectual performance, and tended to have better articulated life goals. Other correlates of the analytic style were increased perceptual vigilance and reduced interference by variable preparatory intervals in a test of reaction time. These data indicate that sorting behavior provides a useful assessment of the child's manner of processing, structuring, and utilizing information about the environment and of the way in which these abilities change over time.

The sorting task we selected was developed and standardized by Rigney (1962). The child was presented with an array of 42 4 × 5 in. cards on which common objects had been painted, for example, a saw, an umbrella, a bird, a clock, and various articles of clothing. These cards were displayed on an easel so that all were visible simultaneously. The child was first asked to identify each picture to be sure that he or she was familiar with all of them. If the child did not recognize or understand any card, he or she was told what it was. The child was then asked to select a group of pictures that were "alike in some way" and to place them on a table. When the child was finished, he or she was asked to explain in what way these pictures were alike. If the child's response could not be scored, the experimenter gave one prompt, for example, "Tell me more about that." The cards were then replaced, and the child was asked to select a different group. Each child was asked to make 10 such groupings. Both the child's rationale and the items belonging in each group were written down by the experimenter. An audiotape of the entire session was made and later compared against the test form to ensure accurate, verbatim recording of each child's responses.

A scoring manual which represented an amalgamation of previous schemes (Tutko & Spence, 1962; Rigney, 1962) was developed to code the children's sorting responses. Each response was categorized as either superordinate, complexive, thematic, or vague. The first three categories were those used by Rigney, with complexive and thematic responses corresponding with those labeled *restrictive errors* by Tutko and Spence. Vague responses were coded separately to represent the *expansive errors* that Tutko and Spence found to characterize reactive schizophrenics. Failures to respond were coded separately, and the quality of the child's verbal facility was discounted as much as possible.

Superordinate responses included those in which items were grouped on the basis of one or more familiar attributes shared by all members of the group (e.g., "All red," "Tools," "Things you wear"). Complexive responses lacked a unifying theme and could take a variety of forms. Like superordinates, they were based on realistic relationships among items, yet no single attribute was described that applied to all the members of the group. For example, one child sorted the apple, pumpkin, candle, and pie together and explained, "You can make an apple pie and a pumpkin pie, and the pies need heat to cook. The candle burns and gives heat." Thematic responses most often included only two items which were related by a functional interaction (e.g., "You use a hammer to pound nails"). Vague responses specified a common attribute that was overgeneralized or contained loose associations to the items. The rationale might either fail to clearly specify any reasonable group of items by being overinclusive or not have any obvious connection to the objects selected. Examples of vague responses were "You can use them," "They're all things," and "They're all things you can hold."

Two copies of each child's test protocol were made and coded by number. Individual items were separated and all groups' responses were mixed together so that each response was coded completely independently and blindly to the parent's diagnosis. Two trained raters independently scored each response. Disagreements were resolved by group decision between the raters after all other scoring had been completed. Reliabilities (number of agreements over agreements plus disagreements) for the coding categories were superordinate, .96; complexive, .66; vague, .71; and thematic, .92.

Referential thinking

Associative and communicative processes are among the most researched topics in adult schizophrenics. Recently, Cohen and his colleagues have used a word-communication task to assess referential thinking in adult schizophrenics. Briefly, the task requires one subject, the speaker, to provide a single, one-word clue that will allow a listener to determine which of two words is the referent. The other subject, the listener, tries to guess, on the basis of the clue, which of the two words is the referent. For example, the speaker might be shown the pair CAR–AUTOMOBILE, with CAR designated as the referent. The speaker's task is to provide a one-word clue to allow the listener to guess that CAR and not AUTOMOBILE is correct. For this pair, clues such as DRIVE and WHEELS would be ineffective whereas HOP and BOX would provide discriminating, helpful information to the listener. In their investigation, Cohen and Cahmi (1967) found that schizophrenics performed more poorly than controls only in the speaker role. Similar results have been obtained in subsequent studies (e.g., Cohen, Nachmani, & Rosenberg, 1974).

In adapting this task for children, the main requirement was forming pairs of words so that the children would understand the words and have sufficient knowledge to provide adequate clues. This was accomplished by drawing on the large literature on word knowledge in children and by pilot testing. The basic Cohen and Cahmi procedure was embellished in two ways. First, drawing on Chapman's theory of verbal behavior in schizophrenia (L. Chapman, Chapman, & Miller, 1964), two types of pairs were constructed. One type had an uncommon (low) meaning associate as the "best" cue, for example, BOWL–DISH – to which a low-meaning but very effective clue is GAME. In the other type of item, the effective cue is *not* a low-meaning response, for example, TENNIS–SOCCER, to which an effective but non–low-meaning response could be RACKET. Based on Chapman's theory, it would be expected that any deficit of the children of schizophrenics would be accentuated when low-meaning responses are required. Second, two versions of the test – free response and multiple-choice – were devised. The multiple-choice version bypasses the process of *generating* associates and requires only the evaluation of the presented alternatives. The low-meaning items in the multiple-choice version also require the subject to be able to "break-set" and recognize the utility of the low-meaning alternative (e.g., YEAR–DATE: TIME-WHEN–FIG). According to the Cohen et al. (1974) perseverative-chaining model of schizophrenic performance in word communication, it is expected that any deficit in the offspring of schizophrenics will be minimal in the multiple-choice version of the test.

A large number of word pairs of all types was constructed and subsequently administered to samples of first, third, and fifth grade elementary school children. The pilot testing allowed items that were either too easy or too hard to be discarded and a 28 item test resulted, 14 free response and 14 multiple-choice items. Half of the multiple-choice items required the use of a low-meaning response. Similarly, in the free response version, half the items could be readily solved with a low-meaning response. But for these items a fully adequate answer could also stay within the high-meaning domain. Responses were scored on a 3-point scale: 0 = inadequate, 1 = adequate, 2 = good. A detailed scoring manual, with extensive examples of different responses, kept interrater reliabilities uniformly above .90. Items were presented to the children with the instructions either to produce or choose a response that would allow another child to know which of the two words was the referent.

Visual search

This task assesses two processes that are thought to be relevant to schizophrenia: the ability to ignore irrelevant input and the ability to maintain attention. Studies of these attentional processes using other tasks have shown that children of schizophrenics perform more poorly than controls. Maintenance of attention has been assessed with a continuous performance task (Erlenmeyer-Kimling & Cornblatt, 1978) and ignoring irrelevant information in a span of apprehension task (Asarnow et al., 1978). Our visual search task, which is tapping similar processes via different operations, should allow some convergent validation of previous findings. The task involves searching down a list of 30 letter strings of four letters each. The lists are mounted on cardboard backing so that they can be inserted into a light-tight box behind a half-silvered mirror. On a ready signal from the experimenter, the child presses a button that illuminates lamps, making the display visible, and activates a clock-counter. He or she then searches down the list and upon finding the target presses the button again. This second buttonpress turns off the lamps and stops the clock-counter. The elapsed time from the first to the second buttonpress provides the index of search time.

Two variables are being manipulated. The first, confusability, relates to the physical similarity between the target and noise letters. In the high confusability condition, the target letter **G** appears with physically similar letters such as **C** and **D**. In the low confusabiliity condition, the target appears with physically dissimilar letters such as **M** and **X**. The second variable is the target location. Each display is considered as having four quadrants and targets appear equally often in each one.

Distractibility

Many researchers have argued that an important component of schizophrenics' attentional deficit is an increased susceptibility to the effects of distracting input (Lang & Buss, 1965; Neale & Cromwell, 1970; Oltmanns & Neale, 1977). One of the first studies of distractibility in schizophrenics was performed by J. Chapman and McGhie (1962). They found that adding a distracting voice to a digit-span test produced a differential deficit in schizophrenics. Other studies (e.g., Rappoport, 1967) soon demonstrated comparable effects but by the mid-1970s it was no longer clear that schizophrenics were especially distractible. The argument, proposed by L. Chapman and Chapman (1973), was that in these studies the distractor condition usually produced a test with greater discriminating power than the neutral condition. Therefore, the greater difference typically observed between schizophrenics and controls in the distractor condition could be due to the differential psychometric properties of the tests.

More recent work, though, has demonstrated that at least some schizophrenics are distractible and that distractibility may be a central aspect of schizophrenic disorder. In the first of these studies, Oltmanns and Neale (1975) formed pairs of neutral and distractor digit-span tasks that were matched for discriminating power. The schizophrenics were still found to be distractible, even with the discriminating power of the two tests equated. A subsequent study (Oltmanns, O'Hayon, & Neale, 1978) replicated these effects and gathered further evidence for the importance of distractibility in schizophrenia. Distractibility was found to be related to thought disorder and it also varied with symptomatology and consumption of psychotropic drugs. With a withdrawal of medication, both symptomatology and susceptibility to distraction increased dramatically in schizophrenics. But performance on the neutral digit-span task was unchanged, suggesting that distractibility is indeed an important aspect of schizophrenia and that such a measure would be valuable in a high-risk study. This possibility is further supported by early results from Erlenmeyer-Kimlings' (1976) project which indicate that a test very similar to the one we are using can discriminate high-risk from control children. As a final reason for including distractibility in our laboratory battery, we should note that it appears to be heritable (Rose, 1976).

In our no-distraction condition, digits are presented at a 1 per 2-second rate and the child tries to report as many as possible after listening to the series. In the distraction condition, the 1 second interval between each relevant digit is filled by an opposite-sexed voice saying an irrelevant digit. Because of the possibility of both ceiling and floor effects being created by the wide variation in our subject's ages, we created four different versions of the test. Using WISC norms, we decided to use three digit tests for 6-year-olds, four digits for 7- and 8-year-olds, five digits for 9-, 10-, and 11-year olds, and six digits for subjects 12 and older.

RESULTS

Means and standard deviations for the information processing variables are presented in Table 1, and results from the deviant responder analyses are presented in Table 2.

Verbal and Performance IQ

For verbal IQ, a one-way ANOVA yielded a significant diagnostic effect, $F(2, 369) = 3.7$, $p < .05$. The children of schizophrenics were significantly lower than those of controls, $t(371) = 2.7$, $p < .05$. For performance IQ, there was also a diagnostic effect, $F(2, 371) = 3.4$, $p < .05$. Children of both schizophrenics and depressives differed significantly from the controls ($p < .01$).

Deviant responder analyses were performed on five data sets (see Table 2): total IQ and on each of the four subscales. The data were standardized and one

Table 1. *Means, standard deviations, and significant* F *ratios for information-processing measures*

	Offspring of					
	Schizophrenics (N = 147)		Depressives (N = 93)		Controls (N = 134)	
	M	SD	M	SD	M	SD
Prorated IQ scores						
Verbal IQ*	92.5	19.7	97.5	19.7	101.5	18.3
Performance IQ*	96.0	16.7	96.5	17.0	103.5	16.7
Sorting responses						
Superordinate*	7.22	2.63	7.57	2.23	7.98	1.83
Complexive**	.87	1.41	.59	1.10	.43	.78
Thematic	.76	1.74	.79	1.70	.42	1.28
Vague	.92	1.10	1.00	1.06	1.04	1.13
Referential thinking–free response						
Low meaning*						
Age 6–10	1.86	1.23	1.85	1.11	2.63	1.09
Age 11–15	3.71	1.64	4.35	1.72	4.05	1.59
Non–low-meaning*						
Age 6–10	12.95	3.41	11.53	2.79	13.96	2.89
Age 11–15	13.17	2.94	13.74	3.02	14.13	3.16
Visual search						
Quadrant 1	16.8	7.1	18.4	7.5	15.3	7.5
2*	18.9	8.3	21.0	8.4	16.3	7.3
3*	24.7	10.6	27.8	13.0	20.9	8.6
4*	35.2	17.4	36.0	17.3	28.4	12.4
Distractibility						
Neutral	.80	.21	.83	.21	.84	.17
Distraction*	.54	.25	.57	.26	.65	.22

*$p < .05$. **$p < .01$.

standard deviation from the mean was selected as a cutoff point. A χ^2 was computed for each of the five distributions. Total IQ, Vocabulary, and General Information were significant ($p < .05$). In each of these cases, the deviant group contained mostly offspring of schizophrenics followed by offspring of depressives and then controls. Thus, in this instance, the deviant responder analysis provided no surprises, replicating, for the most part, the parametric results.

Our finding of lowered Verbal IQ scores relative to Performance IQ scores is

Table 2. *Percentage and significant chi squares of each group falling more than* 1 SD *from the mean in the deviant direction*

	Offspring of		
	Schizophrenics	Depressives	Controls
WISC Scale			
Total*	26	16	8
Vocabulary*	25	18	11
General Information*	21	16	9
Block Design	18	17	12
Picture Arrangement	14	21	14
Referential Thinking[a]			
Free response			
Low-meaning	31.8	28.1	19.9
Non–low-meaning	23.4	26.0	18.4
Multiple-choice			
Low-meaning**	27.1	37.5	17.7
Non–low-meaning*	25.8	31.3	17.0
Visual Search[a]			
Sum of quadrants 3 and 4*	17%	21%	7%
Distractibility[a]			
Neutral*	24	17	11
Distraction*	25	19	12

*$p < .05$. **$p < .01$.

[a]These variables were residualized using age and total IQ. Age was not residualized on the IQ variables because there were no age effects for the children of controls, and sex was not residualized at all since there were no sex differences on these variables for the controls.

consistent with the hypothesis of impaired dominant hemisphere functioning in adult schizophrenics (Shimkunas, 1978; Gur, 1977; Flor-Henry, 1976), and replicates the WISC results from Mednick and Schulsinger's high-risk sample (Gruzelier & Hammond, 1976).

Sorting responses

Between-group differences in either number of items sorted or in failures to respond could confound later analyses. Thus we first analyzed these two variables using 3(Parental Diagnosis) × 2(Age: Young = 6–9; Old = 10–15) × 2(Sex) analyses of variance. The younger children included fewer items in their sorts than did the older children, $F(1, 396) = 13.46$, $p < .01$, and were more often unable to complete the 10 trials, $F(1, 396) = 7.60$, $p < .01$. None of the remaining main effects or interactions was reliable. Therefore we can conclude that between group differences in subsequent analyses are not due to differences in number of objects selected or failures to respond.

Each of the four variables was analyzed using a 3(Parental Diagnosis) × 2(Age) × 2(Sex) analysis of variance. For superordinate responses, there was a main effect of Age, $F(1, 396) = 29.14$, $p < .01$; older children made more superordinate responses than younger children. There was also a main effect of Parental Diagnosis, $F(2, 396) = 4.08$, $p < .02$. Planned comparisons revealed that children of schizophrenic parents made fewer superordinate responses than children of normal parents but did not differ from the children of depressed parents. For complexive responses, there was a main effect for Parental Diagnosis, $F(2, 396) = 7.25$, $p < .01$. Here planned comparisons revealed that the children of schizophrenic parents made more complexive responses than children in either of the remaining two groups. For thematic responses, the only reliable effect was Age; younger children made more thematic responses than older children, $F(1, 396) = 27.09$, $p < .01$. There were no significant effects for vague responses.

Thus there were significant effects of parental diagnosis on two of the sorting categories. But a remaining issue concerns the relationship between diagnosis, sorting responses and intelligence. That is, it is possible that our sorting task is tapping abilities that are highly correlated with IQ. And given the significant differences between the IQs of the groups, the sorting response data may be redundant.

First, we should note that IQ does not share much common variance with either superordinate ($r_{IQ-S} = .19$) or complexive sorts ($r_{IQ-C} = .14$). This information alone, however, does not allow us to conclude that the between-group differences in sorting responses are independent of the between-group differences in IQ. Two procedures have often been used as attempts to "control" third variables like IQ: matching and analysis of covariance. Matching is seriously flawed for a number of reasons (see Meehl, 1970), and Lord (1967) points out that covariance analysis is an inappropriate strategy for trying to "correct" for between group differences in a third variable. Thus, we opted for an alternative procedure, path analysis (Heise, 1975).

There are several different, though statistically equivalent, ways of viewing path analysis; we use the method of flowgraphs (Heise, 1975). With this method, one lists all variables of interest and proceeds to indicate the hypothesized causal relationships among them by drawing arrows from presumed causes to presumed effects (causation need not be unidirectional, but could be reciprocal). The flowgraph for our analysis is presented in Figure 1.

We hypothesize that Parental Diagnosis directly affects sorting and that Parental Diagnosis affects IQ scores, which, in turn, affect sorting. Given the structure indicated by the flowgraph, certain statistical effects should be observed; for example, if path c is operative, then a change in Parental Diagnosis should produce a change in sorting responses. This would be indicated by a nonzero correlation coefficient between variables. However, the path from Diagnosis to Sorting mediated through IQ is not considered in the simple correlation; thus, to take *all* cause-

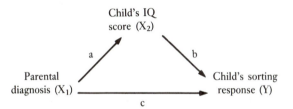

Figure 1. Flowgraph for path analysis for the relationship among parental diagnosis, child's sorting response, and child's IQ score.

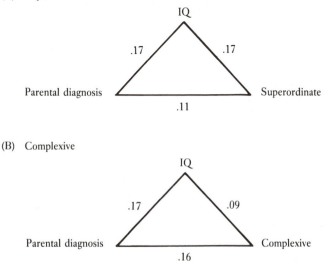

Figure 2. Path analysis for the relationship among parental diagnosis, IQ, and object sorting.

effect paths into account, the path analysis evaluates the variances and covariances for all variables. Then, using the rules of the analysis, weights are assigned to each path which take into account the effects of all other paths. The larger the path coefficient, the greater the causal effect; conversely, a zero path coefficient means the path does not exist at all.

We computed path analyses for superordinate and complexive responses. The coefficient accompanying each path is its standardized path coefficient and, because the system is nonrecursive, the calculations of these path coefficients reduce to correlations. As shown in Figure 2, the coefficients for the two critical paths, Parental Diagnosis → Superordinate Responses (.11) and Parental Diagnosis → Complex Responses (.16) were both significant. Therefore, even in an analysis considering IQ as a causal mediator (diagnosis → IQ → sorting response), Parental Diagnosis continued to exert a reliable effect on sorting responses.

In sum, children of schizophrenics made fewer superordinate and more complexive responses than normals, yet they were distinguishable from children of depressives in only one instance (more complexive responses). These findings hold up even when IQ is taken into account.

Referential thinking

In our analysis of referential thinking, four dependent variables were each evaluated by a 3 (Diagnosis) × 2 (Sex) × 2(Age: less than 11 vs. 11 and over) analysis of variance. The first variable is the frequency with which low-meaning responses were used in the free response version of the test (see Table 1). Significant main effects were found for age ($F = 120.77$, $p < .001$) and diagnosis ($F = 3.00$, $p < .02$). Older children used more low-meaning responses than younger ones, and the children of both schizophrenic and depressed parents gave fewer low-meaning responses than children of controls. Although it appears that only the children of schizophrenics are deviant when the means of the older children are inspected, the age × diagnosis interaction was not significant.

The second variable analyzed was the score on non–low-meaning items of the free response version of the test (see Table 1). Significant main effects were found for age ($F = 53.20$, $p < .001$), and diagnosis ($F = 2.84$, $p < .05$). Older children had higher scores than younger ones, and both the offspring of schizophrenics and depressives were lower than controls. Although none of the interactions were significant, two features of the data should be noted. Among the younger children, the offspring of depressives stand out as a particularly deviant group, whereas among the older children the offspring of schizophrenics have the lowest scores.

The third dependent variable pertained to the non–low-meaning items of the multiple-choice version of the test. Here the only significant effects were age ($F = 64.48$, $p < .001$) and sex ($F = 13.71$, $p < .001$). Older children scored higher than younger ones, and girls higher than boys. The analysis of the fourth dependent variable, low-meaning multiple-choice items revealed only a significant main effect of age ($F = 167.85$; $p < .001$). As expected, older children scored higher than younger ones.

A further examination of the data used a deviant responder strategy. The scores on each dependent variable were residualized using age and IQ, and then were standardized. The percentage of each group falling more than 1 SD from the mean in the deviant direction was noted (see Table 2). Chi-square analyses reveal significant between groups differences on the multiple-choice version of the test. For example, 37.5% of the children of depressives, 27.1% of the children of schizophrenics, and 17.7% of the control children were deviant on the low-meaning items.

Finally, we turned to evaluate the possible impact of IQ on referential thinking scores. IQ was reliably related to each dependent variable (frequency of low-meaning responses: $r = .16$; non–low-meaning free response items: $r = .32$; non–low-meaning multiple-choice: $r = .16$; low-meaning multiple choice: $r = .30$, all ps $< .001$). Because the offspring of patients had lower IQ scores than

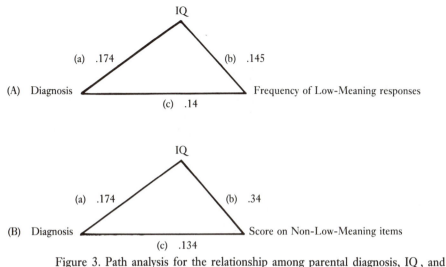

Figure 3. Path analysis for the relationship among parental diagnosis, IQ, and referential thinking.

controls, we attempted to examine the impact of IQ via a path analytic strategy. The analysis evaluates the separate contribution of two causal paths to the dependent variables. The two paths are (a) diagnosis → performance; and (b) diagnosis → child's IQ → performance. Since the parametric analyses revealed a reliable diagnostic effect only for the two dependent variables generated by the free-response part of the test, only these two measures were evaluated. Path *a* is a standardized regression coefficient; paths *b* and *c* are partial regression coefficients (see Figure 3).

Essentially, the analyses allow us to conclude that both paths (diagnosis → IQ → performance; diagnosis → performance) contribute reliably to the variance in each dependent variable. In both cases, the coefficients associated with path *c* (.14 and .134) are statistically significant and indicate that parental diagnosis exerts a direct effect on performance, even with its possible indirect effect (diagnosis → IQ → performance) "controlled."

In sum, the obtained referential thinking results were generally as expected. The children of schizophrenics showed deficits on the free-response version of the test and showed a larger deficit on the items which could be solved using a low-meaning response. The analyses, however, do not allow us to discriminate well between the children of schizophrenic and the children of depressed parents. Only among the older children does there appear to be a schizophrenic versus depressed difference. For example, on the low-meaning responses, the older offspring of schizophrenics have a significantly lower mean than older offspring of depressives. But the overall age × diagnosis interaction was nonsignificant so we cannot conclude that this is a strong finding.

Visual search

A 3(Diagnosis) × 2(Sex) × 2(Age: 6–10 vs. 11 and up) × 2(Confusability) × 4(Quadrant) analysis of variance of search times revealed significant main effects for age ($F = 93.32$, $p < .001$), sex ($F = 8.28$, $p < .004$), diagnosis ($F = 9.69$, $p < .001$), confusability ($F = 342.09$, $p < .001$), and quadrant ($F = 770.34$, $p < .001$). As expected, the highly confusing irrelevant letters slowed search times, and search time increased linearly as targets were located farther down the display. Older children were faster than younger ones, and girls were faster than boys. More interesting, however, is the diagnosis × quadrant interaction ($F = 8.21$, $p < .001$).

Simple effects analyses revealed significant between groups variation at quadrants 2, 3, and 4, with the largest F occurring at quadrant 4. Planned comparisons revealed that the offspring of schizophrenics were significantly slower than the controls at quadrants 2, 3, and 4. Although the offspring of depressives were somewhat slower than the offspring of schizophrenics, those two groups did not differ significantly.

The results of the analysis of variance were corroborated by a deviant responder analysis. A new variable was created, the sum of performance in quadrants 3 and 4. Next, age and total IQ were used in a regression equation and then the residualized visual search scores were standardized. We then examined the percentage of each group that was over one standard deviation above the mean in search time. These percentages were as follows: offspring of schizophrenics, 17%; offspring of depressives, 21%; and offspring of controls, 7% ($p < .05$).

Thus the children of both schizophrenic and depressive parents are slower in visual search than the offspring of controls. This deficit becomes increasingly apparent as the task requires the maintenance of attention for longer and longer amounts of time.

Distractibility

Data were analyzed using a hierarchical multiple regression procedure. Significant main effects were found for Diagnosis ($F = 5.38$), Sex ($F = 5.38$), and Condition ($F = 580.04$). Girls outperformed boys and, as expected, the distractor condition proved considerably more difficult than the neutral condition (see Table 1). The diagnostic effect was further examined at each level of distraction. In the neutral condition no comparisons were significant, while in the distractor condition the offspring of both schizophrenics and depressives were significantly lower than the controls.

A deviant responder analysis was then performed using 1 SD deviation from the mean as a criterion. The data were residualized for age and sex and then standardized (see Table 2). Significant χ^2's were found for both the neutral and distractor conditions. Thus the deviant responder analysis has, in this case, produced sharper results than did the analysis of means. Furthermore, in the deviant responder analysis we achieve some discrimination between the offspring of schizophrenics

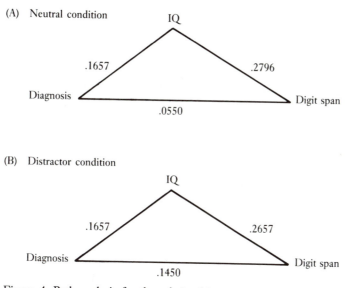

Figure 4. Path analysis for the relationship among parental diagnosis, IQ, and distractibility.

and depressives ($p < .05$. In the distractor condition, deviance obtained for 25% of the children of schizophrenics, 19% of the children of depressives, and 12% of the control children.

Finally, we were again confronted with the fact that IQ was related to performance on this task and so again employed the path analytic strategy described earlier for the object sorting analysis. Results are presented in Figure 4. The path coefficient for Diagnosis → Digit Span was nonsignificant for the neutral condition but significant for the distractor condition. Thus, we can conclude that diagnosis is having a significant effect on performance in the distractor condition.

DISCUSSION

In summary, according to both parametric and deviant responder analyses, children with a schizophrenic parent performed more deviantly than children with normal parents on measures of Verbal IQ, Performance IQ, object sorting, referential thinking, maintenance of attention, and distractibility. Children with a schizophrenic parent were also more deviant than children with a depressed parent in complexive sorting responses and low-meaning referential responses (for older children only). Path analyses indicate that parental diagnosis was related to performance on these tasks irrespective of the influence of IQ.

The analyses further indicate that children with a depressed parent were also deviant on these tasks and, generally, could not be differentiated from children with a schizophrenic parent. What can we conclude from this pattern? First, children with a depressed parent may also be vulnerable. They are at high-risk for adult affective disorder (Winokur, Clayton, & Reich, 1969; Perris, 1973), and for childhood maladjustment (Welner et al., 1977; McKnew, Cytryn, Efron, Gershon, & Bunney, 1979).

A second possibility is that the variables we measured are really not specific to schizophrenia. These variables were among the most salient in the schizophrenia psychological deficit literature, but this literature characteristically reports only schizophrenic versus control differences. Indeed, recent work suggest that some schizophrenic deficits may also be found in other adult psychiatric groups. For example, W. Miller's (1975) review of the literature on psychological deficits in depression indicates that both depressives and schizophrenics exhibit performance deficits on various cognitive, motor, perceptual, and communication tasks, including IQ and time required to inspect a display. If tasks are related to psychosis rather than specific diagnostic categories, and given that children of depressives are at risk, information processing measures may not be discriminating as had been anticipated.

A third possibility is that the causal pathways by which similar performance deficits are produced are different in the different groups. For example, the poor performance of children of schizophrenics on the visual search or distractibility task could reflect an attentional dysfunction, whereas the similarly poor performance of children of depressives could be due to apathy and disinterest in the task.

Finally, we must consider the possibility that our schizophrenic parent group, although reliably diagnosed, may be overly heterogeneous. Indeed, our data indicate that patients who might be diagnosed as schizoaffective according to DSM-II criteria frequent our schizophrenia group. A preliminary reanalysis of our data (Winters, Stone, Weintraub, & Neale, 1980) using DSM-III criteria indicate that the same pattern of results holds up for the children of schizophrenic and unipolar groups, but generally not for the bipolar group.

The issue of deficit specificity is crucial; without a control group of children of parents with nonschizophrenic psychopathology, one cannot properly interpret deficits in children at risk for schizophrenia as being of specific relevance to schizophrenia.

17 *Social behavior of children at risk for schizophrenia*

SHELDON WEINTRAUB AND JOHN M. NEALE

A central feature of the Stony Brook Project is the assessment of general competence behaviors. These behaviors have direct adaptational significance and are supported and rewarded by the environment. Competence plays a significant role in schizophrenia, as indicated both by the schizophrenics' social incompetence and by the fact that measures of competence prove to be the most powerful predictors of course and outcome for adult schizophrenics. Additionally, competence, as measured by teacher and peer ratings, is an effective predictor of later maladjustment.

The schools are a major source in our assessment of childhood competence. Children spend almost half their waking hours in school, the most significant social and psychological arena encountered outside of the family, representative as it is of the competitive, work, and social demands of adulthood. Teachers, as educators and parent surrogates, are in a unique position to assess how a child copes with these demands, and there is considerable evidence that these assessments may be made reliably and validly (Lambert & Bower, 1961; Zax, Cowen, Izzo, & Trost, 1964).

Peers may also provide a sensitive index to a child's adjustment. Peer evaluations are obtained in the rich, nontest context of the child's real-life environment and are based on observations made over extended periods of time by multiple observers who have different personal relationships with the child, and consequently varying perspectives (Smith, 1967). Peer ratings are stable over time, across sex of raters, and over a wide age range (Minturn & Lewis, 1968), and are only minimally influenced by social desirability variance (W. T. Norman, 1963). Peer evaluations have been validated successfully against parental, clinician, and teacher ratings, as well as behavioral observations (Bower, 1969; Wiggins & Winder, 1961; Winder & Wiggins, 1964), and have effectively predicted maladjustment (Roff & Sells, 1968; Cowen, Pederson, Babigian, Izzo, & Trost, 1973; Rolf, 1972).

This research was supported by Grant MH 21145 from the National Institute of Mental Health and funds from the William T. Grant Foundation.

279

METHOD

Teacher ratings and peer ratings were collected in 245 different classrooms on 687 children, including 154 with a schizophrenic parent and 91 with a depressed parent. The preceding chapters provide the distribution of children by sex and school grade and a description of the sampling and diagnostic assessment procedures employed with their parents.

Teacher ratings were obtained with the Devereux Elementary School Behavior Rating Scale (DESB; Spivack & Swift, 1967). It consists of 47 behavior items which the teacher rates either on the basis of frequency or intensity, using a 5- or 7-point rating scale. The 11 scales are:

1. Classroom Disturbance: extent to which child teases and torments classmates, interferes with others' work, is quickly drawn into noisemaking, and must be reprimanded or controlled.
2. Impatience: extent to which child starts work too quickly, is sloppy and hasty in its performance, and is unwilling to review it.
3. Disrespect–Defiance: extent to which child speaks disrespectfully to teacher, resists doing what is asked, belittles the work being done, and breaks classroom rules.
4. External Blame: extent to which child says teacher does not help him/her or never calls on him/her, blames external circumstances when things do not go well, and is quick to say the work assigned is too hard.
5. Achievement Anxiety: extent to which child gets upset about test scores, worries about knowing the "right" answers, is overly anxious when tests are given, and is sensitive to criticism or correction.
6. External Reliance: extent to which child looks to others for direction, relies on the teacher for direction, requires precise instructions, and has difficulty making his own decisions.
7. Comprehension: extent to which child gets the point of what is going on in class, seems able to apply what he/she has learned, and knows material when called upon to recite.
8. Inattentive–Withdrawn: extent to which child does not pay attention, seems oblivious of what is happening in the classroom, and is preoccupied or difficult to reach.
9. Irrelevant Responsiveness: extent to which child tells exaggerated stories, gives irrelevant answers, interrupts when teacher is talking, and makes inappropriate comments.
10. Creative Initiative: extent to which child brings things to class that relate to current topics, talks about things in an interesting fashion, initiates classroom discussion, and introduces personal experiences into class discussion.
11. Need for Closeness to Teacher: extent to which child seeks out the teacher before or after class, is friendly toward the teacher and offers to do things for him/her, and likes to be physically close to the teacher.

Test–retest reliabilities over a 1-week period range between .85 and .91 for the 11 scales, and interrater reliabilities between teachers and teacher aides range between .62 to .77 (Spivack & Swift, 1967, 1973). As regards validity, the scales correlate significantly with grades, controlling for IQ, and discriminate among groups of problem children (Spivack, Swift, & Prewitt, 1972).

Our own cluster analysis of the DESB revealed four clusters: (1) Aggressive–Disruptive (14 items); (2) Cognitive Competence (21 items); (3) Social Competence (8 items); and (4) Achievement Anxiety (4 items). The mean item to cluster correlation was .77 and coefficient alpha for the four clusters is .72, .71, .70, and .77, respectively.

Peer ratings were obtained with a measure we developed, the *Pupil Evaluation Inventory* (Pekarik et al., 1976). The format consists of an item by peer matrix in which the items appear as rows down the left side of the page and the names of the children in the class across the top of the page. The subject checks each child believed to be described by a particular item. This format permits every student to be selected for each item; additionally, all students are rated item by item preventing a possible bias or set that may develop when all items are rated for one person at a time. Only those students of the same sex as the target child are rated by both the boys and girls in the class. The Pupil Evaluation Inventory (PEI) consists of 34 items, and factor analysis has revealed three major dimensions: (1) Aggressive–Disruptiveness; (2) Unhappiness–Withdrawal; and (3) Popularity–Likeability.

Reliability of the PEI, in terms of internal consistency (split-half reliability) and interrater agreement (between male and female raters) on factor scores, is satisfactory. For a sample of third and sixth grade classes tested over a 2-week period, all of the factor test–retest correlations were greater than .80; for the items, the median test–retest correlation was .73.

In order to protect the confidentiality of the children and their families, the reason for our choice of children was concealed from school personnel who had contact with them, and the names of the participating children were not identified to the teacher or the class members. As a further protection, testing was conducted as a class activity, and all of the same-sex classmates of the target child were assessed with the peer and teacher measures.

RESULTS AND DISCUSSION

Teacher ratings

Our first analysis of the Devereux Behavior Rating Scale is according to its clusters: (1) Aggressive–Disruptive (14 items); (2) Cognitive Competence (21 items); (3) Social Competence (8 items); and (4) Achievement Anxiety (4 items). Each of the four clusters was analyzed using a 3(Parental Diagnosis: Schizophrenic, Depressed, Normal) × 2 (Grade Level of Child: 2–5, 6–9) × 2 (Sex of Child) analysis of variance. Means and standard deviations may be found in Table 1. Significant main effects for Sex of Child were found on the Aggresive–Disruptive and Cognitive Competence clusters; boys were rated as more aggressive, $F(1, 658) = 34.24$, $p < .001$, and less cognitively competent, $F(1, 627) = 19.68$, $p < .001$. There were also significant main effects for Grade Level on the Social

Table 1. *Means and standard deviations of Teacher Devereux clusters and scales for children of schizophrenic, depressed, and normal parents*

Devereux clusters and scales	Schizophrenic (N = 154)		Depressed (N = 91)		Control (N = 443)	
	(M)	(SD)	(M)	(SD)	(M)	(SD)
Teacher Devereux clusters						
Aggressive–Disruptive	29.7	13.8	28.8	13.6	27.1	11.3
Cognitive Competence	65.2	24.2	62.3	24.3	58.7	23.4
Social Competence	21.7	7.3	22.4	7.1	24.3	7.6
Achievement-Anxiety	9.5	4.3	9.1	3.7	10.0	4.1
Teacher Devereux scales						
Classroom Disruption	11.0	5.3	10.6	5.2	9.9	4.7
Impatience	11.9	5.5	11.7	5.3	11.0	5.1
Disrespect	7.4	3.9	7.1	4.1	6.5	3.1
External Blame	7.8	4.3	7.6	4.0	7.5	3.7
Achievement-Anxiety	9.5	4.3	9.1	3.7	10.1	4.1
External Reliance	16.2	6.5	15.2	6.3	15.0	6.3
Comprehension	10.6	3.8	10.1	3.7	9.8	3.6
Inattention–Withdrawn	11.5	5.6	11.1	5.5	10.0	5.1
Irrelevant Responsiveness	8.2	3.7	7.7	3.5	7.6	3.4
Creative Initiative	9.3	3.6	9.6	3.9	10.5	4.1
Need Closeness to Teacher	12.4	4.8	12.7	4.4	13.7	4.6

Note: For all clusters and scales, with the exceptions of Creative Initiative and Need Closeness (scales), and Social Competence (cluster), a higher score indicates increased disturbance.

Competence cluster; younger children were rated as more competent, $F(1, 685) = 57.88$, $p < .001$. There were no significant interactions between Parental Diagnosis and Sex of Child or Grade Level. Planned contrasts indicated that children with a schizophrenic parent in comparison with the normal controls were rated by their teachers as significantly more deviant on the Aggressive–Disruptive cluster, $t(657) = 2.28$, $p < .025$; the Cognitive Competence cluster, $t(626) = 2.87$, $p < .005$; and the Social Competence cluster, $t(684) = 3.65$, $p < .001$. Children with a depressed parent in comparison with the normal controls were rated low in Social Competence, $t(684) = 2.16$, $p < .05$; and low in Achievement Anxiety, $t(687) = 1.99$, $p < .05$. There were no differences between children with a schizophrenic parent and children with a depressed parent.

We also conducted a redundant analysis of the Devereux according to its 11 scales, 9 of which consist of four items, 1 of five items, and 1 of three items. Means and standard deviation for the 11 Devereux scales are shown in Table 1. Analyses of variance indicated that teachers rated the children with a schizophrenic parent as significantly more deviant than the normal controls on nine of the eleven

Table 2. *Means and standard deviations (in parentheses) on peer rating factors for children grouped by sex and mother's diagnostic status*

Factor		Boys (N)			Girls (N)		
		Sch	Con	Dep	Sch	Con	Dep
	$N =$	36	77	33	39	76	24
Aggression		24.2	19.0	28.4	18.6	15.2	16.2
		(17.2)	(17.3)	(18.8)	(14.3)	(11.7)	(14.0)
Unhappiness–Withdrawal		15.7	14.8	6.9	20.5	14.5	16.4
		(10.9)	(12.1)	(10.2)	(15.8)	(10.6)	(18.3)
Likeability–Social Competence		25.1	24.3	18.4	23.4	30.0	25.9
		(14.6)	(13.5)	(10.3)	(17.2)	(14.7)	(17.1)

Note: A higher score indicates increased disturbance for all scales except Likeability–Social Competence. (Sch, schizophrenic; Con, control; Dep, depressed.)

factors: (1) Classroom Disturbance; (2) Impatience; (3) Disrespect–Defiance; (4) External Reliance; (5) Comprehension; (6) Inattentive–Withdrawn; (7) Irrelevant Responsiveness; (8) Creative Initiative; and (9) Need Closeness to Teacher. Significant differences between children with a depressed parent and the normal controls were found only on the Achievement Anxiety factor (children with a depressed parent were rated lower). There were no significant differences between children in the two patient groups.

Peer evaluations

We recently reported (Weintraub, Prinz, & Neale, 1978) an analysis of scores on our Pupil Evaluation Inventory for children with a schizophrenic mother ($N = 75$), a depressed mother ($N = 57$), and normal parents ($N = 153$).

Distributions of the percentage scores for items were found to be skewed, so all item scores were transformed by computing the arcsine of the square root of the scores (Winer, 1971). The three factor scores, Aggression, Unhappiness–Withdrawal, and Likeability–Social Competence, represented the average of the transformed scores of the items comprising each factor. Untransformed factor means and standard deviations may be found in Table 2.

Analyses of variance revealed significant main effects for Sex of Child on the Aggression and Likeability factors; boys were rated as more aggressive ($F = 5.81$, $df = 1/273$, $p < .05$) and less likeable ($F = 7.57$, $df = 1/273$, $p < .01$). There were also significant main effects for Grade Level on all three factors; younger children were rated as more aggressive ($F = 14.26$, $df = 1/273$, $p < .001$), more withdrawn ($F = 5.13$, $df = 1/273$, $p < .05$), and more likeable ($F = 3.99$, $df = 1/273$, $p < .05$). For both the Aggression and Unhappiness–Withdrawal factors, analyses of variance revealed no significant interactions between Parental Diagnosis and Grade Level or Sex of Child. Planned contrasts indicated that children of a schizophrenic mother in comparison with the normal controls were rated significantly higher on the Aggression factor ($t(273) = 1.83$, $p < .05$) and the Unhappiness–Withdrawal factor ($t(273) = 1.78$, $p < .05$).

For the Likeability factor, there was a significant interaction between Parental Diagnosis and Sex of Child ($F = 3.50$, $df = 2/273$, $p < .05$); consequently, contrasts were computed separately for boys and girls. Daughters of a schizophrenic mother were rated significantly less likeable than the normal controls ($t(273) = 2.36$, $p < .01$), but not significantly different than children with a depressed mother. No significant effects were obtained for the boys on Likeability.

Because only a small percentage of children with a schizophrenic parent will ultimately become schizophrenic themselves, analyses comparing the means of all target and control children may well fail to detect this subgroup of a high-risk sample. Therefore, in addition to the parametric analyses, a nonparametric analysis of children who were rated as deviant was conducted. The 75th percentile was adopted as a cutpoint for Aggression and Unhappiness–Withdrawal, and the 25th percentile was used for Likeability. The partition of chi-square method for evaluation of multidimensional contingency tables was employed in a four-factor ($2 \times 2 \times 2 \times 2$) analysis (Sutcliffe, 1957; Goodman, 1970).

Two-way, three-way, and four-way interactions for Sex, Grade Level, Parental Diagnosis (Schizophrenic versus Normal), and Dichotomized factor (Extreme Quartile versus Remaining Group) were evaluated. For Aggression, Unhappiness–Withdrawal and Likeability, no three- or four-way interactions were significant. Aggression and Unhappiness–Withdrawal, however, interacted significantly with Parental Diagnosis; significantly more children of a schizophrenic parent scored in the extreme quartile on the Aggression factor and the Unhappiness–Withdrawal factor. Percentages of children in the extreme quartile for each factor are found in Table 3, along with the corresponding chi-square statistics. Finally, the two factors that had produced significant results, Aggression and Unhappiness–Withdrawal, were considered simultaneously; that is, the proportion of children with scores in the extreme quartiles for either Aggression or Unhappiness–Withdrawal was evaluated in the partition of chi-square analysis. This showed that 61.3% of the children of a schizophrenic mother were in the extreme quartile on either Aggression or Unhappiness–Withdrawal, compared to 34.0% of the children of a normal mother ($\chi^2 = 15.4$, $p < .001$). There were no significant differences, however, between children of a schizophrenic parent and children of a depressed parent. For Aggression, Unhappiness–Withdrawal, Likeability, and Aggression or Unhappiness–Withdrawal, the percentage of offspring of depressives falling in the deviant group was 33.3, 31.5, 26.3, and 52.6, respectively.

In summary, our school data strikingly indicate that children with a schizophrenic parent show lowered competence along several dimensions. Teachers rated them as more deviant than their classmate controls on three of the four rational clusters, and 9 of the 11 scales. Children with such a pattern have been described (Spivack et al., 1972) as presenting a major behavioral disturbance. They manifest acting out and impulsive behavior and are in conflict with the

Table 3. *Percentage of children in extreme quartile on peer factors*

Factor	Schizophrenic (%)	Control (%)	Chi square	Significance
Aggression	34.7	19.6	6.16	.025
Unhappy–Withdrawn	38.7	19.6	9.53	.005
Likeability–Social Competence	32.0	22.2	2.53	NS
Aggression or Unhappy–Withdrawn	61.3	34.0	15.40	.001

behavioral demands of the school environment. They seem unable to make productive use of the classroom and achieve poorly. Their peers also perceive them to be different, describing them as abrasive, withdrawn, and unhappy. These children may, indeed, be described as vulnerable.

This picture of lowered competence in the offspring of children with a schizophrenic parent is generally consistent with previous research. We did not, however, find separate behavioral patterns for the boys and girls that were consistent with Watt and Lubensky's (1976) characterization of male preschizophrenics as abrasive and females as withdrawn. Instead, our data reveal a broader range of incompetence in both boys and girls. Perhaps, then, there are multiple developmental pathways to schizophrenia.

Although the children with a depressed parent were not as deviant as those with a schizophrenic parent, they also showed patterns of incompetence and vulnerability. Although there is a paucity of data on the behavioral antecedents of depression, there is evidence that the offspring of depressives are at higher risk for adult affective disorder (Winokur et al., 1969; Perris, 1973), and for childhood maladjustment (Welner et al., 1977; McKnew et al., 1979). There is also the suggestion that social competence may be a relevant dimension of this vulnerability. First, social competence is a relevant variable in predicting the course and outcome of depression (Klorman, Strauss, & Kokes, 1977). Current theories of depression also implicate low social competence as a factor of etiological importance. Lewinsohn (1975), for example, asserts that an inadequate behavioral repertoire can lead to a reduced rate of response-contingent reinforcement, the key variable in his theory of depression. In a similar vein, a low level of social competence could be relevant to acquiring a negative view of the self, environment, and future – Beck's (1967) theory – or to believing that responses and outcomes are independent – Seligman's (1974) learned helplessness theory.

PART VI

The Minnesota High-Risk Studies: 1971–1982

This part is comprised of five brief chapters that together provide a sampling of the theory, methods, and findings of the Minnesota Project. In the first chapter, Norman Garmezy and Vernon Devine very briefly review the history and development of risk research as the project team attempted to define operationally and to establish convergently valid measures for the constructs of *group risk* status, subject *vulnerability*, and developmentally appropriate indices of *competence*. Their selection of five risk cohorts and the relevance of individually matched, randomly selected and stratified normative control subjects are presented in the context of their planned four-stage research plan.

The three chapters following the introductory one represent the final major studies of the Minnesota Risk Research Project. These studies by Keith Nuechterlein, Susan Phipps-Yonas, and Regina Driscoll were, in the Garmezy tradition, separate doctoral dissertations that were planned collectively as a systematic program of collaborative research designed to investigate the occurrence of attentional and informational-processing dysfunction in children characterized by different levels of both risk and peer-rated social competence. In the final chapter of this section, Keith Nuechterlein provides a sophisticated perspective on the potential benefits and pitfalls of future attentional studies with persons at risk for schizophrenia. The reader will find concurrence of opinion in these four chapters and the two describing the McMaster–Waterloo Project.

A final, but very important editorial comment is necessary, and it concerns pertinent information that has been omitted from the description of the Minnesota Project. Many readers of this volume may be unaware of the key roles that Norman Garmezy has played in the shaping and the success of all the projects in the Risk Research Consortium. He, more than any other person, has been responsible for advocating the value of prospective risk research, for establishing the consortium, and for facilitating communication among its members. In the past several years his work, known as Project Competence, has shifted to the detection and description of the attributes of *invulnerable* children among those at high risk.

287

18 Project Competence: the Minnesota studies of children vulnerable to psychopathology

NORMAN GARMEZY AND VERNON DEVINE

The Minnesota studies of children vulnerable to psychopathology had its roots both in the literature of schizophrenia and of developmental psychology. From the former we drew on studies suggesting the importance of early childhood antecedents to the adult disorder; in particular, the literature of prognosis strongly implicated functional competence in childhood and adolescence as being powerfully predictive of recovery from the disorder. Developmental psychology provided a rich and exciting experimental focus on children that pointed to the structure and etiology of many child and adult behavior disorders. It also set forth a literature that emphasized the methodological weakness of using the retrospections of adults to secure data on early life-history factors. Finally, the productive example set by investigators Sarnoff Mednick and Fini Schulsinger gave evidence of the viability of studying children at risk for schizophrenia and related disorders.

In contrast to many of the ongoing studies of risk described in this volume, the Minnesota Project from its inception was narrower in scope and more restricted in the variables that were selected for study.

These differences are evident in four aspects of the basic strategy of research employed in the project. The first was the decision to utilize a cross-sectional rather than a longitudinal design. The second was to use several groups of vulnerable children, two based upon maternal psychiatric status and two others based upon the presence of manifest disorder in the children. In all cases severity of disorder determined the criterion for selection. The third aspect was the utilization of matched and random classroom controls for each of the different groups of targeted children. The fourth was to narrow the variables to be studied by choosing only those of social competence on the one hand and attentional functioning on the other.

The program of research described in this chapter, including the studies of K. Nuechterlein, S. Phipps-Yonas, and R. Driscoll, was supported primarily by the Schizophrenia Research Program of The Scottish Rite 33° A.A., Northern Masonic Jurisdiction. Supplemental support was also provided by the William T. Grant Foundation and by an NIMH Research Career Award MH-K14, 914 to the Principal Investigator, N. Garmezy.

CROSS-SECTIONAL DESIGN

The decision to forego a longitudinal design in favor of a cross-sectional strategy was made realizing that both designs have virtues and shortcomings. Longitudinal studies extended over relatively long periods of time permit an evaluation of ongoing processes of pathological or normal personality development. But to achieve this goal a large sample is needed, and this is difficult to achieve when one is dealing with a low base rate occurrence such as schizophrenic disorder. Even maximizing the likely outcome of schizophrenia by selecting children initially presumed to have a genetic predisposition still results in relatively infrequent expression of the disorder. Furthermore, it can be anticipated that attrition of the subject sample will be heightened as the patterns of disorganization that often characterize schizophrenia-prone families find expression in marked mobility within and across communities, family dissolution, and child placements beyond the environs in which the study is to be conducted. To these potential disadvantages must be added the extended length of the age risk period that characterizes the schizophrenic disorder. To incorporate a time spread to age 45, the terminus of the risk range, requires that the longitudinal study be conducted over a span of decades in order to pick up cases of later breakdown.

In addition there is the ever present issue of selecting variables in childhood that might be expected to have predictive validity for the development of schizophrenia that may occur 10 to 30 years in the future. Even within the relative narrow spans of time within childhood, observational techniques change because there is no single method applicable across the developmental span (Kessen, 1960). How much more difficult then the selection of variables that should traverse the period of childhood and adolescence and extend into adulthood.

These difficulties undoubtedly influenced Baldwin (1960) to suggest a cautious approach to data collection *prior* to embarking on a longitudinal study:

> It should be apparent that a longitudinal study of the effects of one, two, or three variables of childhood experience upon later personality is a big investment for relatively small return – quantitatively speaking. It behooves us, therefore, to precede such an undertaking with careful pretesting, study of cross-sectional differences, and cruder retrospective studies to establish the likelihood of major effects. A longitudinal study is the last, not the first step in a research program. It is an absolutely essential research method if we are to get firm knowledge of psychological change, but paradoxically, it is to be avoided whenever possible. (p. 27)

Our decision, finally, was to move to a series of carefully designed cross-sectional studies of children at risk as an initial strategy for evaluating and describing the developmental attributes of the high-risk versus normal control groups of children at different ages.

THE SELECTION OF VULNERABLE AND CONTROL GROUPS OF CHILDREN

The basic index group in all of the studies were children born to mothers who had been diagnosed as schizophrenic at some prior period in their adult lives. These women were located by screening all female psychiatric admissions to several major public psychiatric facilities. Typically, this screening period covered a brief span of time preceding the initiation of the studies. In the early group of studies case record DSM-II diagnoses were reviewed prior to selecting mothers whose children would serve as the experimental cohort. In later investigations, case records were reviewed and scored independently by clinical judges who then provided a diagnostic judgment. These more careful reviews gave clear evidence of the reliability of the diagnostic assignments of the mothers (cf. Nuechterlein, 1983).

From the very inception of the program we sought to compare the group of children who had been born to schizophrenic mothers with children of less severely disturbed mothers who had received nonpsychotic diagnoses at a number of the same institutions. Our aim was to select a homogeneous sample of affectively disordered mothers. However, in the public facilities in which we worked, a number of the cases selected presented an admixture of symptoms. In the study by Rolf (conducted during 1968–1969) this admixture was one in which the mothers presented *internalizing* behaviors such as "depression, anxiety reaction, and phobic reaction." In a subsequent study by Marcus (conducted in 1972) a large proportion of affective cases in combination with some personality disorders constituted a control group of less severely disordered mothers.

A word about exclusion criteria employed in the earlier studies is necessary. In the case of the selection of the mother groups, exclusion from the study was based on these criteria: (1) evidence of organic pathology; (2) non-Caucasian; (3) beyond the age range 18 to 55; and (4) evidence of mental retardation.

In addition to these two child cohorts that were based upon severity of the biological mothers' psychiatric disorder, it was decided to select for study two additional groups of children who were already showing signs of manifest disturbances that varied in severity. These children were screened by a survey of the intake records of a local child guidance clinic or the clinical evaluation center of the public school system. The case records were then rated for symptoms at intake to derive categories of predominantly externalizing or internalizing symptomatic behaviors that Achenbach (1966) had derived in an earlier Minnesota study. The externalizing children were marked by a predominance of overt acts of aggression, stealing, lying, and bullying behaviors, whereas the internalizing groups reflected behavioral patterns of anxiety, withdrawal, social isolation, and fearfulness.

Reviews (Shea, 1972; Garmezy & Streitman, 1974) of the literature of this well-known dichotomy of children's disorders (which paralleled the findings of Phillips, 1968, and Zigler & Phillips, 1961, in their studies of adult disorder) provided our research group with two additional cohorts of children marked by disordered behaviors that not only reflected variations along a severity dimension, but also were strongly suggestive of differences in their prognostic implications for subsequent adult disorder. Specifically, the literature strongly indicated more favorable outcomes for the internalizing children relative to those with marked externalizing symptoms (Shea, 1972; Robins, 1966).

In the final three studies of *attention* that were performed, as described in separate chapters of this part on the Minnesota Project, the internalizing chil-

Table 1. *Four target groups of children at risk employed in the early Minnesota studies of vulnerable children*

Severity of disorder and prognostic potential	Selection basis	
	Children of disordered mothers	Disordered (clinic) children
Poor to moderate	Group 1–Psychiatric status of mother: Schizophrenia	Group 3–Clinic status of child: Externalizing behavior
Moderate to good	Group 2–Psychiatric status of mother: (Primarily) nonpsychotic; depressive disorders; personality disorders	Group 4–Clinic status of child: Internalizing behavior

dren's group was dropped in favor of a hyperactive group for two reasons: (1) Consistent with our prior hypothesis, the internalizing group performed in a manner that often failed to differentiate them from the normal control children; (2) hyperactive children were deemed to be a far more relevant group to study in investigations of attentional behavior when comparing their performance with the performance of children of schizophrenic mothers. These hyperactive children were not on drugs when studied, nor did they show a predominance of antisocial behavior.

Table 1 show these initial four index groups of children in terms of the basis for their selection and their presumed variation in current competence functioning and prognostic potential.

In addition to these four groups of children at risk, two control groups were also selected for study. When the project began in 1968, we were uncertain as to whether to provide a random or a matched (on demographic variables) normal control child for each index child. The conservative decision was made to provide both in the initial phase of the project.

Accordingly, the following procedure for selecting the normal control children was used: All children in the four target groups were initially located in their respective school classrooms. Teachers in these classrooms were asked to indicate which of the children (including the target child) in her or his class seemed to be getting along reasonably well. The index children who were of specific interest to the investigators were not identified as such to teachers or to school personnel, a procedure that was rigorously observed in the two groups (1 and 2) selected on the basis of maternal disorder. In the case of the children who made up the externalizing and internalizing child guidance clinic groups (3 and 4), teachers (who had often been the original referral source) may have had some awareness as to the status of these children, but the selection basis was never made known to them.

Furthermore, the use of multiple control children who were selected in each classroom served to embed each target child among a more general set of selectees.

Once the teachers had indicated who they considered to be adaptive, the children's cumulative school records were perused to provide a child matched to the target child on the basis of age, sex, grade, social class, family intactness, and, whenever possible, achievement and intellectual level. This child served as the *matched* control child (Group 5). A second child matched only for sex and grade who followed the target child on the class roster served as the *random* control child (Group 6). On this basis the subjects of the study were formed into triads of children (Target, Matched Control, and Random Control) which were distributed over wide-ranging sectors of the city.

The Triad 1 cluster was comprised of all the target children born to schizophrenic mothers, each with his or her own matched and random classroom control. In a similar fashion the Triad 2 cluster was made up of the depressive mothers' children, the Triad 3 group of externalizing children and the Triad 4 group of internalizing children, each also having a Group 5 (matched) and a Group 6 (random) child similarly assigned.

In our early studies we focused on the years of middle childhood by generally selecting children from grades 3 to 6; later seventh and eighth graders were involved in the studies. The numbers of children in each study were quite substantial. In the first study, Rolf (1972) made use of 120 classrooms to provide a total number of 356 children in various triad groupings. In the L. Marcus (1972) study 80 classrooms and 240 children were utilized.

The rationale for the method of subject selection and assignment was complex and logically defensible. Studies of the schizophrenia spectrum disorders (Heston, 1966; Kety, Rosenthal, Schulsinger, & Wender, 1968) suggest that certain forms of psychopathology tend to cohere; other disorders fall outside the spectrum. Although there is disagreement about the spectrum concept, the fact that the nonpsychotic depressive disorders did not appear to be part of the spectrum concept led us to use such a group of mothers for comparison purposes.

Furthermore, the symptom linkage suggested by Phillips (1968) and Zigler and Phillips (1961) also speaks to the inclusion of disorders marked by antisocial activity, for symptoms of "withdrawal from others" and "turning against others" appear to share in common such significant correlates of adaptive insufficiency as poor premorbid adjustment and relatively poor prognosis when compared with patients who exhibit a symptom pattern characterized by "turning against the self." On these grounds it seemed appropriate to attempt to use children born to groups of mothers whose disorders suggested a range of adaptive outcomes, hence the choice of schizophrenia and nonpsychotic depression.

Two factors influenced our choice of already disordered children as additional target groups. The first was our attempt to secure groups of children whose manifest disturbance may have been rooted to a greater extent in psychogenic (i.e., environmental/familial) rather than genetic factors. Second, it was hoped that such children would provide a disordered behavioral baseline against which the children at risk could be compared, just as symptom-free control children would provide a baseline for normal functioning. The second factor involved the predictiveness of long-term outcome based on a childhood disorder.

The utilization of children with externalizing and internalizing symptomatic behaviors for this purpose of prediction was supported by (1) studies of adult outcomes for these two groups as provided by Robins (1966), Shea (1972), and Kohlberg et al. (1972); and (2) for other findings of variations in family disorganization of such children (Achenbach, 1966; Weintraub, 1973).

THE SELECTION OF DEPENDENT VARIABLES

The range of variables being studied by investigators of children at risk for schizophrenia is a broad and encompassing one (Garmezy, 1975). The inclusion of many of these has a clear-cut rationale. This is particularly true of those variables (e.g., information-processing tasks, attentional functioning, psychophysiological measures) that have been shown to differentiate, with consistency, the performance of adult schizophrenic patients from others.

Faced with a similar selection problem in the Danish genetic studies, D. Rosenthal, Wender, Kety, Schulsinger, Welner, and Ostergaard (1968) used a rational basis for selecting an optimal evaluation strategy of the offspring of schizophrenics who had been reared in adoptive homes:

Lacking a clearcut theory, we had recourse to three broad strategies to guide our decisions about what or what not to do. The first was . . . differences found between schizophrenics and normal controls on various psychological and behavior tests. . . .

The second strategy . . . was based on the idea that we should find the same kinds of traits and aberrations in our index group as in the premorbid personality of known schizophrenics. . . .

A third strategy was simply to emulate success (of others) . . . (pp. 380–381)

This formula has been followed similarly by the current risk research groups, although the task is more difficult because the subjects being studied are children and not adults as in the Danish adoption studies.

The Minnesota research group adopted Rosenthal's empirical thrust as the appropriate strategy, but placed a greater emphasis on three factors in selecting variables: (1) their evidential power for differentiating schizophrenic patients from other psychopathological and normal groups; (2) their significance as factors influencing adaptation; and (3) our ability to translate the variable into a form and procedure appropriate for use with children of different ages.

The first and most important priority that the Minnesota Project fixed upon was to devise measures that were indicative of competence. The inevitable search for predictor variables in risk studies assumes that there are available external criteria to evaluate success or failure of adaptation in the children at risk. This first priority – the establishment of measurable childhood components of competence and incompetence – had the strategic objective of providing a needed intermediate criterion of presence or absence of psychopathology in the target children. Such intermediate outcomes are necessary when an investigator must cope with low incidence rates, an undetermined etiology, and a lengthy time period before the appearance of the disorder. Were individuals to become the victims of schizophrenia with a rapid and inexplicable onset in the absence of any precursor signs, investigators would then have to depend solely on an ultimate outcome measure: that is, disorder versus nondisorder. Fortunately, schizophrenia, typically, does not follow such an unpredictable course, and the more malignant processes show clear prodromal indicators. Thus intermediate criteria reflecting competence is a strategically viable procedure for inferring the likelihood of a heightened probability for later negative outcome. However, one must recognize that such predictions will inevitably be subject to an unspecifiable error rate of false positives and false negatives when using these intermediate outcomes as predictors of schizophrenia.

THE FOUR-STAGE STRATEGY OF RESEARCH

The Minnesota Project as originally conceived provided four stages for studying children at risk. Stage I was given over to a search for age-related indices of competence and incompetence. Stage II was seen as one devoted to the discovery of response parameters that could differentiate between the target (i.e., risk) children and their normal control counterparts. Competence variables identified in Stage I studies would then be incorporated in testing the differentiating power of the Stage II variables. In Stage III studies it was hoped that a short-term follow-up study that made use of the Stage II differentiation would compare the adaptation of children at risk and controls. The final Stage IV would be devoted to nontraditional intervention efforts that would be based upon experimental–clinical techniques that would attempt to modify the child's performance on the Stage II variables followed by later evaluations designed to test the effects of behavioral changes on the Stage I competence factors.

This fourth stage was not reached during the decade covered by the project. The results of the studies performed during the course of Stages I to III are discussed in the sections that follow.

STAGE I: MEASURING SOCIAL COMPETENCE: THE ROLF STUDY

The roots of our focus on social competence are manifold. At the level of aphorism there was Whitehorn's observation that the "people who are mentally healthy usually work well, play well, love well and expect well." It translated readily into economic and occupational productivity, interpersonal and sexual competence, and a high level of self-esteem – all of which are hallmarks of the healthy personality. Its counterpart in clinical outcome research was the suggestion by Phillips (1968) that occupational achievement, maturity, and adequacy in sexual and social relationships as exemplified by friendship patterns in childhood, adolescence, and adulthood form the basis for predicting competence after breakdown.

The decision to use sociometry to measure social competence in childhood had a sturdy set of empirical demonstrations in the educational research literature to support the reliability and validity of the method. Subsequently the reports of Cowen et al. (1973), Bower (1969), Lewis and Rosenblum (1975), and Roff, Sells, and Golden (1972) confirmed their appropriateness in risk research. Jon Rolf initiated and carried to a successful conclusion the first study of the Minnesota Program. Preceding the study were two major contributions by DePree (1966) and Weintraub (1973). The former demonstrated the power of the competence variable to transcend social class membership. The latter affirmed the power of a self-control variable for differentiating among externalizing, internalizing, and normal control children; variations in social class status of the children's families occupied a secondary status to the adaptational status of the children.

Rolf set out to translate the emphasis on social, economic, and sexual competence downward to provide types of behavior that would be relevant to children. Thus, he decided to measure social competence by peer acceptance while translating economic competence into performance and work achievement in the school setting. Sexual competence was set aside temporarily as not directly applicable to elementary school children but with a recognition that positive peer play in the context of appropriate sex-typed behavior might presage adequate future sexual adaptation.

To secure age-appropriate measures of social competence, Rolf selected a sociometric measure of peer status, Bower's Class Play (1969) and a more simplified Peer Relations Questionnaire for the younger children in the first and second grades. The latter requires that the respondent indicate who in the class they would and would not like to sit by, work with, and play with. The Class Play requests classmates to take on the role of a casting director and to cast members of the class for different roles in the hypothetical play. The presence of positive, negative, and externalizing roles provided the basis for measuring peer acceptance (Rolf, 1972).

Teachers also provided ratings of each of the triadic groups of children. The 25 items the teacher used were based on Watt et al.'s (1970) rational factoring of Conger and Miller's (1966) teacher's rating scale that had been used successfully to predict delinquency among school children. In addition, the teacher rated the triad of children in her classroom (target child, matched control, and random control) on three 5-point scales designed to measure intellectual potential, overall emotional adjustment, and overall social adjustment.

Rolf's (1972) findings have been summarized by him in this way:

At the *triad* level, the prediction was generally supported that the groups, in comparison with their respective control groups, obtained lower competence scores. At the *target group level* the trend of *peer-rated* competence score ranks indicated that for both males and females the externalizing children were lowest, followed in order of ascending competence by the children with schizophrenic mothers, the internalizing children, and by the children whose mothers had internalizing symptoms. This order was also obtained for the *teacher-rated* competence scores, but only for the girls and not the boys. In the latter case, teachers rated externalizers lowest, and internalizers next lowest, but teachers did not discriminate, with certain exceptions, between the two male target groups with mentally ill mothers and their respective control groups. (p. 241)

The discrepancy between teachers and peers remains an intriguing one. Does it invalidate the peer-liking measure? This is unlikely. There is a substantial literature on sociometry that indicates that peer-liking and peer acceptance can be measured reliably even in the preschool years (Hartup, Glazer, & Charlesworth, 1967). Furthermore, peer-liking measures are stable over time (Master & Morison, 1981) whereas low-liking status is associated with poorer mental health and poor utilization of academic abilities.

There is a challenge posed by the discrepancy between peer (lower) and teacher (higher) ratings of the children born to schizophrenic mothers. Is it a question of the long-cited, but not always substantiated observation that teachers are more insensitive to internalizing children and more attuned to the discomforts provided by disruptive children who, by their classroom behavior, can block the acquisition of social and intellectual skills not only for themselves but for their peers as well? This would account for the peer–teacher agreement with regard to their judgments of the externalizing child and, perhaps, the teacher's nonnegative judgment of the high-risk child. But in that case, why did peers downgrade the risk child? Is it possible that the data simply reflected the moderate correlations that exist between peer and teacher judgments? Or is it possible that the "normal" peer in the course of play perceives aspects of the risk child's behavior that the teacher does not or cannot witness? Are the precursors to ultimate maladaptation to be found in inadequate play patterns, in unresponsivity in play or, perhaps, in subtle negative postures in the course of play? Today, a decade later, the paradox remains unresolved. However, our more recent studies do indicate greater variability in the extent to which peers express their preference (pro and con) for their high-risk peers.

Subsequently a further analysis (Rolf & Garmezy, 1974) was performed on the cumulative school records of these six groups of children. It was hoped that some reconciliation could be achieved by analyzing whether the teacher's ratings would better differentiate between the four target groups of children and their respective controls. In addition, under Rolf's direction, analysis of demographic variables was carried out.

The results of these analyses indicated that: (1) all target groups received significantly lower grades than did their randomly selected controls at some time during grade school. (Of interest also were the findings that the controls matched to these target children were more often late, absent, received poorer grades, and were rated more negatively by peers and teachers when compared with the random controls.); (2) supplementary competence indicators can be adduced from the biographical contents of the academic school record; (3) children of schizophrenic mothers were found on these supplemental measures to resemble more closely the externalizing children; (4) children of nonpsychotic, depressive mothers gave some evidence of behavior disturbance and school difficulties, but these children most closely resembled the control children; (5) the findings for lower socioeconomic status (SES), nonintact, or highly mobile families did not generalize in simplistic ways when applied to children with other backgrounds. For example, those internalizing boys who demonstrated poor social and academic competence were more frequently from intact families that were of more advantaged SES status and had a lower frequency of family moves.

STAGE II: THE STUDY OF ATTENTIONAL FUNCTIONING AND COMPETENCE

The basic focus of the Minnesota studies of risk following Rolf's initial investigation was on attentional phenomena as exhibited by the target and normal control children. As noted in earlier articles (Garmezy, 1977, 1978) the reasoning behind this decision to concentrate on attentional studies was a logical one that was rooted in a series of solid research findings demonstrating that those premorbid levels of competence observed as positive prognostic factors in schizophrenia are essentially representatives of social and occupational skills. Effectiveness in these areas is attainable only under conditions of attentional focusing. Presumably the precursor skills of children similarly reflect the need for an effective attentional substrate.

In an unpublished study Devine and Tomlinson (1975) tested the relationship between competence and attention in 19 elementary school classrooms in the same public school system in which we had conducted our risk studies. They asked teachers to categorize all pupils in their classes into one of four groups ranging from superior adaptation accompanied by a total absence of any signs of problems to the presence of problems that teachers perceived as being sufficiently severe and ubiquitous to require a professional referral.

Following these teacher ratings, trained judges were sent into the classrooms to observe the class for several hours over the span of 1 week. The observation system (Cobb, 1969) used was one of previously demonstrated reliability and validity. The observers did not know of the adaptation ratings that had been provided by the teachers.

The findings strongly supported the presumed relationship between teacher rated competence and observed attention behavior. Across all 19 classrooms the hierarchy of attentional efficiency was concordant with the teacher's hierarchy of the functional adaptation of the children. Furthermore, each competence category contained significantly different levels of attentional effectiveness as exhibited by its student members.

The first attempt to study attentional functioning in groups of target and control cohorts similar to those used by Rolf was conducted by Marcus (1972), who essentially replicated (but with several interesting embellishments) the classical studies of reaction time (RT) in schizophrenic patients conducted by David Shakow and his associates (Rodnick & Shakow, 1940; Shakow, 1946, 1962, 1963, 1979; Cromwell, Rosenthal, Shakow, & Zahn, 1961).

Two hundred and forty children participated in the study; 120 were elementary school pupils in grades 4 to 6 and 120 were junior high school (grades 7–8) students. These children were divided into 80 triads that included 10 drawn from each of the four target groups, one-half composed of boys and one-half of girls. There were 40 triads in each of the two elementary and secondary school groups.

Marcus conducted three related experiments with these 240 subjects. The first was essentially a replication of the Worcester studies, using a *Regular* and *Irregular* RT procedure. Under these two conditions, with sequence rotated for half of each of the groups, the child depressed a response button following a "Ready" signal. With the sounding of a reaction stimulus tone (fed to the child's ear through earphones) the child released the button as rapidly as possible. A 7-second in-tertrial interval was interspersed between each of the 1-, 2-, 4-, and 15-second preparatory intervals (PI). In the *Regular* condition 10–11 trials were presented successively at each preparatory interval, the sequence of the order of presentation of the various PIs being randomized over 20 different orders. For the *Irregular* procedure 50 trials were given with the different PIs presented sequentially in a quasi-random order. Clearly, the Regular procedure was designed to facilitate the child's adaptation to the task, whereas the Irregular procedure added a marked element of uncertainty to the RT task.

The two studies that Marcus added were designed to facilitate the task for the child. The second study was marked by an *Information* procedure. An Irregular sequence was again used but preceding each trial the child was provided, through the medium of a panel of lighted windows, with a qualitative estimate of the PI that was to follow: "very short," "short," "medium," "long," "very long" (cf. Cromwell et al., 1961).

In the third study, defined as a *High Incentive* condition the child essentially selected a desired PI but secured incentive payoffs as a function of the presumed difficulty of the PI that he or she had selected (low payoff for a short PI: high payoff for a long one). Success and failure followed a predetermined payoff matrix. Cooperativeness ratings of the subject were made by Marcus at the conclusion of the testing session.

The basic results of the study are presented in Table 2. These indicate that of the four target groups, only the group of children of schizophrenic mothers failed to reach the performance level of their controls under the basic procedures as well as the two presumably facilitating ones. The externalizing children who performed with relative deficits in two of the procedures showed a significant increment under the Incentive payoff condition. The children of nonpsychotic psychiatrically disturbed women showed an initial performance lag relative to their controls but this difference disappeared with the introduction of the condition in which they were provided with information about the length of the PI as well as in the High Incentive condition. The internalizing children performed in a manner consistent with their controls under all test procedures.

Further analysis of the date indicated, however, that the deficits of the high-risk subjects were not the gross deficiencies characteristic of schizophrenic patients, but were of a far more subtle sort. The children exhibited modifiability and showed themselves to be capable of improvement; they revealed a continued high level of motivation and the retention of a flexible responsiveness. However, the revealed deficit performance was not only evidenced in the younger elementary school groups, comprised of children of schizophrenic mothers and externalizing

Table 2. *Attentional deficits and nondeficits in target groups of risk children relative to their respective combined control groups (matched and random) under the four experimental conditions*

Procedure	Deficit performance Target groups[a] Higher-risk 1	3	Lower-risk 2	4	Nondeficit performance Target groups[b] Higher-risk 1	3	Lower-risk 2	4
Regular	X	X	X					0
Irregular	X	X	X					0
Information (cognitive facilitation)	X	X					0	0
High incentive (cognitive + motivational facilitation)	X					0	0	0

Notes: Deficits measured by significant main (diagnostic status) or interaction (diagnostic status $\times$ PI) effects.

Key to target groups: *children of disordered mothers:* 1–schizophrenic, 2–nonpsychotic; *disordered clinic children:* 3–externalizers, 4–internalizers.

[a]X = Deficit (target > controls).

[b]0 = No deficit (target = controls).

Source: Adapted from Marcus, 1972, p. 181.

children, but in the older junior high school groups as well. This is counter to data obtained with the normal control groups in this study and other studies that detail RT improvements in older children.

In a section of the chapter that follows Susan Phipps-Yonas reports on an effort that she made to replicate partially Marcus's findings. This was not achieved, but there remain sufficient differences between the procedures of the two studies to make uncertain any definitive interpretation of the failure to replicate the previous study.

STAGE III: A SHORT-TERM FOLLOW-UP STUDY

For Stage III it was hoped that a short-term follow-up study would make use of differences observed in Stage II cross-sectional studies by contrasting the subsequent adaptations of the various risk groups with their controls. An effort in this direction was conducted by Herbert (1977) in a summa thesis performed under Vernon Devine's direction.

Herbert sought to determine, 4 to 7 years after completion of the Rolf and Marcus studies, how the children who had participated in those earlier investigations were functioning. The questions she posed were these: What was their progress like in school? Had the differences between the target and control children increased as the subjects matured? What were the relative competence levels of the groups several years after the initial ratings?

To determine the status of the target and control children at the point of follow-up, Herbert returned to the schools where she examined the cumulative school records and interviewed the school counselors, the assistant principals, and the school social worker regarding the children's progress.

The initial effort to locate these children was made by reviewing the central files of the city school system. The original subjects who had not left the city were traced to the schools that they were then presumably attending. A list of all available subjects was prepared with all reference removed as to the original target/control status of the children, and the various schools were then visited. However, as had been the case in the initial studies, many children were not in their assigned classes or even in their assigned schools, and multiple discussions had to be held with school personnel to trace their current location.

Once located, the school records were reviewed to secure the child's grades, attendance, and lateness reports, citizenship grades, and the most recent achievement test scores. In addition, the most knowledgeable school authority, typically the counselor and/or the social worker, who had been assigned to a given student, was interviewed to secure their perception of the child's adjustment, any problems he or she was encountering, as well as indications as to whether the child was outstanding in any way. To retain the school's cooperation and to protect the student's privacy the interviewer emphasized that the project was not seeking personal information but rather the school's judgment about the presence of adjustment problems, if any, and their severity (*mild, moderate, severe*) or any of the child's attainments that were "outstanding." Even with this explanation care had to be exercised in the inquiry to protect the family's privacy.

Usually a team of two interviewers visited the school; while one recorded information from the cumulative record, the other conducted the interviews with school personnel. Subsequently the children's adjustment was rated on a 5-point scale that ranged from "outstanding school leader" through "average," "mild," "moderate," or "severe" problems.

When all data had been recorded, subjects were matched to their original identification numbers in either the Rolf or the Marcus study and the original target and control groups were reassembled for data analysis.

SOME SPECIFIC OBSERVATIONS

Attrition of the original samples. The problem of sample attrition in the central city is a pervasive one. Of the original total of 540 subjects in the two studies combined, 356 (approximately two-thirds of the sample) were followed up. Of Rolf's original groups 172/356, approximately 50%, were located, whereas 183 of Marcus's original of group of 240 (76%) were found. Of the 184 subjects on whom data were not gathered 150 had moved out of the school district and 34 (12 female and 22 male) could not be located. This report is restricted to the children who remained within the city school system.

Unfortunately the children of the schizophrenic mothers' group had the greatest out-of-city mobility compared to their controls (48% versus 26%); mobility was also evident in the externalizer target group (35% versus 22%) and internalizer groups (39% versus 26%). By contrast, the children of the internalizing mother group had a lower mobility rate (16%), a finding made more striking by the fact that its control group showed the greatest mobility of all groups (31%).

"Dropouts." All Target groups except the children of schizophrenic mothers (Target 1s) had higher dropout rates than their combined (matched and random) controls. The externalizing group (Target 3s) showed the highest rate of dropout relative to their controls (24% versus 8%). Surprisingly, the internalizing children (Target 4s) showed a 15% dropout rate compared to 0% for their controls. The children of nonpsychotic mothers (Target 2s) had a 22% rate of school leaving, whereas their control groups showed only a 10% loss. Five percent of the children of schizophrenic mothers versus 12% of their controls dropped out of school. It is possible, however, that the substantial unaccounted for school transfers in the Target 1 group may have cloaked a heavier ultimate dropout count.

Grades. All the control groups had higher average grades than their respective target groups. Of the Target groups the order for grade average was Target 2s (highest), 4s, 1s, 3s (lowest).

Citizenship ratings. Target 3s obtained the lowest citizenship ratings relative to all other Target groups and controls; the Target 1 children had the best ratings and these were commensurate with the ratings teachers had accorded the control children.

Attendance. All Target groups had a higher average absentee rate than the control groups; Target groups 2 and 3 were significantly more absent than were their controls, but this did not hold for the Target 1 children relative to their own control group.

Achievement scores. All Target groups had lower average scores on reading achievement tests relative to their controls with the differences being greatest for the Target 3s and 4s. Nevertheless all Target groups except for the Externalizing children (Target 3) approached mean performance levels on the achievement test.

Positive versus negative outcomes. The category of Positive Outcome was assigned to those students who were in school (or who had graduated) and were rated by three interviewers in the schools as either "average" or "outstanding." Negative Outcome was applied to those children who had either dropped out of school, or had been given ratings of "moderate" or "severe" problems by one or more of the school personnel who had been interviewed. Children whose problems were classified as "mild" or who were not located were excluded from this analysis.

All Target groups when compared with their respective control groups had lower proportions of positive outcomes, but these differences were significant only for the Target 2s, 3s, and 4s. The children of schizophrenic mothers closely approximated the proportion of positive outcomes relative to their controls (60% versus 69%). By contrast these proportions for Target 3s and their respective controls were 31% versus 78%. For Target 2s comparisons revealed proportions of 48% versus 83%, and for Target 4's the respective values for good outcomes were 55% versus 94%.

Thus on follow-up all the Target groups tended, in general, to show poorer adaptation than their controls, with the Externalizing children showing the greatest deficiencies. Although the loss of subjects in Target 1s invites caution in interpretation, the consistency of deficits evidenced in the Target 3 group is confirmatory of a very substantial literature on the maladaptation of such antisocial children.

Herbert (1977) writes:

When we had finished visiting the schools, and were matching the subjects to their identification numbers and diagnostic groups for analysis, we noticed that it was this group which collected all the students about whom we had been given anecdotal "horror stories" by the school personnel who had been interviewed. Time after time, those students on whom we had made notes on information shared by counselors, social workers, and assistant principals on truancy, terrible home situations, delinquency, and various other severe problems proved to be Target 3's. A tentative conclusion – or rather an impression – from this very subjective information is that these subjects are very noticeable in their deviation from the norms of the school and community; they also seem to have as large problems with themselves as they do with the schools and authority in general.

These striking difficulties in adaptation of another group of children at risk suggests the importance of using a variety of potential psychopathological controls as well as normal control groups in studying risk for schizophrenia or related psychopathologies.

PREFACE TO THE FINAL EXPERIMENTAL STUDIES

In the sections that follow the three final major studies of the Minnesota Risk Research Program are presented by the investigators whose doctoral dissertations contributed markedly to enlarging an understanding of the role of attentional functioning in children at risk for schizophrenia.

These studies are marked by several advances in design:

1. They have been completed using the same children as subjects on measures of sustained, selective, and shift attention;
2. They incorporate social competence, both in the Target and Control groups, as an independent rather than as a dependent variable. As such, the studies treat the competence variable as a factor to be related to attentional functioning not only in children at risk, but in normal control children as well; and
3. A new target group – hyperactive children who are not antisocial in their behavior – has been added to these studies. Such children whose attentional dysfunction is markedly evident provide a highly relevant comparison group for evaluating the attentional performance of children who are presumed to be at risk for schizophrenia.

19 Sustained attention among children vulnerable to adult schizophrenia and among hyperactive children

KEITH H. NUECHTERLEIN

As noted in the section describing the background, rationale, and earlier results of the Minnesota High-Risk Project, the study by Rolf (1972) found significant deficits in the peer- and teacher-rated social behavior of children born to schizophrenic mothers as well as in the social behavior of children already identified as having internalizing or externalizing problems. Marcus (1972) followed this study with a demonstration of slowed reaction time among children of schizophrenic mothers and externalizing children, suggesting that a subtle attentional deficit might characterize such children. At the time that the present research was initiated, Erlenmeyer-Kimling (1975) and Grunebaum, Weiss, Gallant, and Cohler (1974) were also reporting preliminary indications of attentional deficits among children of schizophrenic mothers and children of psychotic mothers, respectively.

These early studies suggested the possibility that some children at increased risk for adult schizophrenia might be characterized by deficits in attentional functioning and social competence. At the same time, the studies raised many additional questions. The first question regarding the attentional findings was whether a replicable deficit had been found. A closely related question was whether the deficit was attributable to an attentional dysfunction or to motivational or situational factors. The overall reaction time slowing of offspring of schizophrenic mothers in the Marcus (1972) study was not accompanied by the reaction time patterns as a function of preparatory interval that are characteristic of adult schizophrenia (Nuechterlein, 1977a). Such an increased overall reaction time might be due to motivational, motor, or attentional factors, even though an experimental manipulation of incentives did not result in the disappearance of this deficit.

A similar question regarding the origin of performance deficits reported by

This research was supported by grants from the Scottish Rite Schizophrenia Research Program, NMJ, USA, to N. Garmezy and by a Scottish Rite Dissertation Research Fellowship to K. H. Nuechterlein. The research reported is a portion of a doctoral dissertation submitted to the University of Minnesota (Committee Chairman: N. Garmezy). The author thanks Drs. Erlenmeyer-Kimling and Cornblatt for generously providing information necessary to replicate their playing card version of the CPT. In addition to the author, project personnel involved in initial record review included Regina Driscoll, Susan Phipps-Yonas, Margaret O'Dougherty, David Pellegrini, and Harvey Linder. Symptom appraisal for child guidance clinic children was completed by the author, John Shabatura, and Richard Rexeisen.

Grunebaum et al. (1974) and Gallant (1972) arises, because they found deficits in Continuous Performance Test (CPT) performance only among 5-year-old but not 6-year-old children of schizophrenic mothers. Furthermore, the presence of the mother in the room during testing may have contributed situational performance disruption that is attributable to emotional factors rather than to an enduring attentional deficit.

The positive findings of Erlenmeyer-Kimling and Cornblatt (1978) and Erlenmeyer-Kimling (1975) using an adapted version of the Continuous Performance Test (CPT) with a larger sample of children born to schizophrenic parents, increase greatly the likelihood that a replicable deficit in sustained attention is present among some children born to a schizophrenic parent. However, the playing card adaptation of the CPT employed by Erlenmeyer-Kimling and Cornblatt (1978) differs in several ways from the conventional version used in studies of adult schizophrenics (Orzack & Kornetsky, 1966; Kornetsky, 1972; Wohlberg & Kornetsky, 1973). The playing card version involves a relative rather than an absolute criterion for target stimuli (any two identical cards in sequence), two discrete dimensions of stimulus variation (number and suit), and pairing of successive perceptions. These additional elements would seem to demand more complex cognitive processes, including short-term memory and matching to a continuously changing sample, than the standard CPT and most vigilance tasks (Mackworth, 1970; Stroh, 1971). In addition, pilot testing in Minnesota suggested that this version likely violates, to some extent, an assumption underlying the most straightforward parametric application of signal detection theory analysis (Rutschmann et al., 1977), namely, that the distributions of the effects of signal and noise are normal and have equal variance (Green & Swets, 1966; McNicol, 1972). Thus, an examination of CPT performance of children born to schizophrenic mothers using other CPT versions as well as the playing card version was considered desirable to study further the nature of the suggested deficit in sustained attention.

An additional issue stimulated by the earlier high-risk studies was the extent to which certain attentional dysfunctions may be specific to a vulnerability to schizophrenia or at least to psychosis. Attentional disturbances are prominent in characterizations of certain other forms of psychopathology, in particular, in descriptions of childhood hyperactivity. In fact, DSM-III recognizes the salience of such disturbances in hyperactivity by renaming this condition *attention deficit disorder with hyperactivity* (American Psychiatric Association, 1980). The comparison of attentional functioning in hyperactive children to that in children born to a schizophrenic parent would appear to have special promise for clarifying the nature and specificity of any attentional deficits in these groups.

In the previous study by Marcus (1972) in the Minnesota High-Risk Project, an explicit distinction between hyperactive children and antisocial delinquent children was not made, because the more global division of clinic children into internalizers and externalizers (Achenbach, 1966; Garmezy, 1970) was employed. In the interest of delineating performance differences between these groups, the present research included both hyperactive children and antisocial delinquent children as psychopathological comparison groups.

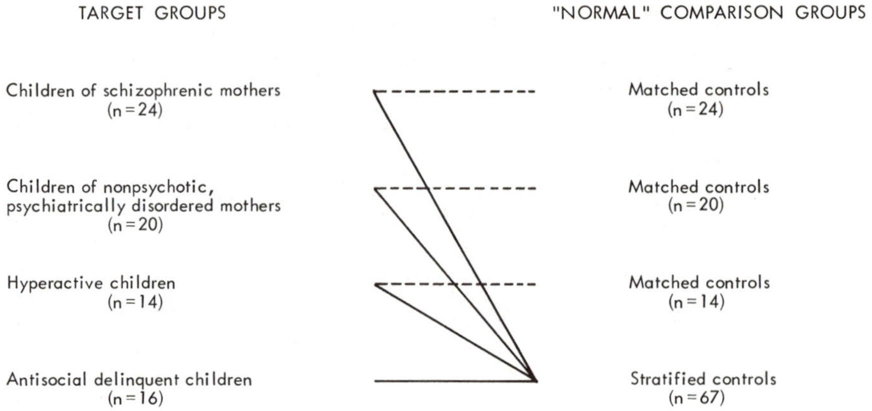

TARGET GROUPS   "NORMAL" COMPARISON GROUPS

Children of schizophrenic mothers   Matched controls
          (n = 24)   (n = 24)

Children of nonpsychotic,   Matched controls
psychiatrically disordered mothers   (n = 20)
          (n = 20)

Hyperactive children   Matched controls
          (n = 14)   (n = 14)

Antisocial delinquent children   Stratified controls
          (n = 16)   (n = 67)

Figure 1. Sample sizes and primary groups to be compared.

SELECTION OF SUBJECTS

This research and the studies by Susan Phipps-Yonas and Regina Driscoll employed four Target groups and four Normal comparison groups that are identified in Figure 1. The mothers having schizophrenic or nonpsychotic psychiatric disorders were identified through a review of psychiatric intake records and hospital charts at two large public hospitals. A total of 1,331 female cases were reviewed, of which 1,259 were excluded at the initial review and 72 were submitted to three diagnostic judges. Most exclusions at initial review were due to the lack of children (496), children being older than 16 years of age (246), children being younger than 9 years of age (108), or patient residence outside the city (129) or unlocatable (113).

Of the 72 cases whose hospital charts were read thoroughly and rated independently by three clinical judges (N. Garmezy, V. T. Devine, and K. H. Nuechterlein), 24 women with a consensus diagnosis of schizophrenia were included among the index mothers, as were 20 women for whom a diagnosis of schizophrenia or *schizophrenia-spectrum disorder* (Rieder, Rosenthal, Wender, & Blumenthal, 1975; Rosenthal, 1975) could be clearly ruled out. Of 24 index schizophrenic mothers, 22 were unanimously given first-choice diagnoses of schizophrenia. The other two index mothers in this group were given first-choice diagnoses of schizophrenia by two of the three judges and a second- or third-choice diagnosis of schizophrenia by the third judge. Most of the remaining women who were excluded after thorough chart review had children in private schools inaccessible to the project, children who were not locatable in the public schools, or were women who had diagnoses judged to be nonschizophrenic psychoses or organic brain syndromes.

The Target groups of hyperactive and antisocial delinquent children were selected from cases seen at either of two child clinics. In addition, additional antisocial delinquent children were recruited from classrooms in two schools for children with behavioral problems. At the two clinics, the charts of 138 cases were evaluated by two raters each, using the Achenbach Symptom Checklist (Achenbach, 1966). The results of a factor analysis of childhood symptomatology (Soli, Nuechterlein, Garmezy, Devine, & Schaefer, 1981) were used to select differentiable samples of hyperactive and antisocial children. Children who scored high on the Hyperactivity factor but not on the Delinquency or Rebelliousness factors (or for females, the Delinquency or Interpersonal Aggression factors) were defined as hyperactive. Antisocial delinquent children were required to have the opposite pattern of factor scores.

In order to ensure case selection consonant with the clinical diagnosis of hyperkinetic reaction, the clear presence of the characteristic symptoms of restless, hyperactive behavior and of poor concentration, distractibility, and short attention span was made an additional criterion for selection of hyperactive subjects.

A total of 14 hyperactive children and 16 antisocial delinquent children were included in the final sample through this process. Children currently taking psychoactive medication were excluded from the final sample, in order to avoid confounding the group differences with known medication effects on attentional task performance (Kornetsky, 1972; Sykes, Douglas, & Morgenstern, 1972). Since the majority of the antisocial delinquent children were recruited 1 year after the rest of the sample and data analysis for these subjects is incomplete, these results will not be presented here.

Each child in the first three Target groups was individually matched to a child in the same classroom on the variables of sex, sociometric status, age, reading achievement scores, and socioeconomic status. (The antisocial children could not be matched individually to classroom comparison children in this way, because the majority were recruited from classrooms for children with behavioral problems. A representative cross-section of peers was not available in these classrooms). Sociometric status was added to the more customary matching variables in order to equate these groups on a known predictor of global level of adult mental health (Cowen et al., 1973; Hartup, 1970; Kohlberg, LaCrosse, & Ricks, 1972). The sociometric index was derived from the number and percentage of negatively toned social roles assigned by classroom peers in an adaptation of Bower's (1960) Class Play procedure, because these measures were found to be most significantly related to later psychiatric contact in a previous study (Cowen et al., 1973). This peer evaluation also served as a measure of the current social competence of each child.

Finally, a large, representative Normal comparison group was selected by stratified sampling within the regular public school classrooms attended by the target children, using sociometric status as the stratification variable. The stratified Normal group for the present research consisted of 67 subjects who did not differ significantly from any of the Target groups in age or vocabulary reading achievement scores, although, as expected, a trend toward lower vocabulary achievement scores was present for the hyperactive sample. The proportion of males and females was quite comparable across groups, with the exception of the hyperactive group, which contained only males. Because the preponderance of hyperactive children are male, the sex composition of this hyperactive sample does not appear to be unrepresentative of this group.

Potential subjects were screened for visual and auditory sensory impairment.

Visual acuity of 20/30 or better, with corrective lenses if necessary, was required for participation. All subjects were between 9 and 16 years of age at the time that testing for sustained attention occurred. The mean age at this testing was 12.9 years.

PROCEDURES

Six versions of the Continuous Performance Test were administered individually to each child. The basic task demands that the subject monitor a quasi-random series of numbers or letters being presented briefly on a small screen at a fixed pace and respond with a button press each time a predesignated target number or letter appears (Rosvold, Mirsky, Sarason, Bransome, & Beck, 1956). In order to further examine previous findings as well as to extend these findings, both old and new versions of the CPT were employed. The session began with the Playing Card CPT, as employed by Erlenmeyer-Kimling, Cornblatt, and Rutschmann (Erlenmeyer-Kimling & Cornblatt, 1978; Rutschmann et al., 1977). The auditory distraction condition was omitted, because early results suggested that it did not contribute strongly to the discrimination between high-risk and low-risk subjects (Erlenmeyer-Kimling, 1975). The second version used was similar to the CPT that Wohlberg and Kornetsky (1973) employed to demonstrate residual attentional deficits among remitted acute schizophrenic individuals. The stimuli were single numerals presented for very brief durations (40 msec for junior high students and 50 msec for elementary school students). The interstimulus interval was 1.42 seconds, identical to that of the Playing Card CPT. The target was the digit "5."

The final four conditions of the CPT involved new adaptations designed to improve detection of certain information-processing deficits. A version of the CPT that provided more difficult discriminations of signal and noise and that met parametric assumptions for convenient signal detection theory analysis was sought. Through signal detection analyses, the ability to discriminate target from nontarget stimuli can be examined independent of differences in biases toward responding in a certain direction (Green & Swets, 1966; Swets, 1973), thereby allowing the processes underlying performance to be isolated more fully.

Pilot testing was completed with adaptations using decreased exposure time, luminance, or cycling time, or including catch trials containing one but not both elements of the targeted stimuli. Finally, stimulus degradation was adopted as the preferred experimental manipulation and was accomplished by blurring the numeral stimuli and superimposing a random pattern of visual noise on these projected numerals.

Piloting showed that the signal detection index, d', yielded quite stable values across different response criterion levels within subjects. In addition, hit and false alarm rates for individual subject's varying criterion levels were converted to normal deviates and plotted on a Receiver Operating Characteristic (ROC) coordinate system (Green & Swets, 1966; McNicol, 1972). Visually fitted lines had slopes that were reasonably close to a value of one, suggesting that the assumptions of normal distributions and of equal variance for the effects of signal and noise were closely approximated. The lower hit rate and higher false alarm rate resulting from the use of more ambiguous stimuli should also allow more reliable determination of signal detection indices than would easier conventional versions.

This adaptation of the CPT, referred to as the Degraded Stimulus CPT, used the same target numeral, interstimulus interval, and exposure times as the preceding more conventional version. Following a condition in which no feedback on performance was provided, each child was administered two versions of the Degraded Stimulus CPT with added auditory feedback immediately following responses to either target stimuli or nontarget stimuli. These feedback conditions correspond to reward and punishment situations, respectively.

The final condition of the CPT required that the child reverse his now overlearned response to the numeral "5" by responding to each numeral from "0" through "9" except the "5s." This Response Reversal CPT was designed to place particular burden on the response selection and organization aspects of information processing, congruent with theories of schizophrenic psychological deficit postulating disproportionate impairment under high response competition conditions (Broen, 1968; Broen & Storms, 1967). Because this condition proved to be quite difficult, the clearly focused rather than the degraded numerals were used in order to avoid lack of individual differences due to floor effects and to allow more direct comparison with the conventional CPT.

During the child's performance of these attentional tasks, the tester rated personality and motivational characteristics on 14 5-point, behaviorally anchored scales.

OVERVIEW OF RESULTS

Analyses were performed to examine both mean differences between groups and presence of disproportionate extreme scoring subgroups. The signal detection indices of d' (indicating signal/noise discrimination) and β (indicating response caution) were calculated for five CPT versions with sufficient error rates to yield reliable signal detection measures. The conventional version of the CPT proved to be too easy to allow reliable signal detection theory analysis.

For the purposes of this chapter, analyses allowing an overview of some major findings will be emphasized. Principal components analysis with direct quartimin rotation was performed on the data from the highly representative, stratified Normal group. These analyses serve to examine the structure of the data derived from related tasks, stabilize the scales of measurement involved by compounding similar indices, and yield summarizing factor scores for further analysis (Gnanadesikan, 1977).

Only the factors from the performance tasks will be discussed in this summary report. Principal components analysis revealed that all d' indices from the five CPT versions loaded on one factor, while all β indices loaded on a separate factor. We will refer to these two performance dimensions, therefore, as CPT d' and CPT β.

The analyses to be presented are intended to be relevant to the underlying assumptions of risk research. Only 10 to 15% of children born to one schizophrenic parent will later develop schizophrenia, and monogenic theories of transmission would suggest that no more than 50% are even prone to the disorder. Even polygenic theory would imply that only some offspring of a schizophrenic parent would be at truly *high* risk for schizophrenic disorder (Gottesman & Shields, 1972; Rosenthal, 1970). Analyses that depend on *mean* differences between children born to a schizophrenic mother and a normal comparison group are unlikely to be most sensitive to vulnerability indices characterizing some proportion of predisposed individuals. In fact, the presence of mean differences without the presence of excessive atypical scorers on some variable might indicate a nonspecific effect of the stresses of having a schizophrenic mother or father rather than a potential vulnerability index or precursor of schizophrenia. Therefore, the search for atypical or extreme scoring subgroups of the offspring of schizophrenics is more likely to be a productive cross-sectional strategy for isolating characteristics that might relate to later schizophrenia and similar conditions.

In these analyses, extreme scoring subjects were arbitrarily defined for each factor as those individuals who fell into the extreme 10% of either tail of the theoretical normal distribution of factor scores. These cutoff scores correspond to upper and lower 10% points for the smoothed distribution of the stratified Normal Comparison group. The number of subjects in each Target group who obtained such extreme scores was compared to the number in the Stratified Comparison group, since this group represents normal performance levels most accurately.

Relative to the Stratified Normal Comparison sample, we found that a significant excess of children born to schizophrenic mothers obtained very low CPT d' factor scores. At the cutting score we arbitrarily selected, 29% (or 7 of 24) of the offspring of schizophrenic mothers as compared to 9% (or 6 of 65) of the normal control children were found to have low CPT d' factor scores. No similar disproportionate number of children born to nonpsychotic, psychiatrically disordered mothers showed low CPT d' factor scores. An excess of children born to schizophrenic mothers was not found for any of the other extreme score analyses of performance factors. Strikingly, the group of hyperactive children were distinguished primarily in these extreme score analyses by a disproportionate number of low CPT β factor scores rather than by low CPT d' scores, relative to the Stratified Normal Comparison group.

In order to investigate further the origin and nature of the excess of low CPT d' factor scorers among the children of schizophrenic mothers, separate analyses of each of the five contributing versions of the CPT were performed. The number of high-risk children who scored lower than the 10th percentile of the stratified controls was tallied for each of the tasks. Although appropriate directional trends were present for three of five conditions, a significantly disproportionate number of the offspring of schizophrenics was found to obtain extremely low d' scores for one condition alone. The condition involved 11.5 minutes of continuous visual monitoring using the Degraded Stimulus CPT without feedback.

Most studies of vigilance within experimental psychology focus on performance decrement over time rather than overall level of performance, because the decrement over time has practical and theoretical implications concerning sustained attention (Broadbent, 1971; Mackworth, 1970; Parasuraman, 1979; Stroh, 1971). Therefore, the group of seven children born to schizophrenic mothers who obtained very low overall Degraded Stimulus CPT d' scores were compared to the remaining 17 offspring of schizophrenic mothers for evidence of differential decrement across the first, second, and last third of trials. Although the cell sizes are rather small, it does *not* appear that the low scoring children show greater d' decrement over time. Rather, they seem to demonstrate consistently lower performance in this low signal-to-noise ratio situation.

DISCUSSION

These data suggest that a disproportionately large subgroup of children born to schizophrenic mothers are characterized by reduced discrimination of relevant from irrelevant stimuli in a sequential stimuli, sustained monitoring task. The performance deficit is apparent chiefly in a situation in which visual stimuli are degraded, thereby creating a low signal-to-noise ratio. This deficit exists in the absence of response bias or criterion differences. This finding is consistent with the possibility that an attentional deficit occurs as a precursor of adult schizophrenia, although follow-up through the period of risk for schizophrenia would be required to examine this issue directly.

The hyperactive children, on the other hand, are distinguished mainly by reduced CPT β, indicating a lack of response caution. Their low β factor scores reflect willingness to respond as if stimuli are relevant even when the sensory evidence for their relevance is rather meager. The performance dysfunction of these hyperactive children appears to be consistent with the impulsive cognitive style of such children, a characteristic emphasized by Douglas (1972). The present data suggest that attentional functioning in hyperactive children and in some children of schizophrenic mothers may differ from normal levels on separate dimensions, thereby lending greater specificity to each type of deficit.

20 Visual and auditory reaction time in children vulnerable to psychopathology

SUSAN PHIPPS-YONAS

Attentional functioning in psychiatrically disturbed patients has been a subject of speculation since before the turn of the century. By far the most popular measure of attention in such populations has involved the reaction time (RT) paradigm, and the results have been strikingly consistent. Following Kraepelin's first report, various empirical studies (Scripture, 1916; Wells and Kelley, 1922; Saunders & Isaacs, 1929; Huston, Shakow, & Riggs, 1937; Rodnick & Shakow, 1940) have demonstrated repeatedly that schizophrenics are characteristically slow responders to both visual and auditory stimuli. Moreover, certain idiosyncratic patterns are associated with their performance on reaction time tasks. For a review of this now extensive literature the reader is referred to Nuechterlein (1977a).

Given the consistency of the relevant data on schizophrenics versus normal adults, the obvious relationship between RT performance and adaptive potential, and the suitability of the measure across most stages of development (Garmezy, 1967), it is hardly surprising to find that the reaction time task was an early choice among risk researchers. Variations on the procedure have been employed in several of the projects described in this volume and in the risk literature (Van Dyke, Rosenthal, & Rasmussen, 1975) in hopes of identifying antecedents of the disorder. As one would expect, given the heterogeneity in general competence expected within vulnerable samples, the results have been mixed. It can be argued that it is unreasonable to look for intergroup differences in risk designs because only a small proportion of the children of schizophrenic mothers are truly vulnerable. A more productive strategy and one which has become increasingly popular (Hanson et al., 1976; Asarnow et al., 1977) would seem to involve searching for atypical subgroups of children within high-risk samples. This latter approach as well as the more traditional examination of group differences was employed in the study described here.

As Garmezy and Devine explain elsewhere in this volume, researchers on the Minnesota Project decided to focus upon three distinct although related aspects of attention and social competence in vulnerable children. When plans for the study reviewed here were formulated, the only available data on reaction time and high-risk samples were those from a study by L. Marcus (1972) that had suggested a fundamental impairment in central attentional processes in the children of schizophrenic mothers. It was with the intention of replicating and extending those

312

findings that this study was undertaken. The decision was made to use only an irregular procedure with both visual and auditory stimuli. Studies of reaction time (Sutton, Hakerem, Zubin, & Portnoy, 1961; Sutton & Zubin, 1965; Sutton, Spring, & Tueting, 1976) had demonstrated that schizophrenics are impaired excessively by a shift in the modality of the imperative stimulus from one trial to the next. To learn whether or not a similar pattern characterized children at risk, we chose to incorporate a modified version of their cross-modal design into our task. In addition, a series of conditions was included to assess the effects of information of varying accuracy regarding the modality of the stimulus. Reaction time studies with normal adults (LaBerge, VanGelder, & Yellott, 1970) have shown that in mixed modality sequences, information regarding modality produces a savings or a reduction in response latencies even when it is correct only 74% of the time. We were interested in determining what would happen with children under similar circumstances and in knowing whether there were any differences among our groups in their ability to profit from the information. A final condition in our RT task involved having the subject predict what the imperative stimulus would be on each trial. Adult data (Hinricks & Craft, 1971) have shown that correct anticipation facilitates responding. Furthermore, Sutton and Zubin's work demonstrated that schizophrenics are affected more adversely by wrong guesses than are controls. We were concerned once again with whether or not guessing would have a varying impact on our subjects. It was our hope that all of these procedural variations might alter differentially the state components of reaction time performance across the Target groups.

SUBJECTS

The groups of children who served as subjects and the methods used to select them were described in the previous chapter on the Minnesota Project by Nuechterlein. With minor exceptions all of the individuals included in his Continuous Performance Test (CPT) study participated in this second phase of our project. The only important difference was the loss of two children of schizophrenic mothers. Given Marcus's (1972) finding of greater impairment among his older subjects, it was unfortunate that the two subjects who did not participate were among the eldest. In each case, the boy and the girl were unavailable for a rather unusual reason compared to the more mundane reasons other subjects, all controls, were lost. Facing a number of criminal charges, the "lost" boy was hiding from the police, and the "lost" girl, having become pregnant at 14, had absconded with a "gypsy." It is impossible to project what their RT performance would have been like. It is noteworthy, however, that one of them did fall into the atypical subset of subjects on the CPT task.

A fourth Target group was included in this and the subsequent study. Our initial strategy, as described in the previous chapter, was to select hyperactive and antisocial delinquent subjects from a child guidance clinic and the child study division of the city public schools. On the basis of the procedures outlined there, 14 hyperactive males and four antisocial delinquents, one female and three males, were chosen. Because this approach did not yield a sufficient number of delinquents, a second sample was recruited from two special schools within the public school system for children with behavior problems. The principals of the schools were asked to describe in detail each of 67 students. Tapes of these interviews were rated independently by three project members using the Achenbach Symptom Checklist (1966). The principals also completed a Checklist for each child. As has been noted in detail elsewhere (Phipps-Yonas, 1978), 12 individuals were classified in this manner as antisocial delinquent (and not hyperactive). Along with the other four children chosen from the child guidance clinic, these subjects constituted the fourth Target group studied. Because of the special status of their schools, it was deemed inappropriate to select matched controls from their classrooms. Consequently none were included in the investigation.

In addition to these changes in the samples from the CPT study, the number of stratified control subjects was increased. Several of the original group of 67 had to be replaced because they had moved out of state. Others were recruited to balance the age and sex distributions of the sample. The final group of stratified subjects involved in the RT study numbered 100, with 48 females and 52 males. They were distributed across the 9 to 16-year-age range in approximately the same proportions as the 131 target and matched control children. Within the stratified sample, there were 33 high sociometric status children, 34 middle range children, and 33 low status children.

It should be noted that all of the subjects were approximately 1 year younger when they participated in the CPT study compared to when they were involved in the reaction time task. The mean age of each group during the latter was about 13 years and 7 months.

PROCEDURES

Throughout the experimental session, which was conducted typically within the child's school, the subject sat in front of an 18 by 19 in. horizontal board with a small lightbulb set behind a 1.5 × 1.5 in. glass window in its center. Ten-inch-wide side panels extended from the board toward the front. In the lower center portion of the right side extension were two 1.5 × 2 in. glass panels set side-by-side. These could be pressed and behind each was a lightbulb. During the latter portion of the session, small white cards were inserted into these panels. One, labeled LIGHT, had a drawing of a lightbulb, and the other showed a set of earphones and read TONE. At the bottom of the board was a 10-in.-wide inclined base in the center of which was the response button. During the task the subject wore headphones through which white noise as well as the auditory stimulus was heard.

There were five basic conditions. In each series a trial began when the side panels lighted up. This was the subject's signal to press the response button. Unbeknownst to him or her, the experimenter recorded the latency of the button press. This was thought to be an unobtrusive index of readiness to begin or general motivation. Following a quasi-random sequence, the imperative stumulus occurred 2, 4, or 7 seconds after the button was pressed. It was the speed with which the child released the button in response to this stimulus that constituted the major dependent variable. Nine percent of the trials were catch trials.

The first two conditions, the order of which was reversed for half of the subjects, involved 33 trials each. For one, the imperative stimulus was a light in the center panel, and for the other, it was a tone heard on the headphones. The third condition, modeled after Sutton and Zubin's procedure, contained 66 trials with the light and tone stimuli intermixed randomly. This was followed by three series of intermixed trials during which the ready signal provided information regarding the modality of the imperative stimulus on each trial. The LIGHT and TONE cards were inserted into the side panels, only one of which lighted up during this condition. For the first 20 trials the modality information provided by the signal was always correct. Before the second set of 20 trials in this condition, the subject was informed that the signal might be wrong "once in a while," as indeed it was 20% of the time. Prior to the third set of 20 trials for which the information was only 50% accurate, the experimenter warned that the signal would now "sometimes be right and sometimes be wrong."

The fifth condition presented a slight departure from the established procedure in that the subject initiated each of the 33 trials by predicting the modality of the imperative stimulus. This was accomplished by pressing either the TONE or LIGHT side panel which then lighted up, as it had in the past, as the ready signal, and the trial proceeded as in the previous conditions. The "guesses" were made to be half "wrong" and half "right" at random. It was emphasized that although subjects should try to guess correctly, the critical measure remained the speed of their reactions.

The basic dependent variables were the median response latencies and the intrasubject standard deviations. In addition various types of anticipatory responses and other extraneous behaviors were scored. The experimental task was followed by a 5 to 10 minute, semistructured interview. This focused on the individual's feelings about the task, on what, if any, cognitive strategies were employed, on attributions regarding perceived success or failure, and on the perceived level of achievement. The experimenter also rated each child for general effort and cooperation.

RESULTS AND DISCUSSION

Series of two, three, and four way analyses of variance constituted the major part of the data analysis. The inclusion of multiple experimental groups differing in size and makeup required a variety of separate comparisons. Each Target group was compared to its matched Control group on each dependent variable. Differences among the Target groups were assessed by a second series of analyses of variance in which they were compared to each other and to the stratified sample. (Because the hyperactive group was entirely male, they were compared only with the other boys.) Final sets of contrasts were drawn between the high, medium, and low status subjects in the stratified sample in order to assess the relationships between the sociometric measure and the dependent variables. Fisher's Least Significant Differences Procedure (Miller, 1966) was used to test specific contrasts.

In order to examine the structure of the data and to obtain summary scores, the reaction time data were subjected to a principal components analysis with direct quartimin rotation. It was hoped that the factors generated by this analysis would identify a subgroup of especially deviant children, but the results were disappointing. Five statistically significant factors emerged, accounting for 51% of the variance. The first of these was a strong, clear-cut speed factor. The second factor, however, was a source of confusion. On it loaded six variables, five of which involved the extent of "savings" in response times attributable to the introduction of accurate modality information or correct predictions. Unfortunately these items loaded in a contradictory manner that defied interpretation. The final three factors, labeled Interest and Motivation, Behavioral Impulsivity, and Starting Speed were much cleaner.

Following the rationale and procedures set out in the previous chapter, we selected as cutoff points for each factor the scores below and above which 10% of the stratified subjects fell. We also examined the Mahalanobis distances. This latter score provides an index of the statistical deviance of an individual from the overall mean of the stratified sample when all of the factors are considered together.

In addition, a second rationally derived approach for identifying atypical children was employed. Nine variables that cut across all of the competence areas in the study were selected for analysis. These included sociometric status, achievement test scores, median RTs, the variability measures, the motivation and cooperation rating, and two summary scores called *Impulsivity* and *Atypical Experimental Behaviors*. A negative cutting score was set for each variable at the value below which 20% of the 159 control subjects scored. Similarly, for six of the variables a positive cutting score was set at the point above which 12% of this group fell. A negative hit on five of the nine variables and an absence of any positive hits were taken as an indication of general deviance. Correspondingly, a positive hit on two or more of the six variables for which such was possible was considered as evidence for general superiority.

The analyses yielded a number of interesting findings with regards to the procedural variations which cannot be presented here. The expected effects of age and of sex did obtain: The boys reacted more quickly and consistently than the girls and the older children outperformed their younger counterparts.

The children of schizophrenic mothers were essentially indistinguishable from their matched controls and remarkably similar to the stratified sample. Despite the large number of comparisons drawn, there were no statistically significant differences between these children and their controls in terms of the speed of their reactions, the individual variability of their performance, or other extraneous behaviors. There was no evidence that as a group these children had any difficulty with the task suggestive of an attentional deficit. Furthermore, all attempts to identify a special subset of markedly deviant children within the group failed. Regardless of the criteria used, it was not possible to select a subset within the sample that was larger, more abnormal, or different in any way from comparable low status subsets within the other groups of subjects. The numbers of extreme cases on the empirically derived factors and the number of deviant Mahalanobis distance scores were comparable to those for the others. Furthermore, the rationally based search identified 3 of the 22 children of schizophrenics as especially deviant, a proportion identical to that found for their matched controls and similar to that overall for the other 209 individuals studied.

In the context of attempting to replicate Marcus's (1972) earlier findings, we were initially disappointed in that the new data were so nonsignificant. Yet we soon realized that the nonsignificance is important. It raises a number of critical questions. The first of these involves our risk sample itself. Although we adopted a more sophisticated and clearly superior procedure for selecting the maternal cohort in this phase of our project (relative to our past reliance on hospital chart diagnoses) and thus probably have a more truly schizophrenic group of mothers, the new sample of high-risk children appears healthier than the old one. Contrary to our expectations based on J. Rolf's (1972) earlier study, the current sample of children of schizophrenics was rated in a very "average" fashion by their peers. Their sociometric status scores fell equally into the top, middle, and bottom thirds of their classrooms. Furthermore, their achievement test scores were at par with those of the stratified controls as well as the city-wide norms, a finding which was unanticipated both on the basis of follow-back studies (Garmezy & Streitman, 1974) and in light of the fact that this group tended to be below average in socioeconomic status.

Because the Minnesota Project has been limited to studying children who attend regular public schools and who thus have achieved a minimal level of adaptation, the range of competence we tap is restricted. It seems likely that a more deviant picture would emerge if a truly representative sample of the entire population of offspring of schizophrenic mothers were examined. This brings us back to the issue of the two subjects who were "lost" since the CPT study, one of whom did extremely poorly on that task. As indicated earlier, it is impossible to know what their RT performance would have been like and whether or not they would have fallen into any deviant subsets. Nevertheless it was the case that both children would have scored negative hits for their poor achievement test scores, and the boy was low in sociometric status as well. Furthermore, the reasons they were unavailable suggest a picture of general deviance, possibly related to impending breakdowns. It may well be then that these individuals were two of the truly vulnerable (preschizophrenic) ones in the sample and that their nonparticipation reflected that very vulnerability. Their absence from this study may explain in part the nonreplication of the Marcus findings as well as the lack of consistency between the CPT and RT data.

The 20 children of women with mixed psychiatric disorders were also basically a very normal group. Although somewhat below average in sociometric status and achievement test scores, they were statistically indistinguishable from their matched controls and from the children of schizophrenic mothers and the stratified groups in their performance on the reaction time task.

In retrospect the 14 hyperactive boys who constituted our third Target group appear heterogeneous. Their scores on many of the variables studied were marked by great intersubject variability. As expected, they were significantly below average in sociometric status and achievement test scores. However in the first three RT conditions, their response latencies were neither slower nor more variable than those of their matched controls. It was only later that their performance became significantly inferior. This may indicate flagging motivation rather than any core attentional deficit, a conclusion consistent with other evidence on similar samples (Kupietz, Camp, & Weissman, 1976). The summary scores for the hyperactive group did reflect considerable impulsivity in some of them, a picture congruent with Nuechterlein's CPT findings.

This pattern of findings led to speculation about the pureness of the hyperactive sample. It may well be that between the date of their initial classification and the time of the RT testing (a period of as long as 4 years), significant developmental changes had occurred. The follow-up literature (Mendelson, Johnson, & Stewart, 1971; Weiss, Minde, Werry, Douglas, & Nemeth, 1971) does suggest considerable changes in hyperactive children as they enter adolescence. Our sample was tested at a relatively old age (for hyperactives), and the heterogeneity observed may reflect the passage of several years during which a group of once similar boys had grown apart in two predictable ways: Some had become increasingly normal, the others increasingly abnormal. Support for this notion was provided by the extreme score analyses which showed a high number of "deviant" boys and surprisingly a disproportionately large number of "superior" individuals. Perhaps the latter group has learned to harness their high energy levels in a productive fashion.

The 16 antisocial delinquents were clearly the most deviant group of subjects. Their reaction times were consistently slower and more variable than those of the other groups. In addition their achievement test scores were very low. It is unfortunate that sociometric scores were not obtainable for most of this group. However the very reason that this was so, their having been expelled from regular classes, suggests that they would not have been popular with their classmates. Besides their poor performance as a group, the delinquent sample contained the highest proportion of generally deviant individuals in terms of both the empirically and rationally derived summary scores. They appear to be in serious trouble on a variety of counts, a prognosis consistent with that suggested in the literature (Robins, 1966).

The power of sociometric status to discriminate between groups of subjects on the basis of the variables studied was striking. Popularity with peers was clearly related to achievement scores and to speed and consistency of responding on the RT task. The subset analyses were particularly enlightening for the stratified sample. Whereas none of the 33 high status children fell into the generally deviant classification, 30% of their 33 low status peers were so identified. Of equal interest was the corollary finding that whereas one-third of the popular group had superior scores on two or more of the general variables, this was true for only two of the subjects in the less popular group. The empirical factor analysis also produced such a pattern. These results, although in need of replication, speak clearly to the value of taking a broad perspective regarding risk.

Efforts are underway to integrate these RT findings with the CPT data reported by Nuechterlein as well as with incidental learning data described by Driscoll in the chapter that follows. We also intend to analyze further the effects of certain maternal variables. It is our hope that in carrying out additional analyses and in interpreting the discrepancies among the three sets of results in hand we may be able to learn more about our high risk sample and about such children in general. As Garmezy (1978) has noted, even in the absence of accurately predicting who within a vulnerable sample will become schizophrenic, high-risk research makes a significant contribution by simply tracking the development of children born to schizophrenic parents. We are optimistic too that our synthesis will shed light on the interrelationships among the processes studied and more generally on that nebulous construct called attention.

21 Intentional and incidental learning in children vulnerable to psychopathology

REGINA M. DRISCOLL

INTRODUCTION

One of the most vigorous areas of current high-risk research focuses on the attentional processes and possible attentional deficits in children of schizophrenic parents.

Zubin (1975) presents a model of an attentional deficit in the adult schizophrenic that places its emphasis on a defect in the ability to shift attention. He discriminates three separate aspects of attention: selection, maintenance, and shift of focus.

Maintenance of attention has been explored in the high-risk child with the Continuous Performance Test (Asarnow et al., 1977; Nuechterlein, 1978b; Erlenmeyer-Kimling & Cornblatt, 1978); shift of focus by such strategies as the cross-modal reaction time study of Phipps-Yonas (1978). Selective attention in these children has been less fully explored. A prevailing feature of this and other models (e.g., McGhie & Chapman, 1961; Broen, 1968) is the emphasis which is placed upon the inability of the schizophrenic to filter out irrelevant stimuli.

This view of selective attention as the process by which one screens out irrelevant stimuli and focuses on task relevant variables has been of interest to the developmental psychologist. The intentional–incidental learning paradigm has been used widely to study the development of strategies of selective attention, particularly by Hagen and his associates (Maccoby & Hagen, 1965; Hagen & Sabo, 1967; Druker & Hagen, 1969).

Incidental learning is defined as that learning which takes place in the absence of a set to learn (Postman, 1964). Postman defines two major categories of incidental learning. In Type I the subject is exposed to certain materials with no instructions to learn. Subsequently, the subject is tested unexpectedly for retention of the material.

In Type II designs, the subject has a specific learning task but is also exposed to materials whose comprehension is not necessary for the performance of the central

This study was financed by the Schizophrenia Research Program of the Supreme Council 33° A. A. Scottish Rite, Northern Masonic Jurisdiction (Dr. Norman Garmezy, Principal Investigator).

task. Later, the subject's retention for this extraneous material is tested. Within Type II incidental learning, two further subdivisions are made. When attributes or features of the learning material are integral to the material but not required for the central task, as, for example, the colors of geometric shapes when the discrimination of shapes is central, Postman labels these features incidental but *intrinsic* components of the experimentally defined learning task. When, on the other hand, the incidental features bear no direct relation to the learning task, then these peripheral items are defined as *extrinsic* components of the experimenter-defined task. An example of this would be when attention is directed to a set of words or a class of pictures for the central task, but additional items (other pictures, digits, geometric forms) are exposed along with the central task materials.

These categories of incidental learning are important but frequently overlooked distinctions among studies in this area.

The definition of incidental learning as the absence of a set to learn presents a subtle problem. Determining conclusively that there was no intention to learn is an effort doomed to failure; one cannot prove the absence of an unseen mental phenomenon. Postman (1964) points out that learning that takes place without overt instructions is nevertheless influenced by implicit demands in the instructions and stimuli. Implicit demands in the learning task itself will also influence the "set" of the learner and can induce covert "intention."

Determining what is actually incidental and what is central in the task is a more complex matter than is superficially apparent. The explicit set is contained within the instructions given by the experimenter. Implicit sets can be easily induced, however. There are unspoken demands within the task to perceive, discriminate, and retain various features of the materials if the task is to be completed successfully. These demands will increase or decrease the probability that attributes of the material will be attended to and will therefore influence the proportion of learning capability which is directed toward the intentional and incidental tasks.

The concepts of set and task demands on the one hand and intrinsic–extrinsic components of the experimental task on the other can be combined to determine what is learned in any given task. If the nature of the task requires that the subject scan the stimulus materials so that the central and incidental features are apprehended, a discrimination made between what is essential for the performance of the central task and what is nonessential, then one may say that all features of the material become intrinsic components of the task perceptually or cognitively. If the task at no time requires that certain features or items be scanned, decoded, or retained, then these items remain peripheral or extrinsic to the task. Thus, the implicit demands of a task can determine whether incidental attributes extraneous to the successful performance of the task are intrinsic or extrinsic components of the task.

The researcher who uses incidental learning to measure selective attention in children defines an intentional (or *central*) task that the child must perform; retention of information unnecessary to the successful completion of the central task is *incidental* learning. Thus, if by the measure of efficiency of performance on some central task over an age range, one may track the development of attention-focusing strategies; then conversely, by measuring incidental learning, one may track the relative abilities of various age groups to screen out irrelevant stimuli.

The attentional strategies of young children are markedly inefficient: Large amounts of relevant information are overlooked, while extraneous information is attended to, to the detriment of performance on the central task (Lehman, 1972; Pick, Christy, & Frankel, 1972; Pick & Frankel, 1974). As the child grows older, he or she becomes better able to select the portions of a stimulus situation relevant to the attainment of a goal and to dismiss competing stimuli (Maccoby, 1969). Selective attention focuses on the intentional nature of a cognitive or perceptual task. There is a motivation or intent to reach some defined goal, and those stimuli that are relevant to the achievement of the goal must be noted, retained, and utilized in the attainment of that goal. Irrelevant information must be dismissed.

Many of the studies of incidental learning in children have used this phenomenon to aid in the definition of the boundaries of attention. A number of these have found that whereas central task performance, that is, intentional learning, invariably increases with age, incidental learning tends to rise and then decline at about age 12 or 13. This is taken as support of the hypothesis that children's selective attentional strategies are somewhat amorphous at younger ages, then gradually become more efficient with increasing years. However, a significant minority of studies find that with the expected positive linear relationship of age and intentional learning, there is a parallel increase over age on the incidental measure, with no decline at later ages.

This discrepancy suggests that the term *incidental learning* used in these studies may cover two separate processes. When incidental features are extrinsic to the central task material, the phenomenon may serve as a measure of diffusion or inefficiency of selective attention. When the subject must attend to various features of the stimuli, make discriminations based on one or more features of the materials, and retain these differences for the successful completion of the central task, then the covert or implicit demand of the task would require that the subject discriminate and categorize stimulus materials along more than one dimension, that is, to maintain a *multiple set* (Plenderleith & Postman, 1956), thus enhancing the discriminability of the items. If the subject can hold this multiple set, then incidental learning of the materials will be increased.

The ability to maintain this multiple set will influence intentional learning as well. Therefore, intrinsic incidental learning and intentional learning should parallel one another as the learning and attentional strategies of the maturing child become not only more efficient, but also greater in breadth and capacity.

INCIDENTAL LEARNING IN THE MINNESOTA SAMPLE OF CHILDREN AT RISK

The present study was designed to determine whether the incidental–intentional learning paradigm could serve as an effective measure of the development of strategies of selective attention and learning in children vulnerable to psychopathology and in normal comparison groups. In the *incidental learning* task, the child sees a series of 15 arrays of three common objects, one of which is always enclosed in a black box. This black box is the central item. The instructions are to learn all the items in the black boxes for later recall. Subsequently the child is tested for recall and recognition of all the items, central and incidental. The incidental items need not be scanned or retained by the child in the performance of the central task. This task provides a measure of extrinsic incidental learning, which is expected to decline at the upper age levels (based on the assumption that older children are more able to focus on the central task).

In the *orienting* task of the second part of the study, the child again sees a series of 15 triads of common objects. None of them is demarcated in any way, and the explicit instructions are that the child must guess which is the central item for later recall. The child indicates his or her guess by pressing a button under the item of choice, and is given immediate feedback about his or her response via a light over the "correct" response. The implicit demand of the task requires that the child scan all the items while seeking the correct response, that he or she discriminate among the items along a dimension of correctness–incorrectness, and that the child choose in favor of a response to some items and against a response to others. Five blocks of 15 triads are again given, and the child is again tested for recall and recognition of all of the items. This task is designed to render all items intrinsic to the central task and therefore to yield a measure of intrinsic incidental learning, which is predicted to increase at the upper age levels (based on the assumption that the older child can better maintain multiple sets).

In this second task, the child listens to a tape of a voice speaking a list of common words which he or she performs the orienting task. This provides an auditory distraction condition and superimposes an extrinsic incidental learning task on the intrinsic incidental learning task. This procedure was included because decrement in performance under auditory distraction conditions in attentional and memory tasks has been shown to discriminate adult schizophrenics from other psychiatric groups and from those with organic brain disease (McGhie, Chapman, & Lawson, 1965a and 1965b; Lawson, McGhie, & Chapman, 1967; Oltmanns & Neale, 1975; Oltmanns et al., 1978). It was predicted that all subjects in this study would suffer in performance under distraction conditions, but that the children of schizophrenic mothers would be affected to a differentially greater degree.

In a separate pilot study employing an independent sample of 60 elementary and junior high school students, tests were made for task order effects. None was found. It would appear that differences in amounts of incidental learning would be attributable to differences in the tasks or the groups themselves.

SUBJECTS

The recruitment of the subjects and their diagnostic confirmations, as well as the selection of control groups, are more extensively described in the preceding chapter by Nuechterlein. Therefore, the subjects will be only briefly outlined here.

Twenty-two of the original sample of 24 children of schizophrenic mothers gathered by Nuechterlein were tested, as were the 20 children whose mothers had diagnoses of nonpsychotic psychiatric disorders. Of Nuechterlein's 14 hyperactive boys, 13 were tested in the incidental–intentional learning study. Control subjects were drawn from the classrooms of each of these subjects, matched on the basis of sex, age, academic achievement, and sociometric ranking by peers. These comprised the original Target groups. A fourth Target group was comprised of antisocial children. Twelve antisocial delinquent children drawn from a special elementary and junior high school for children with behavioral problems were added to Nuechterlein's original four antisocial subjects. Matched normal classroom controls were not available for this group of subjects because their special classrooms were composed of children who had already demonstrated deviant behavior.

A sample of 98 children stratified into the upper, middle, and lower thirds of sociometric ratings by peers was also drawn from the classrooms of the first three targeted groups. This group provided a sample of children spanning all ages, both sexes, and all levels of social acceptance by their classmates. This added another normal sample in case the matched control groups prove to be unrepresentative of the general population of local school children by virtue of having been matched to the targets on several variables, particularly social competence.

The hypotheses about the nature of extrinsic and intrinsic incidental learning presented earlier led to the prediction that the implicit demands of the task would yield more incidental learning in the intrinsic task for all groups. This type of learning was not expected to decline at upper age levels. A decline in intrinsic incidental learning in older children is hypothesized to signal a failure in the child's efforts to scan and discriminate along several dimensions at once. The efficient learner is predicted to show a positive relationship between intentional and intrinsic incidental learning.

Extrinsic incidental learning is a measure of the child's developing ability to attend selectively to task-relevant stimuli. Screening out task-irrelevant stimuli was expected to decline at the upper age levels. Failure of the decline to materialize would suggest that the child was continuing to scan indiscriminately, even when the task did not require such scanning, thus deploying his or her attention in a diffuse, inefficient manner.

Furthermore, if there were a selective attention deficit in children of schizophrenic mothers, one would speculate that these children will show increased extrinsic incidental learning through an inability to focus on task-relevant attributes to the exclusion of peripheral material. Similarly, if these children are developmentally behind their age mates, then they will fail to show the expected decline in incidental learning at the upper age levels.

Of the other targeted high-risk children, the children of mothers with other psychiatric disorders were predicted to resemble their normal controls on these learning measures; the hyperactive boys were expected to show increased extrinsic incidental learning due to their inability to screen out irrelevant stimuli and to show a substantial decline in performance under auditory distraction conditions; the antisocial delinquents were predicted to show generally low levels of performance, as a reflection of their poor behavioral adaptation to their environment.

Contrary to our expectations, the obtained data showed the children of schizophrenic mothers to be a remarkably able group of children. They did not differ from their matched controls or the sociometrically stratified controls. These children prove to be efficient learners who exhibited high levels of intentional and intrinsic incidental learning, consistent with a picture of children who easily maintained their focus on the central task, and who were able to discriminate among stimuli along several dimensions. Children of schizophrenic mothers showed a decline in extrinsic incidental learning at the upper age levels, although the changes over age were not significant for any group. This suggests that this group does not lag behind normal children in their abilities to filter out extraneous material. The expected finding of lower peer acceptance in the children of schizophrenic mothers also failed to materialize: This sample of children represented all levels of sociometric ranking equally.

The only prediction for these children that received support concerned the performance of the children under conditions of auditory distraction. As predicted, all groups showed a decline in central learning in this more difficult situation. However, the children of schizophrenic mothers were the only group who showed a statistically significant ($p < .03$) decrement in intentional learning over the two tasks. This is consistent with the performance of adult schizophrenics under auditory distraction conditions and suggest the possibility of a subtle interference deficit in these children. Beyond this single finding, however, the children of schizophrenic mothers were remarkable for their ordinariness.

The children of mothers with other psychiatric disorders did not differ from their matched or stratified controls, as was expected. The hyperactive boys yielded the most erratic performance and demonstrated a poor ability to focus on the intentional task. Their pattern of learning was characterized by incidental stimuli of both types learned at the expense of the central task items. This group also showed a special sensitivity to the auditorily presented material, yielding a higher recognition memory of auditory stimuli than did any other group. The antisocial delinquent children, again as expected, turned in the most deviant performances. Low rates of learning of every kind were exhibited by this group. This was not thought to reflect an attentional deficit; rather, poor motivation and minimal task involvement were the most likely explanations for this group. The present study was not equipped to investigate the differential performance of the antisocial group under high as well as low motivation conditions. Previous work with similar children (Marcus, 1972) suggests that these children can voluntarily improve their performance on an attentional task when given incentive to do so.

It is not surprising that the present study's sample children of schizophrenic mothers should reveal no differences in mean scores on a variety of attentional measures, because only a small percentage of these will manifest overt disorder in adulthood and since many of those from the original risk cohort were unavailable for testing in this study. Given these limitations, the Minnesota research group attempted to identify a subset of target subjects who had scored in the extreme ranges of performance on the Continuous Performance Test (Nuechterlein, 1978a), the cross-modal reaction time measure (Phipps-Yonas, 1978), and the present intentional–incidental learning study. A factor analysis of the 15 measures drawn from the two incidental learning tasks was derived to facilitate the search for deviant subjects and the comparison of the three studies. The subject pool was the sociometrically stratified normal children. The subtests included all major measures of intentional learning, intrinsic and extrinsic incidental learning, discrimination learning on the training experience of the second task, and auditory stimulus learning. Four major factors were derived, labeled Intentional Learning, Incidental Learning, Auditory Recognition and Triad Recognition (in which subjects were required to identify original triads from the training experiences that were embedded in an assortment of triads deviating in varying degrees from the original).

Subjects who placed in the extreme 10% of the distribution of factor scores were considered to be deviant. Only the antisocial delinquent sample yielded significant numbers of deviant subjects. Forty-four percent of these achieved very low scores on Intentional Learning, compared with 11% of the normal sample. None of the other target groups yielded significant numbers of subjects whose performance fell into extreme ranges on any of the factors.

The Mahalanobis distances from each case to the centroid of all cases in the normative sample for the four factors yielded eight normative subjects (8%) who fell into the extreme 10% of the theoretical normal distribution. None of the children of schizophrenic mothers, the children of the mothers with other psychiatric disorders, or the hyperactive children fell into the extreme range on this global measure of overall deviance on these measures. Only one antisocial delinquent child did so.

The results of the three studies from the Minnesota Project described in these papers suggest that there is no broad attentional deficit that characterizes this sample of children of schizophrenic mothers. The key to such a deficit, if one exists, may be drawn from much more subtle indicators, such as the difficulties these children experience under auditory distraction or the deficits seen on the Degraded Stimulus CPT (Nuechterlein, 1978a). The present study is too complicated by learning and memory factors to provide a pure measure of selective attention; nevertheless, it is clear that these children are efficient and task-oriented learners. The failure of the Minnesota Project to identify a subset of a small sample of high-risk children who demonstrate deviance on these learning tasks may be disappointing to the researcher, but it is a sign of health and competence in a group of children developing under the stress of having a seriously ill parent.

KEITH H. NUECHTERLEIN

The findings from the three recent attentional studies of the Minnesota High-Risk Project suggest that a disproportionately large subgroup of children born to schizophrenic mothers perform poorly on some tasks demanding sustained discrimination of signal and noise stimuli. However, some other measures tapping "attentional" processes apparently do not isolate such a subgroup nor do they produce mean differences between offspring of schizophrenic mothers and normal comparison children. Such a mixture of positive and negative findings across attentional tasks has characterized reports from other high-risk projects as well (Asarnow et al., 1977; Erlenmeyer-Kimling & Cornblatt, 1978). Reflecting on the findings at this point, we feel that additional consideration of certain methodological and conceptual issues might accelerate progress in this promising area.

THE ISSUE OF GENERALIZED DEFICIT

The diversity of performance tasks on which adult schizophrenic patients score more poorly than a normal comparison group is so great that a *generalized performance deficit* has been suggested (Chapman & Chapman, 1973). Because experimental tasks often differ from each other in terms of reliability and difficulty level, an apparent differential deficit for schizophrenics on one task relative to another may occur as a psychometric artifact of the differing discriminating power of the measures rather than as a product of content differences between the tasks (Chapman & Chapman, 1973, 1978). This would appear to be a productive time to consider similar issues in studies of cognition, perception, and attention among children at risk for adult schizophrenia.

Since findings reported thus far by our group and others (Asarnow et al., 1978; Driscoll, chapter 2, this volume; Erlenmeyer-Kimling & Cornblatt, 1978; Grunebaum et al., 1974; Marcus, 1972; Nuechterlein, chapter 19, this volume; Oltmanns, Weintraub, Stone, & Neale, 1978; Phipps-Yonas, chapter 20, this

The preparation of this paper has been supported by a grant from the Scottish Rite Schizophrenia Research Program, NMJ, USA (Co-Principal Investigators: N. Garmezy and K. H. Nuechterlein). The author is grateful to William S. Edell for valuable comments on an earlier version of this chapter.

327

volume) demonstrate that not all performance tasks yield significant differences between children born to a schizophrenic parent and comparison children with normal parents, the likelihood of very severe, wholly generalized performance deficit among offspring of a schizophrenic parent appears slight, even for those children who will eventually develop a schizophrenic disorder. This situation implies that deficits on one task relative to others are not likely to be wholly due to differences in the extent to which each task taps a severe, nonspecific performance deficit.

However, more subtle, relatively generalized cognitive, perceptual, or attentional deficits remain a possibility, especially as the number of tasks reported to show deficits among children born to schizophrenic parents increases. In the case of a subtle, relatively generalized performance deficit among children predisposed to schizophrenia, it appears possible that only tasks *optimizing* discriminating power among normal children would detect deficits to a statistically significant degree relative to normal comparison children. Thus, inattention to the psychometric characteristics of performance tasks in high-risk research might lead to negative findings, whereas in studies of the active schizophrenic state, the multitude of positive findings can easily be interpreted too specifically for the same reason. The primary problem in the high-risk area involves *optimizing* discriminating power, whereas in the study of the active schizophrenic period, *matching* tasks for discriminating power is of principal concern.

In addition to the possibility that selection of tasks with nonoptimal discriminating power may contribute to negative findings in studies of risk populations, variability among tasks in the amount of deviation from optimal discriminating power could result in misleading conclusions regarding the specific source of differences in performance of high-risk children on these tasks. For example, consider a hypothetical case in which two tasks that appear to tap distinct aspects of attention or information processing differ widely (for psychometric reasons) in their approximation to optimal discriminating power for certain variations in performance among normal children. The demonstration of a significant deficit among high-risk children as compared to low-risk children on one task but not the other could be due to either the psychometric or the substantive properties of the tasks or both. In this situation, it would be premature to conclude that children at risk for schizophrenia show deficits in one aspect of attentional functioning or information processing but not in the other.

DISCRIMINATING POWER AND DEVELOPMENTAL EFFECTS

A special and complex case of complications involving discriminating power sometimes occurs in high-risk research in situations in which performance on a task shows significant developmental improvement. Because a fairly wide age range is often present in samples of high-risk children, the scores of both high-risk and comparison children may show significant gains as a function of age. These changes in task difficulty with age may result in much lower discriminating power at some ages than at others. The resulting changes in the extent or existence of score differences between high-risk and normal samples at various ages can easily be misinterpreted as reflecting developmental convergence or divergence of these groups.

One means of correcting this problem is to deliberately eliminate normal developmental trends in task performance by increasing task difficulty with increases in the age of subjects. For example, the version of the CPT using slides of playing cards that was developed by Erlenmeyer-Kimling and Cornblatt (1978) demonstrated significant performance improvement with age. In developing the degraded stimulus version of the CPT, therefore, we employed slightly briefer exposure times for older children than for younger children. This manipulation was pretested on normal children of different ages. Normal developmental effects were thereby successfully eliminated from the later comparisons of the offspring of schizophrenic mothers and the various other groups.

This solution to the problem of changing discriminating power as a function of age must be employed with careful attention to the task variable manipulated, however. Changes in the difficulty level of the task need to be made without significantly altering the psychological functions that the task is designed to measure. In the case of the Degraded Stimulus CPT, for example, changing exposure time from 50 to 40 msec appeared to meet this criterion. In situations in which wide age ranges and large developmental changes in performance are involved, this procedure may demand considerable ingenuity on the part of the investigator. However, the procedure has the advantage of allowing true developmental divergence (or convergence) of high-risk and normal children to be isolated, while apparent but artifactual divergence (or convergence) is eliminated.

CHANGING MODELS OF ATTENTIONAL PROCESSES: THE MEANING OF TASK DIFFICULTY

The impact of task difficulty on the measurement of possible attentional deficits among children at risk for schizophrenia assumes greater importance when viewed in the context of current theories of attentional functioning. The revival of interest in attentional processes within psychology was stimulated partially by structural models hypothesizing a single, limited channel forcing selection between inputs very early in processing (Broadbent, 1958; Welford, 1959). Although the influence of these early selection models persists in some research on schizophrenia, subsequent studies within experimental psychology led to views that the limiting bottleneck occurred in later stages of information processing (Deutsch & Deutsch, 1963; Norman, 1968).

Even more recently, as evidence accrued suggesting greater flexibility in human information processing than the structural bottleneck models imply, increased emphasis has been placed on allocation functions within the individual's overall limitations in processing capacity (Kahneman, 1973) or resources (Norman & Bobow, 1975). Allocation of resources is assumed to be controlled by the individual in response to task demands, up to the point at which competing processing demands or limitations in the individual's relevant processing mechanisms intervene. Some contemporary theorists now use the term *attention* in relation to this resource allocation process. As Keele and Neill recently wrote, "Our overall view of attention has shifted from the notion of limited capacity at particular stages to one of attention as a control process for the flow of information" (1978, p. 42).

What are the implications of these views for attentional studies of high-risk children? The role of task difficulty, rather than being described from a purely psychometric viewpoint, can be phrased in terms of an attentional model (Knight & Russell, 1978). Thus, in a *wholly* flexible allocation model, difficulty level would be a function of the amount of processing capacity, resources, or attention demanded by a task condition. To the extent that tasks are not matched for the amount of global processing capacity required, deficits on one task relative to another may reflect individual differences in overall processing capacity rather than more specific dysfunctional stages or mechanisms. Within a model of wholly flexible allocation of processing capacity, creating performance task measures that are matched for reliability and difficulty level (and thus discriminating power) among normal subjects allows the possibility of rejecting global processing capacity differences as the source of greater deficit on one task relative to another.

ISOLATION OF SPECIFIC ATTENTIONAL OR INFORMATION-PROCESSING DYSFUNCTIONS

One possible interpretation of the current findings of deficits on attentional measures among some high-risk children is that these children have reduced global processing capacity or impaired control functions for allocation of available processing capacity. It would be desirable, however, to isolate more specific information-processing dysfunctions if they are present, because appropriate intervention strategies and theoretical implications would then probably be more specific as well. At least two situations would seem to allow tentative rejection of overall processing capacity as the source of performance task deficits among high-risk children, even without matching tasks on discriminating power.

As has been noted elsewhere (Nuechterlein, 1978b), one of the situations involves tasks that do not tax resource limits. Task difficulty is likely to be a function not only of the amount of global processing resources demanded but also of the quality and nature of the information to be processed (Norman & Bobrow, 1975). Norman and Bobrow (1975) refer to situations as *signal data-limited* if all of the individual's available processing mechanisms have been employed and additional allocation of processing resources does not improve performance. They view the task of recognizing a weak signal in a noisy environment as typical of a signal data-limited process. If one adds an individual differences perspective to their nomothetic model, one can conceive of differences between persons in the fidelity with which specific processing mechanisms are functioning under optimal processing capacity allocation. Thus, for tasks that demand relatively limited processing capacity, individual differences may reflect the existence of ceiling inequality in the adequacy of certain specific processing mechanisms, rather than overall capacity reduction.

Although the reduced processing capacity hypothesis appears to have substantial relevance to schizophrenia, especially given the diversity of performance deficits in the psychotic period, more specific information-processing mechanisms might be better indicators of vulnerability to schizophrenia during prepsychotic and postpsychotic periods. In tasks requiring rather basic perceptual and cognitive processes without competing processing demands, models describing structural processing mechanisms may have greatest relevance. The Degraded Stimulus CPT and other letter or number recognition tasks, for example, may be viewed as involving feature detection and pattern recognition processes (Estes, 1978; Gibson, 1969).

Even when performance on tasks is not influenced by capacity limitations, variations in stimulus quality and complexity would alter the demands on specific processing mechanisms. Optimizing discriminating power may still be necessary to detect subtle deficits. Furthermore, in order to determine whether one specific deficit was present to a greater extent than another, matching of tasks for discriminating power would still be desirable.

A second situation might lead to a more convincing rejection of the hypothesis that cognitive deficits among schizophrenic patients and some persons at risk for schizophrenia are due wholly to global processing capacity reduction. If limitations in overall processing capacity or available resources (i.e., *generalized deficit*) result in individual differences in performance both between schizophrenia-prone (or schizophrenic) and normal individuals and within schizophrenia-prone groups, performance across information-processing tasks requiring substantial processing capacity should be positively correlated to a substantial degree. This correlation should be present in both a mixed sample of schizophrenia-prone and normal (nonvulnerable) persons and within the schizophrenia-prone group. Presumably any global capacity reduction effects should be evident across tasks whenever resource allocations are strained. If uncorrelated cognitive deficits are found within a group of interest despite a reasonable range of scores and high reliability for each measure, more specific sources of dysfunction are indicated. It would be particularly difficult to attribute performance deficits to global capacity reduction (or generalized deficit) if different information-processing deficits were found in different schizophrenic or schizophrenia-prone subjects. A similar situation would involve uncorrelated information-processing measures that tap deficits in different target groups. In this case, the separable dimensions of dysfunction would indicate that the deficits were not wholly due to reduction in global processing capacity in at least one group.

In planning the current Minnesota series of studies, we were conscious of the diverse ways in which the concept of attention has been employed in research on psychopathology (see reviews by Neale & Cromwell, 1970, and Nuechterlein, 1977a, 1977b). This conceptual diversity is consistent with evidence that measures of "attention" among schizophrenic patients are sometimes relatively independent (Asarnow & MacCrimmon, 1978; Kopfstein & Neale, 1972). In order to examine the nature of any attentional disturbances among children born to a schizophrenic parent, we deliberately selected measures that might sample separate processes falling under the broad rubric of attention. Although conceptual attempts to distinguish different attentional components have certain limitations (Garmezy, 1977; Nuechterlein, 1977b), we included promising measures of sustained attention, shifting attention, and selective attention (Zubin, 1975) to allow empirical evaluation of their independence.

Additional analyses will examine correlations and individual patterns of attentional scores across these measures. This approach may help to clarify further the specificity of attentional dysfunctions characterizing certain subjects in the targeted groups. If the measures tapping attentional processes in these three domains are relatively independent, fairly specific deficits rather than global processing-capacity reduction would be suggested. Substantial correlations across tasks, on the other hand, would be compatible with the possibility that the source of positive findings is reduced global processing capacity. Negative findings might then be attributed to nonoptimal task difficulty level. Tasks matched for discriminating power would then be appropriate to resolve the issue of whether specific deficits exist beyond the general reduction in processing capacity.

PART VII

The University of Rochester Child and Family Study: 1972–1982

By far the largest research team in the consortium was organized for the child and family study in Rochester by Lyman Wynne immediately upon his departure from the National Institute of Mental Health. His extensive background of research and theory on family relations and communication disturbances in the families of schizophrenics provided the guiding conceptions for the organization of the project. Diagnostic expertise was brought to the study by John Strauss and John Romano. Alfred and Clara Baldwin designed imaginative procedures to study empirically in the laboratory how family members relate to one another. The ubiquitous Norman Garmezy provided extensive consultation in the early years of the project on experimental design, behavioral measures for the children, and the conceptual rationale for high-risk research. Richard Bell's convergent design for cross-sectional studies of development was adopted as a means to accelerate the pace of longitudinal analysis. Margaret Singer continued her long collaboration with Wynne as a consultant for the interpretation of projective test assessments. And an impressive array of bright, young investigators in psychology and psychiatry has played an important role in planning, implementing, and interpreting the study.

Painstaking care has been taken to describe the clinical symptoms and to classify the subjects diagnostically. The reader may be surprised to find only 18 schizophrenics studied in a project of this magnitude, but that in itself reflects the rigorous precision of diagnosis employed, because 63 of the 145 index patients carried hospital diagnoses of schizophrenia.

The URCAFS Project has emphasized more than any other project the systematic observation of the social ecology of its research subjects, giving special attention to the family system and the school setting. The breadth of these transactional evaluations affords unique opportunities to relate behavior observed in one setting to that observed in others, as well as to important aspects of parental psychopathology. Part VII begins with a conceptual overview of the entire project. Thereafter follow eight circumscribed reports from all aspects of the study. The latter are usually coauthored by at least four investigators and reflect both the magnitude of the labor involved and the collaborative spirit that have characterized URCAFS since its inception.

23   The University of Rochester Child and Family Study: overview of research plan

LYMAN C. WYNNE

This overview will provide a broad perspective of the University of Rochester Child and Family Study (URCAFS), emphasizing the research design and the rationale for choices of samples, methods, and measures. I shall comment especially on those features of the Rochester study that are similar to, and different from other risk research programs, and outline the major variables selected for study. In the chapters that follow, a sample of specific preliminary findings from several teams within the program will be presented.

The central objective of this program was to study concurrently and to follow prospectively children and families with initial differences in three classes of variables: (1) parental mental disorder and psychiatric assessment; (2) family communication and relationship patterns; and (3) child functioning, assessed with psychiatric, psychological, and school competence measures. At initial evaluation, we were interested both in examining correlations among the variables from these three areas and in establishing a baseline from which later, longitudinal changes could be predicted.

We began with a sample in which at least one parent was known to have had a serious disorder requiring psychiatric hospitalization, but in which index sons aged 4, 7, or 10 were not under psychiatric care. In so doing, we deliberately emphasized the parental and family measures as predictor, or *risk*, variables and, for the most part, conceptualized the child measures of *vulnerability* and *competence* as dependent variables. Even though the study was begun when the index children were preadolescent, we expected to find initial differences in the child vulnerability and competence measures.

At initial assessment, the task has been to test whether the relationships between the parents, family, and child variables do fall into theoretically meaningful patterns. The variables were selected and the study was designed to enable us to test competing hypotheses. An example of a set of competing hypotheses that we plan to examine is the following: (1) If current family interaction and communication are relatively healthy, the child's functioning will be competent despite a parental past history of schizophrenia or other psychotic mental disorder; on the other hand, if family patterns are highly deviant, the child's functioning will be disturbed even though parental illness has been nonpsychotic and presumptively carries a relatively low genetic risk. (2) Alternatively, it has been hypothesized that the quality and severity of parental mental illness will predict *both* child functioning and family interaction and that measures of family interaction will add little to the variance in child measures accounted for by the parental psychopathology alone. (3) Still a third hypothesis anticipates that chronicity of mental illness is a key predictor variable, rather than either specific parental diagnosis or family interaction.

At the time of this report, we have just begun to explore such issues across the three areas of parent, family, and child, using the data obtained at the time of initial research evaluation. Relationships between initial data and 3-year follow-up data will be studied in a subsequent stage of data analyses. Here we must be content to describe the research design and some of the variables that we have selected for study, and to report how a few of them are related to one another.

Some of the salient overall features of the Rochester risk program can be summarized as follows:

1. *A concern with both healthy and disturbed child development.* Although the first proposals for this study emphasized child vulnerability to later mental disorder, we very soon balanced this interest in developmental psychopathology with an equal concern about child competence and the precursors and context of healthy development.

2. *The concept of multiple-risk factors.* At the time of the 1969 NIMH Workshop on risk research (Mosher & Wynne, 1970), the focus of most research plans was on the study of offspring of a schizophrenic parent or parents. However, research designs using a *single* risk factor – even the presumably powerful genetic factor associated with parental diagnosis of schizophrenia – began to be questioned as being quite inefficient, in view of the evidence that this single factor is predictive, and randomly at that, of only about 10% of offspring manifesting schizophrenia in adulthood.

With such misgivings in mind, we chose a multiple risk factor strategy when planning the Rochester risk program. To be sure, one of the risk factors incorporated into our design was a parental diagnosis of mental illness, including schizophrenia. We planned a diversity of methods to be used with the parents and with the families as units so that other hypothesized risk factors also could be studied. On the other hand, we chose not to emphasize very broad sociocultural factors, such as poverty and lower-class social status, which may potentiate the emergence of mental disorders and almost certainly help keep their manifestations chronic but which are presumably nonspecific with respect to etiology. Similarly, in examining the intrafamilial environment as well, we chose not to select those factors such as broken homes that are known to have a high frequency in families of non-schizophrenics. Rather, we drew upon our past research with families that suggested that certain patterns of deviant parental communication are found across diverse social classes and cultures and remain consistently more frequent in families with offspring who have already been diagnosed as schizophrenic. Whether or not these deviant family communication patterns are relatively specific for schizophrenia (an unlikely possibility) and whether or not they emerge only after the onset of mental illness in an offspring, as opposed to antedating such illness, were issues that we were eager to evaluate in prospective longitudinal research.

Turning to hypothesized antecedents of schizophrenia within the children (so-called *vulnerability* factors), a number of variables seemed worthy of inclusion in our program, even though none have been established as specific for a schizophrenic outcome. We considered the likelihood that some of these variables, when occurring in combination, might be significant predictors of later developmental changes in the children themselves. Here we drew upon the psychophysiological literature, including autonomic and attentional measures, cortical evoked-response measures of reducing–augmenting (stimulus-intensity modulation), and, later, pendulum eye tracking. Also, we utilized interview and test procedures that would tap soft neurological signs and behavioral precursors of schizophrenia, such as scatter on cognitive tests and externalizing behavior in school and home.

Having developed a multiple-risk factor model going beyond parental diagnosis, we returned to consider the criteria for parental diagnosis. Several points were apparent from a review of the literature. First, it seemed shortsighted to look only for precursors of "typical" schizophrenia in the offspring of "typical" schizophrenics. Not only do typical schizophrenics have offspring with widely diverse outcomes, including high levels of competence, but also patients with seemingly diverse diagnostic features produce typical schizophrenic offspring. Furthermore, the interview procedures and diagnostic criteria that have been used to define genetic risk for any form of schizophrenia turn out to be much less specific and clear than one might assume from reading the literature. The Danish adoption studies suggest that the concept of a broad schizophrenia spectrum may be genetically unifying (Rosenthal, 1975a). On the other hand, the spectrum concept is still loosely defined, and alternative, narrow criteria seemed necessary. Hence, it seemed clear that we needed operationalized and differentiated diagnostic studies of the parent who was initially identified as schizophrenic, as well as similar studies of the spouse who had been largely ignored in the early adoption and risk studies.

Fortunately, our program began at a time when more operationally defined diagnostic typological categories and subtype designations were coming into use, so that the meaning and boundaries of alternative categorizations of schizophrenia could be better specified. Standardized interview evaluation procedures with established reliability had become available through prior research in which we had participated, thus supplementing less structured clinical interview techniques. But, for those investigators eager to build a large sample of children at risk because of parental schizophrenia, we soon learned of the limits imposed by diagnostic rigor: Hospital diagnoses of schizophrenia largely evaporated and later coalesced as affective psychoses.

Another major development in diagnostic practice was the growing attention to specific diagnostic axes, or dimensions. The use of diagnostic axes involves describing each patient in terms of several characteristics, such as chronicity and social functioning, for example, rather than relying on a single, symptom-based label. There is still much controversy regarding whether dimensional methods for assessing patients may be superior to the traditional typological models used in the past to define distinctive patient types, such as schizophrenic or neurotic depressive. The applicability of multiaxial models has been proposed, for example, in studies sponsored by the World Health Organization for the classification of children (Rutter, Shaffer, & Shepherd, 1973) and in a comprehensive approach to adults (Strauss, 1975a).

Because of these developments in the field of diagnosis, we have believed that it is important that risk researchers evaluate parent psychiatric disorders using alternative diagnostic approaches, each of which may have particular validity in relation to various aspects of offspring functioning. In this way, different concepts of schizophrenia, such as narrow versus broad typological criteria and several dimensions of function, can be studied comparatively as parental risk factors within a given sample.

3. *The study of intermediate outcomes.* We have been interested explicitly in intermediate short-term changes in our index children as well as in ultimate, long-term outcomes in adulthood. This emphasis reflects our concern with broad issues of developmental psychology and developmental psychopathology, as well as our clinical interest in children of all ages, both in what they are and what they will be.

4. *A family system concept.* The Rochester program has emphasized, most like the UCLA Family Project, a family system concept in formulating alternative risk variables. Methodologically, this has been expressed in studies of family interaction, and in procedures for sampling direct interaction of family members as a social unit. We have been greatly encouraged in our findings thus far, partially reported in this volume, that family interaction, both independently and in combination with parental psychopathology, is a powerful alternative risk factor predictive of competence levels in the offspring.

5. *Causal models.* Direction of effects (Bell, 1968) is a major long-term interest of the Rochester investigators, although it has been frustrating having to wait for follow-up data to test our hypotheses. Most investigators in our group favor a transactional model of causality that accommodates the multiple domains of our data, and an epigenetic, sequential view of development in which children modify reciprocally the responses of parents, as well as the reverse. Repeat measures are clearly necessary to make such formulations empirically testable. Further exploration of appropriate statistical procedures remains a major task in classifying the research usefulness of transactional models.

SELECTION OF THE SAMPLE OF THE ROCHESTER RISK RESEARCH PROGRAM

Within the broad orientation described above, a number of additional problems needed to be considered in order to create a practical research plan.

Homogeneous diagnostic groupings

A basic dilemma in the high-risk paradigm was discussed by Cromwell and Wynne in a 1976 working paper: If one does not have homogeneous groupings, one cannot determine what the variables are that are relevant to diagnosis; and if one cannot determine what the relevant variables are, one cannot attain homogeneous grouping. As applied to the diagnosis of schizophrenia in high-risk projects, this statement carries the reminder that agreement on diagnostic criteria has not yet been attained, even though considerable progress has been made in the past decade. Earlier, the problem was often hidden under the mantle of arrogant complacency among professionals who responded implicitly: The problems of reaching agreement on criteria and of unreliability between diagnosticians lie in the carelessness of *other* hospitals (clinics, countries). We know what schizophrenia is here, and we are more careful. With the work of the U.S.–U.K. group (Cooper, Kendell, Gurland, Sharpe, Copeland, & Simon, 1972), the WHO International Pilot Study of Schizophrenia (IPSS) (1973), the development of the Research Diagnostic Criteria (RDC), and the evolution of several standardized, reliable interview schedules for rating psychiatric symptoms, the criticism that symptom ratings were unreliable was no longer tenable at the time this study began. A chief instrument for symptom evaluation in this program was an adaptation of the Present State Examination (PSE) that had been used extensively in the WHO studies.

Alternative diagnostic criteria

Even when systematic interview schedules are used to maximize diagnostic reliability, the question of validity remains: Which set of alternative diagnostic criteria are to be used to identify homogeneous groups? Just one example of many studies illustrating the problem of alternative criteria is the report by Strauss and Gift (1977). In a representative sample of 272 patients first hospitalized for functional psychiatric disorders, 122 (45%) of the patients were classified as schizophrenic by at least one set of criteria. Sixty-eight (25%) were diagnosed as schizophrenic by the New Haven Schizophrenic Index, which is similar to DSM-II, whereas 48 (17.6%) were so diagnosed by the Research Diagnostic Criteria, which has some similarity to DSM-III. Especially distressing was their conclusion that the "various systems were not just more or less broad. Although the broader systems included many of the patients diagnosed schizophrenic by the narrower ones, in every comparison of the two systems, there was a considerable proportion of patients classified schizophrenic by each system, whether it was broad or narrow, that was not considered schizophrenic by the other."

Our solution to this problem of conflicting criteria for typological diagnoses was to retain the primary ratings of symptoms in our interview schedules so that *alternative* diagnostic criteria could be applied to these descriptive features. Then, as later evidence emerged favoring one set of criteria versus another, the alternative criteria could be compared in terms of outcome and dependent variables.

Coping with DSM-III

The initial assessments in our study were carried out from 1972 to 1977 at a time when DSM-III had been announced as the forthcoming American standard for psychiatic diagnoses, but the document itself was still undergoing extensive changes. Although at least one-half of our sample had been diagnosed as schizophrenic by one hospital clinician or another, the emerging DSM-III, with a far more narrowly defined category of schizophrenia, left many fewer patients with this diagnosis. In the 1977 version of DSM-III, the important category of schizoaffective disorder was still classified as a type of schizophrenia, in accordance with both American tradition and the then current International Classification of Diseases (ICD-9). Our initial diagnostic classifications were based upon the 1977 version; later these were changed to fit the 1978 DSM-III version in which schizoaffective disorder was placed indeterminately as a "Psychotic Disorder Not Elsewhere Classified."

In this volume, the data analyses were based upon the 1978 version of DSM-III except in the report by Klein and Salzman (see Chapter 27, this volume), which retains the 1977 diagnoses. Interestingly, their data reveal that when the schizo-affective patients are classified with typical schizophrenics, striking contrasts between the children of this broader group and the children of parents with bipolar and unipolar affective psychoses are found. This result may not have emerged with the most recent, final 1980 version of DSM-III in which most patients formerly classified as schizoaffective now fit the broader criteria for bipolar disorder with mood-incongruent psychosis. Currently, we have been updating our diagnostic classifications to fit the 1980 version of DSM-III.

These changes in diagnostic practice have been maddeningly frustrating to many clinicians and investigators. On the other hand, it should be recognized that the changes have come about because of a serious effort to be responsive to recent research findings (see especially Pope & Lipinski, 1978; Procci, 1976; and Brockington & Leff, 1979), and that DSM-III itself is an interim proposal and not the ultimate solution to psychiatric diagnosis. We believe that the application of alternative diagnostic criteria in the risk research field in which families are studied comprehensively and longitudinally has special merit for helping to clarify issues of diagnostic validity.

Parents who are schizophrenic

Even more difficult than this general diagnostic problem is the special problem in selecting index parents for high-risk studies because they are both schizophrenic and parents. Schizophrenics who become parents tend to be a select sample as compared to other schizophrenics, with respect to milder symptoms, later onset, more sexual experience, marital status, and the experience of bearing and raising children. In such persons, diagnostic signs are even less clear-cut than in a random sample of other patients diagnosed as schizophrenic. Thus, simply maintaining stringent criteria is an incomplete answer to this problem of sample selection. The dilemma is that stringent criteria applied when symptoms are mild and variable reduce the number of subjects to the point where few are available for study; but relaxing diagnostic criteria does not provide an acceptable solution either. Although sufficient numbers of cases are then available for investigation, the resemblance of these parents to prototypical schizophrenics may be minimal.

Utilizing diagnostic heterogeneity

The strategy chosen in the Rochester project for dealing with this diagnostic problem was to forego the traditional initial step of separating schizophrenic from nonschizophrenic patient controls. Instead, all parents meeting family and demographic criteria were candidates for the study if they had been hospitalized for a functional psychiatric disorder. Only persons with organic conditions were excluded, that is, if they were alcoholic, organically brain damaged, mentally retarded, or severe drug abusers. A more problematic exclusion group were mothers with a postpartum psychosis within 6 weeks of delivery. Later, we were impressed with the high frequency of patient–mothers (48/106) who had their initial admission or first severe symptoms *later* than 6 weeks postpartum but within a year of the delivery of one of their children; 29 of these 48 mothers had symptoms within a year of the birth of the index son.

Assessment of parental functioning and pathology was made systematically with standard procedures by two diagnostic teams, one headed by John Romano and the other initially by John Strauss, and later by Ronald Kokes (see Chapter 24, this volume). The clinically relevant data have been used used to make assessments and diagnoses from alternative vantage points rather than from a single nosological system. Dependence on the preliminary case record data and on categorical typologic diagnostic agreements was thus avoided.

An affectively disturbed comparison group

Similar issues arise in the selection of diagnostic criteria for comparison groups within the sample. Originally, we considered using a control group of neurotic depressive index parents. We noted that evidence from the Danish adoption studies that serious personality disorders might be within the schizophrenia spectrum, but that depression was outside. We speculated that a psychotic depressive group as a control would yield an older age group and make matching difficult. But as we started to collect our sample, we soon decided that defining boundaries for neurotic depression was even more difficult than for schizophrenia. (Klerman, Endicott, Spitzer, & Hirschfeld, 1979, more recently have argued that the term *neurotic depression* no longer be used because of its vagueness and multiple meanings and criteria.) Therefore, we opted for a strategy similar to that for the schizophrenia-like cluster of patients. We decided to carry out careful and systematic interviews and ratings of affectively disturbed patients so that their symptom features could be stably identified at the same time that alternative classificatory criteria can be applied.

In retrospect, we remain pleased that we have obtained a highly interesting sample of families in which a parent has had unipolar or bipolar affective psychoses, major depression, depressive neurosis, or adjustment disorder with depressive features. As we noted in a 1972 grant application: "The study of the impact of depression in a mother on the development of children is a highly important issue in its own right that has been much neglected in past research. The data on this group of families may well be fresh and provocative. Further, if we find that we can predict severe degrees of maladaptation and incompetence in children of this low-risk group, this finding would be of very special interest."

Dimensional approaches to parental assessment

A major approach to diagnostic evaluation that has gained increasing attention in recent years builds upon the concept of a series of underlying dimensions, or axes, that crosscut the entities and disorders of traditional diagnostic typology. Thus, affectivity can be regarded as a dimension that is ratable in anyone, across all mental disorders. In addition to genetic transmission of affective tendencies, surely the affective lability, expressiveness, and pervasive tone of parents will be relevant to child development. Similarly, we proposed that the dimensions of psychosis–nonpsychosis, of severity, and of episodic versus chronic course should be studied in this program. Such differences in dimensional classifications have been reliably studied and predictive of outcome in 2- to 5-year follow-ups (Strauss & Carpenter, 1972, 1974a, 1974b). From the point of view of multivariate analysis and theory development, the flexibility of this strategy has been attractive. Not only can single variables, small and large generic groupings of variables, and traditional diagnostic classifications be tested for their efficacy in predicting later breakdown, but also classification systems derived later on can be applied to the basic raw data in our files.

Sex of patient–parent

In the interests of homogeneous sampling, at an early stage of planning we considered restricting the sample to families in which mothers but not fathers had been psychiatrically ill. However, we decided to include fathers on the conceptual ground that we could then examine the statistical interaction effects between parental role and psychiatric status. Subsequently, we have been impressed by findings that do show such interaction, for example, see Chapter 28, this volume, by Baldwin et al. In our eventual sample of 145 families, 29 (26.9%) of the index parents were fathers and 106 (73.1%) were mothers.

Sex of index offspring

In 1972 we stated: "Our decision to use only male offspring was supported by the differences observed by Rolf (1972) in his study of competence in male versus female children at risk for schizophrenia, and the subsequent follow-back data provided by Watt et al. (1970) in their analysis of school records of children who developed schizophrenia in adulthood. Also, sex differences in psychophysiologic and other variables are probably significant, especially in the earlier years, and would complicate unduly the task of establishing norms for these measures." Comparable studies of female offspring are still needed.

Age of index offspring

Because adolescence is the age of onset for many schizophrenics, and because other studies (see in this volume, Chapters 2 and 4 by Mednick et al., and Chapter

5 by Rodnick et al.) were beginning with adolescents at risk, we wished to push back the age of our index offspring to preadolescence. We were curious whether testable vulnerability might be less evident or less frequent before a certain age. Because this age may be prenatal, we were pleased at the opportunity to collaborate with Sameroff and Zax who had begun their risk sample with pregnant women and who were planning to follow them at least through the infancy of their children. Now, in 1980, their children are reaching age 10, so that the possibility of comparing samples in the two Rochester studies still is alive and undergoing renewed planning. For these and related reasons, we chose to begin with the age range of 4 to 10 in our index offspring.

A convergence design for accelerating longitudinal studies

A special feature of our design was to try out Richard Q. Bell's suggestion (1953) for accelerating longitudinal research with a convergence design. Although this approach had not been used previously in the study of psychopathology, we were impressed by the proposals by Bell and by Schaie and Strother (1968) that such a design would permit the construction of a composite longitudinal age gradient. Thus, we decided to begin with three cohorts: index sons at age 4, 7, and 10. These three cohorts are then followed up at age 7, 10, and 13. Ages 7 and 10 then become points of potential convergence.

We debated the selection of these particular ages. They were chosen because they permitted the collection of data at strategic times in terms of developmental periods. By age 4, the child has ordinarily acquired language, and failure to talk by age 4 is clear evidence of disturbance in language development. But at age 4, cognitive development is still *preoperational* in Piagetian terminology. Age 7 is marked by operational thinking and conservation in Piaget's terms. This age also provides a good opportunity to assess cognitive and early social functioning in the child.

The age span from 4 to 7 also covers school entrance for the child and separation from the mother and provides an opportunity to detect academic problems at an early stage. Mothering at age 4 involves language and coping with the various problems of negativism, fears, sexual curiosity, and so forth, and is very involving. By age 7, with the child in school, mothering is reduced in amount of direct control, and the child needs new skills to cope with peer relations and academic expectations. At age 10, the child nears the period of formal operations and preadolescence. Ages 7 to 10, we believed, are not marked by any pervasive change in mother–child relations, but the shift from ages 10 to 13 is marked with formal operational thinking and emergence of teenage problems.

At present (March, 1980), we are about to complete the 3-year follow-up data collection. Only after analysis of these data is completed will we be able to assess convergence. On the whole, we are still satisfied that these age points are interesting, and we are pleased that Anthony's group has joined with us in giving special attention to these ages.

Social class and race

A decision to eliminate Social Class V was dictated largely by the practical consideration that this group would have greater difficulties in cooperating on both economic and psychological grounds; therefore, it seemed prudent first to obtain experience with middle-class subjects. A decision not to include non-Caucasians was linked to the social class issue. We wished to avoid a likely sample skew in which Class V, black schizophrenics would be compared with middle-class white neurotics. Anthony's difficulties with this problem were helpful in making this decision about our sample. If the social class range within our sample was large, we expected that interaction of the social class variable with other variables would make interpretation difficult for findings involving such variables as child social competence and family interaction. Nevertheless, we have carefully assessed the actual social class levels of the families. As subsequent chapters will indicate, this decision to make the sample relatively homogeneous with respect to social class appears supported by clear relationships among other variables that are not accounted for by social class variability.

Intact families

We decided to restrict our sample to families in which the marriage was intact at initial research evaluation and in which an index biological child was being reared by these parents. Mednick (1978) has pointed out the hazards of Berkson's fallacy: Because of inevitable biasing of small, selected samples, one can easily overgeneralize in interpreting the findings. Data from risk samples having only intact families will illustrate the problems, as Mednick points out. We, too, have had misgivings about the difficulty of working only with intact families. To be sure, the quality of the marriages in the sample has varied considerably, and 19% dissolved during the first 3-year follow-up. But intactness at initial evaluation was important because we were interested in holding at least some family relationship and interaction variables reasonably consistent within the sample as a whole. This goal was comparable to obtaining a certain minimal homogeneity in individual parental diagnoses while proceeding to allow, and to study, the substantial diagnostic diversity that remains.

In summary, it will be recognized that exclusion of cases to achieve homogeneity may successfully restrict the influence of a number of presumably extraneous variables that could potentially affect the dependent variables. At the same time, the population to which the results of the study can be generalized becomes increasingly limited as each factor is controlled.

A trade-off of gains and losses was clearly anticipated from this strategy of subject selection. In the interest of broad investigative planning, it has been hoped that some high-risk projects would follow a tests-and-measurement logic with a still broader population sampling. In this way, the potential difference in results with and without major exclusion criteria can be understood more easily. One firm conclusion is that one project cannot solve all questions, and the importance of other high-risk projects with systematic differences in design is evident. This collaborative goal was proposed at the 1969 NIMH Workshop on risk research (Mosher & Wynne, 1970) and has remained as an objective of the Risk Research Consortium.

AREAS AND DOMAINS OF URCAFS VARIABLES

As a device to help us organize and conceptualize our variables, we have grouped them into three *areas:* parent, family, and child. We view each area as having several *domains,* for example, the domain of school functioning in the child area. Each domain, in turn, has *components,* such as teacher ratings and peer ratings in school functioning. As a strategy of data analysis, we examine each method and component first in its own right, then build composite variables for the domain, and eventually (not yet) we may be able, though only for certain limited purposes, to have composite measures for each of the three major areas.

Schematically, the domains and their major components in our study are as follows:

I. *Parent area*
    Domains
        A. Diagnostic typologies (alternative criteria compared, including DSM-III)
            1. Structured interviews (modified PSE)
            2. Semistructured interviews
        B. Clinical dimensions of individual parental functioning
            1. Severity (Global Assessment Scale, GAS)
            2. Chronicity
            3. Psychosis scales
            4. Schizophrenc and paranoid symptom dimensions
            5. Affectivity and emotional expressivity dimensions
            6. Work and social functioning
            7. Dichotomized ratings of 59 clinical variables from videotaped interviews
        C. Psychologic dimensions
            1. Delta Index and Thought Disorder Index (Rorschach)
            2. Developmental level (Rorschach)
            3. Field dependence–independence (Rod and Frame)
            4. Intellectual functioning (WAIS)
            5. Pendulum eye tracking
            6. Personality functioning (MMPI)
            7. Latency and deviance of associations (Goldstein Word Association Test)
            8. Affective and cognitive functions (Gottschalk Five-Minute Speech Samples)
        D. Historical assessment
            1. Premorbid adjustment ratings of index parent
            2. Medical, psychiatric, and developmental history of each parent

II. *Family area*
    Domains
        A. Communicational–Cognitive–Attentional variables
            1. Communication Deviance/Healthy Communication
            2. Acknowledgment code

3. Who-to-whom patterns
4. Focus of speech codes
5. Relationship codes
6. Clarity code
7. Agreement–disagreement code
8. Laughter codes
9. Interruptions/simultaneous speeches code
10. The "product" of consensus
    Items 1–10 are scored from the following procedures:
    a. Individual parental Rorschach
    b. Individual parental TAT
    c. Spouse Consensus Rorschach
    d. Family Rorschach
    e. Plan-something-together (family)
B. Affective–Relational variables
   1. Warmth (Family Free Play)
   2. Positive and negative relationship codes (consensus procedures)
   3. Anger and other affective states (individual Rorschach)
   4. Affective attributions (TAT)
C. Structural–Contextual
   1. Object relations schemata
   2. Balance, activity, and hierarchy in:
      a. Family Free Play (parents–index child triad)
      b. Family Consensus Rorschach (whole family)
      c. Spouse Consensus Rorschach (couple)
      d. Family Cleanup Procedure (whole family)
   3. Referential communication
   4. Extrafamilial context; supports provided by:
      a. Extended family
      b. Social class
      c. Ethnic and religious affiliation
      d. Community and neighborhood social network
      e. Accessibility of "helping" agencies: general, medical, psychiatric, social agencies, church, and other groups
D. Historical variables
   1. Family history of psychiatric and medical illness; pedigree data
   2. Stages of family life-cycle at time of parental episodes of illness
   3. Family rally versus disturbance in response to impact of parental illness

III. *Child area*
Domains
A. Views of the child in school:
   1. Peer ratings
   2. Teacher ratings
B. Views of the child by parents: Rochester Adaptive Behavior Interview (RABI)
   1. Global ratings (RABI-1)
   2. Quantification of item ratings (RABI-2)
C. Views of the child by health professionals:
   1. Obstetrical
   2. Neurological

3. Psychophysiological
   a. Cortical evoked responses
   b. Pendulum eye tracking
   c. Autonomic functioning
4. Psychological
   a. Intellectual (WISC)
   b. Projective, cognitive, and achievement (Rorschach, TAT, Human Figure, WRAT, Bender)
   c. Piagetian measures
   d. Censure–praise assessment
   e. Attentional measures (auditory and visual scanning and sensory integration)
5. Clinical psychiatric
   a. Diagnostic typologies
   b. Global competence evaluations
   c. Q-sort evaluations

24 Diagnostic, symptomatic, and descriptive characteristics of parents in the University of Rochester Child and Family Study

RONALD F. KOKES, DAVID HARDER,
PATRICIA PERKINS, AND JOHN S. STRAUSS

The University of Rochester Child and Family Study (URCAFS) comprehensively evaluated 145 families that, in summary, fulfilled the following criteria: (1) intact family with mother, father, and children living together and including; (2) one parent who had been hospitalized for a functional psychiatric disorder (excluding primary diagnoses of alcoholism, drug addition, mental retardation or organic brain disease); and (3) one son aged 4, 7, or 10. All the families were Caucasion and English speaking. All but two of the families were in social classes I–IV (Hollingshead, 1978). With eight exceptions, the families were evaluated no sooner than 3 months after the last hospitalization of the index parent; the assessment occurred at a mean duration of 3.9 years after the parent's most recent hospitalization. In 39 of the families, the father was the previously hospitalized or index parent; in 106 of these families, the mother was the index parent.

After a family was selected for study on the basis of hospital records, the initial URCAFS clinical assessment of both parents was carried out separately by each of the two teams. One team was headed by John Romano, the other initially by John Strauss, and later, at the time of this report, by Ronald Kokes. A psychological test team of Barry Ritzler and Margaret T. Singer studied parental functioning independently. The present report describes the procedures and preliminary findings of the Kokes–Strauss team.

These assessments of the index parents were based upon data from two points in time: the last hospitalization (called *key admission*) and the initial URCAFS evaluation. Psychopathology at the time of the interview was assessed by this team with the Psychiatric Assessment Interview, an adaptation of John Wing's Present State Examination (Wing, Birley, Cooper, Graham, & Isaacs, 1967) and the Katz Adjustment Scales, R-1 and R-2 (Katz & Lyerly, 1963). Social and work functioning were assessed with the structured Social Data Interview from the World Health Organization's International Pilot Study of Schizophrenia (IPSS, 1973). Parental psychopathology for the time of key admission was assessed with the Standard Psychiatric History, a structured interview from the IPSS and the Case Record Rating Scale (Strauss & Harder, 1974), which collects symptom information from the hospital records parallel to that collected in the Psychiatric Assessment Interview.

The spouse of each index parent was evaluated using the Spouse Background

348

and Social Data Interview, also adapted from the IPSS. In nine families, after the identification of the index parent, it was discovered that the spouse also had had a psychiatric hospitalization. In these cases, hospital records were reviewed and clinical research assessments were made. These spouses all were diagnosed as having had either an alcoholic or a nonpsychotic depressive illness, in some cases in addition to a personality disorder. Follow-up evaluations of the parents are currently underway. These take place approximately 3 years after the initial research evaluations when index children have become 7, 10, or 13 years of age, in keeping with the convergent longitudinal design. Data collection instruments from initial evaluation have been adapted to collect data on current and 3-year follow-up interim functioning regarding symptomatology, treatment (including re-hospitalizations and medications), social and work functioning, changes in family structure, and status of the marriage.

Based on all data available at the time of interview, each index parent was given a primary diagnosis according to the DSM-III criteria of January, 1978, and placed in one of the following 10 diagnostic categories: (1) schizophrenia; (2) schizophreniform, reactive, and paranoid disorders; (3) schizoaffective disorder; (4) bipolar affective disorders; (5) unipolar depressive disorder, psychotic; (6) unipolar depressive disorder, severe; (7) unipolar depressive disorder, moderate; (8) adjustment disorder with depression; (9) anxiety disorders and conversion reaction; and (10) histrionic and other personality disorders. The diagnostic categories will change somewhat with use of the later, 1980 DSM-III criteria that we are in the process of implementing. It is particularly noteworthy that the schizoaffective group is expected to be appreciably smaller.

By combining these 10 diagnostic groups in different ways, several traditional diagnostic comparisons can be made. For example, in the second column of Table 1, the diagnostic categories are grouped so that functioning of families with an index parent who has had a psychotic disorder can be compared to families with index parents whose illness has not been psychotic. Other combinations allow different diagnostic comparisons, such as schizophrenia versus nonschizophrenia, schizophrenia versus all affective versus remaining diagnoses. In the third column of Table 1, the breakdown allows for comparisons among families with a schizophrenic parent, families where the parent has had a severe or psychotic affective disorder, including schizoaffective, and families where the disorder has been nonpsychotic. This grouping ($N = 138$) omits seven families in the study in which the index parent was psychotic but did not fit clearly into either the schizophrenic or affective group. However, because this distinction has been of particular interest to some investigators, and because it is stable and unlikely to change significantly as we review our diagnoses using final DSM-III criteria, we will use it for descriptive tables in this chapter.

The distribution of families by diagnosis of index parent by sex of index parent by age of index child is presented in Table 2. There was a significantly larger number of index mothers than index fathers, 103 versus 35, with more index mothers in all diagnostic groups except schizophrenia (Mo = 5; Fa = 10).

Characteristics of the index parents in each diagnostic group are reported in

Table 1. *University of Rochester Child and Family Study: DSM-III (1978 version) diagnoses of index parents*

1. Schizophrenia	15			Schizophrenia	15
2. Schizophreniform, reactive and paranoid disorders	7	Psychotic disorders	68	Omit	
3. Schizoaffective disorder	20				
4. Bipolar affective disorders	20			Severe and psychotic affective disorders	60
5. Unipolar depressive disorder, psychotic	6				
6. Unipolar depressive disorder, severe	14				
7. Unipolar depressive disorder, moderate	34	Nonpsychotic disorders	77	Nonpsychotic hospitalized disorders	63
8. Adjustment disorder with depression	7				
9. Anxiety disorders and conversion reaction	10				
10. Histrionic and other personality disorders	12				
Totals	145		145		138

Table 2. *University of Rochester Child and Family Study: case distribution by parent diagnosis, sex of parent, and age of child*

Parent diagnosis	Age of index child						Totals
	4		7		10		
	Father	Mother	Father	Mother	Father	Mother	
Schizophrenic	3	1	2	3	5	1	15
Severe and psychotic affective disorders (including schizoaffective disorder and unipolar severe)	2	9	3	17	7	22	60
Nonpsychotic disorders (all with hospitalization)	4	18	2	17	7	15	63
Totals	9	28	7	37	19	38	138

Table 3. *University of Rochester Child and Family Study: diagnosis of index parent by parental IQ, parental age, and social class at initial evaluation*

Diagnosis of index parent	Mean IQ		Mean age		Mean social class
	Index	Spouse	Index	Spouse	
Schizophrenia (N = 15)	108	113	35	36	2.9
Affective psychoses (N = 60)	107	114	39	40	3.1
Nonpsychotic (N = 63)	110	114	34	35	3.1
Totals (N = 138)	108	114	36	38	3.1

Table 3. The mean IQ of all parents was 111. Differences across groups were nonsignificant. The mean age of index parents at URCAFS interview was 36. The mean social class level was 3.1 on the Hollingshead (1978) Four-Factor Scale; again, the differences across groups were not significant.

Hospitalization and episode of illness data of the index parent are reported in Table 4. The mean number of hospital admissions for the index parents prior to study was 2.7, with the means across the groups ranging from 1.8 for the nonpsychotic disorders to 3.5 for the severe and psychotic affective disorders. The total mean duration of all hospitalizations for 138 index parents was 20.0 weeks. Parents with affective disorders had the longest total duration of hospitalizations, an average of 35.7 weeks. The nonpsychotic patients had the shortest duration of hospitalization, an average of 5.5 weeks, with the schizophrenics (18.1 weeks) midway between the nonpsychotic and affective disorders.

Course of illness rating is reported as a single episode, episodic, or chronic. A *single episode* is a single psychiatric hospitalization that took place more than 2 years before initial URCAFS evaluation. An illness is called *episodic* if there was a 2-year symptom-free period at any time after the first hospitalization, followed by a later relapse. Illness is called *chronic* if there were no such symptom-free 2-year periods after first hospitalization. The rating is not made if the patient's first hospitalization was recent, that is, less than two years prior to their URCAFS evaluation. Most notably, as shown in Table 4, the affective psychotic group has the highest percentage of parents with an episodic illness, thus defined. The schizophrenic group has the highest proportion (67%) of chronic parents. However, more than 40% of the patients in the other two categories also have a chronic illness.

Ratings of level of social and work functioning were assigned to both index parent and spouse for time of URCAFS interview and are being assigned for time of follow-up. Ratings are based on both quantity and quality of social relations and work. Ratings range from 0 (no useful work or no social relationships) to 4 (continuous full-time competent employment or a number of close or gratifying relationships).

Mean scores in Table 5 indicate that schizophrenic index parents have the

Table 4. *University of Rochester Child and Family Study: chronicity and hospitalization measures of index parent by diagnosis of index parent*

Diagnosis of index parent	Single episode	Episodic	Chronic	Recent	Mean number hospitalizations	Mean total weeks in hospital
Schizophrenia (N = 15)	2	1	10	2	3.0	18.1
Affective psychoses (N = 60)	6	18	25	11	3.5	35.7
Nonpsychotic (N = 63)	12	3	28	20	1.8	5.5
Totals (N = 138)	20	22	63	33	2.7	20.0

Table 5. *University of Rochester Child and Family Study: mean social and work functioning scores of parents at time of initial evaluation*

Diagnosis of index parent	Index parent		Spouse	
	Social functioning	Work functioning	Social functioning	Work functioning
Schizophrenia	2.5	2.9	3.4	3.8
Severe and psychotic affective disorders	3.1	3.4	3.1	3.7
Nonpsychotic	3.2	3.6	3.1	3.7

lowest social functioning ($\bar{x} = 2.5$), and the lowest work functioning ($\bar{x} = 2.9$). The most striking quality, however, of the social and work functioning scores is the generally high level of the ratings. The schizophrenics, with the lowest mean ratings on both scales, still had some moderately close relationships of moderate frequency; that is, they met with friends more than once a month and they were employed on the average about half the time and with at least moderate competence. Because family intactness is one of the criteria for inclusion in the study, it may have resulted in selection of patients who tended to function fairly adequately in other aspects of their lives also.

The index parents also were assigned a rating from 0 (symptoms not present) to 100 (symptoms definitely present and severe on each of 32 symptom dimensions constructed by Strauss, Carpenter, and Bartko from the World Health Organization International Pilot Study of Schizophrenia data. The dimensions range from psychotic types, that is, hallucinations, delusions, and bizarre speech, to affective types to neurotic types such as depression and anxiety. Work is currently in progress to identify clusters of these symptoms that might be predictive of child functioning.

Every family in the URCAFS sample contains by definition at least one parent who has been hospitalized for a psychiatric disorder. The affective psychotics and the nonpsychotics predominate, but there also are a small group of people who meet strict criteria for the diagnosis of schizophrenia. The sample as a whole consists of intact, mostly middle-class families with middle-aged parents who have above average intelligence. Close to one-half of the patient parents have been psychotic and close to one-half suffer from an illness that is chronic. Despite this, on the average their social and work functioning is not severely impaired.

25 A strategy and methodology for assessing school competence in high-risk children

LAWRENCE FISHER, PAUL SCHWARTZMAN,
DAVID HARDER, AND RONALD F. KOKES

Garmezy (1975a) has suggested that *competence* and the mastery of basic life tasks be used as the primary concept for the assessment of the child at risk. A cluster of competence variables can be used both to clock current and intermediate outcomes in the development of the child at risk and to predict later outcome in adolescence or adulthood.

Our model of assessment of competence in the school setting is based on the assumption that all behavior is displayed within the context of a social system. Because such behaviors are judged, evaluated, and sanctioned positively or negatively by that system, it is the system itself that defines what is competent and what is incompetent behavior by means of selective reinforcement in everyday interactions. It is the researcher's task to identify the norms and values within the system that define competent behavior.

With this goal, we began by tape-recording teacher and student discussions about competent and successful functioning in school, as well as incompetent and unsuccessful school functioning. These discussions were carried out with teachers of academic subjects and with random groups of students in elementary school and junior and senior high schools in the Rochester area. Each recording then was reviewed to obtain verbatim descriptors of competent and incompetent behaviors that later were used as items in rating scales. These items were then submitted to a large number of teachers of students and their ratings were factor analyzed within school level by grade and sex. These were replicated on independent samples of urban and suburban and rural school settings, and test–retest reliabilities were obtained (Rubenstein & Fisher, 1974).

The Rochester Teacher Rating Scale emerged from this process as one of two final instruments used in the study of the elementary school competence of UR-CAFS children (Fisher, 1980). Four factors or dimensions as rated by the teachers are scored for each child:

> Factor 1 – Social compliance;
> Factor 2 – Social competence indicating the child's effective functioning with his peers;
> Factor 3 – Cognitive competence; and
> Factor 4 – Motivation or involvement in academic activities.

355

The second instrument, the Rochester Peer Rating Scale, is a sociometric technique (Rubenstein, Fisher, & Iker, 1975). All the children in the classroom are asked to select a classmate who fits the role described in the item, for example, "A boy or girl who is well behaved in school." Four factors emerged from the analysis of the judgments of peers in grades 1 through 6, and similar dimensions describe the 7- and 10-year-old URCAFS children:

Factor 1 – Brightness–compliance;
Factor 2 – Intrusiveness;
Factor 3 – Dullness; and
Factor 4 – Friendliness.

The decision was made to use each classroom as the reference group to which the URCAFS child was compared. For the teachers' ratings, each male student was scored on each of the dimensions and placed in a within class t-distribution with a mean of 50 and a standard deviation of 10. For the peer judgments, the number of nominations for each role for the child was taken as his raw score. Because of the distribution of these scores, the median and the semiinterquartile range was used rather than the mean and standard deviation. A given student score on each dimension could be compared with those of his male classmates, and also with students from different classrooms in terms of deviation from the home classroom as the reference point.

One of the attractive features of these school ratings is that they are completely independent of any of the other measures of the child and they are uninfluenced by the fact that the child has a parent who has been psychiatrically ill. Neither the teacher nor the peers knew that there was an URCAFS child in the classroom; only the school administrator, who gave permission for the study, knew that a child was part of the URCAFS research program.

A different instrument was developed for children in the junior and senior high schools, which will be used in follow-up studies; but these instruments are not relevant for this report on the 7- and 10-year-old children.

The test–retest reliabilities of the ratings were obtained by repeating the measurement on a sample of classes after a 4-week interval. The reliabilities of the teachers' ratings of the four dimensions are as follows:

Social compliance = .80;
Social competence = .79;
Cognitive competence = .71; and
Motivation = .75.

The reliabilities of the peer ratings are:

Brightness–compliance = .85;
Intrusiveness = .88;
Dullness = .88; and
Friendliness = .68.

The teachers' ratings consistently show lower test–retest reliabilities than the peer ratings.

So far, we have presented procedures for the assessment of school competence at a dimensional level. However, many types of analyses require more global indices of competence based on totals of several factors or on profiles of performance. With this in mind, we have developed an assessment ladder for the elementary school child that designates scores at four measurement levels, as presented in Table 1.

Level II of the assessment ladder represents an a priori rational grouping of teacher and peer dimensions into three behavioral domains: Academic competence, Social/emotional behavior, and Compliance behavior. These three measures are not independent: Brightness–compliance is included in two of the three clusters, and Intrusiveness in a different pair of clusters (see Fisher & J. E. Jones, 1980). This level of analysis has been particularly helpful in testing specific hypotheses requiring both teacher and peer judgments. Also at this level, although not represented in Table 1, are the mean teacher and mean peer ratings. These ratings summarize the teacher and peer views of the index children's competence. Before aggregating the four components of each measure, the direction of the Dullness and Intrusiveness scales were reversed.

Level III represents a statistical clustering of the entire profile of eight teacher and peer dimensions. For a sample of 100 children, not including any URCAFS children, each child's profile was correlated with every other child's profile, and the resulting intercorrelation matrix was analyzed by several different clustering programs. The same matrix was also factored by the method of principal components, followed by a varimax rotation. The seven clusters shown in Table 1 emerged from this analysis. Each of the clusters was replicated over different clustering methods for each of two independent, non-URCAFS samples, and thus they appear to be highly stable (Fisher, 1980). The profile of each URCAFS child then was assigned to one of the seven clusters by two independent judges. It was possible to assign 80% of the children to these seven clusters. In Level IV, these seven profiles, or clusters, were grouped into two broader ratings of competence. The Competent–Incompetent score reflects a 2-point classification of the profiles, as indicated in Table 1, and the Global Rating categorizes the profiles along a 4-point Competence dimension. In order to agree with the direction of other global ratings of the children, a high score of 4 represents the most incompetent children, and 1 is supercompetent (better than average).

The Rochester Teacher and Peer Rating scales have been related to several measures of the parent and the family (Fisher, Harder, & Kokes, 1980; Fisher & J. E. Jones, 1980; Harder, Kokes, Fisher, & Strauss, 1980; Kokes, Harder, Fisher, & Strauss, 1980; and Fisher, Kokes, Harder, & J. E. Jones, 1980). For the purposes of this report, we can summarize briefly the major findings by saying that child competence in school is related to psychopathological features of the patient parent in an interestingly complex manner. An example of the results is shown in Table 2.

Most strikingly, the 7- and 10-year-old sons of the parents with the psychotic and severe affective disorders (frequently episodic) consistently function more competently than the sons of the less severely disturbed but more chronic non-

Table 1. *Scales and levels of analysis of elementary school children*

Level of analysis	Scale — Peer dimension	Scale — Teacher dimension
I. Dimensional	Brightness/compliance; Intrusiveness; Dullness; Friendliness; Social compliance	Social competence; Cognitive competence; Motivation
II. Integration	Academic competence (Brightness/compliance, dullness, cognitive competence, motivation); Social/emotional behavior (Intrusiveness, friendliness, social competence)	Compliance behavior (Brightness/compliance, social compliance, intrusiveness)

	Peer dimension				Teacher dimension		
III. Profile	Supercompetent	Competent	Incompetent	Bright/shy	Noncompliant	Dull	Assertive
Sample A (N = 100)	12	13	16	12	5	21	7
Sample B (N = 100)	14	12	15	7	10	17	5
% Total sample	13	12.5	15.5	9.5	7.5	19	6
IV. Global							
1. Competent (+); incompetent (−)	+	+	−	+	−	−	+
2. Global rating (1 to 4)	1	2	4	2	3	4	2

Note: Of the 200 profiles, 8 were assigned to two profile groups and 26 were not clearly classified statistically, leaving a total of 166, or 83% of the sample, included in the present format.

Table 2. *One-way analyses of variance of child competence variables by parent DSM-III diagnosis (1978 version)*

	Child competence variables for 7- and 10-year-olds	
Parental diagnosis	Peer rating (*M*)	Teacher rating (*M*)
Schizophrenia (*N* = 11)	45.52	45.95
Severe and psychotic affective disorder (*N* = 49)	53.93	53.25
Hospitalized non-psychotic disorders (*N* = 41)	49.20	47.71
Mean of classmates	50	50
F	5.25	5.65
p-Values	<.01	<.005

psychotic patients. Less surprisingly, there is a consistent trend for the sons of the schizophrenics to be rated as least competent. Because the final 1980 version of the DSM-III diagnoses are not yet available, and because there are many complex components of parental functioning, the full implications of the association between parental and child features remain to be examined.

26 A clinical research approach to the assessment of adaptive function in children at risk

STEPHEN MUNSON, ALFRED L. BALDWIN,
PAMELA YU, CLARA P. BALDWIN, AND
DEBORAH GREENWALD

The children of psychiatrically disturbed parents develop in an unusual and often puzzling environment. In addition to the usual diversity of temperamental characteristics, these children may bring to their environment some special qualities determined by their genetic heritage. The transaction among these factors results in a great variety of experiences and behaviors in these children, which, over time, develop into recognizable patterns of personality style and coping ability. This chapter will focus on the attempts of the Child Clinical Assessment Team at Rochester to understand these children at discrete points in their development.

The Child Clinical Assessment Team was organized halfway through the data collection of the initial sample of URCAFS families. In this sample we have therefore studied a subsample of 56 children who have parents with a variety of disorders, including schizophrenia, schizoaffective psychosis, affective disorders, and other psychotic disorders and nonpsychotic syndromes. The children are all boys: Fourteen were age 4; 27 were age 7; and 17 were age 10. In addition to this subsample at initial assessment, our group has nearly finished collecting data on the entire 3-year follow-up sample ($N = 110$).

The tools we use to study these children were derived from the experience of other investigators, notably E. James Anthony (1969b) and Clarice Kestenbaum (Kestenbaum & Bird, 1978). We collect the history of perinatal events, developmental achievements and medical difficulties in a single structured interview with both parents. In a second interview, the parents' description of the child's adaptive behavior is collected through Fredric Jones's (1977) structured Rochester Adaptive Behavior Interview (RABI). Also, a neurological examination is conducted, as well as a standard psychological testing battery focusing on intelligence, neurological integration, school achievement, and personality functioning of the child. All of this material is reviewed and summarized by a child clinician who then meets with the parents in a nonstructured interview to clarify the inevitable discrepancies and ambiguities that result from data collected from such a variety of procedures.

Following this, the same clinician meets with the child. For the 4-year-old children, a semistructured playroom interview is conducted (Simmons, 1974). For older children, we conduct a verbal interview, focusing on family relationships, school functioning, peer relationships, fantasy life, and the child's self-concept. This meeting usually takes 1 hour and is recorded on videotape.

These procedures result in a fascinating array of data. For purposes of comparison with the data of other investigators in the program, we have organized the material in three ways. First, following the example of many similar studies, we make a global assessment of the child's adaptive functioning using a scale adapted from Glidewell, Domke, and Kantor (1963):

1. – *Above average adjustment:* A happy child who tends to be superior in his relationships with others and in his accomplishments. Minor problems are overshadowed by his considerable strengths.

1.5 –

2. – *No significant problems:* A child who is generally happy and accomplishes reasonably well the things that usually go with his age and level of development. A few slight problems may be present, but he handles them adequately.

2.5 –

3. – *Subclinically disturbed:* A child who is not so happy as he might be; has moderate difficulties getting on. Growing up represents something of a struggle.

3.5 –

4. – *Clinically disturbed:* A child who has, or, at his present rate is likely to have, serious problems of adjustment, and needs clinical help because of such problems. Certain aspects of his relationships with others and/or his accomplishments are markedly deficient in spite of some compensating social assets.

4.5 –

5. – *Seriously disturbed:* Extreme or bizarre behavior, problems of adjustment that are intense and overshadow social skills which are limited and generally inadequate.

Initially, we used a 5-point scale; however, with experience we found our clinicians adding intermediate points, making 9 possible points for rating. Each child is rated by two independent raters who review all the data. The average Pearsonian correlation between these two independent raters is .90.

The global rating is useful but reduces the information to a bare minimum. Therefore in a second procedure we are reviewing all child cases for diagnosis according to DSM-III. Only 13 (22%) of this sample of 58 children had sufficiently distinctive symptoms to qualify for a DSM-III diagnosis.

Our third procedure results from a desire to describe and classify the children in a comprehensive, yet meaningful, way. Following the advice of Norman Garmezy, a group of us decided to investigate the usefulness of a Q-sort analysis of our clinical data. We consulted with Jeanne and Jack Block who have published the California Q-sort for Children (Block, 1961). With this consultation and the considerable inventiveness of Clara and Alfred Baldwin, who joined the team for this purpose, we devised the Rochester Adaptation of the California Child Q-sort.

This instrument consists of 84 items that describe characteristics of the child's thinking, the rater's perception of the child's responses to his environment, the rater's inferences about the child's perception of himself and his world, the quality of the child's interactions with others, and an assessment of the child's appeal to other people.

Two child clinicians, working independently, review all the clinical data on each child and then assign each Q-sort item to one of nine categories, ranging from category 1 for items that are least salient for the child, to category 9 for most salient

Table 1. *Distributions of Child Overall Psychiatric Evaluation (COPE) ratings*

Global COPE rating	Absolute frequency	Percentage of cases
1	4	6.9
2	15	25.9
3	27	46.6
4	9	15.5
5	3	5.2
Total	58	100

and aptly descriptive items. At least nine items are assigned to each category; the remaining three may go in any three categories.

The Q-sorts of the two independent raters are then combined to provide a composite Q-sort for the child. This composite has the standard properties of the original Q-sort. The reliability of the composite can be estimated from the correlation between the two raters using the Spearman–Brown correlation. If the original correlation is less than $r = .60$, a third, independent judge is asked to perform a third Q-sort, and all three are then combined to provide the composite score for the child. The average reliability of the composite Q-sort for the first series of cases was $r = .88$, with a range from .75 to .97.

There are several advantages to the Q-sort procedure. Because the score for each item is based upon the relevance of the item to a particular child, there is no necessity to judge the children in relation to the distribution of children in the population. In this largely nonpathological group of children not (yet) seen for clinical care, it is a special advantage not to be limited to symptoms and evidence of psychiatric disturbance and to be able to assess strengths and competencies. The required distribution of items across all categories allows one to correlate any two Q-sorts without concern about differences in standard deviations. Hence, we can assess interrater reliabilities and can compare children on the basis of their similarity in patterns of item distribution.

For the first of the three tools, we have preliminary results for all 58 cases seen in the initial sample. For computer analysis, we have labeled our global rating COPE (Child Overall Psychiatric Evaluation). The COPE ratings fall into a normal distribution with a mean score for all ages combined of 2.93, a range of 1 to 5, and a standard deviation of 1.35 (Table 1).

Alfred Baldwin has taken the major responsibility for reducing statistically the 84-item Q-sort to a smaller number of summary variables that described the qualitative differences among the children. Because each child's Q-sort has the same mean and standard deviation, the similarity of two children is well described by their correlation. Using the Johnson Hierarchical Clustering Program (Johnson, 1967), seven groups of children were identified in a subsample of 49 cases on whom Q-sort data were available for computer analysis. This arrangement of

Table 2. *Q-sort clusters of URCAFS children*

Group	Qualitative descriptors	*N*	Mean COPE score
1	Open, trusting, curious	13	1.95
2	Reflective, conforming	6	2.40
3	Worrying, responsive	4	2.75
4	Helpful, stable	4	2.50
5	Disobedient, overactive	8	3.85
6	Shy, anxious	5	3.15
7	Constricted, depressed	5	3.40

seven clusters leaves four children outside any cluster. Once the clusters were described statistically, we were able then to discover the common clinical characteristics which define the cluster by inspecting the Q-sort items that have mean ratings for the cluster at the extreme ends of the item placement scale. In other words, each cluster of children will have a group of items whose mean value will be either very high or very low. These items will represent the attributes that are most and least salient of the group.

The groups identified by this method are qualitatively interesting (Table 2). Group 1 consists of 13 children. They are healthy, as evidenced by the fact that the mean COPE score of this group is 1.95 (on a 5-point scale in which 2 denotes average, "good" adjustment. These are vital, happy, curious children with high self-esteem and an open and trusting attitude toward others. Group 2 has six children with a mean COPE rating of 2.4 (that is, less well adjusted but not needing clinical care). These children have high need achievement, are reflective, and conforming to adult expectations. Group 3 has four children with a mean COPE score of 2.75 (less healthy than the first two groups). These children are responsive to adults. They brood and worry but cope reasonably well and are not depressed. They are not inclined to express hostility and they withdraw under stress. Group 4 has four children who are especially helpful, empathic, stable, and not anxious. Their average COPE score is 2.5. Group 5 has eight children and has a mean COPE rating of 3.85 (the least healthy of any cluster). These are physically active children who overreact to minor frustration. They have difficulty attending to a task and are unable to delay gratification. They have rapidly shifting moods, are disobedient, and insecure about their parents' love for them. Group 6 has five children and a mean COPE score of 3.15. They are highly obedient and very involved with their family. They are emotionally constricted and shy, anxious, and fearful and often express this with bodily symptoms. They brood and worry, but are intelligent and able to attend to tasks. Group 7 has a mean COPE score of 3.4 and has five children. These are neither bright-eyed nor energetic and vital. They have low self-esteem, withdraw from tasks under stress, and seem unable to persist at tasks. They are constricted, emotionally bland and, in a word, depressed.

An analysis of variance comparing the COPE scores of these Q-sort groups shows that the clusters are highly differentiated by COPE. However, most of the difference is between Group 1 (our healthiest group) and all the other groups. Also, there is a significant difference between Cluster 2 and Cluster 5. Although many of these groups sound like clinical syndromes, each group contains some children who are judged by clinicians to be functioning well. Thus, with these groupings, we appear to be describing qualitative differences that need not reflect pathology or health in a global sense. These descriptors may prove to be useful in predicting future patterns of adjustment. Follow-up Q-sorts will indicate the stability of these groups and the persistence of the characteristics in individual children.

Another strategy useful in the analysis of Q-sort data is the comparison of individual and group Q-sorts with a standard Q-sort. Three clinicians in our group independently sorted the items in an attempt to describe a hypothetical healthy, relatively invulnerable child. Our interrater correlations on this sort ranged from .82 to .89. The composite Q-sort of these raters was then compared with the Q-sort groups described earlier. The Pearsonian correlation with the healthiest group (Group 1) was .83.

If one compares individual Q-sorts with this ideal Q-sort, one finds a distribution of the correlations across a range from $-.59$ to $+.80$, with small numbers of children present at every intermediate level.

Once we have clustered the full set of cases, we propose to use, as summary variables for each child, the correlation of his sort with the composite Q-sort for all the children in each cluster. Thus the clusters provide Q-sorts that characterize each type of child. The children who belong to a particular cluster will have higher correlations with the average of that cluster; but each child may well have quite diverse correlations with the averages of the *other* clusters.

This summary describes in some detail the procedures we are using to collect data about children who experience the genetic and environmental risks of having psychiatrically disturbed parents and some of the techniques that are useful for organizing and understanding clinical data about such children. We believe these techniques will allow us to describe these children in a way that is valid and that will allow statistical analyses of transactions between the children, their families and their extrafamilial context.

27 Child competence as assessed by clinicians, parents, teachers, and peers

PAMELA YU, ROBERT PRENTKY,
LAWRENCE FISHER, ALFRED L. BALDWIN,
DEBORAH GREENWALD, STEPHEN MUNSON,
AND CLARA P. BALDWIN

Efforts to provide quantifiable data on child competence have generally focused on the child's adjustment in various specified domains, according to judgments made by qualified individuals within those domains. Separately, such efforts might be likened to the attempt of the six blind men to describe the elephant.

Within the University of Rochester Child and Family Study (URCAFS), assessments of child competence have been derived from four rich and independent data sources: (1) psychiatric evaluation (Munson et al., Chapter 26, this volume); (2) teacher and (3) peer judgments in the school setting (Fisher et al., Chapter 25, this volume); and (4) parental report (F. Jones, 1977; Prentky, 1979). Each of these investigative areas have generated a global score to reflect the index child's functioning. One major aim of the URCAFS will be to derive an integrated composite of these global scores as an overall index of the child's functioning across various life domains.

The psychiatric evaluation of the child has generated three separate measures, described by Munson et al. in the preceding chapter. The present chapter reports comparisons of one of those measures – the Child Overall Psychiatric Evaluation (COPE) – with teacher, peer, and parental report measures. We sought to gauge empirically the interrelationships of these four judgments of competence, each of which stands on its own as a unique source of information about the child.

The data are based on the sample of 58 children on whom we have COPE ratings from the time of initial URCAFS evaluation. This sample consists of 14 4-year-olds, 27 7-year-olds, and 17 10-year-olds. It is representative of the URCAFS sample as a whole in demographic and parental diagnostic characteristics.

MEASURES

Clinician ratings (COPE). As described in Chapter 26 of this book, each child was independently rated by two clinicians using a global scale, adapted from Glidewell et al. (1963), ranging from above average adjustment (1) to seriously disturbed (5).

Parental report measures: Rochester Adaptive Behavior Inventory (RABI). The RABI is an assessment of parental perceptions of the child's socioemotional functioning, both inside and outside the home (F. Jones, 1977). It is administered as a structured clinical interview to both parents together, in the form of specific, behaviorally oriented questions. The five parallel forms of the RABI (for ages 2.5, 4, 7, 10, and 13) were designed for use in longitudinal research; each form contains 136–138 items.

RABI-1 scoring (F. Jones 1977) yields an index of overall adjustment on a 1–5 scale following the same continuum as COPE. Ratings were made by the research technicians who administered the interview; therefore, the RABI-1 ratings in part reflect subjective interviewer judgments, which might be gleaned from subtleties of parental behavior in the interview. Scores are available for all 58 children compared in this chapter with the COPE ratings.

RABI-2 scoring (Prentky, 1979) is based on a systematic quantification of each of 70 nonredundant RABI items, rated on continua from pathology to health. RABI-2 scores also differ from RABI-1 scores by excluding items concerned with school and achievement behavior. This was done to eliminate, as much as possible, overlap of parental report and school measures. Ratings consist of an overall rating of adjustment (summation of item scores) and three empirically derived factor scores, as follows:

> *Factor 1:* Expressiveness, Compliance/Cooperativeness, Socialization, (lack of) Antisocial and Immature Behaviors;
> *Factor 2:* Somatization and Fear; and
> *Factor 3:* Motivation and Obsessiveness.

Higher scores on RABI-2 rating and factors reflect better adjustment. Scores are available for the 7- and 10-year-olds ($N = 42$).

School ratings by teachers and peers. The school-based measures are the Rochester Teaching Rating Scale and the Rochester Peer Rating Scale reported earlier in this volume (Fisher et al., Chapter 25).

RESULTS

Professional clinical judgments of overall child competence are highly and significantly correlated with peer, teacher and parent judgments, as shown in Table 1. For the sample as a whole, the strongest relationship is between clinican (COPE) and parent (RABI-1) ratings ($r = .61, p < .001$). The parent ratings (RABI-1 and RABI-2) are, expectedly, highly correlated ($r = .77, p < .001$). However, an interesting difference between the two is reflected in the significant relationship of teacher rating with RABI-1 ($r = .42, p < .05$); it is minimally associated with RABI-2 ($r = .17$). (RABI-2 excludes parental judgments of the child's school behavior.) Neither of the parent measures is significantly correlated with peer ratings.

The correlations of COPE with the other four measures vary with the age of the child. Whereas clinical and parental judgments are robustly correlated at ages 4 and 7, these relationships are lower at age 10 (Tables 2 and 3). On the other hand, the correlation of clinical and teacher ratings is not significant for 7-year-olds (r

Table 1. *Correlations among child competence assessments, ages pooled for 4-, 7-, and 10-year-olds* (N = 58)

| Competence measures | School | | Parents | |
	Mean peer rating (*N* = 38)	Mean teacher rating (*N* = 37)	RABI-1[a] (*N* = 58)	RABI-2 (*N* = 42)
COPE[a]	.44**	.45**	.61***	.52***
Mean peer rating		.57***	.25	.13
Mean teacher rating			.42*	.17
RABI-1[a]				.77***

Note: For 4-year-old group, only COPE and RABI-1 ratings exist. COPE × RABI-1 *r* = .77*** (*N* = 14).
[a]Scale reversed for presentation purposes; low scores reflect pathology and incompetence.
*p < .05.   **p < .01.   ***p < .001; all two-tailed.

Table 2. *Correlations among child competence assessments, 7-year-olds* (N = 27)

| Competence measure | School | | Parents | |
	Mean peer rating	Mean teacher rating	RABI-1[a]	RABI-2
COPE[a]	.40	.26	.69***	.67***
Mean peer rating		.46*	.45*	−.12
Mean teacher rating			.44*	−.10
RABI-1[a]				.79***

[a]Scale reversed for presentation purposes; low scores reflect pathology and incompetence.
*p < .05.   ***p < .001; all two-tailed.

Table 3. *Correlations among child competence assessments, 10-year-olds* (N = 17)

| Competence measure | School | | Parents | |
	Mean peer rating	Mean teacher rating	RABI-1[a]	RABI-2
COPE[a]	.49	.69**	.42	.25
Mean peer rating		.74**	.19	−.16
Mean teacher rating			.37	−.27
RABI-1[a]				.71***

[a]Scale reversed for presentation purposes; low scores reflect pathology and incompetence.
**p < .01.   ***p<.001; all two-tailed.

Table 4. *Correlations of child competence variables with social class*

Competence measure	Social class		
	4-, 7-, and 10-Year-olds ($N = 58$)	7-Year-olds ($N = 27$)	10-Year-olds ($N = 17$)
COPE	.30**	.32*	.31
RABI-1 rating	.17	.33*	.01
RABI-2	.07	−.04	.26
Mean teacher rating	−.25	−.23	−.31
Mean peer rating	−.27	−.18	−.32

*$p < .05.$ **$p < .01.$

$= .26$), but is highly significant for 10-year-olds ($r = .69$, $p < .001$). One can speculate that these differences may arise because the clinician can obtain more information directly from the older children and may rely more on information from the parents in assessing the less verbal younger children.

When the clinician COPE judgments are correlated with the specific factors in the teacher ratings, peer ratings, and the RABI-2, COPE is more highly related to factors with a cognitive component in both school ratings than to other factors. COPE also is more highly correlated with Factor 1 (Expressiveness, Compliance, etc.) in the parental RABI-2 than with the other RABI-2 factors. We have not yet studied the relationships of certain clusters in the Q-sort with specific factors obtained with the other procedures.

Social class effects

Even though the sample selection in URCAFS deliberately limited social class variation, the experience of other risk research programs makes legitimate the question of whether child competence from various domains might be explained by variation in familial social class. In order to rule out a potential social class effect, we examined the zero-order correlations of social class membership (as per the Hollingshead criteria) with the child competence variables from all four sources. As seen in Table 4, moderate relationships of social class with these child variables do indeed exist. Although only the correlation of clinicians's rating (COPE) and social class reaches significance ($r = .30$, $p < .01$), the data from parents, teachers and peers all approach significance with some variation by child age.

More crucially, we have considered whether the relationships among the child variables are simply a function of social class. Hence, we examined the intercorrelations of the child competence ratings with social class controlled, or partialed out. Tables 5 to 7 show that controlling for social class does *not* affect the relationships among child competence ratings. In fact, not only do all significant correla-

Table 5. *Correlations among child competence assessments with social class partialed out; ages pooled; 4-, 7-, and 10-year-olds* (N = 58)

Competence measure	Peer (*M*)	Teacher (*M*)	RABI-1[a]	RABI-2
COPE[a]	.39**	.40**	.60***	.57***
M Peer		.54***	.22	.15
M Teacher			.39**	.19
RABI-1[a]				.79***

[a]Scale reversed for presentation purposes.
**p<.01.   ***p < .001.

Table 6. *Correlations among child competence assessments with social class partialed out; 7-year-olds* (N = 27)

Competence measure	Peer (*M*)	Teacher (*M*)	RABI-1[a]	RABI-2
COPE[a]	.37*	.21	.65***	.69***
M Peer		.44*	.42*	.12
M Teacher			.40*	.09
RABI-1[a]				.82***

[a]Scale reversed for presentation purposes.
*p < .05.   ***p < .001.

Table 7. *Correlations among child competence assessment with social class partialed out; 10-year-olds* (N = 17)

Competence measure	Peer (*M*)	Teacher (*M*)	RABI-1[a]	RABI-2
COPE[a]	.44	.65**	.44*	.36
M Peer		.71**	.20	.27
M Teacher			.38	.38
RABI-1[a]				.74***

[a]Scale reversed for presentation purposes.
*p < .05.   **p < .01.   ***p < .001.

tions remain so at the same level of significance, but most associations are even stronger.

DISCUSSION

Comparisons of the relationships among clinician, parent, teacher, and peer judgments of child competence yield substantial interjudge agreement for this sample of 58 children at risk for psychiatric dysfunction. The nature of these relationships, however, are complex and age dependent.

The intercorrelations among judgments of child functioning from different settings suggest that the child's overall level of adjustment can be reliably assessed across settings. The fact that no pair of judgments shares more than 58% of the variance points to considerable uniqueness in the judgments made in different settings: judgments agree, but only in part. This finding supports the value of obtaining multiple measures of child competence in research, and augurs well for the utility of an eventual composite index of competence to reflect the child's functioning across different domains. The child who does poorly across settings is likely to be at greatest risk; as F. Jones (1974) and others have observed, the presence of marked incompetence in many areas of functioning is highly stable over time and a most ominous sign of vulnerability.

Within this sample, social class does not seem to act as a biasing factor for these data. However, it should be noted that the URCAFS sample was selected to be relatively homogeneous with respect to socioeconomic status, and does not include the lowest social class (Class V). Social class does share a moderate proportion of variance with child competence data from different domains. However, the convergence of data from those domains, as well as the patterning of that convergence, derives from nonoverlapping sources of variance. We can conclude that social class effects do not explain our findings.

28 Response-contingent learning in children at risk

ROBERT H. KLEIN AND LEONARD F. SALZMAN

In addition to the clinical, school, and parental-report approaches to the child's functioning, the Rochester risk-research program has studied the child's efficiency in learning paired associates under conditions of praise and censure.

According to the social censure hypothesis (Rodnick & Garmezy, 1957; Garmezy, 1966), the performance deficit observed among schizophrenics derives from their extreme sensitivity to censorious stimuli. These stimuli presumably mobilize disruptive anxiety, often lead to withdrawal or to irrelevant or inappropriate responses, and generally cause an interference with more adaptive behavior. This hypothesis has provided the impetus for theory about the etiology of schizophrenia and for considerable research into the stimulus factors relevant to performance and deficit in schizophrenia.

Results from this research, however, have been inconsistent and have proven difficult to integrate into a coherent theory (Atkinson & Robinson, 1961; D. Cavanaugh, Cohen, & Lang, 1960; Garmezy, 1952, 1973; Johannsen, 1964; Losen, 1961; and Webb, 1955). In an effort to clarify this literature, Klein and Salzman (1978) recently reported that 10-year-old children of schizophrenic parents performed significantly more poorly than children of nonschizophrenic parents on a nonsense syllable discrimination task administered under conditions of response-contingent social reinforcement. When reinforcement was provided by the children's mothers, schizophrencs' offspring made approximately twice as many errors as did offspring of controls under *both* praise and censure conditions. These results did not confirm the social censure hypothesis. Instead, they were interpreted as suggesting that either form of social reinforcement administered by the mother, or merely the mother's voice itself, had a uniquely disruptive effect on the learning efficiency of schizophrenics' offspring.

The present study extends these preliminary findings by including offspring at two different age levels, adding a normal control group, and distinguishing between the diagnostic groups of nonschizophrenic parents. Specifically, we tested the children of schizophrenics, affective psychotics, neurotic depressives, and normal controls on discrimination-learning tasks in which social reinforcement was provided by the child's mother. We sought to determine to what extent the functioning of schizophrenics' offspring would resemble that of adult schizophrenics performing under conditions of social censure. We hoped to establish whether

371

such schizophrenics' offspring would demonstrate a unique pattern of differential sensitivity to various forms of social reinforcement.

METHOD

Subjects

The subjects for this study were a subsample of the children investigated in the University of Rochester Child and Family Study (URCAFS) and an age-matched normal control group of children recruited from a local public elementary school. These subjects were 52 10-year-old and 31 7-year-old male URCAFS children, plus 16 normal control children. The number of children at each level according to index parent (identified patient) diagnosis or normal control status is summarized in Table 1. Diagnostic classifications were based upon 1977 DSM-III criteria (Spitzer, Endicott, & Robins, 1978). The 1977 version of DSM-III classified schizoaffective disorder as a subtype of schizophrenia. Offspring of parents with borderline, atypical, or questionable schizophrenic symptoms were excluded from this data analysis. Parents with a diagnosis of affective psychosis manifested either unipolar psychotic depression or bipolar depressive psychosis with both manic and depressive features; those parents with nonpsychotic disturbances were characterized by neurosis or personality disorder. Thirteen of the index schizophrenic parents, 20 of the affective psychotic, and 28 of the nonpsychotic index parents were female.

Procedure

The experimental task involved discrimination learning of a list of nonsense syllable pairs matched for association value (Glazer, 1928). Ten pairs of syllables were presented with one member of each pair designated by the investigator as the correct syllable to be learned. The child was not informed in advance as to which syllables were "correct," and his initial responses had to be guesses. Criterion was achieved when subjects selected the correct syllable from each pair on the list two times in succession. Syllable pairs were assembled by inspection so as to minimize any random homophonic similarity between two syllables in the same pair. Three equivalent form lists with 10 pairs of syllables in each list had previously been constructed via preliminary testing.

The apparatus consisted of an electronically operated console on which pairs of stimulus syllables were presented one above the other by a rear screen projector, the syllable position corresponding spatially with two response keys available for subjects. Tape-recorded auditory reinforcement messages were delivered to subjects through high-fidelity earphones. Errors and trials to criterion were recorded by the experimenter.

The task was administered under each of three conditions: baseline information feedback, and the two response-contingent reinforcement conditions: praise and

Table 1. *Mean scores across reinforcement conditions for errors and trials to criterion*

Diagnostic group		N	Neutral		Praise		Censure	
			M	SD	M	SD	M	SD
				Errors				
Age 7	Schizophrenics' offspring	7	25.57	21.65	39.00	26.55	48.57	31.29
	Affective Psychotics' offspring	10	35.80	33.62	35.90	36.55	28.00	27.82
	Nonpsychotics' offspring	14	37.00	29.91	44.71	27.79	49.86	30.98
	Normal Controls' offspring	8	26.13	17.06	24.63	13.31	20.00	9.61
Age 10	Schizophrenics' offspring	12	20.67	14.23	37.33	26.11	37.00	29.85
	Affective Psychotics' offspring	18	16.00	11.85	20.28	18.69	19.33	12.26
	Nonpsychotics' offspring	22	15.86	7.69	22.23	15.57	25.91	14.76
	Normal Controls' offspring	8	19.88	7.00	16.00	6.26	20.38	10.24
				Trials				
Age 7	Schizophrenics' offspring	7	12.00	5.83	14.00	6.19	15.28	4.68
	Affective Psychotics' offspring	10	12.40	6.36	11.10	6.51	10.40	6.52
	Nonpsychotics' offspring	14	12.71	5.82	14.71	5.25	15.86	5.91
	Normal Controls' offspring	8	11.88	5.38	10.13	2.64	11.50	5.07
Age 10	Schizophrenics' offspring	12	10.42	5.47	13.00	6.13	13.17	6.52
	Affective Psychotics' offspring	18	8.53	3.58	9.74	4.87	9.63	4.61
	Nonpsychotics' offspring	22	8.73	3.86	10.32	4.42	11.95	4.54
	Normal Controls' offspring	8	9.75	3.01	7.50	2.39	10.13	3.23

censure. The specific list to be learned in each condition was selected randomly for each subject.

In the baseline neutral information feedback condition, the correct syllable for the preceding pair appeared on the console screen immediately after the subject's response, and subjects simultaneously heard the syllable letters spelled by a female technician with whom the child had worked in earlier experiments. In the response-contingent reinforcement sessions, the correct choice again appeared subsequent to each response. Rather than hearing the syllable spelled aloud by the technician, however, the subjects heard one of a number of tape-recorded messages spoken by their mother. In the praise condition subsequent to a correct response, subjects heard, "Yes, that was right," or "Yes, you got that one right," but heard nothing following an incorrect response. Conversely, under conditions of censure, subjects heard, "No, that was wrong," or "No, you got that one wrong," following an incorrect response, but heard nothing following a correct response.

In order to obtain the actual parental reinforcement messages, mothers recorded a series of such messages, several of which were selected for use in the experiment on the basis of auditory clarity. Two successive experimental sessions were required to complete the three tasks. The neutral condition was presented during Session 1 and the praise and censure conditions were presented in counterbalanced order during Session 2.

RESULTS

Preliminary analyses established that there were no signficant differences in IQ between diagnostic groups. Raw error scores and trials to criterion were transformed to square root of errors and log-trials, respectively, to control for heterogeneity in variances, and these data were analyzed in a 4 (diagnostic group) × 3 (reinforcement condition) ANOVA. Table 1 presents the means and standard deviations of errors and trials to criterion for all subjects.

Analysis of the error scores revealed, as expected, a significant main effect for age $[F(1, 91) = 8.66, p < .005]$ in which older children made fewer errors than younger children. In addition, there was a significant main effect for reinforcement conditions $[F(2, 182) = 6.72, p < .002]$, and a trend toward a significant main effect for diagnosis $[F(23, 91) = 2.30, p < .09]$.

More importantly, a significant interaction was found between diagnosis and type of reinforcement $[F(6, 182) = 3.63, p < .002]$. Therefore, two post hoc sets of comparisons were made using Newman–Keuls tests: (1) between diagnostic groups within each condition; and (2) between conditions within each diagnostic group. The contrasts between groups revealed that there were no significant differences between the four diagnostic groups under the neutral condition. Under censure, however, both the Schizophrenics' and Nonpsychotics' Offspring made significantly more errors than did Affective Psychotics' $(p < .05)$ or Normal Controls' Offspring $(p < .05)$. There were no differences under censure between Schizophrenics' and Nonpsychotic Patients' Offspring, nor between Affective Psychotics' and Normal Controls' Offspring. Similar analyses of performance under the praise condition yielded the same general pattern of differences but the results failed to reach levels of statistical significance.

Comparison between conditions within each diagnostic group indicated that Schizophrenics' Offspring made significantly more errors under praise $(p < .05)$ or under censure $(p < .05)$ compared to the neutral condition. Nonpsychotic Patients' Offspring also performed less effectively under praise $(p < .05)$ and under censure $(p < .05)$ compared to the neutral condition. There were no differences in performance for either group when praise was compared to censure. In contrast, there were no significant differences in performance between any conditions for either the Affective Psychotics' or Normal Controls' Offspring.

DISCUSSION

The results point clearly to the disruptive effects of social reinforcement upon performance in the offspring of schizophrenics (including schizoaffectives) and nonpsychotic psychiatric patients. This is particularly evident in their performance under the censure condition. In contrast, there were no differences between children of parents in the four diagnostic groups when the response to their performance is simply neutral information feedback. The inclusion in this study of normal controls, and the separation of the nonschizophrenic parent controls into Affective Psychotic and Nonpsychotic Parent groups has revealed that the interference with learning from social reinforcement is not limited specifically to the children of schizophrenics; this disruptive effect is also found in the offspring of the nonpsychotic parents who were psychiatric patients. Moreover, the performance of the offspring of the affective psychotic and the normal control parents was similar to one another and differed from both the other two groups.

Two factors might account for the similarity in performance of the children of the schizophrenics and the nonpsychotic patients: (1) chronicity; and (2) comprehensibility of the parents' illness. Specifically, these offspring might be more disrupted by parental messages because they may have been more routinely exposed to consistently anxiety arousing experiences with parents who are chronically disturbed. Parents with chronic disturbances, whether a schizophrenic, neurotic, or personality disorder, are unlikely to have periods of remission marked by an absence of emotional tension and anxiety. Their typical chronic life-long patterns of maladjustment may have an enduring disruptive effect upon their communications and relationships with their children. In contrast, parents with an affective psychosis are likely to manifest an episodic course of illness; when not undergoing a psychotic episode, they may appear relatively free from disturbance. These alternating periods of health and illness may have a less disruptive effect upon the nature of their communications and their relationships with their children.

A second related factor, that of the comprehensibility of the parents' illness may also be relevant here. Namely, it is possible that the children of affective psychotic parents may be able to comprehend the illness as episodic and view disturbed behavior more readily as something that waxes and wanes, independently of whatever they do, and from which recovery with few residual unpleasant effects is likely.

It is important to note that the children were grouped entirely on the basis of a risk factor presumed to induce vulnerability, but without reference to the children's clinical adjustment or competence. No children in the sample were under psychiatric care, and they were well below the age of risk for schizophrenia. Clinical evaluations of the children and of their social and emotional adjustment have been conducted, so that direct measurement of the relationship between important personality characteristics and performance on our task will be possible. The present results, however, may already have pointed to experiences within the family system that may shape the children's vulnerability to disruption during learning.

29 Free Play family interaction and the behavior of the patient in Free Play

CLARA P. BALDWIN, ALFRED L. BALDWIN,
ROBERT E. COLE, AND RONALD F. KOKES

The next three chapters report on the family interaction variables. Family interaction was observed in two settings, a Free Play session and a Consensus Rorschach.

THE FREE PLAY SETTING

The mother, father, and the index child were observed in a free play setting in the laboratory. The playroom contained a variety of toys, adapted to the age of the index child. The toys were selected with the following criteria in mind.

1. They should be interesting to the index child, but complicated and difficult enough that the child might well need parental help and the parent might well be induced to help the child. On the other hand they did not require the child to ask for help. He or she could play with the toys on his own.

For example, a Skaneateles Train Set was included. A 4-year-old can run the engine along on the floor with no trouble. On the other hand if he wants to hook the cars together, he may need some help. The track sections can be connected together but some children have difficulty in connecting them. To construct a track that forms a closed loop requires some planning, and many 4-year-olds need parental help in the design. Some asked for it; more frequently the parent volunteered help or even imposed it on the child. Thus the train stimulated interaction, but allowed the child to play by himself and have fun.

2. The toys should also be interesting enough for the parent to play with them by herself/himself. Thus for the 7- and 10-year-olds there was a Shoot-the-Moon game and a Multi-Rollaway. Both of them are difficult enough to challenge any adult, but 7-year-olds can also succeed and have fun.

3. No strictly adult pasttimes were provided. There was no stack of adult magazines which might provide either parent with an easy refuge from interaction with the rest of the family. To be sure, one parent brought his own magazine and read it throughout the session, but we did not make it easy.

The instructions were as follows:

You can see all the toys in this room. We are interested in how families interact with each other and how children learn about a new playroom. You can each of you do anything you want, but we would like you to play with _____ as you might at home if you had a half hour without any interruptions. As you can see from the microphones we are recording every-

376

thing that goes on because we cannot take notes fast enough to keep up with everything that goes on.

These instructions were planned to permit freedom of choice but to encourage the parents to play with the child. Most of the parents gave the child free choice about what he/she wanted to play with, and played with the child if he/she needed any help. Almost no parents allowed the child to wander aimlessly about the room. On the other hand if the child was absorbed in some play, many parents felt free to play independently of the child.

THE DATA COLLECTION AND DATA REDUCTION

The interaction of the family in the Free Play was recorded on videotape and audiotape to facilitate the preparation of a verbatim transcript of the interaction. The interaction was also described by an observer in an ongoing running narration. This narration was coded by a computer program to be described shortly and the output of the program are the data reported in this study. The videotape and the verbatim transcript are available and have been analyzed in several specific projects, but none of those results will be presented here.

The decision to use the observer's narration as the basic raw data for the study and to develop a computer program for coding it was based upon a number of considerations. The two major alternatives were to code the interactions from a careful inspection of the videotape, or to design a checklist of possible behavioral acts and code the behavior as it occurred in the playroom.

We decided that a careful analysis of the videotape would be too time-consuming and inefficient. We decided against an on-the-spot checklist because it seemed more incomplete than we wanted. To allow time for coding we would have to time-sample the interaction, and the checklist of specific behaviors that is short enough to be feasible was not sufficiently detailed for our purpose.

THE NARRATIONS AND CODING

A verbal narration in ordinary language is a partially coded record of the interaction. When the narrator says, "The mother asks the child to connect the two tracks," he is coding the act as a *behavior request*. What he actually heard might have been: "Would you please put the tracks together?" One of the major rules for narrators is to interpret the verbal and nonverbal action and describe it in a simple affirmative sentence in ordinary language. The narrator's sentence also codes the behavior in other ways. It states that the actor is the mother and the child is the recipient and that the act is verbal since the word ASKS is used.

It is the narrator's responsibility to include affective terms in his narration if they are appropriate. He may use the adverb WARMLY or PLEASANTLY or AFFECTION-ATELY or in some interactions the affect may be conveyed by the content of a verb such as PRAISES, or by nonverbal content such as HUGS or CARESSES.

The narrator is asked to report whether or not there is a response if the preceding act is response-demanding (as with a question). If an act is not response-demanding but a response nevertheless is made, that response is included in the narration.

In summary, the narrator does have certain rules to follow, but he is given great freedom in the particular words he uses and we try to provide him with a vocabulary that is helpful.

The computer program consists of four parts: The first is Lanal II (1971), a programming language for writing coding rules. The second is a dictionary of the words commonly found in narrations. This dictionary was compiled by an actual survey of the narrations of several narrators observing several families. In the dictionary each word is defined by a set of features that are inherent in the meaning of the word. Thus the definition of MOTHER is:

> MOTHER: Animate, Person, Label, Noun.

The definition includes both semantic and syntactic features. The syntactic features are used in the coding program; the semantic features represent the output of the coding. The dictionary definition of each word represents a consensus of two "lexicographers"; disagreements were resolved in a full group meeting.

The third component of the program is a set of rewriting rules. Each sentence of the narration is rewritten to delete uninformative words, to assign features to words that depend upon the context of the word in the sentence, to shift the semantic features of adjectives and adverbs to the noun or verb they modify and to delete the modifier. The output of this program is a rewritten transcript in which each sentence is reduced to a sketetal form with each word marked by a set of features. For example, the following sentence would be rewritten as shown in the illustration.

> Original sentence: The child asks the mother something about the balance beam.
> Rewritten sentence
> C: Animate, Person, Actor, Label, Noun
> Ask: Verbal, Seek, Information Act, Verb, S-Form
> M: Animate, Person, Recipient, Label, Noun
> Something: Uncertainty, Noun
> Balance beam: Inanimate, Label, Noun

The fourth part of the program is a set of counting rules. Each rewritten sentence is processed by each counting rule and if the sentence meets the criteria of the counting rule, it is tallied. The output of each rule in the counting program is a count of the number of sentences in the narration that meet the criteria for that rule. There are 556 such counting rules in the counting program. These frequency counts are the raw data for the analysis of the free play interactions.

What actually happens is that the observer dictates an on-the-spot narration of the interaction. This narration is transcribed in rough draft and returned to the observer for editing. When editing, the observer makes sure that the narration says what he intended and that it is acceptable to the program. This edited narration is then transcribed and entered into the computer program.

Table 1. *Internarrator reliability for selected variables* (N = 51)

Variable	Correlation
Total social acts	
Mother-to-child	.88
Child-to-mother	.75
Father-to-child	.90
Child-to-father	.70
Mother-to-father	.75
Father-to-mother	.77
Initiations	
Mother-to-child	.85
Child-to-mother	.69
Father-to-child	.90
Child-to-father	.71
Mother-to-father	.78
Father-to-mother	.73
Rate	
Mother-to-child	.91
Father-to-child	.92
Proportion	
Mother-to-child	.66
Father-to-child	.61
Family warmth	.68

RELIABILITY OF NARRATIONS

Table 1 shows the interobserver reliability of the major variables reported in this study. These correlations (Pearson r) are between two observers independently narrating the family interaction. Such reliability correlations are expectably affected by the standard deviations of the measures. Thus events that occur rarely, such as expressions of hostility, show lower interobserver correlations. Also indices which are quotients tend to be lower in reliability because of their dependence on the reliability of both the numerator and the denominator.

THE GENERAL PATTERN OF FAMILY INTERACTION

1. Rate of parent–child interaction. One important descriptor of a family's interaction is the amount of interaction. A family with no interaction is obviously not function-

TOTAL NUMBER OF SOCIAL ACTS

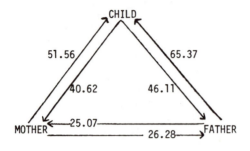

RATE OF INTERACTION: TOTAL NUMBER OF
ACTS BETWEEN MEMBERS OF DYAD

MOTHER AND CHILD	FATHER AND CHILD	MOTHER AND FATHER
92.13	112.24	51.34

PROPORTION OF INITIATIONS

MOTHER TO CHILD	FATHER TO CHILD	MOTHER TO FATHER
.57	.60	.51

FAMILY WARMTH = 56.53

Figure 1. Average values for URCAFS sample for selected variables ($N = 146$).

ing as a family in this setting. There are settings, like doing homework, where lack of interaction is quite appropriate. Hence, one cannot assume that more interaction is better but within a given context the amount of interaction is an important variable.

In these families, the total number of social acts by each family member directed toward each other family member is shown in Figure 1. Most of the social interaction in these families is between parents and children. The amount of interaction between the two parents is about half the amount between either parent and the child. The setting and the interactions encourage the parents to play with the child.

Furthermore, there is a high correlation between the social acts within each

Table 2. *Correlations within dyads for warmth*

	M to C	C to M	F to C	C to F	M to F	F to M
M to C	X	.39	.32	.24	.30	.30
C to M		X	.04	.42	.41	.37
F to C			X	.38	.15	.33
C to F				X	.40	.40
M to F					X	.62
F to M						X

dyad. The number of social acts the mother makes to the child is correlated (r = .78) with the number of social acts the child makes to the mother. And the same is true for the father–child (r = .73) and the father–mother dyads (r = .80). These reciprocal correlations are shown in Table 2 for total social acts. The correlations between dyads are much lower. We have, therefore, summed the social acts within each dyad to obtain a variable called *rate of social interaction*. The rate for the mother and child is the sum of the social acts by the mother to the child and by the child to the mother. Thus we have three rate variables, *mother–child rate, father–child rate* and *mother–father rate*. The rate between the parents will not be discussed here.

The correlation between mother–child rate and father–child rate is −.27. When the total rate for a family is about one social act every 7 seconds, an increase in one dyad's rate tends to be at the expense of another dyad.

2. Proportion of initiations. A second important variable describing the interaction between any two people is the relative dominance of one person in relation to the other. In this Free Play situation we see from Figure 1 that there are more acts by each parent toward the child than by the child toward the parent. We could use this ratio as a measure, but we decided to refine it slightly. If one person initiates all the social acts and the other person never does anything but respond, that is a kind of dominance even if the number of initiations by one and the responses by the other were equal in number.

Therefore we have chosen to measure proportion from initiations only. The mother–child proportion is the number of initiations by the mother to the child divided by the total number of initiations by either member of the pair (i.e., mother–child initiations plus child–mother initiations). We also have a corresponding father–child proportion and a mother–father proportion. The average values of these proportions for the whole sample are shown in Figure 1. The correlation between the mother to child proportion and the father to child proportion is significant (r = +.42). This correlation suggests that the two parents behave consistently toward the child and the child behaves consistently toward the mother and the father.

Table 3. *Age changes in family interaction*

	Age 4 (N = 37)	Age 7 (N = 47)	Age 10 (N = 62)	Significance of age change
Rate of social interaction				
MC	121.00	79.55	84.45	$p < .001$
FC	120.07	123.55	99.00	$p < .05$
Proportion of initiations				
MC	.62	.56	.55	$p < .05$
FC	.65	.60	.57	$p < .01$
Family warmth	49.66	56.87	60.61	n.s.

3. Family warmth. A third important descriptive variable is the expression of affect within the family. Warmth is coded when there is a direct statement of approval or liking by one person for another, and also when the social act is performed in a warm way like physical hugging, playful teasing, telling a joke, or accompanying a request by a warm smile. The narrator is responsible for including warmth in his description of the behavior, usually as the adverb, WARMLY. All such evidences of warmth are coded by the computer program. The reliability of warmth is not so good as the more objective features of the act but still is satisfactory.

When the warmth variable is correlated across the dyads, we find that unlike social acts, there is a moderate correlation between every dyad and every other dyad (generally in the 30s and 40s). See Table 2. Thus we decided to sum the total warmth score for the whole family. By so doing we improved the internarrator reliability and obtained a major variable, *family warmth.*

AGE DIFFERENCES IN FAMILY INTERACTION

The URCAFS sample of index children consists of 4-, 7-, and 10-year-olds. On the basis of our previous studies of mother–child interaction and the evidence from other sources we expected that the rate of interaction would decrease with the age of the child, and that the proportion of initiations made by the parent would approach .50. In other words as the child becomes older the balance of the child's and his/her parent's initiations approaches equality.

Table 3 shows the results. There is a very clear and statistically significant decrease in rate of interactions both for the mother–child and the father–child dyad from age 4 to age 10. Table 4 indicates, however, that the mother declines most from age 4 to 7, whereas the father's decline comes primarily between the ages of 7 and 10.

The proportions of parental initiations for both the mother–child and the father–child dyad also declines with age. The decline is highly significant statistically from the low 60s at age 4, to the middle 50s at age 10. The mother and the father show about the same proportion of interactions. In fact, the father–child

Table 4A. *Patient–spouse difference in interactions with children*

	Patient	Spouse	Difference	Significance
Rate	91.55	113.01	27.46	$p < .0001$
Proportion	.57	.61	.04	$p < .001$

Table 4B. *Rate of interaction*

	Mother	Father	Total
Patient	87.24	103.79	91.55
	($N = 108$)	($N = 38$)	
Spouse	106.75	115.22	113.01
	($N = 38$)	($N = 108$)	
Total	92.32	112.24	102.28

Table 4C. *Proportion of initiations*

	Mother	Father	Total
Patient	.56	.59	.57
	($N = 108$)	($N = 38$)	
Spouse	.60	.61	.61
	($N = 38$)	($N = 108$)	
Total	.57	.60	.59

proportion is correlated .30 with the mother–child proportion, even with age held constant.

All of these trends are quite understandable. The young child is less able to sustain his/her attention on a task and requires more interaction with the parent to maintain play activity; younger children also require more parental suggestions and questions and initiations because they need more help. With increase in age the amount of play interaction declines. Furthermore, the older child initiates more interactions. For example, from age 4 to age 7 the mother declines in initiations from 55 to 35, while the child's initiations to the mother drops only from 31 to 28. Family warmth tends to increase with age but the age change is not significant.

EFFECTS OF PATIENT STATUS ON FAMILY INTERACTION

In each of these families one parent has been hospitalized some time in the past for a psychiatric disorder. In order not to study the immediate effects of parental separation, we established the policy of admitting families to the research study not less than 3 months after discharge from the hospital.

The remainder of this chapter will examine the relation of the following characteristics of the index parent (whom we will call the patient) to his or her role in the family interaction: diagnosis at key admission; mental health at the time the family was observed and the recency of hospitalization.

We have been guided throughout this analysis by the general hypothesis that mental illness reduces the patient's resources for dealing with problems outside of his or her own preoccupations. Thus, we expect that the illness will reduce the patient's investment in family interaction and his/her involvement in it. Furthermore we hypothesize that the sicker the patient, the more this is true; psychotic patients will show this effect more than nonpsychotic patients, and recently discharged patients will exhibit this withdrawal more strongly.

We make this hypothesis, knowing that for some patients it must be wrong. We know that some patients are very active in the Free Play but on the average we expect less interaction, a lower proportion of initiations and less expression of affect. The results generally confirm these expectations.

Patient–spouse and sex differences

If we contrast the patient in each family with the healthy spouse, we find a very clear and statistically significant difference (see Table 4A). The spouse is more socially interactive with the children than the patient, and the spouse has a higher proportion of initiations than does the patient. This clear finding becomes more complex upon closer scrutiny.

First, there is a much bigger difference when the mother is the patient and the father the spouse, than when the father is the patient and the mother the spouse. Table 4B summarizes the findings. Fathers are more active than the mothers, when patient or spouse status is held constant; and the spouses are more active than the patients, whether they are fathers or mothers. Within a family, when the mother is the patient and father the spouse, the sex effect and the patient–spouse effect combine to produce very large differences, whereas in the families where the father is the patient, the two effects cancel each other and result in a very small patient–spouse difference. The same phenomenon shows up in the proportion scores, although all the differences are less striking (see Table 4C).

Effect of diagnosis

Table 5A shows the variations in patient–child interaction associated with the diagnosis of the patient–parent. Table 5B shows the results between the patient and the child. The diagnosis of the patient, the age of the child, and the sex of the parent–patient are the independent variables. The results confirm the findings on age and sex differences, but in addition they show a consistent and significant difference between the diagnoses. The three diagnostic categories are schizophrenia (which excludes the schizoaffective diagnosis); affective psychoses, including schizoaffective diagnoses as well as the usual affective psychoses; and the nonpsychotic disorders. For both mother and father patients, and for each age of

Table 5A. *Rates of interaction*

Parental diagnosis	Father as patient	Mother as patient	Average
Schizophrenia (N = 15)	81.00 (N = 10)	67.20 (N = 5)	75.69
Affective psychosis (N = 60)	99.46 (N = 12)	78.68 (N = 48)	83.18
Nonpsychotic disorder (N = 63)	105.80 (N = 13)	97.04 (N = 50)	98.80
Total (N = 138)	97.30	86.92	89.50

Table 5B. *Analysis of variance*

	df	Sz	Mean Sq	F	p
Age of child	2	19872.9	9936.45	7.57	<.001
Sex of index parent	1	7279.87	7279.87	5.548	<.05
Dx. of index parent	2	9048.92	4524.46	3.448	<.05
Age × Sex	2	13642.8	6821.4	5.199	<.01
Age × Diagnosis	4	2475.87	618.97	.472	<.50
Sex × Diagnosis	2	30.90	15.45	.012	<.50
Sex × Dx. × Age	4	4688.64	1172.16	.89	n.s.
Error	115	150890.98	1312.09		

child, the schizophrenics are least active, the affective psychotics next, and the nonpsychotic patients most active. This difference is significant at the 5% level, and there are no interactions involving diagnosis. There are no significant differences in proportion of interaction or family warmth related to these diagnostic categories.

Global mental health of the patient

We have available the Global Assessment Score (rated by John Romano) for the general adequacy of functioning of the patient at the time of initial URCAFS evaluation. Following our general line of reasoning, we hypothesize that patients with GAS scores less than 60 will have a lower rate of interaction of the patient and the child and a lower proportion of initiations and the family will show lower warmth. The results are shown in Table 6. The differences are all significant in

Table 6. *Relation of mental health and recency of hospitalization on family interaction*

	Patient–child rate	Significance	Patient–child proportion	Significance	Family warmth	Significance
Patient GAS < 60 (N = 36)	75.14		.52		48.27	
		$p < .01$		$p < .01$		$p = .05$
Patient GAS ≥ 60 (N = 110)	96.09		.59		59.37	
Recency ≤ 180 days (N = 26)	77.46		.55		63.47	
		$p < .02$		n.s.		n.s.
Recency > 180 days (N = 120)	93.83		.57		55.15	

the predicted direction, for rate and proportion ($p \leq .01$) and for family warmth ($p = \leq .05$).

Recency of hospitalization

Once discharged from the hospital the patient faces problems in resuming a normal role in the family. The recently hospitalized person may feel inadequate because of his/her mental illness and the family may cast the person in the role of a sick person. All of these considerations lead to the hypothesis that patients less than 6 months after discharge from the hospital will be less active, show lower proportion of initiations and less warmth than patients who have been out of the hospital for a longer period. Recency and GAS scores are independent. There is no tendency for patients recently discharged to have lower GAS scores than those discharged earlier. The results on rate, proportion and warmth are shown in Table 6. Patients recently discharged are significantly lower in rate, but not for proportion or warmth.

SUMMARY

We have discussed the general features of the family interaction in the Free Play situation: the high rate of interaction with the child, and general predominance of parental initiations in the parent–child interaction, the high correlation among all dyads on warmth. This led to the selection of three variables for study, rate of patient-child interaction, proportion of parental initiations to the child, and family warmth.

1. There are major differences in family interaction depending on the age of the child.
2. The patient's rate of interaction with the child and proportion of interaction is lower than the spouse's rate. This holds for the 4- and 10-year-olds separately but not for the 7-year-olds.
3. The rate of patient–child interaction is highest for nonpsychotics, lower for affective psychotics, and least for schizophrenics.
4. Patients with a low Global Assessment Score have lower rates and lower proportions of interaction with their children and less warmth than patients with a higher GAS score.
5. Patients who have been recently hospitalized have a lower rate than those hospitalized longer ago.

30 *A cross-setting assessment of family interaction and the prediction of school competence in children at risk*

ROBERT E. COLE, MANHAL AL-KHAYYAL,
ALFRED L. BALDWIN, CLARA P. BALDWIN,
LAWRENCE FISHER, AND LYMAN C. WYNNE

INTRODUCTION AND DESCRIPTION OF THE PROCEDURES

One aspect of social development that interests us is the development of transactional styles, in particular, whether and when children freely engage their environment, are assertive in seeking help, information, and support, and are generally warm and invite others to respond. There are reports (Hartup, Glazer, & Charlesworth, 1967; Charlesworth & Hartup, 1967) that children who make frequent positive overtures toward others more frequently receive them and are more fully accepted by their peers. White and Watts (1973) emphasize the ability of competent children to gain the attention of others and to use others as resources. In addition, Zigler and Trickett (1978) include in their definition of social competence a host of variables related to friendly assertiveness and outer-directedness. Finally, Cowen et al. (1973) present evidence that peer judgments of antisocial behavior link to later psychiatric disturbance.

Certainly, the development of a friendly, outgoing interpersonal style depends in part on behavior modeled upon and rewarded by a child's family. An examination of the frequency, reciprocity, and warmth of social interaction in families with children at risk should help us understand why some of the children in our study are more competent than others.

We are fortunate in the URCAFS Project to have a number of opportunities to observe our subject families working and playing together. Included among our research procedures are both structured and unstructured tasks that involve various constellations of family members. This report presents some of the data from two of these procedures, the Free Play and the Family Rorschach.

The Free Play is an unstructured task in which a subgroup of the family, the mother, father, and index child are asked to play together for 30 minutes as they might at home. This is the only task assigned. The Free Play situation is described more fully by Baldwin et al. (see Chapter 29, this volume).

The Consensus Rorschach (Loveland, Wynne, & Singer, 1963) is a structured task conducted in two phases, first with the marital pair, then with the whole family. In the first phase, the Spouse Rorschach, the parents, while alone, are given a Rorschach card and are asked to examine the card and reach a consensus about what the card looks like to them. Having completed this task, the parents are then instructed to explain the task to the children and to achieve consensus, as a family, about what a new card looks like. Thus, the Family Rorschach, the second phase, includes clearly structured tasks: (1) parents teach the children; (2) family members solicit responses from one another; (3) family reaches consensus.

The combined data from two such different settings provide a much more complete understanding of interaction in families than do data from only one setting and improve greatly our predictions of how the children in these families will perform in school.

School ratings

The dependent variables in these analyses are the teacher and peer ratings of the competence of index children in school (see Fisher et al., Chapter 25, this volume). For these analyses, we modified the peer scales. The peer data are collected by having each child in the classroom nominate one child for each item, rather than rating all of the children as the teachers do. Occasionally, one of the children in our sample receives an extreme score. For example, if the index child is the *only* child in his classroom who is seen as intrusive he will be nominated by nearly all his peers and his score will be very high (sometimes as high as 10 standard units above the mean). If two or three children are nominated as intrusive, then the resulting scores, although still high, will not be unusually high. Seven percent of the children were rated more than two standard units above or below their classroom median by their peers, compared to only one child (1%) when the children are rated by their teachers. For this reason the peer ratings have been trichotomized at .5 standard units above or below the classroom median. As reported elsewhere (Cole & Al-Khayyal, 1981b), this does not change the overall pattern of results, but should make the results more stable. This is particularly important when we study the data with multivariate analyses.

Free Play results

We have developed a model of appropriate family behavior in the Free Play task that has been presented elsewhere (Baldwin, Baldwin, & Cole, 1982). In brief, after observing a family play together, we ask three questions about each parent–child dyad: (1) Do the parent and child play together or, more specifically, is the total rate of social interaction in the dyad at least moderate? (2) Is there a balance of interaction between parent and child or is the distribution of acts skewed? (3) Do parent and child appear to enjoy playing together and express warmth toward one another? When the answers to all questions are "yes," we view the dyad as active and warm and believe that the family members are rewarding one another for interaction that conveys warmth.

In the absence of a large pool of normative data, we had no a priori standards for acceptable levels of interaction and warmth, or of balance in the number of parent-initiated and child-initiated acts. We had no exact criteria that specified at what point interaction becomes so infrequent or so devoid of warmth that it could be said parent and child do not interact, reward, or support each other. We divided our sample of families into two subsamples so that we could use the data from one, the criterion sample, to establish our criteria, and then use the data from the other, the replication sample, to test the validity of our classification. We examined the criterion subsample scatter plots and compared each of the family interaction variables with the overall teacher and peer ratings.

From these scatter plots, we established what we believe to be minimally acceptable levels of interaction and warmth and acceptable ranges of parent–child balance. Separate criteria were established for mother–child and father–child interaction at each child age. In the criterion sample, we found that children in families who fell below these minima, or outside these ranges, were more likely to fall below their classroom averages on the teacher and peer rating than were children in families within these guidelines. We then used these criteria to classify the families in the replication sample – without recourse to the school data. We could then use the replication sample to test our hypotheses. This procedure is a revision of the procedure originally used to classify these families.

To summarize our results, the number of active, warm parent–child dyads (0, 1, or 2) within a family is related to both the mean teacher rating ($r = .62, p \leq .004$, $N = 23$, criterion sample; $r = .48, p \leq .009$, $N = 33$, replication sample) and the mean peer rating ($r = .46, p \leq .044$, $N = 23$, criterion sample; $r = .51, p \leq .005$, $N = 33$, replication sample) in both samples. These correlations are statistically significant only in the families of 10-year-old children, and only these data are presented. Family activity/warmth is related to social class in the criterion sample ($r = .60$) but not in the replication sample ($r = .20$).

If a family is active and warm, then we can say, from what we have observed in Free Play, that they seem to function well together, they interact frequently and warmly, and they apparently respond to each other's social initiations. Yet we have no evidence that our classification of a family's transactional style is stable and would be the same in other settings. For example, we are as yet unable to predict how the family might appear when given a *task* to do. For this reason, it was essential that we observe these families in a relatively structured setting.

The Family Rorschach

The Family Rorschach is unlike the Free Play in two major ways: (1) there is a specific task to be accomplished to which all in the family must simultaneously direct their attention; and (2) the task includes both parents and all those children living at home, ranging in age from 4 to 19. Controlling for the effect of the presence of varying numbers of children of varying ages on a family's total amount of interaction and the distribution of acts is a challenging but necessary task.

There is clear evidence in group interaction literature (Shaw, 1976) that in large groups (and, we would add, groups with young children) the task leaders exercise greater authority than the leaders of small groups, as measured by the percentage of total speeches the leaders make or by the percentage of time they speak. Because the percentage of speeches made by a parent is an important element in our classification of family interaction, and because it depends upon the number and ages of the children present, we must correct this percentage for these family configuration variables. We describe what we believe to be a productive and successful approach to this problem elsewhere (Cole & Al-Khayyal, 1981a). Because the family now must operate as a unit, it seems appropriate to classify the behavior as a unit, rating the whole family as active and warm or not. Furthermore, with all members of the family present, there is insufficient interaction between the index child and each parent to classify these relationships separately. To receive the designation of active and warm the family must be (1) reasonably active; (2) reasonably warm; and (3) demonstrate reasonable equity in the percentage of speeches made by each person; specifically, the ratio of parent/child speeches, mother/father speeches and the variance in the percent of speeches made by each of the children must all suggest equity in the opportunity to speak. The exact criteria for each of these indices are presented in Cole and Al-Khayyal (1981a).

Family Rorschach results

We again divided our sample of families into two subsamples so that we could use the data from one, the criterion sample, to establish our criteria for active, warm interaction.

Our classification of family interaction in the Family Rorschach task is related to the teacher and peer ratings. As with the Free Play results, these relationships are statistically significant only in the 10-year-old subsample, and only these data are presented. The Family Rorschach classifications are related to the mean teacher ratings in both samples ($r = .60$, $p \leq .009$, $N = 22$, criterion sample; $r = .32$, $p \leq .03$, $N = 33$, replication samples) and to the mean peer ratings in the criterion sample ($r = .60$, $p \leq .009$, $N = 22$, criterion sample; $r = .20$, n.s., $N = 33$, replication sample). In the replication sample, the Family Rorschach classification is related to two of the individual peer scales, bright/compliant student ($r = .31$, $N = 33$, $p \leq .05$) and dull ($r = -.29$, $N = 33$, $p \leq .05$), but not to the overall score. The Family Rorschach classification is not related to social class, although as reported elsewhere (Cole & Al-Khayyal, 1981b), the family interaction–school correlations are much stronger in the lower social classes (III, IV, & V) than in the higher social classes (I & II).

Combining data from the two procedures

The most interesting and powerful analyses compare family behavior in one task with behavior in the other task and then combine this information. If we compare classifications of families across the two tasks, the Free Play and Family Rorschach, we discover that the two sets of classifications are indepentent ($\chi^2 = 1.19$, n.s.). Knowledge of the families' behavior in one task provides little information about their behavior in the other task. Because both family variables relate to the children's school functioning and are themselves unrelated, we expect both to contribute independently to the explained variance of the school ratings.

To test this notion both family variables were included in multiple regression analyses of the two summary school variables. At first, only the data from the replication sample are presented. The two family variables together account for 28.3% of the variance in the teacher ratings ($r = .53$, $F(3, 29) = 3.82$, $p \leq .02$) and 28.1% of the variance in the peer ratings, ($r = .53$, $F(3, 30) = 3.27$, p $\leq$ .03). Both the Free Play variable and the Family Rorschach variable make significant contributions to the variance in the peer rating, but only the Free Play variables makes a significant contribution to the teacher rating. Knowledge of the families' behavior in both settings improves significantly our prediction of the teacher ratings. However, if we wish to assess the potential benefits of a second interaction procedure we must also look at the results from the analyses of the criterion sample. In the sample *both* the procedures make a significant contribution to the variance in *both* school measures, independent of which variable is entered into the equation first. The two variables together account for 69% of the variance in the teacher ratings and 51% of the variance in the trichotomized peer ratings. It is also interesting to examine the relationships between the family variables and the eight individual teacher and peer ratings in the two samples. Both family variables do not contribute to the variance in all eight individual scales. Although no clear patterns emerge in both the criterion and replication samples, the Free Play measure seems to be more strongly related to the cognitive school measures. The Free Play measure and not the Family Rorschach measure contributes to the variance in the teacher rating of cognitive competence and peer rating of dull student, regardless of order of entry into the equation, in at least one sample.

DISCUSSION

Our classification of family behavior does reliably relate to the teacher and peer ratings of the children's school performance and accounts for one-quarter of the variance in these ratings, at least in the sample of 10-year-olds. Our hypothesis that it is a family's transactional style that accounts for the school success or failure of their children requires an analysis of the actual transactions among the members of the family. This analysis is now underway. There is evidence however, presented by Baldwin et al. (see Chapter 29, this volume), that children in active/warm families are themselves interpersonally active and warm. In Free Play the rate of mother–child initiations is highly correlated with the rate of child–mother initiations and the rate of father–child initiations is highly correlated with the rate of child–father initiations. Furthermore, warmth expressed by any family member is correlated with warmth expressed by each other family member. In sum, there is evidence to support our hypothesis that the link between family interaction and the school ratings is indeed the children's transactional style and that children in families in which active and warm interpersonal interaction is common are more likely to engage their environment actively, and to be outgoing and friendly than children from families where such interaction is not common. A knowledge of the modal pattern of interaction within a family will help us identify those children at risk who are likely to develop serious behavioral or emotional disorders because of their inability to engage others successfully.

31 Predicting current school competence of high-risk children with a composite cross-situational measure of parental communication

JAMES E. JONES, LYMAN C. WYNNE,
MANHAL AL-KHAYYAL, JERI A. DOANE,
BARRY RITZLER, MARGARET T. SINGER, AND
LAWRENCE FISHER

In the URCAFS program, communication is one of three domains of parental functioning that we have studied with multiple methods. A matrix of domains and methods is presented schematically in Table 1. Findings with the structural variables of balance and activity, and the affective variables of warmth and relationship statements, have been presented in the preceding chapter. Wynne, Jones, and Al-Khayyal (1981) have made a preliminary report of relationships of parental variables across domains. Here we shall focus on the communicational domain.

Communication Deviance (CD) is a construct referring to a class of verbal transactions that make it difficult for a listener to follow the meaning intended by a speaker or to share a common focus of attention. Such communication creates difficulties for any listener, but it is presumed that particularly ominous difficulties arise for a child who already has cognitive or attention deficits. Communication Deviance includes several varieties of odd language, for example, arbitrary disruptions of the transaction, ambiguous references, and partial disqualifications. Communication Deviance has been shown to be a significant characteristic of the parents of schizophrenic patients and has been identified in a variety of parental speech samples: Individual Rorschach (Wynne, Singer, Bartko, & Toohey, 1977; Singer, 1967; Singer, Wynne, & Toohey, 1978); Object Sorting Test (Wild, Singer, Rosman, Ricci, & Lidz, 1965); Family Rorschach (Doane, 1977); Thematic Apperception Test (F. Jones, 1977); and family therapy tapes (Morris & Wynne, 1965). A number of other studies documenting disturbances in the communication of parents of schizophrenics speak to the issues of CD, for example, Lerner (1965), Behrens, Rosenthal, and Chodoff (1968), and Beavers, Blumberg, Timken, and Weiner (1965). The UCLA Family Project has shown that the presence of CD in the Thematic Apperception Tests (TATs) of parents of disturbed but nonpsychotic adolescent boys is significantly associated with schizophrenic spectrum outcomes 5 years later (Goldstein et al., 1978; Doane, et al., 1981). In the UCLA study, the nonpsychotic disturbance of the adolescents was the initial basis for sample selection, whereas in the URCAFS Project a parent, but not the child, has been diagnosed as having a mental disorder.

This chapter reports a test of the hypothesis that current parental CD is associated with *current* competence or incompetence of the child, as measured at school.

393

Table 1. *Multiple method variables for three domains of parental functioning*

| Methods | Domains of parent functioning | | |
	Communicational/ cognitive/attentional	Structural/ contextual	Affective/relational
Family Free Play	—	Balance and activity	Warmth
Family Rorschach	Parental Communication Deviance Parental Healthy Communication	Balance and activity	Positive and negative relationships statements
Parents' individual Rorschachs	Communication Deviance	—	DeVos affective scales
Parents' individual TATs	Communication Deviance	Kinship content	Affective attributions

Follow-up data will be used to test the hypothesis that current parental communication difficulties predict to future child functioning.

The URCAFS Project has been in the fortunate position of being able to measure parental communication variables with a variety of methods. The first indication of the efficacy of the multiple method measurement of the CD construct came from Doane's dissertation (1977) at Rochester. In a preliminary sample of 62 7- and 10-year-olds, she found that the mother's total CD in the Family Rorschach and in the individual Rorschach makes independent and important contributions to the prediction of the index child's incompetence, as indicated in ratings by peers, teachers, and parents. The father's CD did not contribute, and neither did either parent's CD during the Spouse Rorschach (Doane et al., 1982).

We now have data on additional children and also two more measures of parental communication: parents' Healthy Communication (HC) on the Family Rorschach, and parental CD on the individual Thematic Apperception Test.

METHOD

Sample

For the purposes of this analysis, we are using data from the families of 55 10-year-olds for whom there are both complete school data (see Chapter 25 by Fisher et al., this volume) and complete data on parental communication across measures. As the report by Yu et al. shows (Chapter 27, this volume), there appear to be differences in school measures at the 7- and 10-year-old levels that make pooling of these age groups inadvisable.

Dependent variables

The index child's competence at school was measured through ratings by his peers and teachers (Fisher, 1980). For this analysis, five indices of school functioning were used: (1) cognitive–academic abilities; (2) social–emotional behavior; (3) rule following/norm compliance; (4) mean peer rating; and (5) mean teacher rating.

In addition, an overall school competence score was constructed from these five scores in the following way. The distribution for each of the five scores was trisected into a group with high competence (assigned $+1$), medium competence (0), and low competence (-1). For each child these five resulting scores were summed and 6 was arbitrarily added to yield an overall competence score with a possible range of 1 to 11 (i.e., with no negative scores).

Four measures of parental communication

Communication Deviance in individual Rorschachs. Margaret Singer and Barry Ritzler scored the individual four-card Rorschachs of every URCAFS parent, using Singer's 1973 revision of the 1966 Singer–Wynne CD manual. The mother's total CD has repeatedly predicted the competence of the index child better than the father's total. In the present analysis, the mother's individual Rorschach CD is defined as *high* if her total is greater than one-half standard deviation above the mean, and *low* if lower than one-half standard deviation below the mean.

Communication Deviance in Family Rorschach. Doane (1977) found that the mother's total CD in the Family Rorschach was the best predictor of child competence. In the present analysis, the mother's total CD on the Family Rorschach was considered high if greater than one-half standard deviation above the mean, and low if lower than one-half standard deviation below the mean.

Healthy Communication in Family Rorschach. Al-Khayyal (1980) developed a manual that scores the converse of CD in the Family Rorschach, namely parental *Healthy Communication* (HC) that is clear, easy to follow, and facilitates the children's staying on the task. Al-Khayyal used one split-half to develop a best prediction and then tested its stability in the other half. The best predictions were obtained from a profile of the parent couple's functioning in five areas. The couple's profile is defined as healthy (30% of the sample) if they do a relatively good job in (1) clearly and completely teaching the task to the children; (2) structuring and supporting on-task behavior; (3) presenting percepts clearly; (4) reaching a consensus; and (5) closing the task in a clear, complete manner. Conversely, the opposite prediction is made when the couple shows relatively poor functioning in the five areas (24% of the sample).

Communication Deviance in individual TAT. The parents' individual three-card TATs were scored for total CD by Jones and a research assistant, Kathleen Mullaney, using the manual developed by F. Jones (1977).

A composite measure of parental communication

A combined parental communication measure was produced by tabulating the number of times parents were high on the three CD measures and showed poor functioning on the Al-Khayyal HC measure, and then subtracting the number of times that parents were low on CD measures and had a healthy profile on the HC measure. This produced a variable with 9 points (from +4 to −4). In order to do analysis of variance, this variable, namely, the composite parental measure was trichotomized (+4 to +1; 0; −1 to −4) into low, intermediate, and high levels of deviance.

RESULTS

Table 2 shows that for the 10-year-olds, all associations between the parental composite communication variable and child competence in the school setting were very highly significant. These findings are especially remarkable in light of the fact that the school ratings of the index children by teachers and peers were obtained entirely independently of the family assessments carried out in the hospital research setting with the family. As described by Fisher et al. (Chapter 25, this volume), index and control children in the same classroom were rated comparatively by peers and teachers who did not know of the presence of the index child in the group. Across all the areas of child functioning, cognitive/academic, social/emotional, and rule following/compliance, and for ratings by both teachers and peers, the children of parents with a high level of Communication Deviance were rated consistently as less competent. Furthermore, a consistent linear relationship across the three levels of parental communication was maintained with respect to each child measure. In addition, it can be noted that parental Communication Deviance was not related to social class.

In contrast, the school ratings for the sample of 7-year-old index children showed only nonsignificant trends when correlated with the composite parental communication measure, most positively in the cognitive/academic area ($p = .07$). This negative finding is similar to other results concerning the school ratings of the 7-year-olds. In Chapter 27 (this volume) Yu et al. noted a marked difference between school-related and nonschool-related reports by the parents about the index 7-year-old children. Further analyses, especially with follow-up data, will be required to clarify whether the differences for the 7-year-olds, compared to the 4- and 10-year-old samples, reflect developmental, age-related changes, or one of several other possible explanations.

DISCUSSION

The findings presented here strongly support the hypothesis that deviant parental communication patterns are reflected in incompetent functioning of their 10-year-old sons. We do not yet know at what age this association between a measure of family functioning and an extrafamilial measure of child functioning first can be

Table 2. *Average level of child functioning: 10-year-olds rated by teachers and peers for three levels of parental Communication Deviance*

Composite parental Communication Deviance	N	Child variable					
		Cognitive/ academic	Social/ emotional	Rule following/ compliance	Mean peer	Mean teacher	Overall competence
Low	27	2.96	2.04	2.85	54.9	55.8	6.74
Intermediate	9	2.67	1.44	2.11	52.5	52.3	5.67
High	19	1.21	1.05	1.63	44.7	43.4	3.58
$F(2, 52)$ Linear test		17.79	11.68	9.31	11.75	29.14	23.58
p (One-tailed)		<.0001	<.0006	<.0018	<.0006	<.0001	<.0001

found. Other nonschool measures of the children at different ages also need to be studied in relation to the parental measures.

Methodologically, this chapter presents one way of combining multiple measures of a parental communication construct. We also are using other methods of exploiting the power of cross-situational measurement, such as multiple regression analysis, to identify various combinations of variables and their possible interactions. (See Wynne, Jones, & Al-Khayyal, 1982, for such a report.)

The results from Doane's dissertation (1977) on multiple measures of Communication Deviance provoked a new viewpoint about this construct. Originally, Singer and Wynne hypothesized that CD may be an enduring style likely to be found consistently across situations (Singer & Wynne, 1966). This hypothesis is supported for the parents of children who are doing poorly; those parents tend to have high CD across situations. Conversely, the children who are doing well tend to have parents who are consistently free of CD across procedures. For these two extreme groups, CD does appear to be a consistent cross-situational style. However, for intermediate cases and the sample as a whole, Doane found little correlation between CD measures across situations. This relative independence of the measure across situations suggested the potential value of a composite variable in which different communication measures contribute together to predict criterion variance in the child. Hence, we advise anyone wanting to measure communication variables to do so with multiple, short procedures rather than rely on a single, long procedure, such as using only a 10-card Rorschach or only a set of TAT cards. A strategy of multiple methods capitalized on the enhanced predictive power gained from combining the separate CD measures.

PART VIII

The McMaster–Waterloo High-Risk Project:
1972–1982

In this section, the McMaster–Waterloo High-Risk Project's history, achievements, and future plans are presented by the project team in the first of two chapters. In the second chapter, Joan Asarnow outlines the findings of a series of investigations into the basic determinants of peer-rated social competence in high- and low-risk children. In both these chapters, the authors are careful to nest their risk research in the larger context of the current state of the art of clinical and basic research. Considerable attention is given to the methodological difficulties inherent in attempting to measure reliably basic underlying markers of vulnerability across developmental stages and throughout the premorbid to postmorbid course of a psychological disorder. The reader will discover that the McMaster–Waterloo project's focus on attentional and social competencies is similar to that of the Minnesota project. The similar findings of attentional and social deficits by these two projects in their different risk groups provides some cross validation of their hypotheses. It is important to note that the McMaster–Waterloo Project has made the difficult but necessary step of using peer-rated social competence as indices of intermediate outcome. In this regard, they will be able to contrast their "premorbid outcome" data with the Minnesota, Rochester, and Stony Brook projects.

32 The McMaster–Waterloo High-Risk Project: multifaceted strategy for high-risk research

R. A. STEFFY, R. F. ASARNOW, J. R. ASARNOW,
D. J. MacCRIMMON, AND J. M. CLEGHORN

OVERVIEW

The McMaster–Waterloo High-Risk Study uses a longitudinal, prospective research design. Typical of most of the other projects in the Risk Research Consortium, our work has adopted a parental (mother's) diagnosis of schizophrenia as the risk marker, intends to test samples differing in risk levels on a battery of measures over the years of risk, and is awaiting evidence of differential outcome in our samples. In this chapter, we review briefly the rationale, results, and conclusions drawn from the first phase of our study (reported in detail elsewhere: Asarnow, MacCrimmon, Cleghorn, & Steffy, 1978, 1979; Asarnow, Steffy, Cleghorn, & MacCrimmon, 1977; and MacCrimmon, Cleghorn, Asarnow, & Steffy, 1980). We then describe revisions in the test battery adopted for a follow-up assessment and a network of other research that complements the prospective high-risk study. This latter phase of our work was organized to refine our study of attentional processes and to develop a peer assessment technology to be used with children at risk. The chapter concludes with the discussion of a number of guiding principles that have underwritten our program of research.

INITIAL ASSESSMENT

Rationale for the McMaster–Waterloo High-Risk Project

Distinctive advantages. As new comers to high-risk research, our organizational efforts in 1972 adopted a longitudinal, prospective research design similar to the work of others in the consortium. To make a unique contribution, we added two special features to our research design that seemed likely to provide new insights.

The authors of this work wish to make known their appreciation for financial support of this work provided by the Ontario Mental Health Foundation, including Grants No. 387 to Cleghorn and MacCrimmon, 512-74B to Asarnow and MacCrimmon, 408-72D, 735-77/78, 757-78/80, and 802-80/81 to Steffy. A Social Science and Humanities Leave Fellowship (No. 451-80-1730) and a grant from the Child Abuse Program of the Ontario Ministry of Community and Social Services to Steffy assisted in the preparation of this chapter.

401

First of all, samples of foster children were used in order to investigate children at biological risk who were not under the immediate social influence of mentally disturbed parents. On the average they were tested at the age of 16 and had left their biological parents at 9 years. Although this choice does not provide the elegant environmental control of many adoptee studies, the approach handled some of the unknown variance associated with stress levels and modeling effects that ordinarily might obscure understanding of vulnerability. Our investigation provided a control for "hard knocks" (i.e., the social disadvantages of being moved from one foster family to another) by adding a Low-Genetic-Risk foster group. A randomly selected community control sample was added to provide normative data for our measures and also to assess the effects of being raised in foster homes, per se.

The second special feature of our project was to use a set of measures demanding various types of attentional functioning. In a recent, unpublished review of the literature on high risk for schizophrenia (Steffy, 1980b), we found only 29 out of 220 measures used in 18 projects investigated the types of information processing and perceptual–motor skills that have substantial attentional requirements. In the early 1970s, only the New York Project had a strong emphasis on attentional functioning, using, for example, such measures as the Continuous Performance Test, reaction time, evoked response, and attention span. Our decision to emphasize measurement in this area was based on (1) the central position of attentional dysfunction in many contemporary theories of the schizophrenic disorder (Chapman & McGhie, 1962; Cromwell, 1975; Shakow, 1962; Venables, 1964; Zubin, 1975); (2) the exceptional sensitivity of attentional tasks in discriminating schizophrenics from normals (Holzman, Levy & Proctor, 1976; Rodnick & Shakow, 1940; and Steffy, 1978); (3) the highly reliable relationships between measures of schizophrenic functioning and external criteria (Bellissimo & Steffy, 1972; Cancro, Sutton, Kerr, & Sugerman, 1971; King, 1954; Rosenthal, Lawlor, Zahn, & Shakow, 1960; and Steffy & Galbraith, 1975); and (4) accumulating evidence indicating that attentional dysfunction in children may be a marker of risk for later pathology (Offord & Cross, 1969).

Design limitations. The attempt to fashion a high-risk study with these two features, foster children subjects and a heavy emphasis on attentional functioning, was not done without cost. From an initial pool of nearly 900 potential mothers whose children had been removed to foster homes, the number of mothers with an unambiguous schizophrenic diagnosis (satisfied the criteria of agreement between the two project psychiatrists, Cleghorn and MacCrimmon) was only 28 with a total of 33 eligible, high-risk, foster children. As reported elsewhere (Asarnow et al., 1977), the final number of high-risk foster children actually available for testing was only 9; consequently, our results are likely to suffer from an ascertainment bias. It was also the case that the children in our sample have had life stresses unique to fostered children. Although a Low-Risk Foster Children group gave a control for these factors, nevertheless our results must be interpreted with caution because of possible unknown influences that the combination of schizophrenic heritage and fostering practices may produce in interaction.

Another selection bias in our research resulted from the emphasis on attentional functioning to the neglect of other domains of measurement. Although a narrow focus has benefits of precision and operational clarity of measurement, it is important to note that there is no one acceptable definition of the attention construct; there probably are many different types of attentional functions (e.g., Moray, 1969; Zubin, 1975). Noting that various attentional measures show weak intercorrelations (Kopfstein & Neale, 1972; also Nuechterlein, Chapter 22, this volume), it is necessary to provide a test battery that samples a variety of different information-processing and perceptual–motor challenges in order to feel that this complex construct has been adequately assessed. With this in mind, eight different measures, yielding 25 separate indices and five attentional factors, were chosen to represent this domain.

The results of initial testing

The results from the first phase of this project which have been reported elsewhere (e.g., Asarnow et al., 1977), will be reviewed briefly here.

Attention battery results. Despite the small sample size (9 high-risk, 10 foster control, and 10 community control children) three of the eight measures showed statistically significant differences on those subconditions that placed the greatest demands on information-processing capacity. This sensitivity was found in: (1) complex levels of the Concept-Attainment Test, a concept-formation procedure; (2) the more complex levels of the Span of Apprehension Test which tested selective attention and/or rate of information processing for tachistoscopically presented visual targets amidst visual noise; and (3) the complex condition of the Reitan Spokes Test that requires a visual search for numbers and letters. In particular, measures of the Span and Spokes Test performance were intercorrelated. An examination of the pattern of scores showed a pattern of deficit in some children on both of these particular measures. This led to a cluster analysis to isolate the children whose patterns of performance on factor analytically distilled scores were similar to each other. We found that one cluster was made up mainly of the community control children who gave the best scores overall, another cluster heavily represented the Foster Control group, a third cluster of four subjects was formed by 3 of the 9 high-risk children and one foster-control child. Members of the latter cluster had particularly poor levels of performance on the Spokes and Span Tests and a few other tests with distracting conditions. Considering the demands for selective attention exacted by these tests and the fact that the more complex high-distraction conditions accounted for the cluster differences, the children in this third cluster were considered to suffer a *perceptual overload* problem. In addition, a fourth cluster was composed of one high-risk child who was distinguished by poor scores on virtually all measures and who clinically appeared to be a multiply handicapped individual.

In conclusion, this cross-sectional research was successful in isolating a subset of high-risk children who seemed to show a special attentional problem similar to the sort identified by a number of theorists as a particular problem for schizophrenics. In fact, the Span of Apprehension performances of Cluster 3 and 4 children were identical in pattern and absolute level to samples of acutely ill and of remitted schizophrenics, and significantly different from the other children and from adult normal controls (Asarnow et al., 1979).

Furthermore, this pattern of results is congruent with findings of measured attentional problems reported by other members of the consortium, some of whose reports are summarized in this volume. In particular, the work of Erlenmeyer-Kimling and Cornblatt (1978); Grunebaum, Weiss, Gallant and Cohler (1974); and Nuechterlein (1983) using the Continuous Performance Test (CPT) with various types of distractor or degraded stimulus conditions has shown significant differences among high risk and control children.

Social adjustment differences. As reported by MacCrimmon et al. (1980), four of the five children in the attentional deficit clusters in the initial testing were found to have *t*-scale scores on the Schizophrenia (Sc) scale of the Minnesota Multiphasic Personality Inventory (MMPI) above 70. Furthermore, from evaluations of the separate scores of the Psychiatric Status Scale (PSS; Spitzer et al., 1970), highly significant differences among the three risk groups were observed in the scores on the Student or Trainee Role measure. We observed that the high-risk children had more difficulty in successfully meeting the challenges of school, such as attendance, deadlines, and concentration. They reported greater conflict with others and a general dislike of school. Furthermore, items measuring tendencies toward Social Isolation also yielded significant differences. As one might suspect, the children with the attentional problems and also the higher scores on the Sc and Pt scales (*t*-scores greater than 70) of the MMPI were the ones showing high scores on the student role and social isolation factors of the PSS.

This finding corroborates impressions that children at greater risk for schizophrenia have particular difficulties in their social and school adjustment. Basic to the definition of the process schizophrenic (Becker, 1959; Kantor, Wallner, & Winder, 1953; and Wittman, 1941) or the poor premorbid schizophrenic (Zigler & Phillips, 1960), is an attribute of poor social and heterosexual relationships during the adolescent years. Watt and his colleagues found that the school histories of children to be later diagnosed as schizophrenics contained teacher reports of difficulties in social and school adjustment (Watt et al., 1970).

In view of the power of school and peer adjustment in predicting concurrent and later psychiatric problems, as well as the discriminating power of the school role index from the PSS Interview measures in our Phase I data, the McMaster–Waterloo Project has given special emphasis to the investigation of these social abilities in the follow-up investigations as well as in its network of related research.

THE TEST BATTERY TO BE USED IN THE FOLLOW-UP PHASE

Because the subjects of our study are now between 20 and 21 years of age, the measures chosen for the follow-up investigations can use techniques validated with adult populations. As indicated in Table 1, the tests selected for the battery

Table 1. *Test battery employed for initial assessment and 5-year follow-up for the McMaster–Waterloo High-Risk Project*

	Initial assessment	5-Year follow-up
I. Attentional assessment		
Span of apprehension[a] (complex items)	X	X
Reaction time indices	X	X
Average latency	X	X
Latency variability	X	X
Redundancy–deficit	X	X
Drift		X
Time-linked impairment		
Continuous Performance Test (CPT)	X	X
Standard	X	X
Degraded		X
Spokes Test[a]	X	X
Competing voices	X	X
Digit Symbol Substitution Test	X	X
Stroop	X	X
Trail Making Test		X
II. Cognitive Assessment		
Communication deviance scores (Rorschach)		X
Delta index (Rorschach)		X
Genetic level (Rorschach)		X
Rattan–Chapman Vocabulary Test		X
Bannister–Frisella Grid Test		X
Cohen Referential Communication Test		X
Concept-Attainment Task[a]	X	X
III. Neuropsychological assessment		
WAIS–Short Form		X
Reitan Battery-Selected Tests		X
Tapping Test		X
Tactual Performance Test		X
Speech Perception Test		X
IV. Assessment of psychiatric status		
PSS (trainee and social isolation)	X	X
Gunderson "borderline syndrome"		X
Anhedonia measure		X
MMPI[a] (Sc and Pt Scales)	X	X
Strauss–Carpenter Outcome Scale		X
V. Assessment of environment		
Life experience survey		X
Social support interview		X

[a]Significantly discriminated high-risk children from controls.

will again emphasize heavily the study of attentional functioning and several measures used in the initial battery will be included in the follow-up. The overlap of items provides an opportunity to compare new results with the results obtained on the initial testing 5 years ago.

The addition of new measures reflects a growing sophistication in the assessment of attentional functioning; they also reflect our wish to broaden the range of functions to include particular measures of conceptual and social functioning. The measures of social functioning will be used as predictors for future judgments of outcome and also as intermediate outcome criteria to evaluate the predictive efficiency of our early measures. Some special features of the revised test battery will be described in the following sections.

Measures of attention. The Span of Apprehension and the Spokes Test measures have prominent positions in the Phase II test battery because they were among the most discriminating tools in the first phase. As noted in an earlier section, the Span of Apprehension Test is widely used in the study of high-risk children and in investigations with schizophrenically ill patients at various stages of illness, that is, acute, chronic, and remitted (Asarnow & MacCrimmon, 1978). This task has been extensively studied (Neale, 1971; Neale, McIntyre, Fox, & Cromwell, 1969), and in recent unpublished work has been found to have excellent sensitivity in discriminating between schizophrenics and manic-depressed patients (Asarnow & MacCrimmon, 1980). It is a task ideally suited to the assessment of selective attention and has been accepted in the new battery in almost the identical form that was used with the children 5 years ago.

The reaction time measures also are an important part of the test battery. The measures chosen for the first test of the groups did not have a strong discriminating power, but they did show modestly strong loadings on an Overload factor obtained in the factor analysis. Beyond the results of that study, however, there are compelling reasons for following the lead of Mednick (1966) in including reaction time measures in batteries selected to study children at risk for schizophrenia. Marcus (1972) in the Minnesota project found reaction time (general latency) deviance in high-risk children. Marcus's lead was followed up by Phipps-Yonas (Chapter 20, this volume) who compared reaction time and peer-rated social competence. DeAmicis and Cromwell (1979) found 40% of their non-ill relatives of schizophrenic patients to show redundancy deficit (a derived latency index) on the reaction time procedure.

The Stroop Test (Wagner & Krus, 1960), the Competing Voices Test (Rappaport, 1968), the Digit Symbol Substitution Task from the Wechsler Adult Intelligence Scale (WAIS) and the Continuous Performance Test (Kornetsky & Orzack, 1978) were used in the previous study and showed some small but interesting relationships to the group Overload factor and the performance of children in the overload pattern cluster. These tests also will be included in the follow-up.

Control measures: intellectual and neuropsychological assessments. The initial phase of our study did not devote sufficient attention to the study of general and specific abilities in these children. The new battery will include measures aimed at detecting differential deficits in intellectual and neuromotor functioning, using estimates of verbal and nonverbal intelligence from the WAIS, as well as certain items assessing neuropsychological functioning taken from the Reitan battery (Reitan & Davison, 1974). In light of the discriminating power of the Spokes Test in the earlier testing, and recent reports of soft neurological signs in the high-risk children studied by Fish and Hagin (1973) and Marcus (1974), we also consider these tests to measure important and potentially predictive functions in their own right.

Cognitive abilities: measures of thinking disorder. In light of the earlier discriminating power of the Concept-Attainment Test (a somewhat complex and unwieldy procedure that has been dropped from the revised battery) and because of the obvious importance of thinking disorders to the definition of the schizophrenic disorder, the following well-established procedures will be used to examine cognitive functions. Following the lead of the Rochester URCAFS Project (Chapter 31, this volume), the Rorschach Inkblot Test will be used to obtain samples of problem-solving speech to evaluate communication deviance, genetic level (Steffy & Becker, 1961) and the delta index of thinking disorder (Watkins & Stauffacher, 1952). The Bannister–Fransella Grid Test (Bannister & Fransella, 1967) and the Rattan and Chapman (1973) multiple choice test of vocabulary (providing control for strength of association within the multiple alternatives) permits the study of subtle signs of thinking disorder that might not be apparent from the psychiatric interview or self-report measures.

We also are curious to note how cognitive–perceptual deficits might become manifest in social behavior. Tasks requiring decentration and relatively high-level communicative behavior, such as the Cohen Referential Communication Task (Cohen et al., 1974) might be expected to be particularly sensitive to impaired cognitive–perceptual functioning. It is possible that the communication tasks will provide some hints as to possible links between impaired attention and social dysfunction.

Psychiatric assessment. Because the major criterion for high-risk research is the presence or absence of psychiatric disability during the adult years of the sample, the project psychiatrists will give, as before, the structured Psychiatric Status Schedule, PSS (1970), in order to compare directly the current symptomatic status of the subjects with their previous status. The MMPI also will be readministered and the Chapman Anhedonia Scale (Chapman et al., 1976) will be added to assess personality dispositions.

Measures of social outcome. Using outcome scales developed by Strauss and Carpenter (1972) to measure social and vocational adjustment, and life stress scales (e.g., Sarason, Johnson, & Siegel, 1978), we shall evaluate the quality of life of our subjects. This is because any judgments of functional impairment must first take into account the influence of stressful life events as they are likely to moderate the predictive relationships between measures of vulnerability and outcome.

COLLATERAL RESEARCH

Although currently satisfied with the choice of items for the new battery, there is no doubt that limitations in the choices will become apparent. Probably, 5 years hence we shall be arguing for yet another "definitive" battery. We know well the limitations of all of the measures. Not only are there complexities among the subjects, but the measures are little understood. This insight has prompted our team to chose measures with great caution (e.g., Corning & Steffy, 1979; Steffy, 1977). Elsewhere this concern with respect to measures used in the high-risk work has been discussed in a paper entitled "Tools of the Trade," a review of the measures used in the high-risk universe (Steffy, 1980b). Although the members of the consortium collectively have used a sound sampling of measures in their work, the factorial complexity of measures, and the problems with reliability, validity, and coverage remain perennial obstacles in the way of understanding. To obtain greater interpretive power from the testing results applied to vulnerable populations, both individual differences in the subjects and the measures should be investigated methodically (see also Nuechterlein, Chapter 22, this volume). To accommodate this requirement, the McMaster-Waterloo High-Risk Project has established an interrelated series of cross-sectional and longitudinal studies. We investigate attention/information-processing functions and social competence in a wide range of actively disturbed psychiatric patients, patients in remission, normal adults and children. These studies have focused on attempts to identify markers for schizophrenia and to isolate the process tapped by the markers. Table 2 provides an overview of these studies.

Studies of attentional functioning in adults

It is accepted generally that schizophrenics have a problem processing their perceptions of information (Cromwell, 1975; McGhie, 1969; Nuechterlein, 1977a; Shakow, 1962; Venables, 1964; and Zubin, 1975). Our laboratory research with schizophrenic patients has explored a number of methodological and theoretical issues pertaining to the deficient attentional and perceptual performances in schizophrenics. This work has been reviewed elsewhere (Cromwell, 1975; Steffy, 1978), so it will be appropriate here only to indicate the major investigative themes.

The first concern is with the *specificity of the dysfunction.* There is good evidence for the power of various reaction time paradigms and the Span of Apprehension Test (Asarnow & MacCrimmon, 1980) to discriminate between schizophrenics and nonschizophrenics. These tasks have shown sensitivity to various dimensions of pathology such as chronicity, presence of paranoid symptoms, and the process-reactive dimensions (Steffy, 1980b).

The second concern pertains to the *stages of illness* in individuals who have validly diagnosed schizophrenic disorders. For a measure to be considered a bona fide, robust marker of schizophrenia it ". . . should be sensitive to dysfunction across the course of the disorder; in particular such a measure should be able to detect dysfunction in individuals who are vulnerable to schizophrenia but who are not symptomatic" (Asarnow & MacCrimmon, 1980). As an example, the same

Table 2. *Overview of McMaster-Waterloo High-Risk Project*

To identify markers of schizophrenia	To isolate processes tapped by markers

Studies of children
Attentional assessment of high-risk children (longitudinal)
    R. Asarnow, R. Steffy, D. MacCrimmon, and J. Cleghorn
	Development of attention/information processing in normal children (cross-sectional study)
	    M. List
	
	Social competence risk markers
	    J. Asarnow, L. Butler, E. Wagner, and D. Baar
	
	Neurometric, neuropsychological and attention/information processing assessments of children with behavior problems (cross-sectional)
	    W. Corning, R. Steffy, and D. Crowne

Studies of adults
Follow-up of grown high-risk children
    R. Steffy, R. Asarnow, J. Asarnow, D. MacCrimmon, and J. Cleghorn
 	
Longitudinal study of attention/information-processing in schizophrenics from acute disturbance to the postpsychotic stages
    R. Asarnow, D. MacCrimmon, and R. Steffy
 	
Studies of schizophrenic patients during the postpsychotic stages (cross-sectional)
    R. Asarnow, R. Steffy, and D. MacCrimmon
 	
The prediction of outcome in schizophrenic patients using attention/information-processing tasks
    R. Steffy
	Parametric studies of the span of apprehension in partially recovered schizophrenics
	    R. Asarnow and D. MacCrimmon
	
	Backward enhancement studies
	    R. Asarnow and D. MacCrimmon
	
	Parametric studies of reaction time in process schizophrenics
	    R. Steffy, K. Galbraith, A. Bellissimo, R. Kaplan, and D. MacCrimmon

pattern of Span of Apprehension performance was obtained in children at risk for schizophrenia as in groups of remitted and disturbed schizophrenics. We also have observed that general latency and variance of reaction time performance are more readily bound to stage of illness than are derived measures of redundancy deficit (Steffy & Galbraith, 1980).

In addition to individual difference comparisons, *parametric investigations* of the various signal and response properties of these tasks have been conducted to increase their sensitivity. This aspect of the research sometimes provides theoretical contributions (e.g., Steffy & Galbraith, 1974), and at other times a "fine-tuning" of the measurement properties of the task (Bellissimo & Steffy, 1975). The refinement of these procedures should increase their sensitivity to pathological processes, and their predictive strength. In this manner, their predictive value is extended not only to the measurement of high-risk children, but it is also relevant to estimating outcome of adult individuals already carrying a psychiatric diagnosis. That is to say, these measures may have utility in accounting for long-term outcomes. In recent work, process schizophrenics who scored poorly on an aggregate score of reaction time deficits were observed later to have a deteriorating course of hospitalization (progressively greater lengths of stays) than did individuals with less deficient aggregate scores even though they had been matched for other typical prognostic factors (Steffy, 1980a).

The use of attentional test batteries with children

Two projects are currently underway with children of various ages and measure sets. These projects collectively provide an estimate of attentional functioning from age 7 through adolescence.

(1) In a recently completed study, List (1980) tested normal children of 7, 10, and 13 years of age on the Span of Apprehension, the CPT, and the Trail-Making tests. This research provided developmental data on the response to various signal/noise levels or other types of distractor stimuli in tests of selective attention. The findings gave evidence of shifts with age in attention/information-processing abilities. Although CPT was insensitive to developmental differences, the Span of Apprehension scores indicated a difference between 7 and 10 years. In addition, correlational analysis revealed that the different attention and information-processing tasks shared neither variance among themselves nor with the measures of intelligence and cognitive tempo. However, the pattern of attentional test performances across ages was in accord with the gross body movement and eyes-off-target measures obtained from systematic behavioral observation during testing. List concluded that the relationships between the behavioral and individual test data confirmed the correlational and developmental data indicating that CPT and Span of Apprehension Tests measure different information processing abilities.

A similar insight can be drawn from examining the effects of distraction procedures at different developmental levels. List found that a distraction condition added to the standard CPT task had no effect at any of the three age levels. In contrast, the distraction conditions (noise levels) in the Span of Apprehension Test had a significant effect at all three age levels, and differentially affected the performance of the 7-year-olds.

The List study holds promise of helping us to refine our initial, somewhat vague concept of overload. It provides a bridge between our studies of the attention/information-processing abilities of children at risk for schizophrenia and theory and research concerned with the development of perceptual–cognitive abilities in normal children.

(2) An investigation by William Corning in collaboration with Douglas Crowne and Richard Steffy has begun to study neurophysiological functioning of children between the ages of 7 and 14 with a variety of behavioral problems, such as delinquency, learning disabilities, or classroom behavioral problems. In this study a survey of physiological and psychological functions is being assessed in order to apply *taximetric strategies* (Corning & Steffy, 1979). In this research we use measures of standard intelligence (the WISC-R), items from the Reitan Neuropsychological Battery, measures of attentional functioning, and a neurometric battery of EEG measures (John et al., 1977). The neurometric measures provide a spectral analysis of the EEG functioning assessed separately on the various traditional electrode sites as well as a study of the intercorrelations of activities at homologous and adjacent sites. At present, this work is something of a fishing expedition in which we are looking for clusters within each measure set as well as an agreement across measures in order to find distinctive natural groupings within a heterogeneous group of children with behavioral problems. To date, we have found cluster analyses of EEG data to correspond to intelligence test scores (Corning, Steffy, & Chaprin, 1981). Ultimately, this research gives us an opportunity to learn if there are distinctive patterns in brain activity in children who show attentional deficits on our measures.

Taken collectively, these studies provide a developmental base for measures of attentional functioning, and their specificity for children vulnerable to schizophrenia relative to children with other types of disturbed functioning (learning disabilities, behavioral disorders, and the broad variety of problems associated with socioeconomic status, school failure, etc.).

Studies of interpersonal competence

At the University of Waterloo a number of students have completed thesis research in which the structure, reliability, and validity of peer assessment procedures were investigated. Four separate studies have investigated the Bower Class Play, a task which has been found to be an especially good risk marker (Cowen et al., 1973; Rolf, 1972). Our work with peer assessment techniques has identified children who are marked by negative and positive peer nominations, and then contrasted the patterns of their behavior in various situations. Postive- and negative-scoring children interacting with teachers and peers in the classroom or in other school-related activities (such as recess) have been investigated in studies by Joan Asarnow (1980) and Lynda Butler (1979). Esther Wagner (1978) examined the behavior of positive- and negative-scoring children in both competitive and cooperative dyadic play, and a study of family interaction in children with aggressive behavior disorders has been conducted by Deborah Baar (1979). The studies by Asarnow and Butler also examined cognitive mediational styles (i.e., typical self-statements) and interpersonal problem-solving skills in these children.

Several of the Waterloo studies have employed sequential or time series analyses to examine differences in the patterning and predictability of behavior sequences. Analyses of temporal sequence consistently provided information that was not apparent from analyses of response rates alone. Since an account of these studies is given in the chapter by Joan Asarnow to follow, only general impressions of the results will be given here. Briefly, the negatively evaluated child's school behavior is generally maladaptive. Rather than attending to academic tasks, they tend to spend more time than their positively evaluated peers daydreaming, tuned out, off-task, and involved in negative teacher and peer contacts (Asarnow, 1980; Butler, 1979). They tend to be less dominant, less appropriately assertive, and to engage in more hostile–submissive behavior (J. Asarnow, 1980; E. Wagner, 1978).

The finding of relatively high rates of tuned-out and off-task behavior in negatively peer-evaluated children is intriguing in light of the impaired attentional and social functioning found in some of the high-risk children. (This issue is discussed in depth in this volume by Nuechterlein, Chapters 19 and 22; Phipps-Yonas, Chapter 20; and Driscoll, Chapter 21.) It is also interesting to note from a prevention perspective that Joan Asarnow found the behavioral differences between positively and negatively evaluated boys to be more pronounced in sixth graders than fourth graders, suggesting that maladaptive behavior patterns become more entrenched with increasing age and thereby merit early attention.

CONCLUDING REMARKS

In this chapter we have reviewed the rationale and the results of the first phase of the McMaster–Waterloo High-Risk Project with particular attention to the advantages and design limitations, and also have introduced the test battery to be used in follow-up work.

A variety of different research interests and projects have been spawned by the original McMaster–Waterloo study. The overall program of research may be depicted as a multimeasure, multisubject (age and problem) matrix. In our estimation this network of diverse investigations is a necessary complement to the traditional longitudinal, prospective research design for investigating the life history of the schizophrenic disorder.

A number of principles have guided the direction of our varied research interests. First of all, schizophrenia has been considered to be a set of disorders characterized by primarily episodic manifestations, whereas vulnerability to the disorder is relatively enduring. Deficits in attention/information-processing abilities may be markers of vulnerability to schizophrenia. Our general research strategy (e.g., R. F. Asarnow & MacCrimmon, 1978) evaluates the extent to which a task taps vulnerability to schizophrenia by seeing if it is sensitive to dysfunction in a variety of individuals who are vulnerable to schizophrenia and who may or may not be symptomatic.

Second, developmental influences need to be taken into account in measures of psychological functioning. Could children at risk for schizophrenia show deficits on tasks sensitive to adult schizophrenia for different reasons than adult schizophrenics show deficits? To answer this question the development of attention/information-processing abilities in normal children must be investigated systematically.

A third principle pertains to the importance of research into the psychological processes that underlie our tests. For the most part we have been empirically minded in our selection of measures, choosing tests on the basis of their yield in previous research. Discriminating power in a given psychological test, however, does not automatically confer clear understanding of the underlying processes. Psychological tasks are complex, as has been argued elsewhere (Corning & Steffy, 1979; Steffy, 1977). Therefore, the test battery chosen for assessing the high-risk group must be used in testing other populations with clear criteria-defining attributes (psychosis, EEG anomolies, behavioral disorders, chronological age differences, etc.) in order to sharpen understanding of these measures.

A fourth principle pertains to an exploration of the relationship between attention/information-processing abilities and social competence. In the original study some of the children with the most profound deficits in attention–information were found to be socially isolated and had difficulty functioning in school and in modulating anger. It is likely that communication deviance and transactional style deviance involve difficulties in maintaining a shared focus of attention, excessive distractability, and other perceptual problems. It is likely that successful interpersonal functioning (reflected in demands for communication, task orientation, cooperation, affiliation, etc.) requires intact attentional functioning. If this be the case, one might expect attentional dysfunctions to be primary in accounting for some portion of interpersonal difficulties. Following this reductionist viewpoint further, one also might expect that a neuropsychological and a neurophysiological substrate would be basic to both the attentional and interpersonal functions. The sensitive discrimination of the Spokes Test in the initial phase of the MacMaster–Waterloo Project and the reports of Fish (Fish & Hagin, 1973) and Marcus (1974) that soft neurological signs have been observed in children at risk, indicate the need for an assessment in this area in future work.

These several investigative assumptions have been influential in suggesting new directions, and perhaps explain the diverging quality of our research program. In a recent newsletter of the consortium we linked this diverging strategy to a "middle-aged spread" in thinking; viewed more kindly, this diverging research strategy is an attempt to develop a nomological network of associations among measures and thereby a better insight into the natural history of schizophrenic disorders.

33 The Waterloo studies of interpersonal competence

JOAN ROSENBAUM ASARNOW

As outlined in the preceding chapter, several investigators at the University of Waterloo have been conducting research in the areas of interpersonal competence and social adjustment. The present chapter summarizes findings and highlights major methodological features from four recent studies. Although the four studies had somewhat different concerns, aims, and procedures, several findings were replicated across studies. These findings suggest a picture of the behavioral styles associated with different patterns of social adjustment and/or levels of social competence.

The studies described here employed what are believed to be behavioral markers of psychiatric risk. Three of the studies targeted children on the basis of receiving negative evaluations on the Class Play (Bower, 1969), a peer assessment measure that has demonstrated power in identifying children with overt symptoms as well as children destined for subsequent mental health difficulties (Cowen, et al., 1973; Rolf, 1972). The fourth study defined risk on the basis of residential placement for aggressive behavior problems. All four studies included control groups of comparable but more adequately adjusted children.

This strategy of contrasting high-risk children exhibiting low levels of social competence with more "competent" controls served several functions. It helped identify areas of functioning critical to the attainment of social competence, and provided information necessary for designing intervention programs aimed at enhancing social adjustment. This strategy also yielded normative developmental data, which is relatively scarce for older children. Furthermore, the use of subject selection procedures designed to detect both overt and incipient behavior problems (e.g., the Class Play) provided a means of generating information about the onset and course of children's behavior problems as well as optimal times and foci for intervention.

Preparation of this manuscript was conducted while the author was a NRSA–NIH postdoctoral trainee under the direction of Michael Goldstein and Eliot Rodnick. The author wishes to thank Donald Meichenbaum for his contributions during all phases of the research, and Michael Goldstein and Eliot Rodnick for their assistance with the preparation of this manuscript.

414

RESEARCH ON BEHAVIORAL PATTERNS

As noted previously, three of the Waterloo studies employed negative peer evaluations on the Class Play measure to select high- and low-risk samples from classrooms. This measure asks children to pretend to be directors of a hypothetical class play and to nominate classmates for a series of positive (e.g., "class president") and negative (e.g., "cruel boss") roles. Subjects in the Waterloo studies were selected by means of a negative perception measure derived by dividing the number of nominations for negative roles by the total number of nominations for each person. Children at the extremes of their classroom distributions on this measure were selected for the positive and negative peer perception groups.

Although there were commonalities between studies, there were also procedural differences. Briefly, J. Asarnow (1980) examined the behavior of fourth and sixth grade boys in a variety of school settings using an event based sequential observational procedure. Butler (1979) studied the school behavior of a fifth grade mixed-sex sample using a time sampling procedure. Coding categories employed by Asarnow and Butler were similar to those employed by Gottman, Gonso, and Rasmussen (1975) that focused on the affective tone of peer and teacher interactive behavior (i.e., positive, neutral, or negative) as well as the child's task orientation in the classroom. Asarnow extended the Butler categories to allow recording of assertive and aggressive behavior. Wagner (1978) used an event-based sequential coding procedure to assess the behavior of fourth through sixth grade boys involved in competitive and cooperative games. Wagner's coding categories were based on those used by Carson (1969) in which behavior could be coded for dominance as well as affective tone (i.e., friendly versus hostile).

Both Butler and Asarnow found that negatively evaluated children spent more time engaged in tuned-out or off-task behavior and less time on-task relative to their controls who had been more positively evaluated by peers. This finding is interesting in light of evidence emerging from the McMaster-Waterloo Project (R. Asarnow et al., 1977; Steffy et al., chapter 32, this volume) and other consortium projects (Erlenmeyer-Kimling & Cornblatt, 1978; Nuechterlein, 1983) indicating attentional disturbances in subsets of genetic risk samples. Although the relationship between classroom and laboratory attentional problems as well as between genetic and behavioral risk samples requires clarification, it is noteworthy that attentional and social problems emerge as discriminating variables in studies using such diverse methodologies and subject selection procedures.

Examining teacher and peer interactive behavior, Butler and Asarnow found that children with negative peer ratings initiated and received significantly more negative peer and teacher contacts than positively evaluated children. Wagner's data also indicated more negative and fewer positive peer interactions for these children. Collectively, these data portray the academic task and socially interactive behaviors of these children as being generally negative and maladaptive. Rather than attending to academic tasks, children with negative peer ratings appear to be spending more time than their positively evaluated peers daydreaming, tuned-out, and involved in aversive or avoidant teacher and peer interactions. This pattern of school behavior would be likely to interfere with both optimal academic progress and the enjoyment of school, an expectation that is supported by the higher school dropout rates (Roff et al., 1972; Garmezy & Devine, chapter 18, this volume) and lower high school success (Gronlund & Holmlund, 1958) found in follow-up studies of children with poor peer relations.

Other findings from the Waterloo studies suggest that children with negative peer ratings may have difficulties with assertiveness. J. Asarnow (1980) found that these children received more assertions from classmates than children with positive peer status. Moreover, if one adopts Patterson's (Patterson, Littman, & Bricker, 1967) view of aggression as the negative end of the assertiveness dimension, the finding of high rates of playful aggressive responses in these negatively evaluated children (J. Asarnow, 1980) suggests that they may have difficulty modulating assertive behavior. For example, when they attempt to respond in a strong assertive manner, they may do so in an aggressive and somewhat inappropriate way. Further evidence of problems with assertion is provided by Wagner's findings of more hostile–submissive behavior in boys with negative as opposed to positive peer status.

Results from Baar's (1979) analyses of family interaction patterns in boys placed in residential treatment for aggressive behavior problems suggest that this high-risk population may also have difficulties with assertiveness. Baar found the largest differences in the behaviors of aggressive and nonaggressive boys to occur in the hostile–submissive category, with aggressive boys initiating significantly more hostile–submissive behaviors than nonaggressive controls. Although Baar's subject selection criteria clearly differed from those in the normal classroom peer studies, the finding of a strong correlation between negative peer perception on the Class Play measure and aggression ratings (J. Asarnow, 1980) suggests some behavioral similarities between these samples with low social competence.

Several of the Waterloo studies used lag sequential analyses (Sackett, 1977) to detect patterns and sequences in social interaction. This procedure involves selecting a behavior as a criterion and examining the probability of other behaviors following the criterion at specified *lags*, or steps, in the sequence of behaviors. A sequence is considered *probable* if the conditional probability of the consequent following the antecedent event exceeds the unconditional probability of the consequent. Stated somewhat differently, a sequence is considered probable if knowing that an antecedent occurred at a prior lag adds significantly to the ability to predict the occurrence of a consequent. A z-score statistic can be derived as an index of the extent to which observed frequencies of various consequents following targeted antecedents exceed expected frequencies. Positive z-scores indicate that a consequent is more likely after the antecedent than at other times, while negative z-scores indicate that the probability of a consequent is less likely than would be expected from base rates. It is generally suggested (Gottman, Markman, & Notarius, 1977) that as z-scores approach 1.96 they can be interpreted as reflecting probable sequences. Often observations are pooled across subjects in order to obtain more stable estimates of sequential dependencies. Because this pooling procedure does not control for individual differences in the frequency distributions of observed behaviors, such results require cautious interpretation and replication.

Although it is beyond the scope of this chapter to present a full description of the methodology of sequential analysis (see Bakeman & Dabbs, 1976; or Gottman et al., 1977), some of its uses can be described. First, sequential analyses permit the identification of probable sequences of social interaction. For example, lag-1 sequential analyses of children's reponses to assertive behavior from peers in Asarnow's fourth grade sample revealed that the most predictable response to receiving a neutral or friendly assertion was the initiation of a neutral or friendly assertion respectively. Moreover, z-scores for these antecedent–consequent combinations exceeded the 1.96 level for both the positive and negative peer-perception groups, suggesting that this tendency to respond assertively to the assertive behaviors of a peer constituted a probable sequence of interaction for both groups of fourth graders.

A similar pattern was evident for playful aggressive responses. The probability of the child's initiating a friendly, playful aggressive response after receiving a friendly playful aggressive response from peers was significantly above base rate levels. In addition, children with high peer-rated social competence were more likely than would be expected from base rates to respond to neutral playful aggression with a reciprocal neutral, playful aggressive response.

A second use of sequential analysis is the study of *differential patterning* of responses between target groups. The sequential analyses complemented the previously described response rate data by demonstrating differences (z-scores differed by 1.96 or more) as a function of peer status in the patterning of interactive sequences involving assertive responses. As noted previously, the response rate data suggested that children with negative peer status may have difficulties with assertiveness. Consistent with this notion, the sequential analyses demonstrated that boys with positive peer status were more likely than expected from base rates to respond in a friendly assertive manner after receiving a friendly assertion from classmates than were boys with negative peer status. In contrast, boys with negative peer status were more predictably friendly but unassertive than positive status boys after receiving a friendly assertion. Similarly, after receiving neutral assertions from peers, negative status boys were more likely than expected from base rates to respond in a neutral but unassertive manner, whereas positive status boys tended to respond with neutral or friendly assertions as well as some negative responses. Thus, consistent with the hypothesis of problems with assertiveness in negatively evaluated children, boys with positive peer status were more predictably assertive after receiving assertions from peers than boys with negative peer status.

Results concerning responses to playful aggression also supported the hypothesis of problems with assertiveness in children with negative peer status. Positively evaluated fourth graders, relative to negatively evaluated classmates, were more likely than expected from base rates to respond in a playful aggressive manner to playful aggressive initiations from peers. This finding, combined with the response rate data suggests that in spite of an overall pattern of more playful aggressiveness,

Table 1. *Clusters identified on the basis of commonalities in peer perception*

	Proportion of subjects in each cluster	
Cluster	Grade 4	Grade 6
Aggressive	.24	.09
Disliked	.07	.10
Stars (Liked–Visible)	.18	.13
Average	.40	.56
Aggressive–Disliked	.03	.02
Neglected–Disliked	.04	.05
Aggressive–Disliked–Visible	.03	.02

Source: J. Asarnow (1980).

children with negative peer status are more likely to back down when confronted with playful aggressive responses from peers.

Another issue addressed by Asarnow was that of differentiating various forms of peer adjustment. Although peer problems have demonstrated promise as a non-specific predictor of mental health difficulties, there is little information concerning the specific correlates and diagnostic outcomes of different types of peer problems. As a first step in addressing this issue, Asarnow employed cluster analyses to construct an empirically derived classification system for identifying types of children's interpersonal functioning. Three major dimensions along which peer adjustment problems could be defined were identified: (1) the extent to which a child is liked; (2) the extent to which a child is perceived as aggressive; and (3) the extent to which a child is visible as opposed to neglected or ignored by the peer group. Peer ratings of these dimensions were obtained using likeability, aggression, and visibility scales from the Peer Rating Sociometric (Hymel & Asher, 1977), Peer Nomination Inventory (Wiggins & Winder, 1961), and Class Play (Bower, 1969), respectively, and subjected to hierarchical cluster analysis. Separate analyses were conducted for samples of fourth and sixth grade boys to determine whether cluster structures could be replicated across grades.

The cluster analyses resulted in seven types of children classified on the basis of commonalities in peer perceptions emerging in both the fourth and sixth grade samples. These clusters or types of children were as follows: (1) Aggressive; (2) Disliked; (3) Stars (liked and visible); (4) Average; (5) Aggressive–Disliked; (6) Neglected–Disliked; and (7) Aggressive–Disliked–Visible. Cluster names indicate the variables on which each cluster showed profile elevations. If subjects in a cluster showed elevations of one standard deviation or more on a variable, that variable appears in the cluster name (e.g., children in the Aggressive cluster were over one standard deviation above the mean in perceived aggressiveness but within one standard deviation of the mean on the likeability and visibility variables). Table 1 summarizes the proportions of the fourth and sixth grade samples found in each cluster.

Interestingly, an extreme cluster of Aggressive–Disliked–Visible children emerged in both grades. These children were the most extreme children in their respective samples in the extent to which they were both disliked and visible, as well as being over two standard deviations above the mean in aggression ratings. Due to the optimizing nature of the statistical operations employed in cluster analysis, these findings should be interpreted cautiously until they are cross-validated. Even so, children in this cluster would appear to be particularly interesting from the vantage point of risk research, because these children most closely resemble the subtype of aggressive children with inadequate peer relations that has been described as showing particularly poor concurrent and later adjustment (Morris, Escoll, & Wexler, 1956; Rolf, 1972; and Shea, 1972).

CONCLUSION

What is the potential contribution of studies of interpersonal competence to risk for schizophrenia research? First, the fact that social competence measures have been shown to be predictive of course and outcome for adult schizophrenics (see Garmezy, Masten, Ferrarese, & Nordstrom, 1978; and Goldstein, 1980) suggests the need for continuing research on the developmental aspects of social competence in high- and low-risk children. Basic studies of social competence can provide the necessary data base for the development of intervention programs aimed at enhancing social competence. Such intervention programs may yet prove to be one of the more effective avenues for preventing and/or minimizing the negative outcomes associated with forms of schizophrenia characterized by poor premorbid adjustment patterns.

Second, given the trend to use social competence measures as intermediate outcome criteria in risk research, it may be important to specify the behavioral and cognitive–mediational styles contributing to different levels of social functioning. In addition to the research presented in this chapter, other studies conducted at the University of Waterloo have focused directly on evaluating the relationship between social problem-solving skills and peer adjustment (J. Asarnow, 1980; Butler, 1979).

It should be acknowledged that social competence measures such as peer and teacher ratings may lack the specificity required to identify unique patterns of social dysfunction specific to the schizophrenic process. For instance, fine-grained analyses of behavior patterns may be required to highlight particular attentional or regulatory problems that distinguish the social behavior of preschizophrenics from that of children destined for alternative psychiatric problems. The Waterloo studies of interpersonal competence are offered as a body of research that can assist in interpreting the findings emerging from risk research and suggest additional research questions.

PART IX

High-Risk Studies of Infancy and Early Childhood

Most of the projects presented to this point have sought candidates for high-risk research among school-age populations. The justification for this is both plausible and practical. Considering that the median age for onset of schizophrenia is in the early twenties, the follow-up required for school-age cohorts would range from 5 to 25 years with an average around 12 to 15 years. If the criterion for risk is a schizophrenic parent, then by the time the offspring reach school age the parents will have had ample "life space" to manifest schizophrenic disorder, thus increasing the breadth of the research dragnet.

It is tempting, though less practical, to study children at risk for schizophrenia from preschool age or from birth or even from the time of gestation. The scientific leverage from such research designs is obvious, but the period of longitudinal pursuit must be extended by 5 to 18 years, which means that the investigators must, in effect, grow old following the research subjects. Research designs calling for one or two decades of persistent follow-up to reach payoff are rare enough; those calling for three decades or longer demand nothing less than professional heroism. For this reason the authors of the following six papers deserve special commendation.

Barbara Fish began her study of young infants of schizophrenic mothers in 1952 and has followed their subsequent development steadfastly for 30 years, despite a change of her residence (from New York to California). Joseph Marcus and his colleagues were able to take advantage of an NIMH project organized in Israel to obtain neurological assessments of a sample of infants at risk there. Thomas McNeil originally became interested in this field of research through his dissertation adviser, Sarnoff Mednick, and was able to pursue this interest by resettling in Lund, Sweden, where he has collaborated for more than a decade with Lennart Kaij in studying schizophrenic women during pregnancy and at delivery. The project in Lund has the distinction of following children at risk for schizophrenia from the earliest point in life: before birth. Arnold Sameroff and his colleagues undertook a similar investigation at about the same time in Rochester, New York. Responding largely to the stimulus of some controversial findings reported by the Danish Project, Gunnel Wrede organized a study in Helsinki, Finland, of pregnancy and birth complications for a high-risk sample of Finnish children. Jon Rolf developed a preschool project in Vermont focusing on children with a more general psychiatric risk.

It is natural for high-risk studies of infancy and early childhood to concentrate

421

especially on neurological and other organic processes that may be either tell-tale or functional precursors of schizophrenic and other psychiatric disorders. Much attention has also focused on the psychological experience of mothers during pregnancy and delivery, which presents an approach to the important issue of emotional bonding in the earliest part of life. As readers, we must wait patiently for the full implications of these important investigations. The intermediate reports here cover only the first act of a long and probably complicated drama.

34 Characteristics and sequelae of the neurointegrative disorder in infants at risk for schizophrenia: 1952–1982

BARBARA FISH

BACKGROUND, THEORY, AND RATIONALE

This study was designed to test the hypothesis that specific neurointegrative disorders in infancy predict vulnerability to later schizophrenia and schizophrenia-related psychopathology. The basic hypothesis has been that there is a considerable genetic contribution to schizophrenia, a contribution probably mediated by a neurointegrative deficit; this neurointegrative deficit, interacting with environmental factors, as described by Meehl (1962) and others, leads to schizophrenia in some of the vulnerable individuals (Fish, 1957). Neurointegrative disorder in infancy, severe enough to be measurable on behavioral developmental tests, was hypothesized to be the antecedent primarily of early onset, poor premorbid chronic schizophrenia, of which childhood schizophrenia was considered to be the most severe variant (Fish, 1977).

We drew the parameters to be measured (physical growth, physiological symptoms, state behavior, and neurological maturation), as well as the criteria used to define severe neurointegrative disorder, from Bender's histories of irregular development in the infancy of several childhood schizophrenics (Bender, 1947; Bender & Freedman, 1952). Gesell testing was chosen as the best available measure of both normal and "uneven" neurological maturation. Thus, what was later abbreviated as Pandysmaturation (PDM) (less accurately called pandevelopmental retardation in some earlier papers) was diagnosed on the basis of (1) an abnormal profile of function on a single examination, analogous to the intratest scatter on psychometric testing of adult schizophrenics; (2) an abnormal longitudinal pattern, with retardation and loss of function succeeded by acceleration, analogous to the cognitive regression and return of function seen in the onset and recovery of acute adult schizophrenics; and (3) dysmaturation that involved central nervous system

This research was supported, in part, by Public Health Service Research Grant MH-31653 from the National Institute of Mental Health, and by grants from the Harriett Ames Charitable Trust, New York: the William T. Grant Foundation, New York; the Scottish Rite Schizophrenia Research Program, N.M.J., U.S.A.; and the Stephen R. Levy Research Fund.

423

(CNS) organization at all levels, from physical growth and control of homeostasis to higher cognitive functioning, as opposed to more focal organic disorders of single systems.

It was hypothesized that such PDM serves as an early marker in infancy for the inherited neurointegrative defect in schizophrenia and that the severity of PDM would predict the vulnerability to later schizophrenia. Whether a particular vulnerable child would become psychotic, or compensate as a schizotypal personality disorder, was thought to depend upon an interaction between the severity of PDM and the individual's experiences (Fish, 1959). A genetically determined biological vulnerability can be exaggerated by a destructive or impoverished environment and can be compensated for by a constructive one.

In 1952, we began to study vulnerability to later schizophrenia in infants born to disadvantaged mothers. Fourteen infants of 14 such mothers were studied, and 2 of these mothers were later chronically hospitalized and diagnosed as schizophrenic (Fish, Shapiro, Halpern, & Wile, 1966). This study was intended to be a pilot study to test the feasibility of the method. However, the critique of a 1958 proposal to study 100 infants born to schizophrenic mothers and 100 normal controls, beginning at birth, stated that "no one believed the 1957 report," detailing how "Peter's" vulnerability to schizophrenia was predicted at 1 month. The study section further advised omitting the schizophrenic offspring. Instead, we continued, without funding, to study 10 more infants born in 1959–1960 to hospitalized schizophrenic mothers. These 12 offspring of schizophrenic mothers, the high-risk subjects, and 12 offspring of nonpsychotic mothers (controls) have been followed from that time to the present day.

The predictions of vulnerability consisted of ranking the infants according to the severity of PDM between birth and 2 years. The diagnosis of PDM required a lag in physical growth as well as a lag in gross motor and/or visual–motor development. Based on the analogy with neurologic disorders that result in mental retardation, neurointegrative disorder was considered to be more profound if it affected more "primitive" CNS functions, such as physical growth and gross motor development. Similarly, earlier and more profound retardation and actual loss of a previously acquired function were considered to be signs of greater severity.

The entire course of psychobiological development after 2 years was considered to be the test of these predictions. It was predicted that:

1. The infants with PDM would develop schizophrenia or borderline schizophrenia later.
2. The later severity of this mental disorder would be related to the severity of PDM in infancy.
3. Severity of the later schizophrenic disorder would be reflected in more poor premorbid *process* features, including earlier onset, greater cognitive and social impairment, and a flattening of affect (not florid, acute schizophrenic symptoms).
4. The more severe the PDM, the less likely that individuals could compensate in positive environments (Fish, 1960).

However, in a small intensive clinical study, such as this, we can only hope to gain some clues as to the effects of different types of rearing experiences on infants with different developmental profiles.

METHOD

Sample

The selection of the 24 subjects is described above. They now range from 23 to 30 years of age. Their demographic characteristics are given in Table 1. Six of the high-risk infants grew up in carefully selected, stable, adoptive homes, three were reared by grandmothers, and three had intermittent and chaotic rearing by their psychotic mothers, broken by periods spent in institutions or multiple foster homes. Ten of the schizophrenic mothers have been hospitalized from 2 to 27 years (median, 5 years); five were rehospitalized for additional periods of unknown duration.

Measures and procedures in infancy

The analysis of infant development was based on Gesell (1947) tests and physical measurements, repeated at key ages 10 times between birth and 2 years. Subjects were examined at birth, 3 days, monthly for 4 months, and then at 6, 9, 13, 18, and 24 months. Separate developmental quotients (DQs) were obtained for gross motor, visual–motor, and language development. Visual–motor items were analyzed for specific integrative functions (Fish & Hagin, 1973). The analysis of the serial DQs in different functions is comparable to following serial changes in IQs in older individuals. Height, weight, head circumference and overall body growth (*Auxodrome*) were plotted on the Wetzel (1946) grid.

In the 1959–1960 cohort, in order to measure the apathy observed in the 1952 preschizophrenic infant, behavioral state was recorded through 4 months of age for 2 hours, during the presentation of a standard series of stimuli and the Gesell examination (Fish & Alpert, 1962, 1963). Caloric vestibular responses were also tested in this cohort (Fish & Dixon, 1978) at Colbert's suggestion, after he found they were decreased in schizophrenic children. The maximal stimulus of 1 minute of cold air at 10°C was used, which is equivalent to instilling 30 ml of ice water for 1 minute (McNally & Stuart, 1953). The duration of nystagmus or tonic deviation after the end of the stimulus was measured in seconds and analyzed according to the initial state of arousal and the infant's age.

Measures and procedures on follow-up examinations

Follow-up examinations were conducted at 10 years, 15 to 16 years, and 20 to 22 years. The blind, independent psychological and psychiatric assessments when the children were 10 years old included a DSM-II diagnosis, psychiatric symptom ratings, global severity ratings, and ranking of psychopathology; the Wechsler

Table 1. *Demographic characteristics of 12 offspring of schizophrenic mothers and 12 controls*

	Offspring of schizophrenic mothers	Controls
Birth cohorts		
Born 1952–1953	2	12
Born 1959–1960	10	0
Boys	7	3
Ethnic background		
White	5	7
Puerto Rican	3	4
Black	4	1
Biological mother's SES		
III	3	3
IV	2	4
V	7	5
Rearing family's SES		
II	2	0
III	3	6
IV	6	6
V	1	0
Composition of rearing family		
Stable two-parent home	6	7
One-parent or intermittent father	6	5
Emotional climate of rearing family		
Positive: warm, supportive, encouraging	8	7
Overprotective and/or demanding	0	2
Stable, but open derogation of child after 6 years	1	3
Chaotic, rejecting, abusive (Schizophrenic mother and social agency)	3	0
Obstetrical complications (severe or moderate)		
(Schizophrenic = 1, PDM unknown; controls = 4, with no PDM)	1	4

Intelligence Scale for Children (WISC), the Rorschach, Thematic Apperception Test (TAT), Human Figure Drawings, Bender–Gestalt, and a perceptual–motor battery.

In 1974 to 1976, when the youngest cohort was 15 to 16 years old and the oldest was 22 years old, this battery was expanded to include the SADS and a Borderline

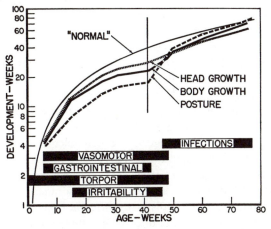

Figure 1. Relationship between mean postural–motor development, physical growth, and clinical disturbances of preschizophrenic infant (Peter). Body Growth indicates auxodrome on Wetzel (1946) grid. Development-weeks indicates age at which postural–motor performance occurs in normal standardization sample: "normal" curve produced when development-weeks equals chronological age in weeks, from Fish (1959).

Schedule, Goldstein's Word Association Test (WAT), and the MMPI. Interviews and psychological testing were audiotaped from 1974 on, for subsequent verbatim analysis and evaluation. This expanded battery has now been administered to the 10 youngest subjects at 20 years. (The expanded battery was developed in consultation with Michael J. Goldstein, Margaret T. Singer, and James E. Jones.)

RESULTS

Characteristics of Pandysmaturation (PDM) in infancy

Analysis of the development curves revealed a major disorganization of neurological maturation in eight infants. This involved postural–motor, visual–motor, and physical development as early as the first month of life. There was no fixed neurological defect, but rather a disorder of the timing and integration of neurological maturation.

Several features distinguish this from the usual forms of retardation and precocity. First, there was an unusual fluctuation in the rate of development, with marked retardation being succeeded by marked acceleration. This was most severe in Peter (Fig. 1) (Fish, 1977). His postural–motor development dropped to 45% of normal at 9 months of age and then, without any change in his external circumstances, it suddenly accelerated to 250% of normal in the next 2 months, and reached normal levels by 13 months (Fish, 1959). Other features differed from the usual patterns in chronic organic brain syndromes. Sometimes there was a temporary loss of a previously acquired ability. At times, they showed a reversed cephalocaudal gradient of postural development, with head control lagging months behind the control of trunk and legs. At times, a "higher" function, such as visual–motor ability, remained relatively intact at a time when postural–motor ability was severely retarded. This is the reverse of the pattern in diffuse, chronic brain damage (Paine & Oppe, 1966). In infants with brain damage, higher cognitive functions are usually affected first, whereas postural development and physical growth become retarded only when the damage is more severe.

During the periods of PDM there was also marked intratest scatter within the gross motor items and within the visual–motor items; that is, the infant would fail items normally passed at a very much younger age and simultaneously pass items at, or months above his/her chronological age. The erratic functioning of these infants is analogous to the disturbance of older schizophrenic patients, who fail easy items on an intelligence test and then succeed on more advanced items during the same session. This erratic pattern was distinctly different from simple acceleration, seen in three control infants, and the brief, simple motor lags seen in three control infants who had moderate to severe pregnancy and birth complications (Fish et al., 1965).

In adult schizophrenics it is difficult to determine which aspects of their peculiar test performance might be disturbances in attention or cognitive function that are specific to schizophrenia, and which might be nonspecific results of anxiety or disturbed motivation (Shakow, 1963). However, when one sees this disorganized pattern in the first month of life, it is clear that such temporary states of poorly integrated CNS functioning can occur in high-risk infants, long before complex motivational and defensive behaviors have developed.

By definition, this Pandysmaturation involved physical growth as well as gross motor or visual–motor development or both. It was sometimes associated with apathy and physiological disturbances (Fig. 1). Bender's histories of preschizophrenic infants had led us to expect some disturbance of growth, but we had not expected that the physical growth curve would parallel the psychomotor developmental curves as closely as they did.

PDM related to genetic risk, not obstetrical complications

There was a higher incidence of PDM in the offspring of schizophrenic mothers (χ^2, $p < .05$) (see Table 2), but PDM was not related to obstetrical complications, nor to sex, ethnic background or the socioeconomic status (SES) of biological or rearing parents. Three-fourths of both our schizophrenic and control mothers were from SES classes IV and V. In this small sample the high-risk infants actually were exposed to fewer severe to moderate pregnancy and birth complications than the controls (see Table 1). Complete antepartum records for the first trimester were not available for several mothers in both groups. None of the children with PDM had had any pregnancy or birth complications. Only one of the children with pregnancy or birth complications showed a mild regression of development and a peculiar pattern of scatter (at 4 months), but none had PDM, with an overall

Table 2. *Relation between maternal schizophrenia, incidence of pandysmaturation, and disorders at 10 years*

Mother's diagnosis	Number with PDM (0–2 years)	Number and severity of psychiatric disorder at 10 years (blind evaluation)	Number with reading disability at 10 years (blind evaluation)
Schizophrenia	7 PDM	4 Severe (2 schiz.)	3
		3 Moderate	2
	4 None	2 Moderate	1
		2 Mild or none	1
	1 ? PDM	1 Severe	1
No psychosis	1 PDM	1 Severe	1
	9 None	2 Moderate	0
		7 Mild or none	1
	2 ? PDM	2 Mild or none	0

Note: PDM = pandysmaturation; ? PDM = unknown. For the offspring of the 12 schizophrenic mothers the frequencies of 7 with PDM, 10 with severe or moderate disorder at 10 years, and 8 with reading disability at 10 years were all significant by χ^2 test. Among the 8 children with PDM the frequencies of 8 with severe or moderate disorder at 10 years and 6 with reading disability at 10 years were also significant and nearly significant, respectively.

retardation of physical growth and postural or visual–motor development. Obstetrical complications in the controls were followed (in three) by brief lags in early head control, of a mild degree, that then returned to normal. Therefore, in individual infants, as well as in the group data in this study, PDM was significantly related to a genetic history of schizophrenia, but not to pregnancy and birth complicatons.

PDM related to psychiatric morbidity at 10 years

PDM also was related to the independent blind evaluations of severe to moderate psychopathology at 10 years. PDM had been most severe in the two children diagnosed as schizophrenic at 10 years, and was most extreme in Peter (Fish, 1977). His onset was earlier and his subsequent cognitive and perceptual disturbances were more severe than Linda's. Children in whom PDM was milder and shorter were ranked just below the schizophrenic children in the severity of their psychiatric disturbance at 10 years (Table 2). Children who had no associated retardation of physical growth had still milder psychiatric disorders at 10 years. The offspring of schizophrenic mothers therefore had a higher incidence both of PDM and of the subsequent severe to moderate psychopathology at 10 years (Table 2).

Abnormally quiet state

In addition to PDM, three other abnormal patterns in the first months raise neurophysiological questions. The first was an *abnormally quiet* state found in four offspring of schizophrenic mothers. As measured in the 1959 cohort, these infants differed from the others between birth and 4 weeks of age in their ability to maintain an unbroken state of quiet visual alertness for 15 to 80 minutes, without a pacifier, as early as 18 hours of age (Fish, 1963; Fish and Alpert, 1962). In contrast, the normally active infants spontaneously cried when awake and could remain alert only for 2 to 5 minutes without a pacifier while under 2 months of age. The abnormally quiet infants did not cry in the first month, even with vigorous postural manipulation, unlike the others, although their responses to visual, auditory, and tactile stimuli were normal or increased. Their spontaneous activity was decreased in amount, speed, and vigor.

These features had been observed clinically in the first preschizophrenic infant, Peter, in 1952. In the 1959–1960 study these differences in spontaneous activity and in responses to stimuli were measured under standard conditions. These quiet infants also had extreme underactivity, flaccidity, and overextensibility of the joints. Their muscle tone was as doughy as that of infants with Down's syndrome. This hypotonia was apparently of central origin, as their deep tendon reflexes were two+ to three+, loose, and pendular.

The quiet infants also differed following caloric stimulation in the first month. Their mean nystagmus when awake was only .5 seconds, compared to 37.2 seconds for the active infants. Decreased nystagmus is a very sensitive indicator of slight decreases in arousal (Collins, 1963; Pendleton & Paine, 1961). But in these abnormally quiet infants, the decrease in nystagmus, spontaneous motor activity, and the response to manipulation all occurred in the presence of normal or increased visual fixation and following. The abnormally quiet state was characteristic of these infants between examinations, as well. It appeared therefore to be a sustained, but relatively focal depression of CNS functioning in the first month, limited to gross motor, proprioceptive, and vestibular systems.

In three of the four quiet infants, this abnormally quiet behavior was a precursor of severe psychopathology at 10 years. But Linda, who became grossly psychotic by 6 years of age, had appeared normally active in her first month. She and two other high-risk infants (one "slightly quiet," one "sleepy and irritable") were apathetic only *after* the first month, and two of these showed severe psychopathology later.

Decreased vestibular responses

Absent or decreased (1- to 10-second nystagmus) vestibular responses did *not* predict later psychopathology. However, they were associated with the periods of PDM between birth and 2 years of age, with the abnormally quiet state in the first month, and with the failures of bimanual skills in the fourth and seventh months (Fish & Dixon, 1978). The transitory nature of the absent responses rules out the possibility of an organic lesion of the vestibular system. Instead, it appeared to be a sensitive indicator of periods when several different CNS functions manifested integrative disorder. This suggests that transitory states of decreased CNS activity, which depressed gross motor, proprioceptive, and vestibular functions, but not vision, accompanied periods when CNS integration was disrupted.

On most of these occasions there were no overt behavioral changes to suggest the presence of a decreased arousal, which might have explained the failures in performance and the decreased nystagmus. The infants usually appeared visually intent and focused in their attention to the performance materials. The hypoactivity of the abnormally quiet babies in the first 4 weeks, which was accompanied by decreased nystagmus, has been discussed earlier. There were also four occasions when waking infants who had decreased nystagmus showed some degree of behavioral apathy. Although they were visually alert on these four occasions, three infants did not cry during the 60 seconds of cold air (10°C) stimulation that usually produced crying. They also showed complete absence of nystagmus on these occasions. This exceptional underresponsiveness occurred only in the three infants of the 1959–1960 cohort who were seriously disturbed at 10 years. Furthermore, these four instances occurred at the age when PDM was most severe in these infants. The absence of the usual irritability with caloric stimulation suggests some covert state of decreased arousal. However, the association of this state with the periods of the worst PDM, when physical growth was maximally retarded, testifies to a cumulative phenomenon that had begun one or more months before. This means that the poor central nervous system integration at these times was not a momentary phenomenon, but part of a continuing, profound process.

Visual–motor disorders in infancy: failures of integrated bimanual skills

Visual–motor performance showed several severe disturbances that will not be reviewed in detail here (Fish, 1957, 1960, 1971a, 1976a; Fish & Hagin, 1973). These included delays in visual fixation on objects held in the infant's own hand, in contrast to normal attention to surrounding objects, severe delays in reaching and manipulation in the first year; apraxia and retarded form perception in the second year.

Only one item, failure of hand-to-hand integration, was correlated with the presence of later severe to moderate psychiatric impairment ($p = .022$, Fisher's test) (Dixon & Massey, 1969). This integrated functioning of one hand with the other at the midline normally begins with mutual fingering of one hand by the other at 16 weeks, followed by the transferring of objects from one hand to the other at 28 weeks, and finally at 40 weeks to the simultaneous grasp of one object in each hand and approximating them. In the 1959 cohort, failure in these specific bimanual skills occurred in all eight of the children rated as having severe to moderate psychiatric impairment at 10 years, but they were not failed by either of the two children rated as having mild to no impairment.

There was also a significant relationship between the times when midline bimanual skills were failed and when vestibular response was reduced on one or both sides. This relationship was significant at 16 weeks ($p = .008$, Fisher's test). It declined at 28 weeks ($p = .071$) and appeared at random at 40 weeks. The preschizophrenic infant, Linda, had the most severe retardation in these hand-to-hand items and in the associated vestibular hyporeactivity. Although finger dexterity developed normally, her hands did not engage at the midline like a normal 16-week infant, even when she was 28 weeks old, and she did not transfer objects like a 28-week-old, even when she was 58 weeks of age.

Soft neurologic signs at 10 years

Another sequel of early developmental disorder, in addition to severe psychopathology, was the occurrence of specific reading disabilities with perceptual disorders at 10 years of age. These were usually associated with failure on the block-design subtest of the WISC and failures on the perceptual battery, including high Koppitz scores and distortions on the Bender–Gestalt Test, poor fine coordination, and defective finger schema. These perceptual defects also occurred significantly more often in the offspring of the schizophrenic mothers (see Table 2), similar to the findings of Marcus (1974) and Erlenmeyer-Kimling's much larger studies.

Our infant data indicate that antecedents can be found before 2 years of age for some of the perceptual symptoms seen at 7 to 10 years. Failure on the block-design subtest of the WISC at 10 years correlated significantly with failure on the formboard at 1.5 to 2 years of age. The occurrence of reading disability and perceptual disorders at 10 years showed a trend toward a relationship with PDM in infancy which was not quite significant at the .05 level ($\chi^2 = 3.54$) (see Table 2; six of the eight infants with PDM showed such disorders at 10 years). However, the four instances of severe perceptual disorders, which were reflected in WISC Performance IQs below 80 at 10 years, all occurred in high-risk infants with PDM.

High Koppitz "developmental scores" on the Bender–Gestalt result from several different types of visual–motor disorders (Fish & Ritvo, 1979). Lauretta Bender evaluated the 10 year Bender-Gestalts of our subjects, without any other information available. Of the eight high-risk subjects with reading disabilities, she considered five to show signs typical of schizophrenia, one resembled an organic brain disorder, and two were indistinguishable from the Bender-Gestalts of ordinary dyslexic children.

Incidence of psychiatric disorders at 20 to 22 years

Blind, independent diagnoses of the subjects will be obtained later in the course of this project. At this stage we have only Fish's nonblind diagnoses and Gottesman's blind evaluations of the 1974–1976 MMPIs. As one might expect, the clinical diagnoses are more conservative than psychometric evaluations made in the absence of any case history information. The clinical diagnoses must be considered highly tentative because of the age of the subjects, the incompleteness of the adult data at this stage of the project, and the fact that the diagnoses were made by Fish, nonblind.

Fish has tentatively diagnosed six of the high-risk subjects as having severe schizophrenia-spectrum disorders. Edwin was hospitalized at 19 years for paranoid and homicidal preoccupations associated with visual hallucinations, as well as suicidal ideation (Fish, 1982). The hospital staff independently diagnosed him as "schizophrenia, schizoaffective, depressed type." His psychosis met the DSM-III criteria for schizophrenia; he had met the criteria for schizotypal personality disorder since he was 15 years of age. The other five disturbed high-risk subjects currently meet DSM-III criteria for schizotypal or schizoid personality disorder, including the two independently diagnosed as schizophrenic at 10 years. Gottesman evaluated the MMPIs of these six subjects as schizophrenia or borderline schizophrenia (four), borderline schizophrenia or schizoid (one), and possible cyclothymic personality disorder in the schizoaffective spectrum (one).

These six subjects have been treated for 4 to 14 years (mean, 8.5 years) by others, independent of the research; two are still in treatment. Three have had 5 months to 3 years of hospitalization, followed by continuing (one, currently), or extended (6 to 7 years) residential treatment (two). One of the latter two is the only one of the six ill subjects who was self-supporting at 20, and she worked as a dishwasher. All six of these schizophrenic, schizoid or schizotypal subjects had PDM in infancy and severe to moderate psychiatric disorders at 10 years (including the two diagnosed as schizophrenic). *If* they were confirmed subsequently, these six diagnoses of schizophrenia, schizoid or schizotypal personality disorder would be related significantly to PDM, to high-risk status and to the blind evaluations of severe psychiatric disorders at 10 years.

If confirmed, this high incidence (50%) of severe spectrum disorders would require some explanation. First, these were very chronic schizophrenic mothers, resembling Mednick's population and very different from the New York and Rochester samples. Furthermore, the father of one ill subject was hospitalized and possibly schizophrenic. Eliminating this individual would yield an incidence of 45% (5 of 11 high-risk subjects). This resembles the incidence of spectrum disorders in Mednick's 1976 data reported to this conference (42% to 48%, according to diagnostic criteria used).

Five of the controls had diagnosable mental disorders at 22 years (according to Fish, nonblind). Three had depressive disorders (two chronic, one episodic) and two had personality disorders (one antisocial, one borderline i.e., unstable type). Gottesman's blind evaluations of their MMPIs agreed with Fish's nonblind diagnoses in four of these five subjects; one hysteroid young woman appeared psychotic on her MMPI. Five of the six controls whom Fish diagnosed as having no mental disorder also appeared normal on their MMPIs. Only one control has not yet achieved an independent vocational adjustment; he also was the only control infant who had PDM and severe psychopathology at 10 years.

DISCUSSION

Neurointegrative defect in infants at risk for schizophrenia: a dysregulation of maturation at all levels

Gross motor delay was one aspect of the PDM observed in about half of our high-risk infants. This recalls the large-scale controlled studies of preschizophrenic children by O'Neal and Robins (1958), Watt (1974), and Ricks and Berry (1970). In these studies, difficulty in walking, or severe organic handicaps, including neurologic disorders or slow motor development, significantly differentiated pre-schizophrenics from their controls. In retrospective studies of disturbed children and adults, only the most severe motor retardation is recalled, and therefore these histories obtained in childhood cluster in the most chronically ill adult schizophrenic patients.

Delays in the development of infants genetically at risk for schizophrenia have now been reported by other investigators. In their second H-R study, S. Mednick et al. (1971) found that retarded motor development at 5 days and at 1 year differentiated the infant offspring of schizophrenic fathers and mothers from controls, and we related this to our data (Fish, 1971b). In their reports for this conference, Marcus and Sameroff documented the significantly poorer sensorimotor development which both investigators found in their schizophrenic offspring in the first year (at 4 and 8 months or 4 and 12 months of age). As in our study, these delays were not associated with pregnancy or birth complications.

Our study, which used more frequent measurements in the first 2 years, revealed a disorganization which is far more complex than simple sensorimotor retardation or acceleration. Our infants with PDM had periods when several different CNS functions manifested a profound integrative disorder. The biological disorder during these periods disrupted the normal timing, sequences, and spatial organization of development. It was a disorder of the overall regulation and patterning of the orderly progress of maturation, not a disorder of isolated traits or functions. The normal temporal pattern was changed in a disorderly fashion so that the rate alternated between being excessively slow and excessively fast; it even went into reverse, with a loss of previously acquired abilities. The spatial patterning was disrupted, as seen in the temporary reversal of the cephalocaudal gradient and the failures of midline integration of the hands. The peculiar scatter in functioning resulted in a profile of successes and failures on any single examination, unlike what is seen in chronic brain syndromes. This pattern also differed from the simple retardation or acceleration of gross-motor or visual–motor DQs seen in several control infants.

Lastly, this integrative disorder affected many systems under control of the CNS, including physical growth, gross-motor, visual–motor, vestibular functioning, and possibly arousal. The biological disorder in preschizophrenic and vulnerable infants appears to be a disorder of the total organism. Repeated failure of performance on developmental tests might conceivably be due to decreased atten-

Table 3. *Neurointegrative defect in infancy: signs of dysregulation of maturation in many systems*

Periods of decreased CNS integration
Retarded development followed by acceleration
Regression of development; loss of function
Reversed cephalocaudal gradient
Failure of integration of midline bimanual skills
Profile of failures unlike chronic brain syndromes
Continuous visual alertness (15–80 min, vs. 2–5 min) with minimal vestibular and
    motor responses (abnormal "quiet" state, 0 to 1 month)

Involvement of many systems
Retarded physical growth with most severe, overall retardation (pandysmaturation)
    (PDM)
Decreased muscle tone, activity, crying ("quiet" state)
Decreased response to proprioceptive stimuli ("quiet" state)
Retarded postural–motor development followed by acceleration
Decreased caloric nystagmus (.5 sec vs. 37.2 sec) (decreased "arousal"?) with "quiet"
    state, failed midline bimanual skills (4 and 7 months) and PDM (0 to 24 months)
Disorders of visual–motor development
Fluctuating cognitive development

Severity of neurointegrative defect related to outcome
Pandysmaturation (0 to 24 months) related to schizophrenia and severe to moderate
    personality disorders (10 yr) ($p < .01$); PDM related to WISC Performance IQ below
    80 (10 yr) ($p < .025$)
Failed midline bimanual skills (4, 7, or 10 months) related to severe to moderate
    psychopathology (10 yr) ($p = .022$)
Visual–motor retardation (form board, 18 to 24 months) related to visual–spatial deficit
    (block design, 10 yr) ($p < .05$).

tion and initiative, but the associated lag in physical growth was obviously cumulative over weeks to months (see Table 3).

We have hypothesized that these periods of severe dysmaturation reflected the fluctuating level of integrative disorder in the central nervous system, which was considered to be the essence of the schizophrenic disorder in infancy and possibly later also (Fish, 1975). The periods of most severe developmental regression and disorganization in infancy would then be analogous to the acute exacerbations of psychosis in adult schizophrenics, both being signs of increased "activity" of the schizophrenic process. The periods of accelerated development and return to normal levels in the infants would represent remission of the schizophrenic activity. In the 1959 study, the periods of severe developmental regression, presumably the periods of increased schizophrenic activity, were accompanied by repeated decreases in nystagmus and by severe apathy and underresponsiveness in the three infants who had severe psychopathology at 10 years. This suggests that there may have been a covert depression of arousal that accompanied the periods of most profound integrative disorder. The association of disorders of arousal, physical growth, tonus, motility, and vasovegetative functions suggested a dysregulation involving hypothalamic, neuroendocrine, and reticular activating systems during the infancy of preschizophrenics (Fish, 1960).

It is important to emphasize the transitory nature of these developmental disorders, since the larger high-risk studies have had to rely on less frequent infant tests. Furthermore, the other high-risk infant studies have used the Bayley, which omits early stages of motor control, and is therefore less sensitive than the Gesell to neurointegrative disorder. (When we rescored our data using the Bayley, only the two individuals with the most retarded *visual*–motor development were identified.)

It seems necessary to reiterate that we never consider simple variability in infant development to be a pathological phenomenon. In 1957 we differentiated the pandisorganization of development in the vulnerable infants from the three non-vulnerable infants who showed simple retardation or acceleration of gross-motor or visual–motor DQs on one or more examinations. In these latter infants, the variability in DQ was limited to a single function; it did not result in an unusual profile of functioning, and deceleration was not accompanied by a lag in physical growth. In 1957 these relatively benign instances of variability in development were contrasted with the pandysmaturation of the two "most vulnerable infants," Peter and one control. Only in these two were "the lags and accelerations in other areas accompanied by parallel lags and accelerations in body and cranial growth." This pandysmaturation was subsequently found in six additional high-risk infants in the 1959 cohort.

So far, no other high-risk infant study has yet analyzed the profiles of functioning during developmental delays, nor has anyone looked for an associated lag in physical growth to identify the pandysmaturation that we found. It was only this more severe, *pan*developmental disorder, which was related to psychiatric morbidity at 10 years (and possibly to schizophrenia spectrum disorder at 20 or 22 years) in our sample.

E. James Anthony asked why I thought other infant researchers "have not seized upon the organizing potential of the PDM concept." It is gratifying that now, in retrospect, the accumulating longitudinal data on our 24 children seems more convincing to others. But in 1965, when Mednick and Schulzinger's first report sparked the current series of high-risk studies, the 10 year follow-up of only our first cohort had been published; that of our second cohort appeared in 1973, followed by analyses of both cohorts in 1975. Although neurointegrative disorder in schizophrenia was central to the organizing hypotheses of Erlenmeyer-Kimmling, Nuechterlein, and Asarnow et al., the suggestion in our early papers that PDM might be an analog in the neurological maturation of preschizophrenic *infants* probably seemed farfetched to a generation unfamiliar or unimpressed with Lauretta Bender's neurological conceptualizations of childhood schizophrenia. In any case, the next generation of high-risk infant studies was inspired less by theories of PDM and infant neurointegrative disorder than by Mednick's postulate that pregnancy and birth complications were antecedents of schizophrenia. In part, this may explain why other infant studies ignored physical growth and used the Bayley (because psychologists prefer its standardization), instead of the Gesell, which is preferable for evaluating neurological maturation. It did not help matters that our scoring system was not readily available and that we advocated 10 tests in the first 2 years, an expensive design for a large sample. But these problems could have been resolved if PDM had been considered important enough, for example, to include in the 1967 Dorado Beach discussion of high-risk research. Why it was not, I leave to more objective observers.

Impact of environment on PDM

We assumed in 1952 that even if PDM should prove to reflect a genetic vulnerability to schizophrenia, it could be exaggerated by a destructive or impoverished environment and could be compensated for by a constructive environment. In a small sample such as ours, suggestions that this occurred are anecdotal rather than conclusive. It was our clinical impression that some of the earlier and milder developmental symptoms could be modified by early intervention. A few brief examples have been reported in earlier papers. It appeared that the impact of different patterns of nurturing was different in vulnerable infants with different degrees of vulnerability, and with different profiles of other developmental assets and liabilities. A depressed or withdrawn mother may have a more devastating effect on an apathetic infant than on an oversensitive, irritable one. An agitated, tense, or chaotic mother may be more disorganizing for the latter type of infant.

If we knew more about the mechanisms whereby the early motor, perceptual, and cognitive handicaps were produced, one could study the effects of specific early interventions on specific developmental impairments, as White and Held (1967) have done in institutionalized infants. Our data suggest that modern techniques for measuring arousal, focused attention, early pattern recognition, bilateral eye–hand control, interhemispheric integration and neuroendocrine regulation of growth might elucidate some aspects of the clinical disorders we observed.

If early interventions could be developed that could prevent, arrest or compensate for the perceptual and cognitive impairments that our high-risk infants often showed before 2 years of age, I believe that one might interrupt the sequence of cumulative academic and vocational failure that makes for a more chronically disabled schizotypal child and adult.

CURRENT STATUS OF THE RESEARCH

In 1979–1980 the same standardized interview and battery of psychological tests was given to our youngest subjects, at age 20, which had already been administered to the oldest cohort at age 22. We are continuing to follow our subjects by telephone and personal interviews. The increasing psychopathology and maladaptation, especially in the 23-year-olds, has necessitated doing this more frequently.

We are currently putting together the mass of information collected over the past 23 to 30 years into full life-history narratives, and coverting handwritten notes and audiotaped interviews into a usable data form. We believe that our essential contribution will be to provide an in-depth study of the life histories, from birth to young adulthood, of these 24 subjects who have a high incidence of psychopathology.

Subsequently, we will obtain independent diagnostic evaluations of these 24 individuals by five experts, Irving Gottesman, David Rosenthal, Ming Tsuang, Lyman Wynne, and Gabrielle Carlson, who will be blind to risk status, Fish's predictions, and previous diagnoses by the research team. As an additional approach to rating the severity of schizotypal symptoms in relatively well-compensated subjects who are diagnosed clinically as schizoid or paranoid personality disorders, we will obtain expert, blind, independent assessments of deviant thinking and communication on psychological test responses. Hollis Johnston will rate the WISC/WAIS and Rorschach responses using the Thought Disorder Index, a revision of the Delta Index which she developed in collaboration with Philip Holzman. Margaret Singer and Jeri Doane will rate Communication Deviance on the Rorschach and Proverbs Tests and Jeri Doane will rate Communication Deviance on the TAT.

Elsewhere we have reviewed in detail the changing manifestations of neurointegrative disorder with maturation, from retardation of gross-motor, visual–motor, and speech development in infancy to subtle defects on tests of motor integration, the Bender–Gestalt, the block design subtests of the WISC/WAIS, and subtler evidence of thought disorder in borderline schizophrenic patients and in many relatives of schizophrenics. Now that our subjects are young adults, we can test the initial hypothesis that in infancy "these early neurological disturbances may merely be more primitive manifestations of the same underlying disorder of integration that is manifested in adult schizophrenics by the disorganization of complex psychological functions" (Fish, 1960). We selected the measures of schizophrenic thought disorder and communication deviance developed by our collaborators, in order to study integrative disorder of higher cognitive functions, and to determine whether neurointegrative defect in individuals at risk for schizophrenia does indeed show a continuity from birth to adulthood in affected individuals.

Only very global analyses of the infant data have been possible up to now, for example, mean gross-motor and visual–motor developmental quotients (DQs), the range of basal-to-ceiling performance, and descriptions of irregular profiles (passing advanced items and failing earlier ones). The initial ranking of the PDM was based on such gross measures, weighted in importance according to somewhat arbitrary rules.

We therefore plan to do more detailed quantitative analyses of the infant data to provide leads for designing a proper, and hopefully more economical, replication. When other investigators have asked for an explanation of our scoring system we only had a makeshift handout, supplemented by extensive correspondence and discussions. We plan to spell out these "rules" in proper sequence and in sufficient detail, testing the program on our own data, so that the scoring could be done readily in larger populations. Other investigators have also asked which ages seem most critical, and which exams could be dropped with the least loss of information. We have additional questions, such as which aspects of neurointegrative disorder are most critical and which are the simplest ways of measuring them; and could more frequent physical measurements substitute for some of the repeated developmental tests. We hope to derive some tentative leads regarding these questions from our own data, which would permit one to pose more precise questions and design more definitive studies of vulnerable infants in the future.

In a new study we would still use PDM as a gross marker for the inherited neurointegrative defect in schizotypal infants. But we would like to see more recent and sophisticated measures added to a new study, particularly to assess arousal, affective responses and early bonding, focused attention, early pattern recognition and cognitive functioning, bilateral hand control, interhemispheric integration, and the neuroendocrine regulation of growth. The abnormalities seen in our subjects suggest the need for more study of these parameters from birth to 2 years. Electroencephalographic measures of arousal would be more specific for this function than a repetition of the vestibular testing. The examination of behavioral state probably could be abbreviated. It is most critical between 1 and 4 weeks, when one can identify the abnormally quiet state.

We believe that PDM may identify not only the most vulnerable infants, but also the periods of "schizophrenic activity." It could therefore be useful in interpreting data from more high-powered measures, if studied simultaneously in the same subjects. A series of 2-year studies could identify the most promising measures to evaluate specific preventive interventions for the handicaps we observed before 2 years, and also to follow their evolution into their sequelae at 7+ years.

35 Infants at risk for schizophrenia: the Jerusalem Infant Development Study

J. MARCUS, J. AUERBACH, L. WILKINSON, AND
C. M. BURACK

During the last decade, substantial data have accumulated to support the existence of a congenital neurointegrative deficit that characterizes the prepsychotic state of schizophrenics. Evidence of neurological, neurophysiological, perceptual, and attentional deficits in these patients can be found in the work of numerous investigators (Asarnow et al., 1977; Fish & Hagin, 1973; Fish, 1977; Gamer, Gallant, Grunebaum & Cohler, 1977; Grunebaum, Weiss, Gallant et al., 1974; Hanson et al., 1976; Holzman et al., 1976; Heston & Denny, 1968; Quitkin, Rifkin & Klein, 1976; Mednick et al., 1971; Rieder et al., 1977; Erlenmeyer-Kimling, 1975). J. Marcus (1970, 1974) in a collaborative study with Rosenthal (1971, 1972) and others (to be designated for the purpose of this report as the Israeli School-Age Study) found similar deficits in a subgroup of children born to schizophrenic parents. These children performed poorly in areas of fine motor development, motor and visual–motor coordination, and auditory integration. This subgroup comprised roughly half of the offspring ($N = 50$ offspring of schizophrenics). Five

This chapter is a modified version of an article with the same title published in *Archives of General Psychiatry*, *38*, 703–13, 1981.

The project was supported by grants from the U.S.–Israel Binational Science Foundation (Grant 598); the Chief Scientist's Office of the Israel Ministry of Health; The Olivetti Foundation; the Center for the Study of Human Sciences of the Hebrew University; the Department of Psychiatry, University of Chicago; Forest Hospital Foundation; and Mrs. Harry Jacobs. In addition, this work was supported in part by National Institute of Mental Health Psychiatry Education Branch, Grant MN06300–22, and by National Institute of Drug Abuse, Grant PHS 5 R18 DA–01884.

Amalia Mark and Vera Peles of the social work staff of the Jerusalem Mental Health Center recruited and interviewed the parents, and Sheila Maeir examined many of the infants. Louis Guttman and Ruth Guttman, Israel Institute of Applied Social Research and the Hebrew University, gave theoretical guidance and consultation. The staff of the Maternal and Child Care Centers of the Municipality of Jerusalem cooperated throughout this project. Milton Rosenbaum, Director of the Jerusalem Mental Health Center, helped launch this study. Jean Endicott and her staff at Biometrics Research, Inc. performed the computer analysis of the protocols of the Current and Past Psychopathology Scales. Arnold Sameroff, Illinois Institute of Developmental Disabilities, contributed to all phases of the project. The following persons provided help in data analysis and technical assistance: Alisa Maeir, Werner Wothke, Sandra Gruba-McCallister, Rita Jeremy, Sydney Hans, and Tamera Bultemeier.

440

of the children in this subgroup have subsequently shown early signs of psychotic breakdown; four of them have been hospitalized. These findings suggested the possibility that poor functioning in motor and perceptual areas might be an indicator of the hypothesized neurointegrative deficit and that this deficit might represent a genetically determined vulnerability to schizophrenia, as proposed by Rosenthal in his version of a diathesis–stress model (1963).

To test the viability of a genetic model for the transmission of schizophrenia, several preliminary questions had to be addressed. Could these neurointegrative deficits be identified in infancy? Are they specific to schizophrenia? Are they due to genetic causes, perinatal insults, or a combination of these factors? Could these findings be replicated in similar subgroups chosen from different populations? Would such a replication add support to a genetic model for the transmission of schizophrenia?

Our attempt to investigate such issues led to the establishment of the Jerusalem Infant Development Study in 1973. Here we report our initial findings from that study. We have tried to address three other questions that derive from them. (1) When attempting to assess and compare the development of infants, how should one deal with the variability inherent in early development? (2) How does the heterogeneous nature of schizophrenia affect the interpretation of findings from risk research in this area? (3) What methodological approach is most appropriate for analyzing these issues?

METHOD

Subject sample

From 1973 to 1976 we recruited pregnant women attending Maternal and Child Care (MCC) Centers of the Municipality of Jerusalem whose husbands or who themselves had had a history of schizophrenia. Seventy percent of the pregnant women in Jerusalem use these centers, and we screened a majority of them. Other women were recruited to form comparison groups. These women or their husbands had a history of affective disorders, personality disorders, neuroses, or had no history of mental illness. Most of the women were referred to the project by neighborhood MCC Centers. Six subjects diagnosed as schizophrenic were referred by local psychiatric services. Consent was obtained from each couple after the project had been explained both orally and in writing.

Over a 4-year period from January 1973 until April 1977, a total of 54 couples and their infants participated in the study. The following four diagnostic categories were formed (with each couple counting as 1 case): schizophrenic (17 cases), affective disorders (6 cases), personality disorders and neuroses (13 cases), and no mental illness (18 cases). Of the 17 cases diagnosed as schizophrenic, 9 were considered chronic, 2 acute, 1 schizoaffective, and 5 questionable. One of the 9 cases of chronic schizophrenia consisted of a mother and a father who were both chronic schizophrenics, so there were 10 chronic schizophrenics who participated in our study. The chronic schizophrenics could not be classified as "back ward" patients. They were married and lived with their families most of the time. Two of the chronic schizophrenics were hospitalized during part of their pregnancies. The mother of subject 6 was hospitalized from the beginning of her pregnancy through the fifth month and again after she gave birth. The mother of subject 4 was hospitalized for 3 weeks at the beginning of her pregnancy. All mothers were receiving prenatal care in MCC Centers. Table 1 gives diagnostic information and ages of parents in the schizophrenic group. Subject numbers were assigned to the infants rather than to their families; because some families had more than one infant, there are more subject numbers (19) than family cases (17).

Each woman in the No-Mental-Illness group was matched with a woman from one of the Psychopathology group on the basis of age, ethnic background, years of education, and gravidity. It is unfortunate that not enough women were recruited into the No-Mental-Illness group to allow for case-by-case matching with each woman in the Psychopathology groups. However, analysis of these demographic variables yielded no statistically significant differences among the groups.

Diagnosis

Before delivery, 54 women and 44 husbands were given a clinical interview based on the Current and Past Psychopathology Scale (CAPPS) developed by Endicott and Spitzer (1972). Seven women and 14 husbands refused, either actively or passively, to be interviewed with the CAPPS. To interview orthodox religious Jews, several items about sexual behavior had to be omitted. Initially, consensual diagnosis for each husband and wife was made by a team consisting of a psychiatrist, two psychologists, and two social workers. The team used all material available, including the clinical interview, psychiatric case histories, and the CAPPS computer diagnosis. The initial diagnoses were based on DSM-II (1968). These initial diagnoses were later revised using updated information and the Research Diagnostic Criteria (RDC) (Spitzer & Endicott, 1975; Spitzer et al., 1975).

Infant assessment procedure

A questionnaire about the pregnancy was given during the clinical interview. This questionnaire covered current health and medication, previous pregnancies and births, and selected background data such as subjects' perceived desirability of the pregnancy. Obstetric records were reviewed for information about prenatal, perinatal, and postnatal difficulties. The Rochester Obstetrical Scale (Zax, Sameroff, & Babigian, 1977) was used to score each area of difficulty. Sixty-seven infants were born to the 54 couples during the course of the study, but data from only 58 infants were used. The reasons for excluding data from 9 of the infants included lack of consensus on parental diagnosis, parents diagnosed as having a primarily organic disorder, twin births, loss of contact with the mother, or death of the infant. The final sample of infants included 19 born into schizophrenic families (3 of these from the same family), 6 into affective-disorders families, 14 into personality disorders–neuroses families (two of these in the same family), and 19 into families with no mental illness (two of these in the same family).

The infants were assessed at 3 and 14 days of age with the Neonatal Behavioral Assessment Scale (NBAS) (Brazelton, 1973) and at 4, 8, and 12 months of age with the Bayley Scales of Infant Development (BSID) (Bayley, 1969). At 4 and 8 months of age, the infants' mothers were interviewed about the temperament of their babies using the Carey Temperament Interview (Carey, 1970). The families were again interviewed about the development of their infants and the status of the family when the infants were between the ages of 1 and 4 years. A more extensive follow-up is planned after the children enter school.

The NBAS consists of two 6-point scales of initial and predominant states, 27 behavioral scales, and 18 reflex items. The state of the infant, ranging from sleep to alertness to crying, plays a crucial part in both the administration and scoring of the test. The behavior items are 9-point scales measuring motor reactivity, ability to habituate to stimulation during sleep, ability to orient to auditory and visual stimuli, and ability to cope with other kinds of stimulation. The test measures both neurophysiological functioning and interaction with the care giver.

The BSID was used to measure mental, motor, and social–behavioral development after the neonatal period. The Mental Scale includes pass–fail items measuring visual and auditory development, reaching, object permanence, imitation, language acquisition, and object relations. The Motor Scale consists of pass–fail items assessing fine and gross motor behaviors. Social behavior is assessed via the infant's reaction to the examiner and to the test situation and materials. This last set of 9-point scales is called the Infant Behavior Record.

The Carey Temperament Interview consists of 70 items assessing the infant's adaptability, mood, threshold, persistence, distractibility, rhythmicity, activity levels, and tendency to approach during sleep, feeding, bathing, play, and new situations. The mother's responses to the questions are used to construct a global rating of temperament on a continuum from easy to difficult. The questionnaire is based on the work of Thomas, Chess, Birch, Hertzig, & Korn (1963).

RESULTS

Examiner bias

After each testing session, the infant examiner guessed the group membership of the mother and rated her for various symptoms (depression, anxiety, etc.). This was done to determine if the infant examiner, who was supposed to be unaware of the diagnosis of the parent, was, in fact, able to identify correctly the mother's classification and if the examiner had systematic impressions of the mother that could have affected infant ratings. In general, no statistically significant examiner biases were found.

Pregnancy, birth, and early health information

Basic nutrition and prenatal care were good in all groups. The majority of women had a normal labor and delivery. Medication was given sparingly, usually less than 50 mg of an analgesic. The babies born to women in the Schizophrenic group

Table 1. *Parents and infants in schizophrenic group*

Subject number of infant	Diagnosis		Age (years)		Sex of infant	Birth weight (g)	ROS[a] score, total/prenatal
	Mother	Father	Mother	Father			
1	Chronic schizophrenia	Chronic schizophrenia	29	34	F	2,440	5/2
2	Schizophrenia (questionable)	Personality disorder	28	30	M	3,350	3/1
3	Normal	Schizoaffective	36	36	F	2,300	5/1
4	Chronic schizophrenia	Personality disorder	31	29	F	3,000	0/0
5	Normal	Acute schizophrenia	36	—	M	3,320	3/1
6	Chronic schizophrenia	Personality disorder	—	—	M	2,440	—
7[b]	Chronic schizophrenia	Normal	22	23	M	2,380	3/1
8	Chronic schizophrenia	Reactive depression	41	48	M	—	2/2
9	Schizophrenia (questionable)	Normal	38	49	M	2,820	3/2

10	Schizophrenia (questionable)	Normal	26	26	F	3,600	—
11	Chronic schizophrenia	Paranoid personality	28	36	F	2,730	2/0
12[b]	Chronic schizophrenia	Normal	25	26	M	2,790	4/1
13	Normal	Chronic schizophrenia	29	43	M	3,250	1/0
14	Chronic schizophrenia	—	24	—	M	3,230	1/0
15	Chronic schizophrenia	Normal	28	30	M	2,950	1/1
16	Schizophrenia (questionable)	Normal	26	34	F	3,180	2/0
17	Acute schizophrenia	Normal	22	23	F	3,230	3/0
18[b]	Chronic schizophrenia	Normal	23	24	F	3,560	2/1
19	Schizophrenia (questionable)	Personality disorder	33	35	M	3,120	2/2

[a]ROS indicates the Rochester Obstetrical Scale.
[b]Subjects 7, 12, and 18 are from the same family.

were somewhat lighter (mean = 2,982 g) than the babies born to women in the other groups (Affective Disorders, M = 3,290 g; Personality Disorders–Neuroses, M = 3,398 g; No Mental Illness, M = 3,180 g), although the differences were not significant (F(3, 45) = 2.59, p > .05). The findings of lower birth weights for infants in the schizophrenic group are not unique to this study. Similar results have been reported by Sameroff and Zax (1978) and Mednick et al. (1971).

The role of perinatal complications as primary, secondary, or interactive factors in the etiology of vulnerability to schizophrenia has been of special interest since the 1968 report of Mednick and Schulsinger. The results of numerous studies have produced an equivocal picture, which has been summarized by McNeil and Kaij (1978). In our sample there was no clear relationship between perinatal complications and the occurrence of poor motor and sensorimotor development.

Rochester Obstetrical Scale (ROS) scores were determined for 47 of the 54 mothers in our study. (The ROS reports of 7 mothers were burned in a fire in the records room of Hadassah Hospital.) There were no significant differences (F[3, 43] = 0.35, p > .05) between diagnostic groups on the scale (Schizophrenic, M = 2.5; Affective Disorders, M = 2.2; Personality Disorders–Neuroses, M = 2.8; No Mental Illness, M = 2.1). In the Rochester Developmental Psychopathology Study (Zax et al., 1977) the mean ROS scores for diagnostic groups ranged from 3.5 to 4.8, indicating that more risk factors were present in the Rochester sample than in our Jerusalem sample. Based on our recent intensive experience with both Israeli and U.S. inner-city newborns, we are quite confident that the low-risk scores of the subjects in the Jerusalem samples were due to the fact that prenatal care is more easily available in Israel than in the United States and that the general nutritional and environmental status of our participants may be superior to that of people from a similar social class in the United States. These two factors may also account for the lack of fetal and neonatal deaths in our samples as compared with the Rochester sample or with the sample reported by Rieder et al. (1975). Table 1 gives the ROS scores (total and prenatal) of the infants in the schizophrenic group.

Analyses of group differences

Initially, to compare our data with the findings of other risk studies of schizophrenia, we used a group-differences approach to statistical analysis to examine the four diagnostic groups on the NBAS and BSID. However, after we present our analyses of group differences, we will present an individual-differences approach to statistical analysis that we believe is more appropriate for risk research on schizophrenia and for other research examining heterogeneous psychiatric populations.

Analyses of variance (ANOVAs) between diagnostic groups on the NBAS showed no significant differences at 3 and 14 days of age. Several significant differences were found on the BSID at 4 and 8 months. The mental development index (MDI) of the BSID Mental Scale indicated significant differences among the groups at 4 months of age (F[3, 52] = 3.05, p < .05), although all of the groups scored within the normal range. The mean values were as follows: Schizophrenic,

$M = 92.6$; Affective Disorders, $M = 99.8$; Personality Disorders–Neuroses, $M = 102.4$; No Mental Illness, $M = 103.4$. There were no significant group differences on the 4-month Psychomotor Development Index (PDI) of the BSID Motor Scale.

At 8 months of age, the MDI also revealed significant differences among the groups: $F(3, 53) = 4.10$, $p < .05$. The mean values were 82.4, 100.7, 108.6, and 104.8 for the four groups, respectively. On the 8-month PDI there were significant differences as well: $F(3, 53) = 3.31$, $p < .05$. The means for the four groups were 78.1, 91.4, 92.4, and 103.6, respectively. For the 12-month MDI and PDI scores, the means were of the same relative magnitudes as for the 8-month scores, but were only marginally significant.

Analyses of individual differences

We believe that statistical analyses of differences between diagnostic groups are inappropriate because the behaviors indicating vulnerability to schizophrenia should be present only in those infants with a genetic loading for schizophrenia. A genetic model would predict that only a subgroup of infants born to schizophrenic parents have the genetic predisposition to the illness, and therefore early markers would be present only in this subgroup. Buchsbaum and Rieder (1979) demonstrated "the limited power of measurements obtained from groups of patients and controls" and that "group comparisons of schizophrenics vs controls are prone to overlook biological deviations in schizophrenics if the illness is heterogeneous." Thus, a group-differences approach is inappropriate when the index group is heterogeneous. Dawes and Meehl made a similar point in 1966. The analysis of individuals gains even a greater importance when it is recognized that important content often lies with the "outliers," as has been so clearly expressed more recently by Kidd and Matthysse (1978) and Boulding (1980).

The analysis of individual differences presented two problems. First, most of the variables available for our analyses involved rudimentary, nonmetric scales. The NBAS, for example, consists of a few observational categories for assessing each behavioral modality. In some cases, such as the activity variable, these categories are not even ordered in terms of pathology. Second, although modes of functioning (e.g., perceptual, motor) can be specified independently of developmental level, the behaviors that represent them are age- or stage-specific. Behavioral indicators of perceptual functioning in a newborn, for example, are necessarily different from those in an older child, even though both may involve the same neurological substrates. Theoretical continuity thus requires a statistical procedure for tracing developmental paths through multiple indicators of the same constructs.

Several statistical procedures have been proposed for solving these problems. Linear models such as regression analysis, linear discriminant function analysis, and factor analysis have been used to reduce observations on multiple attributes to relatively simple representations. However, with typical psychiatric and behavioral data, these representations are difficult to interpret. Often the categories of attributes are not ordered on a theoretical dimension or do not comprise known intervals on a scale. Even when scaling assumptions are appropriate, linear models are overly influenced by outliers or extreme values (Hampel, 1974; Wainer & Thissen, 1976) and nonnormal distributions. Finally, various cluster-analysis models have been proposed to solve these problems. However, cluster analysis requires prior assumptions concerning distance metrics and scaling of variables. Different assumptions can lead to totally different clustering solutions. To resolve these problems, we used a method developed by Guttman (Lingoes, 1973) called *Multidimensional Scalogram Analysis* (MSA).

Multidimensional Scalogram Analysis

This method requires that each subject can be described by a profile. This profile consists of several attributes on which the subject is measured, for instance, a set of observations made by a clinician about a particular person. These attributes may be quantities or even unordered categories. For example, subjects can be described by attributes of sex, age, birth weight, and type of delivery (normal, breech, cesarean, etc.). The method arranges the subjects in a dimensional space such that subjects with similar profiles are placed close together and subjects with dissimilar profiles are placed further apart. In other words, subjects who are plotted closest to each other have the most attributes in common, and those plotted farthest apart have the least.

The MSA program provides a solution (spatial representation) that contains the simplest structure obtainable. This simple structure shows the distribution of subjects on all the attributes jointly as well as on each attribute separately. One can determine which attributes show a clear grouping or simple ordering of categories and whether several attributes that are linked theoretically show similar patterns of groupings, or orderings. Attributes that exhibit clear groupings or orderings usually account for most of the overall variation between subjects. Attributes that exhibit similar patterns of groupings account for the variations between subjects in similar ways. These similar attributes comprise a set of facets that describe subjects in a lower dimensional space. Thus, complex profiles of attributes describing a set of subjects can be reduced to a simple set of theoretical facets. Unlike many other statistical procedures, MSA allows the clinician to examine the profiles of individual subjects directly in the final representation. In fact, MSA organizes data in a manner similar to the way in which a clinician organizes the data he or she collects from the anamnesis, roentgenograms, laboratory findings, and physical examination to arrive at an individual diagnosis. Multidimensional Scalogram Analysis and other Guttman theories and techniques are described more fully in a comprehensive survey by Shye (1978).

Motor and sensorimotor scales

Based on findings in the 1965 Israeli School-Age Study, it was hypothesized that the infants' motor and sensorimotor functioning should be related to parental diagnosis. Measures were available for the analyses of functioning in these two domains at ages 3 days, 14 days, 4 months, 8 months, and 12 months. For the 3- and 14-day time points, items representing motor and sensorimotor functioning were selected from the NBAS; for the later points, such items were selected from the BSID. To identify the set of items that had enough variation to be useful indicators, a Permutation Scalogram Program developed by Wilkinson (1979) was run on the NBAS and BSID data at the various time points. Items were chosen on which at least 10% of the infants (six or more) had scores different from the modal score. (Items not included because of low variability were reexamined separately to determine if they contained any meaningful, nonrandom structure.) Items representing areas of functioning other than motor and sensorimotor development, like language and social development, were eliminated from these analyses. Thus, at each time point, a set of items that measured the infants' age-appropriate motor and sensorimotor abilities was chosen. Motor development was represented by items involving a direct motoric response, either gross or fine. Sensorimotor development was represented by items involving a motoric response to sensory or cognitive processing (Table 2). After all the NBAS and BSID motor and sensorimotor items were selected, two additional judges were used to sort the items again into the two categories of functioning (motor and sensorimotor). The intraclass correlation between all three raters was .86 for the NBAS items and .88 for the BSID items.

The final analysis of individual differences involved separate scalings of all the subjects on these items for each time point. Five MSAs were computed for this purpose. The MSAs revealed that two-dimensional solutions were adequate for representing each of the five time points. In each case, the representation had a simple structure, the dimensions of which corresponded to the hypothesized motor and sensorimotor domains. Subjects' performance was ordered from poor to good on the two dimensions jointly. The results of these MSA analyses allowed a simple representation of the subjects' performance. Global motor and sensorimotor scores were computed for each subject by summing the subjects' scores on the individual items. Three items on the NBAS required rescoring before summing. General Tonus and Activity were rescored as follows: 5 − (absolute value of [score − 5]); this was done because in the MSA they showed a U-shaped relation to healthy functioning. The MSA analyses revealed that Tremulousness was related inversely to healthy functioning, so the scoring procedure for this item was reversed.

Figures 1 through 5 show scatterplots of these global scores. The axes have been standardized to allow comparisons across the five time points. Figure 6 differentiates most clearly the poorly performing infants in the Schizophrenic group from the others. This figure plots the mean of each infant's five motor and five sensorimotor scores and thus shows the average performance of each infant during the first year of life.

As Figures 1 through 6 show, 13 infants (8 of whom had at least one parent who was a chronic schizophrenic) in the Schizophrenic group repeatedly performed poorly on the motor and sensorimotor measures (jointly) during the first year of

Table 2. *Infant behaviors representing motor and sensorimotor functioning*

3 and 14 Days (NBAS)[a]	4 Months (BSID)[a]	8 Months (BSID)	12 Months (BSID)
Motor functioning			
General Tonus	Manipulates Table Edge Slightly	Sits Alone, Steadily	Holds Crayon Adaptively
Motor Maturity	Carries Ring to Mouth	Scoops Pellet	Pulls to Standing Position
Pull to Sit	Picks up Cube	Sits Alone, Good Coordination	Stands up by Furniture
Defensive Movements	Retains 2 Cubes	Cube: Complete Thumb Opposition (Radial–Digital)	Stepping Movements
Activity	Hands Predominantly Open	Prewalking Progression	Walks with Help
Tremulousness	Cube: Ulnar–Palmar Prehension	Early Stepping Movements	Sits Down
	Sits with Slight Support	Pellet: Partial Finger Prehension (Inferior Pincer)	Pat-a-Cake: Midline Skill
	Turns from Back to Side	Pulls to Standing Position	Stands Alone
	Effort to Sit	Raises Self to Sitting Position	Walks Alone
		Stands up by Furniture	Stands up: 1
		Combines Spoons or Cubes: Midline	Throws Ball
		Stepping Movements	
		Pellet: Fine Prehension (Neat Pincer)	
		Sits Down	

Sensorimotor Functioning

Inanimate Visual	Reaches for Dangling Ring	Manipulates Bell: Interest in Detail	Fingers Holes in Peg Board
Inanimate Auditory	Follows Ball Visually Across Table	Pulls String Adaptively: Secures Ring	Stirs with Spoon in Imitation
Animate Visual	Head Follows Dangling Ring	Rings Bell Purposively	Attempts to Imitate Scribble
Animate Auditory	Head Follows Vanishing Spoon	Uncovers Toy	Unwraps Cube
Animate Visual–Auditory	Closes on Dangling Ring	Fingers Holes in Peg Board	Pushes Car Along
Alertness	Turns Head to Sound of Bell	Picks Up Cup: Secures Cube	Puts 3 or More Cubes in Cup
	Turns Head to Sound of Rattle	Stirs With Spoon in Imitation	Uncovers Blue Box
	Reaches for Cube	Looks at Pictures in Book	Turns Pages of Book
	Manipulates Table Edge Actively		Pats Whistle Doll, in Imitation
	Eye–Hand Coordination in Reaching		Dangles Ring by String
	Regards Pellet		Puts Beads in Box (6 of 8)
			Places 1 Peg Repeatedly
			Removes Pellet from Bottle
			Blue Board: Places 1 Round Block
			Builds Tower of 2 Cubes
			Spontaneous Scribble
			Puts 9 Cubes in Cup
			Closes Round Box

*a*NBAS indicates Neonatal Behavioral Assessment Scale; BSID, Bayley Scales of Infant Development.

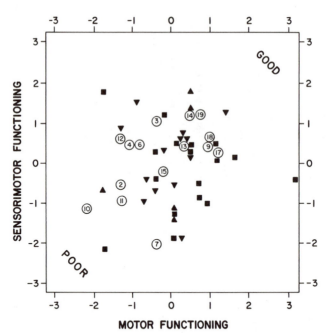

Figure 1. Infants' scores on motor and sensorimotor scales at age 3 days. At ages 3 and 14 days, scales are comprised of selected items from Neonatal Behavioral Assessment Scale; at ages 4, 8, and 12 months, scales are comprised of selected items from Bayley Scales of Infant Development. Circle with number indicates Schizophrenic group and subject number; triangle, Affective-Disorders group; inverted triangle, Personality Disorders–Neuroses group; and square, No-Mental-Illness group.

life (subjects 1 through 13). The remaining six infants born to schizophrenics, as well as most of the infants in the other diagnostic groups, repeatedly performed well during the first year. At any given time point there were several infants in the nonschizophrenic groups who performed poorly; however, the poor performers at any one time point tended to be different from those at other time points. Only nine (of 39) infants in nonschizophrenic groups repeatedly performed poorly throughout the first year of life; these were scattered among the three diagnostic groups, indicating that their performance was not attributable to their diagnostic group. Note that for clarity of presentation, subject numbers have been assigned only to infants in the Schizophrenic group. Subject numbers in all figures and tables have been assigned to the infants based on their overall level of functioning (from bad to good) as seen in Figure 8 (which will be explained). Also note that a few cases are missing at some of the time points due to missing data. To ensure that relevant content areas were not overlooked, we examined separately motor and sensorimotor items that had been rejected because the infants' scores on these items showed minimal variability. Several of these items did in fact serve to further distinguish the subgroup of poor performing infants born to schizophrenics from

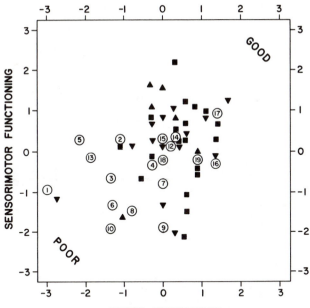

Figure 2. Infants' scores on motor and sensorimotor scales at age 14 days. See Figure 1 for explanation of scales and symbols.

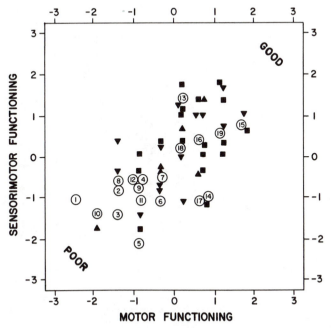

Figure 3. Infants' scores on motor and sensorimotor scales at age 4 months. See Figure 1 for explanation of scales and symbols.

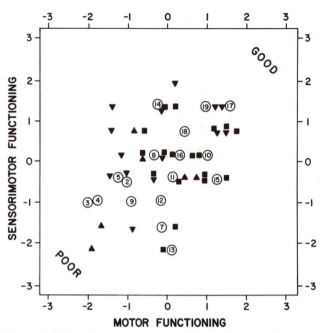

Figure 4. Infants' scores on motor and sensorimotor scales at age 8 months. See Figure 1 for explanation of scales and symbols.

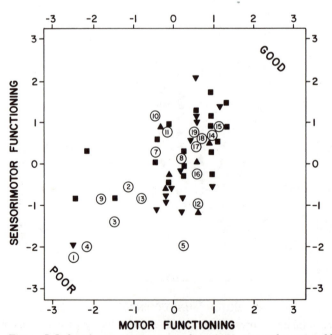

Figure 5. Infants' scores on motor and sensorimotor scales at age 12 months. See Figure 1 for explanation of scales and symbols.

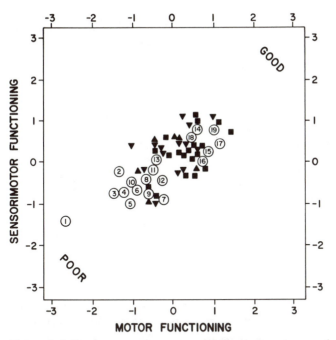

Figure 6. Infants' scores of average performance on motor and sensorimotor scales over five time points (Figures 1 through 5). See Figure 1 for explanation of scales and symbols.

the other infants. These items primarily involved even greater deficits in gross and fine motor development.

Variability

An important area of investigation in risk research in schizophrenia and other child development research concerns the issue of variability in behavior during early development. This is seen as normal and typical by some (Emde, Gaensbauer, & Harmon, 1976) and as possibly pathognomonic by others (Fish, 1977). Even though the BSID is generally considered a very reliable test (the reliability of the NBAS over time has been questioned by Sameroff, 1978b), infants do show much variability across age in their test performance. Therefore, we decided to examine carefully the relationship in our sample of diagnosis to variability in performance. We constructed an index to assess the average amount of variability in performance across the five time points. An index score was computed for each infant by calculating the distance between his/her position on Figure 1 (Day 3 NBAS score) and his/her position on Figure 2 (14 days NBAS score), repeating this calculation for all possible pairs of figures and taking the average of all these distances. It was found that almost all of the infants in our study, regardless of parental diagnosis, evidenced a relatively high degree of variability in performance during their first year of life. It is interesting that the four least variable performers were infants of

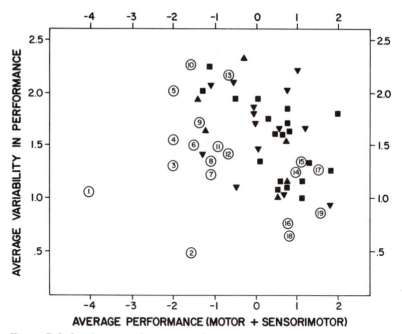

Figure 7. Infants' scores of average performance (motor + sensorimotor scores) vs. scores of average variability in performance. See Figure 1 for explanation of scales and symbols.

schizophrenics whose mean performance scores were relatively extreme. One was a repeatedly poor performer (subject 2) and three were repeatedly good performers (subjects, 16, 18, and 19). When we compared the distribution of average variability scores of infants in the Schizophrenic group with the scores of infants in the nonschizophrenic groups, the former showed significantly less variability (Schizophrenic group, $M = 1.35$; nonschizophrenic groups, $M = 1.60$; $t(56) = 5.0$, $p < .001$). Also, poor performing infants of schizophrenics were less variable than poor performing infants of nonschizophrenics, and good performing infants of schizophrenics were less variable than their counterparts born to nonschizophrenics. In general, poor performers showed greater variability than good performers (see Figure 7).

For closer comparison with other risk studies in this area, we examined those infants whose MDI or PDI scores (i.e., Bayley developmental quotients [DQs]) fluctuated by 30 or more DQ points from one testing session to another. There were eight infants whose MDI scores fluctuated by 30 or more points; four of these were infants in the Schizophrenic group and four were in the non-schizophrenic groups. Eight infants had PDI scores that fluctuated by 30 or more points; three of these were infants in the Schizophrenic group and five were in the nonschizophrenic groups. These findings indicate that extremely high variability in mental and motor development during the first year of life is not specifically

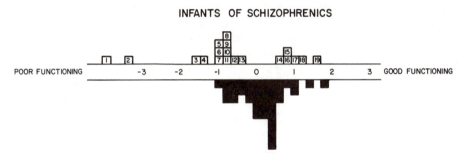

Figure 8. Distribution of infants' scores on index of the ratio of average performance to average variability in performance for Schizophrenic vs. nonschizophrenic groups. Subject numbers are in squares.

characteristic of the offspring of schizophrenics in our study. Also, no infants passed a series of items at an earlier time point but failed them at a later time point; and only one infant (subject 12) showed scatter within a specific time point (12-month Motor Scale) by passing a series of easy items, failing a series of more difficult items, and then passing an even more difficult series.

Ratio of average performance to average variability in performance

We thought that it was important to look at the infants' average motor and sensorimotor performance using a weighting procedure that gives less weight to extreme observations that are variable (Andrews, Bickel, Hampel, Huber, Rogers, & Tukey, 1972). We constructed a new index that was computed in the following manner. An average performance score was calculated for each infant by summing the motor and sensorimotor standard scores shown in Figure 6. This score was then divided by each infant's score on the index of average variability in performance. Figure 8 shows the distribution of scores of the Schizophrenic and nonschizophrenic groups on this new index of the ratio of average performance to average variability in performance. The infant in the Schizophrenic group who exhibited the poorest performance over the five time points, based on this index, was called "subject 1," the next poorest performing infant "subject 2," and so forth. The infant in the Schizophrenic group who exhibited the best performance during the first year of life was called "subject 19." (All references to subject numbers in this chapter are based on Figure 8.)

Examination of Figure 8 reveals that there were two major gaps in the distribution of infants in the Schizophrenic group, between subjects 2 and 3 and between subjects 13 and 14. These gaps were shown to be significant ($p > .05$) by the Tukey gap test (Wainer & Schacht, 1978), indicating that the three groupings of infants (subject 1 and 2, 3 through 13, and 14 through 19) showed significantly different performance. This means that the distribution of infants in the Schizophrenic group was essentially bimodal, but with two infants (subjects 1 and 2) comprising a set of extreme outliers. Close inspection revealed that subject 1 had one of the largest combinations of prenatal, perinatal, and postnatal insults.

In this chapter we have designated subjects 1 through 13 (as well as any infants of nonschizophrenics performing as poorly or more poorly) as the repeatedly poor performers, and subjects 14 through 19 (as well as infants of nonschizophrenics performing as well or better) as the repeatedly good performers. The distribution of infants of nonschizophrenics did not reveal any significant gaps and approached a normal distribution. From this result, there appeared to be a subgroup of 13 infants born to schizophrenics who repeatedly performed poorly during their first year of life and were clearly different from other infants born to schizophrenics and from most infants born to nonschizophrenic parents.

It is important to point out that when we speak of "good" or "poor" performance, we are speaking in relative terms. There is some degree of arbitrariness in saying that subjects 1 through 13 are the poor performers and subjects 14 through 19 the good performers. Certainly the distribution of subjects in Figure 8 suggests some kind of dividing line between subjects 13 and 14, although it is probably more judicious to say that a gray area exists from approximately subject 7 to subject 13, where performance is only marginally below the overall sample mean.

The range of poor performers could be attributable to genetic factors, perinatal and postnatal factors, or to a combination of these. Therefore, we will now take a closer look at individual differences in performance in light of these factors.

Perinatal complications and low to low-normal birth weights

Only three infants in the Schizophrenic group had moderate to high ROS scores (1 or more *SD* above mean; i.e., score $\geq$ 4). These infants were among the subgroup of 13 poor performers. In contrast, 9 of the 39 infants in the nonschizophrenic groups had moderate to high ROS scores, but none of these infants showed poor performance. These results indicated that there was not a greater incidence of perinatal complications (as evidenced by high ROS scores) in the subgroup of poor performing infants of schizophrenics than in the other groups, and when perinatal complications did occur, the infants of schizophrenics were somewhat more likely to be adversely affected by them. This second inference suggested that these fetuses/neonates in the Schizophrenic group may have been especially vulnerable to external insults.

Although our sample had minimal perinatal complications, we found an interesting result concerning birth weights. Seven of the 13 poor performing infants of schizophrenics had low to low-normal birth weights (between 2,300 and 2,900 g). Four of these had a mother and one had a father and a mother who were chronic schizophrenics. The latter infant had one of the lowest birth weights and also was the poorest performer in our study. One of the seven infants was only 35 weeks' gestational age at birth (premature), and one was described as small for date, but none had been placed in an intensive-care unit. None of the good performers in the schizophrenic group had birth weights less than 2,900 g. In contrast, nine infants in the nonschizophrenic groups had birth weights less than 2,900 g, but only three of these showed poor performance during the first year. Thus, as was the case for high ROS scores, low birth weights were associated to some degree with subsequent poor performance, primarily for a subgroup of infants born to (chronic) schizophrenics.

To determine if the low birth weights were related to prenatal complications, we examined the prenatal scale of the ROS separately. Only two infants (both in the nonschizophrenic group) had severe prenatal problems (toxemia). The remaining prenatal problems were mild to moderate (a score of 1 or 2 on the prenatal scale). Five of the seven infants of schizophrenics with low birth weights had had mild to moderate prenatal problems. All five of these performed poorly. There were six infants of schizophrenics with birth weights greater than 2,900 g who also had mild to moderate prenatal problems. Three of these showed poor performance. In contrast, none of the eight infants of nonschizophrenics with birth weights below normal had prenatal problems. However, there were 10 infants of nonschizophrenics with birth weights greater than 2,900 g who had mild to moderate prenatal problems. Only two of these showed poor performance. These results suggested that there was a greater association between prenatal problems and birth weights, and between prenatal problems and subsequent poor performance, for a subgroup of infants of schizophrenics than for the infants of nonschizophrenics and the remaining infants in the Schizophrenic group. However, although prenatal problems may have contributed somewhat to the finding of low birth weights in four of the infants in the schizophrenic group, two infants in this group without prenatal problems also had birth weights less than 2,900 g, indicating that etiological factors other than those measured by the ROS Prenatal Scale may have been operating. There were also eight infants of nonschizophrenics without prenatal problems who had birth weights below normal, but these cases were scattered throughout the three diagnostic groups, indicating that their birth weights were not attributable to their diagnostic group. Other as yet indeterminate factors may have been responsible for these birth weights.

First, then, we see that prenatal and perinatal problems and low birth weights tended to be associated with poor performance primarily for a subgroup of infants of schizophrenics (subjects 1 through 13). Second, prenatal and perinatal problems did not occur more often in this subgroup of poor performing infants of schizophrenics. Third, more low birth weights were found in this subgroup of offspring of schizophrenics. In every case, low birth weight in an infant of a schizophrenic was associated with poor performance during the first year, and in only a few cases was it possible that these birth weights were affected by prenatal complications. Considering that all of the mothers in the study were known to have had good prenatal care and nutrition, the most plausible hypothesis to account for this birth weight finding is the existence of some type of mild intrauterine growth retardation associated with CNS dysmaturation, as suggested by Fish (1977). Fourth, we have shown that prenatal and perinatal complications could not be the only factors influencing the poor performance of the subgroup of infants of schizophrenics, although these problems clearly add insult to injury for the developing fetal brain. It is interesting that in a little-known Russian study (Vartanyan & Gindillis, 1972) the brains of aborted fetuses of schizophrenics and normal mothers were studied in vitro, and explants from the former were shown to have a lower rate of viability, less mitotic activity, and, in a few cases, more chromosome aberrations. Although this study has not been replicated (to our knowledge), it raises interesting theoretical issues for investigation, especially the hypothesis of a genetically determined vulnerability of fetal brains of offspring of schizophrenics.

Institutionalization and multiple separations

Several infants in our study had been placed in institutions, and others had experienced multiple separations from their mothers. Six infants in the Schizophrenic group and one in a nonschizophrenic group were institutionalized for a major portion of their first year of life. Five of these infants of schizophrenics showed poor performance during the first year (even prior to institutionalization), whereas the other infants showed good performance even though they were in the same institution. Two infants of schizophrenics and four infants of nonschizophrenics had multiple separations from their mothers during their first year of life. Of these, one infant of a schizophrenic and two infants of nonschizophrenics showed poor performance. Thus, institutionalization and multiple separations may have had some effect on performance irrespective of diagnosis, although the infants of schizophrenics may have been more vulnerable to these postnatal insults.

It is important to add that there were two infants of schizophrenics who had no perinatal and prenatal complications, were not institutionalized, and did not experience multiple separations, yet repeatedly performed poorly during the first year of life. There were also three infants of nonschizophrenics who did not have these insults, yet performed poorly. However, these latter cases were not concentrated in a particular diagnostic group, implying that diagnosis was not a factor in their performance.

In summary, we found that (1) a specific subgroup of infants born to schizophrenics (subjects 1 through 13) showed repeatedly poor motor and sensorimotor performance during the first year of life; (2) prenatal, perinatal, and postnatal complications could not account fully for the poor performance of this subgroup or explain its size; (3) such insults had a more adverse effect on this subgroup than on the other infants; and (4) only a few infants of nonschizophrenics performed poorly, and these were scattered among the three diagnostic groups. A parsimonious explanation that would seem to account for the poor performance in this subgroup of infants born to schizophrenics would be some genetically determined neurointegrative deficit. In several cases this deficit seemed to be further complicated by additional insults. This would suggest that the primary deficit made these infants especially vulnerable to external insults.

Clinical profiles

To gain a better clinical picture of the poor performers in this subgroup, we examined their performance on individual items from the motor and sensorimotor scales at each of the time points. At 3 and 14 days of age, most of the infants in this subgroup showed weakness in upper-body muscle control (Pull to Sit), varying degrees of jerkiness and deficits in free-flowing limb movements (Motor Maturity), and a tendency to moderate or elevated muscle tone (General Tonus). None of the infants showed hypotonicity. A few infants evidenced occasional tremulousness in the alert state, and a few showed occasional tremulousness in the nonalert state. The level of activity of these infants was in the normal to low-normal range. The infants were in the normal to low-normal range for visual-orientation items (Animate Visual, Inanimate Visual), in the normal range for auditory–orientation items (Animate Auditory, Inanimate Auditory, Animate Auditory–Visual), and in the lower range for alertness. None were hyperalert.

At 4 months of age, almost none of these infants exhibited visually guided reaching or age-level hand coordination (Reaches for Cube, Manipulates Table Edge Slightly–Actively, Eye–Hand Coordination in Reaching, Picks up Cube, Retains Two Cubes, Closes on Dangling Ring). Many showed visual tracking with the head (Follows Ball Visually Across Table, Head Follows Dangling Ring, Head Follows Vanishing Spoon), but most did not search for unseen, audible stimuli (Turns Head to Sound of Bell, Turns Head to Sound of Rattle).

At age 8 months, most of these infants could not raise themselves to a sitting position, pull themselves to a standing position, or stand up holding onto furniture. Most had not achieved the fine motor coordination necessary for picking up small objects (Pellet: Partial Finger Prehension – Inferior Pincer), nor had they achieved midline coordination (Combines Spoons or Cubes). Almost all of the infants made no attempt to search for disappearing objects (Uncovers Toy, Picks up Cup–Secures Cube, Looks for Contents of Box).

At age 12 months, most of these infants had gross motor difficulties in that they could not stand up from a supine position (Stand up: 1) or stand alone. Many could not walk with help, and a few still could not make stepping movements or sit down. Also, a few lacked fine motor control in grasping small objects (Pellet: Fine Prehension – Neat Pincer), and had still not attained midline coordination (Pat-a-Cake). Most of the infants seemed to have achieved some elements of object permanence in that they searched for disappearing objects (Looks for Contents of Box). However, many failed to retrieve objects whose retrieval required longer time, more complex motor behavior, and longer memory (Unwraps Cube). Many showed some ability to perceive and imitate certain human behaviors (Stirs with Spoon in Imitation), but most failed when these behaviors were more complex (Attempts to Imitate Scribble).

DISCUSSION

In this chapter our primary focus has been to examine the hypothesis that neurointegrative deficits can be found in a subgroup of offspring of schizophrenics and that these deficits suggest some kind of genetically determined vulnerability to schizophrenia. We reasoned that several preliminary questions had to be addressed first. Could neurointegrative deficits be identified in infancy, prior to important postnatal environmental influences? Yes. We found a subgroup of infants born to schizophrenics who repeatedly showed poor motor and sensorimotor performance in the first days and throughout their first year of life. Seven of these infants also had low to low-normal birth weights.

Could such deficits be found in other mental disorders, or are they specific to schizophrenia? Deficits in motor and sensorimotor performance were found in several infants born to mothers with other mental disorders and in a few infants born to normal mothers. These deficits were not associated with a specific non-schizophrenic diagnosis; the deficits were concentrated in a subgroup of infants of schizophrenics.

Were such deficits due to genetic causes, perinatal insults, or a combination of these factors? Our analysis of group and individual differences indicated that prenatal, perinatal, and postnatal insults could not account completely for the low birth weights or for the motor and sensorimotor deficits. However, the subgroup of infants born to schizophrenics may have been more vulnerable to these insults, when they occurred. The infants of schizophrenics who seemed to be impervious to these insults and who generally performed well throughout the first year may be a cohort of *invulnerable* infants referred to in the literature. All these findings together are not inconsistent with the hypothesis that the motor and sensorimotor deficits increased vulnerability to insults, and low birth weights observed in the subgroup of infants of schizophrenics were genetically determined.

Genetic models for the transmission of schizophrenia (Rosenthal, 1963; Kidd, 1978) all postulate that a schizophrenic parent would transmit to his or her offspring a genetically determined constitutional vulnerability. One focus of risk research in schizophrenia has been to define the characteristics of this inherited vulnerability, both to understand the etiological factors in schizophrenia and to describe specific functions that might be considered biological or behavioral genetic markers. However, any model, either a multifactorial or a single-major-locus-threshold model, would recognize these markers for only a subgroup of offspring of schizophrenics. In the simplest model, that of a single dominant gene, this subgroup would consist of half of the offspring of a single schizophrenic parent, as suggested by Rosenthal (1963).

Although the inevitably limited sample size of longitudinal studies does not lend itself to the clarification of specific genetic models, it is worthwhile noting the recurrence (in our study and in other studies among first-degree relatives of schizophrenics) of subgroups with neurointergrative dysfunctioning that represent approximately half of these relatives. Grunebaum et al. (1974) found attentional deficits in three of five 3-year-old offspring. Asarnow et al. (1977) found a cluster of attentional deficits in four of nine offspring. Ragins, Schachter, Elmer, Preisman, Bowes, & Harway (1975) found 4 of 10 children of schizophrenics who exhibited delayed reflex maturation. Fish (1977) reported on neurointegrative dysfunctioning in approximately half of the offspring seen by her. Holzman et al. (1976) found disturbed smooth-pursuit eye movements in approximately 45% of first-degree relatives. Rutschamnn et al. (1977) found a subgroup of offspring of schizophrenics with poor performance on a test of sustained attention. Finally, Marcus, Hans, Mednick, Schulsinger and Mikkelson in an as yet unpublished

MSA reanalysis of data from the Danish High-Risk Project (Orvaschel et al., 1979) found a subgroup of approximately half of the children of schizophrenics (matched with controls having identical perinatal histories) who showed poor coordination, reciprocal coordination, posture and gait, and other motor impairments.

The repeated identification of similarly sized subgroups with neurointegrative impairments (in some cases clearly not related to perinatal factors) in different populations would appear to support the hypothesis of a genetically determined vulnerability that represents at least one component of "endophenotype" or "schizotaxia" (Meehl, 1962, 1972). Nonetheless, the exact nature of a genetic model for the transmission of schizophrenia can be determined only through the design and execution of appropriate multigenerational pedigree studies.

When attempting to assess and compare the development of infants, how does one deal with the variability inherent in early development? The issue of variability in infant development has been discussed by Emde (1978), who pointed out that the apparently poor stability of the NBAS test "documented the dynamic complexity of development itself." He argued that variability and range of behavior are highly adaptive in that they increase opportunities for "matching or synchronizing such behavior" with an unpredictable caretaker environment. Because an infant enhances his own organization by interaction with specific caretakers, it is logical that developmental stability of individual differences would not be expected. The poor stability may be accounted for also by the major biobehavioral shifts that occur in infant development. We found that almost all of our infants, regardless of parental diagnosis and overall average performance, showed a high degree of variability in motor and sensorimotor performance during their first year of life. Yet, even within this variability we were able to identify distinct subgroups of poor and good performers.

Fish (1977) has postulated that high variability in neurological development during infancy may be an early neurophysical expression of schizophrenia. She described a pattern of erratic development of preschizophrenic infants that was characterized by fluctuation in the rate of development from marked acceleration to marked retardation. However, in our study the subgroup of poor performers born to schizophrenics showed even less variability than did other infants. This apparent discrepancy might be accounted for by the fact that Fish had a somewhat different sample and used different statistical methods. She also examined somewhat different modes of functioning (including physical growth) and saw the children more frequently.

One cannot discount the problem of heterogeneity in schizophrenia. Being defined as schizophrenic by RDC criteria does not clearly define a homogeneous pathological entity (Meltzer, 1979). Whereas there does appear to be some degree of homogeneity in our study in that a large number of infants in the Schizophrenic group were born to chronic schizophrenics, this still does not ensure a truly homogeneous cohort. One might look for more definitive biological markers and neurophysiological dysfunctions in the patients themselves and use these as part of the definition of the cohort. If one finds continuity of basic biological markers or neurophysiological dysfunctions between clinically defined parents and their offspring, one will be in a much better position to theorize about the importance and sequence of these markers and dysfunctions. In fact, several investigators (Quitkin et al. 1976; Tucker, Campion, & Silverfarb, 1975; Rochford, Detre, Tucker, & Harrow, 1970) have identified subgroups of schizophrenics with increased signs of neurological and behavioral impairments. Thus, it is possible that our sample contained a large number of parents with such impairments and that the subgroup of infants showing neurointegrative deficits were born to those schizophrenic parents with neurological impairments. However, this would be surprising because our sample of schizophrenic parents was drawn from a large and probably diverse universe of schizophrenic patients in the city of Jerusalem.

In a subsequent follow-up, we would like to do this type of reassessment of the parents. We recognize the need for a more complex genetic model to guide the design of future studies as well as a more complex (multidimensional) model for data analysis that takes into account a larger number of possible subgroups, genetic–environmental interactions, and paths of development.

Finally, what methodological approach is most appropriate for analyzing the issues we have raised? We have attempted to show that both theory and data suggest that an individual-differences approach to data analysis like MSA is most appropriate because it permits the identification of subgroups (when they exist) and makes it possible for the clinician or researcher to observe and monitor any person, or subgroup of persons, identified as being at risk. Such approaches also enable one to examine outliers as well as various types and directions of functioning.

The profile of infant functioning reported here should by no means be seen as clinically diagnostic. These initial research findings need further replication and longitudinal study. They should not be misconstrued as signs that can presently allow the clinician to predict the outcome for any particular infant born into a schizophrenic family. This is especially true because we have not yet completed the analyses of our development data. It is possible that additional variables will improve the predictions we have developed so far.

We do not attribute the development of clinical schizophrenia to a single factor. There are certainly multiple factors involved in the determination of the final expression of schizophrenic behaviors (Cloninger, Christiansen, Reich, & Gottesman, 1978). One of them is likely to be the vulnerability inherent in the neurointegrative deficit. However, this deficit must interact with other, as yet undefined, variables to produce a clinical schizophrenic psychotic state.

36 Offspring of women with nonorganic psychoses

THOMAS F. McNEIL AND LENNART KAIJ

with Ann Malmquist-Larsson, Barbro Näslund, Inger Persson-Blennow,
Nancy McNeil, Gösta Blennow, and Curt Borgenstam

This study is based on a genetic model (Garmezy, 1972) and constitutes a prospective, longitudinal high-risk project on the offspring of pregnant index women who have (had) psychoses of a nonorganic nature. At least one demographically matched pregnant control woman was chosen for each index woman, and the control mother and offspring were studied in a manner identical to that for the index case. The study was conducted in southern Sweden; subjects were sampled in an area with a population of about 1,230,000 persons and extending approximately 120 × 130 miles. All research personnel who actively studied the mothers and offspring were, as far as possible, kept blind as to the index–control status of the mothers, and all were blind as to the project's diagnosis of the index case.

The first phase of the study began during pregnancy and continued until the offspring reached 2 years of age. The complete research program during this first phase included 11 research contacts with each case. For practical reasons, this research program had to be restricted for some subjects in the outlying geographical areas. The major study areas consisted of two interviews during pregnancy regarding the mother's life situation and experience of pregnancy; testing of fetal heart-rate responsivity; study of maternal psychiatric status from pregnancy through 2 years after delivery; investigation of somatic pregnancy and birth complications, including personal observation of the labor, delivery, and immediate postnatal condition and behavior of the neonate and parents; assessment of neonatal neurological and somatic condition; standardized observation of mother–infant interaction and interview with the mother on six occasions; investigation of offspring temperament at three ages; and study of offspring physical health course during the first 2 years of life.

The second project phase, currently in progress, assesses the offspring and their environments at 6 years of age. This assessment includes Griffiths' Developmental Scale, Children's Apperception Test, Continuous Performance Test, study of neuromotoric development, a modified Rochester Adaptive Behavior Inventory

This research has been supported by Grants No. 3793 and 6214 from the Swedish Medical Research Council, by Grant No. MH18857 from the National Institute of Mental Health, and by an award from the Grant Foundation, Inc. During the course of the study, McNeil was also associated with Lafayette Clinic, Detroit, Michigan.

465

Table 1. *Diagnostic group and sample size*

Diagnostic group	Index group			Control group		
	Invited (N)	Rejected (N)	Final (N)	Invited (N)	Rejected (N)	Final (N)
Schizophrenia	18	1 (6%)	17	23	1 (4%)	22
Cycloid psychosis	18	3 (17%)	15	20	1 (5%)	19
Affective illness	17	2 (12%)	15	18	0	18
Total endogenous	53	6 (11%)	47	61	2 (3%)	59
Psychogenic psychosis	6	0	6	7	0	7
Postpartum psychosis	18	0	18	18	0	18
Other psychoses	17	0	17	20	0	20
Total nonendogenous	41	0	41	45	0	45
All subjects	94	6 (6%)	88	106	2 (2%)	104

(RABI) interview, clinical judgment of the child's mental status and characteristics, investigation of temperament and attachment by questionnaire, and an interview regarding the home and family situation.

DIAGNOSIS

The criteria used for sampling and for diagnostic group placement were determined in advance of the study. Subjects were included in the index sample if they presented psychotic symptoms of any duration, that is, gross disturbance in reality testing, including delusions and/or hallucinations, and absence of insight into the unreal nature of these experiences. Schizophrenia and endogenous affective illness could be diagnosed even in the absence of these psychotic symptoms. Subjects were excluded for: (1) psychotic onset preceded by alcohol or drug overuse or by clear somatic disease or injury, excluding pregnancy and childbirth; (2) preexisting chronic alcoholism or drug dependency; (3) signs of more than just a minimal lesion or a disease of the central nervous system; or (4) mental retardation since childhood.

In accordance with European tradition, clouding of consciousness (i.e., twilight states and confusion) was not, a priori, regarded as a sign of organicity and was thus not per se a criterion for exclusion from the study. The nonorganic psychotic index sample included for study (Table 1) was further categorized according to the diagnostic system summarized below.

Endogenous psychoses

Schizophrenia. This diagnosis was used in a restrictive manner, based on Bleuler's *primary symptoms.* In practice, this usage is in close agreement with the description of *process schizophrenia* proposed for the DSM-III (Spitzer et al., 1978). In addition to the psychotic forms of schizophrenia, pseudoneurotic and nonregressive (Nyman, Nyman, & Nylander, 1978) forms were accepted in the study, provided that the Bleulerian criteria were fulfilled. The criteria for inclusion were: insidious onset; any degree of autism, splitting of affect, thought, and/or volition (ambivalence); flattening or loss of affect, anhedonia; loosening of associations and formal thought disorder; and disturbances in perception including dishabituation. In addition, all but two subjects diagnosed as schizophrenics in the current sample exhibited secondary symptoms such as delusions and hallucinations. The criterion for exclusion was clouding of consciousness.

Cycloid psychosis (Leonhard, 1961). *Cycloid psychosis* is best described as a hereditary variety of schizoaffective psychoses, usually with clouding of consciousness. The criteria for inclusion were: recurrent course (at least two episodes); acute onset and complete recovery between episodes; *all* of the following: prominent mood disturbances, clouding of consciousness, hallucinations, delusions; and homotypical heredity.

Endogenous manic-depressive and unipolar affective illnesses. These diagnoses were used in a sense generally agreed upon in psychiatry. Episodes of the disorders did not need to be of psychotic severity. The criteria for inclusion were: in the presence of homotypical heredity, at least two depressive episodes or one manic episode; in the absence of homotypical heredity, at least three depressive episodes or two manic episodes or one manic and one depressive episode. The criteria for exclusion were: clouding of consciousness; or all episodes related to obvious mental trauma.

Nonendogenous psychoses

This category includes nonorganic psychoses that did not clearly fulfill the criteria for any of the endogenous psychoses. Because the project's original interest concerned primarily the endogenous psychoses, the nonendogenous psychoses category was, prior to sample selection, viewed somewhat as an "other" category. With the restrictive diagnostic criteria employed, the Nonendogenous group ($N = 41$) came to comprise almost one-half of the total index sample (Table 1). For descriptive and analytic purposes, the total Nonendogenous group was further divided into the subgroups, Psychogenic Psychosis, Postpartum Psychosis, and Other Psychoses.

The classification of subjects within the Nonendogenous Psychoses group was based on the circumstances surrounding onset, and not on symptom picture. The symptoms are kaleidoscopic, with a variety of paranoid and other delusions, hallucinations, sometimes clouding of consciousness, panic, fear, and mood disturbances, as shown in Table 2.

Psychogenic psychosis. This diagnostic category is often termed *reactive psychosis*, and we have chosen the term *psychogenic* as indicating our specific intention for the

Table 2. *Symptom characteristics for the nonendogenous psychoses subsample*

| | Nonendogenous psychoses subgroup | | | |
| | Psychogenic Psychosis (N = 6) | Postpartum Psychosis (N = 18) | Other Psychoses (N = 17) | Total (N = 41) |
Characteristic	N (%)	N (%)	N (%)	N (%)
I. Symptoms				
Mood disorder	6 (100)	16 (89)	16 (94)	38 (93)
Clouded consciousness	3 (50)	12 (67)	11 (65)	26 (63)
Panic states/attacks	3 (50)	15 (83)	7 (41)	25 (61)
Formal thought disorder	1 (17)	1 (6)	2 (12)	4 (10)
Sensory hallucinations	3 (50)	7 (39)	14 (82)	24 (59)
Paranoid attitude/delusion/system	5 (83)	8 (44)	13 (76)	26 (63)
Depressive thoughts/delusions	4 (67)	13 (72)	7 (41)	24 (59)
Grandiose ideas/delusions	0	0	3 (18)	3 (7)
Suicidal thoughts/acts	2 (33)	1 (6)	2 (12)	5 (12)
Hypochondriasis/dys-morphophobia	3 (50)	2 (11)	1 (6)	6 (15)
Highly aggressive behavior	1 (17)	2 (11)	2 (12)	5 (12)
Neurotic symptoms	0	1 (6)	0	1 (2)
II. Psychotic onset				
Acute	5 (83)	17 (94)	13 (76)	35 (85)
Subacute	1 (17)	1 (6)	4 (24)	6 (15)
III. Disease course				
Discrete	4 (67)	12 (67)	6 (35)	22 (54)
Recurrent	2 (33)	6 (33)	11 (65)	19 (46)

category. The diagnostic category has only recently been accepted as a separate entity outside Scandinavia (McCabe, 1975). In the present sample, all three forms were found, that is, affective, confusional, and paranoid types of psychogenic psychosis. The criteria for inclusion (Jaspers, 1965) were: onset in close temporal relation to obvious mental trauma other than pregnancy and childbirth; trauma mirrored in the content of thoughts, delusions and hallucinations; remission when the trauma subsides.

Postpartum psychosis. The criteria for inclusion were: psychotic onset within 6 months after a previous delivery (*not* the current delivery); mental symptoms, problems, and disturbance of a nonpsychotic nature can exist at other times outside the postpartum period. The criterion for exclusion was: psychosis during a postpartum period but which constitutes an episode or exacerbation of an endogenous psychosis as defined above.

Other nonendogenous psychoses. This was a residual category containing all non-organic nonendogenous psychoses not classifiable as psychogenic or postpartum psychoses.

SAMPLING

Index subjects

The final project sample consisted of 192 cases, 88 index and 104 controls. During a 4.5-year period (from about January, 1973 through June, 1977) 53,540 names of pregnant women registered at the prenatal clinics in the geographical areas of Skåne, Blekinge, and Halland as far north as Falkenberg were checked against a list of approximately 5,800 women in the fertile age range (born after December 31, 1929) who had been admitted since January 1, 1945 to eight psychiatric hospitals and six inpatient psychiatric clinics in a larger geographical area including and surrounding the pregnancy-sampling area, and who had hospital diagnoses suggesting a nonorganic psychosis. This list was updated for newly hospitalized cases at least once every 6 months during the collection of the sample.

A total of 262 pregnant women were found in this psychiatric list during the approximately 4.5-year sampling period. This figure does not include the 33 cases found during sampling but with expected dates of confinement after the project sampling cutoff date of June 30, 1977, nor the 69 cases with first psychiatric hospitalization during sampling but after the pregnancy in question. Of these 262 cases, 119 (45.4%) were categorized as nonorganic psychoses by project psychiatrists on the basis of all known psychiatric records for the woman and her relatives, when relevant.

Among the 119 pregnant women who were diagnosed as nonorganic psychotics, 98 fulfilled the remaining criteria for acceptance into the index sample, namely: (1) still pregnant at admission to the sample (i.e., not aborted and not delivered); (2) not themselves a physician or physician's wife (relevant to one case); and (3) able to speak Swedish, Danish, or Norwegian. Among the 98 cases accepted into the index sample, 91 (93%) accepted participation and began the study (Table 1).

After completion of the first phase of the study (2 years of age), at least 2 years after identification of the last index case and prior to data analysis, all known psychiatric records – including new records and entries – were again independently reviewed and judged by the project diagnosticians for all cases accepted for study. The same diagnostic criteria were used as at the first assessment. No data collected in the project were available to the diagnosticians for this rediagnosis, which was based solely on psychiatric records. Three index subjects who had been studied in the project were judged at final diagnostic assessment not to qualify as nonorganic psychotics, and these three subjects were removed from the sample. (One of these had also rejected participation at her second reproduction.)

The final total Index group thus consisted of 88 cases (88 reproductions for 83 women), whose specific diagnostic distribution is shown in Table 1.

For simplicity of expression, the subjects in the Index group are referred to as Schizophrenics, Cycloids, Affectives, Psychogenics, Postpartum Psychotics, and Other Psychotics.

Control subjects

For each index subject chosen for active study, one pregnant control woman was chosen on the basis of the following sampling criteria: (1) consecutive admission from the same (or a demographically equivalent) prenatal clinic; (2) Swedish-, Danish-, or Norwegian-speaking woman; (3) woman and the fetus's biological father residents of Sweden since about 15 years of age; (4) woman and the fetus's biological father free from a history of treatment for psychosis as diagnosed by a project diagnostician based on any existing psychiatric records; and (5) matched with the index case on parity (0, 1, 2+), maternal age, social class (1, 2, 3) and, when possible, marital status at pregnancy identification. One live-born control child born to a mother participating through delivery was included for each index case who began and continued participation in the project.

Among the 106 control subjects asked to participate, 98% accepted and began the study. The final control sample consisted of 104 cases (104 reproductions for 98 women). The surplus of control cases resulted from several factors, and the extra controls were used to improve further the specific index and control groups' comparability on demographic characteristics.

The Specific Control groups were very highly comparable to their Index groups on parity and maternal age at delivery. Social class was also quite similar for the Specific Control and Index groups. For some entirely unclear reason, the Index groups generally tended to produce more male offspring, whereas the Control groups had comparatively more female offspring.

PROCEDURE

The index and control subjects who actively participated in the study and who became pregnant again within the sampling period were offered participation for a second time. Such double reproductions constituted small proportions of both final index and control samples (6%), and the double reproductions were well distributed over the specific diagnostic groups.

With the extensive geographical area covered by the project, the degree of financial support available, and the limited research personnel available to cover these cases, some restrictions had to be made in the extent of the measures employed in the outlying areas. In order to obtain data on the diagnostic groups that were of greatest interest from a genetic-risk viewpoint and provide comparable control-group data, it was decided that all subjects in the central project area would be offered the full study program, but that both index cases with nonendogenous psychoses (as diagnosed at entrance to the study) and their matched controls who lived in the outlying geographical area (defined as those not delivering in Malmö or Lund) would be excluded from the neonatal neurological and pediatric assessment and from the home observations. This restriction affected 18 index and 19 control subjects who otherwise participated in the study.

Pregnancy interviews

McNeil conducted a semistructured interview with the 192 actively participating women at one of their prenatal clinic visits, or in a few cases at an obstetrical department for hospitalized cases. All were interviewed after quickening, and 84% of the sample was interviewed between the 21st and 32nd week of pregnancy. No notable relationship was found between timing of the interview and the scores obtained on selected variables.

Prior to the interview, the interviewer was informed only of the mother's name, birthdate, and expected date of confinement. The mother's medical and psychiatric history was discussed only to the extent that she spontaneously volunteered such information during the interview.

The general purpose of the interview in the longitudinal study framework was to provide information regarding current pregnancy factors of a psychological, psychosocial, and interpersonal nature that are hypothesized to be of importance for the subsequent development of the mother–child relationship and the psychological and somatic development of the child (either directly or via obstetric complications). The following were hypothesized to constitute negative general prognostic factors: (1) negative maternal life situation and poor external support for the pregnancy; (2) negative maternal attitude toward the pregnancy and/or the baby; (3) strong maternal fears regarding the near future; (4) active maternal mental disturbance during pregnancy; and (5) strongly experienced stress during pregnancy.

Analyses presented here compare the Index and Control groups on the data from the pregnancy interview, and thus address the question of whether the Index groups, as contrasted with the Controls, evidenced more of the hypothesized negative prognostic factors during pregnancy.

Labor, delivery, and early postnatal condition

The labor, delivery, and early postnatal condition of the subjects were studied both through medical records and through the personal, standardized observation by one project researcher (McNeil). Parental permission was obtained for this observation. The deliveries took place over a 4.5-year period at 11 hospitals in 11 different cities widely spread through the geographical area.

Among the 185 deliveries to mothers participating in the project, observation of the case was done before partus or within 2 hours postpartum in 83% (154/185) of the sample. The observer arrived in time for the delivery in 70% ($N = 130$) of the cases; in 17 additional cases, he arrived within 1 hour postpartum, and in 7 other cases between 1 and 2 hours postpartum.

Negative parental attitude toward the researcher's presence at the birth was strongly related to index status; 85% (11/13) of those who during pregnancy were either negative ($N = 5$) or somewhat uncertain regarding his presence ($N = 8$) were index cases, and the four mothers who did not allow the observer to enter into or remain in the delivery room after arriving at the hospital were all index cases.

The data regarding the births and immediate condition of the subjects are quite extensive, and will thus be presented elsewhere.

Neonatal neurological assessment

A neonatal neurological assessment was included in the current study because of previous findings suggesting the relevance of neurological deviation for the development of chronic schizophrenia as well as other forms of pathology.

The neurological assessment was developed for use in the project, with special consideration given to previous high-risk findings, and it comprises an integration of the items, techniques, and scoring systems from other research groups and projects. The methods, scoring systems and results are presented more extensively in Blennow and McNeil (1980). In addition to the common neurological assessment items such as reflexes, response patterns, and neurological syndromes, special attention was paid to muscle tone, changes in arousal and wakefulness, sensitivity to touch and stimulation, and activity level. The examiner was attentive to subtle neurological deviations that would not generally be of interest in ordinary clinical pediatric studies; such marginal or minor deviations were labeled and analyzed separately from certain, clear neurological abnormalities.

The examinations were conducted at the puerperal wards at 11 different hospitals by Blennow, an experienced pediatric neurologist. An attempt was made to examine the neonates on the third or fourth day after delivery and at about 2 hours after feeding. The practical circumstances attending the study and its subjects led to deviations from these optimal times in some cases, but such deviations appear to have had little effect on the results of the assessment. The examiner was blind as to the experimental and diagnostic status of the case, as well as to the case's obstetric history; this blindness was of special importance when engaging in a search for possible subtle deviations, because the risk for overdiagnosis exists.

In total, 126 neonates received neurological assessment, these representing 85% of the neonates intended for examination. Cases were missed for a variety of reasons, such as untimely discharge from the puerperal ward, failure of notification of the birth, and examiner unavailability.

For data analysis, Psychogenic Psychosis and Postpartum Psychosis were combined into one group, yielding the following offspring samples: Schizophrenia Index: $N = 13$, Control: $N = 19$; Cycloid Psychosis Index: $N = 12$, Control: $N = 15$; Affective Index: $N = 11$, Control: $N = 14$; Psychogenic/Postpartum Psychosis Index: $N = 10$, Control: $N = 16$; and Other Psychoses Index: $N = 9$, Control: $N = 7$. The total Index group thus consisted of 55 cases and the total Control group of 71 cases. The small group sample sizes and the relatively low frequency of clear neurological abnormality generally hindered meaningful calculation of the statistical significance of group comparisons; statistical significance was thus calculated when potentially meaningful, and results are otherwise generally presented in terms of percentages.

Temperamental evaluation of the offspring

One of the study's important measurement areas concerns offspring temperamental characteristics and response tendencies early in life. Measurement of infant/child temperament seemed especially appropriate for the project because Thomas and Chess's (1963, 1968) work had shown that dimensions of theoretical interest to the project (e.g., sensory threshold, approach, adaptability, distractibility) could be measured at an early age in all infants, and that temperament patterns identified early in the child's life appeared to have some predictive value for later mental disturbance. Carey's (1970) experience with constructing parental questionnaires for the effective measurement of offspring temperament served as the model in the current project, and three parental questionnaires were developed by project researchers for measurement of nine temperament characteristics (Thomas et al., 1963) in children at 6 months, 1 and 2 years of age (Persson-Blennow & McNeil, 1979, 1980). The questionnaires were tested on a demographically representative standardization sample and were found to be appropriate for all parents and to yield broad ranges and balanced distributions of scores on the temperament variables. Gender, birth order, and social class were found to have little influence on individual differences in temperament at these ages (Persson-Blennow & McNeil, 1981).

The three questionnaires were used in the current high-risk study and completed by the parents of 163 offspring ($N = 158$ at 6 months, 149 at 1 year, and 147 at 2 years).

Home visits and observations of mother–child interaction

Home visits were conducted by project researchers Näslund and Persson-Blennow on six occasions during the child's first year of life. The purpose of the visits was: (1) to observe longitudinally mother–child interaction; (2) to study the child's attachment to the mother and stranger anxiety at 1 year of age (these representing a measure of the child's emotional development); (3) to study the child's language and motoric development; and (4) to study the child's social environment during the first year of life.

It was hypothesized that attachment forms the basis for an individual's relationship to other people. The study of the development of the child's attachment to the mother was conducted through longitudinal observation of the interaction between mother and child, with special emphasis on what have been termed *attachment behaviors* (Ainsworth, 1964; Bowlby, 1970).

Experience in a pilot study (Näslund, Persson-Blennow, & McNeil, 1974) led to the development and refinement of an observation schedule consisting of 65 5-point scales for the study of mother–infant interaction in two observation situations, the feeding situation and the play situation.

The variables represented in the observation schedule were grouped into four categories, primarily on the basis of Ainsworth's work (1964): (1) mother's social behavior (e.g., smiling, eye contact, verbal contact); (2) child's social behavior (e.g., smiling, babbling, eye contact); (3) reciprocal behavior (e.g., smiling, eye contact, verbal contact); and (4) mother's sensitivity toward the child (e.g., sensitivity in feeding).

In addition to the study of the interactional and attachment variables by observation, the mothers were also interviewed at each visit regarding the child's physical health, eating and sleeping habits, and social and motoric development (in terms of developmental milestones). The way in which the mother experienced the child was also discussed.

The visits were made at the maternity ward at 3 days of age and at home at 3 weeks, 6 weeks, 3.5 months, 6 months, and 1 year of age, because those ages were considered interesting from a developmental and nurturance point of view. In the current project, 142 mother–child pairs (index and control combined) were observed at the visits at the maternity wards and in the home. Of the 852 planned visits, 749 (88%) were conducted. Missed visits were due in most cases to mental illness in the mother.

Stranger anxiety. The presence and strength of the child's stranger anxiety was studied upon the observer's arrival at the home at 1 year of age (per Schaffer & Emerson, 1964), and was defined in terms of the child's immediate reaction to the observer (e.g., fear, whining, whimpering, crying, active avoidance of the observer, clinging to the mother).

Attachment. The child's emotional relationship to the mother was studied in two standardized situations (by Ainsworth's method): (1) mother's separation from the child for a maximum of 3 minutes; and (2) reunion: mother's return. The child's score for total attachment to the mother was defined as the sum of the child's points from both situations.

The general hypotheses to be tested were that differences in the child's stranger anxiety and attachment to the mother should be found between Index and Control groups, and further that differences in attachment and stranger anxiety should exist among different Index diagnostic groups.

Vocabulary (Näslund & Persson-Blennow, 1979). The measure used for the child's verbal development was the mother's report of the child's vocabulary at 1 year of age, that is, the number of words used and which words they were. The range of scores for vocabulary within the entire sample was very large (0–15 words), and some children even used two-word sentences. On the basis of a grammatic and semantic analysis of the data collected, the children were categorized into three different language groups (Nelson, 1973): Those using primarily socially expressive language (familiar persons and animals, words for emotions and needs), object-oriented language (nonfamiliar things and animals), or action-describing language (activity and change). The hypothesis tested was that Index and Control groups would differ from one another on language development, both regarding vocabulary size and language form and content.

RESULTS

Pregnancy

External supports for the pregnancy. Index cases, as compared with controls, reported significantly and clearly less interpersonal support for the pregnancy; they had poorer relations with their husbands and parents, and these significant persons were more often negative toward the pregnancy. This was true for every Index diagnostic group, although for Affectives, this concerned a small proportion of subjects with a very bad situation. Index cases also had significantly more total external stresses, reflected in a generic score composed of reported problems with housing, finances, work, and a generally poor environment (bad town, living alone, etc.). These stresses were especially frequent for Schizophrenics, Psychogenics, and Other Psychotics.

Attitude toward the pregnancy. Highly significantly more index (33%) than control (9%) reported having not intended to become pregnant. The mother's initial reaction upon learning she was pregnant was significantly more often reported as negative in index (16%) than control (3%). Those Index diagnostic groups showing the most frequent negative initial reaction were Psychogenics (33%), Other Psychotics (24%), and Schizophrenics (19%). Fourteen mothers reported having considered a legal abortion, and 10 of these were index cases (all diagnostic categories except Postpartum Psychotics). Significantly more index cases reported the pregnancy as currently unwelcome or unpleasant at the time of the interview, and this was especially true for Psychogenic Psychotics (50%) and Schizophrenics (24%). Clear and unmistakable denial of pregnancy was found in only five cases in the total sample, all of these being index cases (two Schizophrenics, one Affective, two Other Psychotics).

Fears about the near future. More than one-third of the total sample reported no fear at all about the coming delivery, and this did not differ for index and control samples. Significantly more index (20%) than control (7%) mothers reported being panicked about the delivery; differentially high rates of panic were found in Schizophrenics (31%), Other Psychotics (35%), Psychogenics (33%), and, to a lesser extent, Postpartum Psychotics (22%). In contrast, as many controls as index mothers (57%) reported being very worried or panicked about whether the baby would be malformed, damaged, or ill in some way. Significantly more index (19%) than control mothers (3%) reported being concerned about their own mental health in the near future, and not surprisingly the Postpartum Psychotics were the subjects expressing the most concern about this (44%). No significant difference was found in the proportion of index (30%) and control (23%) women expressing concern about being a good mother to the coming child.

Table 3. *General Psychopathology Scale*

Category 1. Healthy. Has no known symptoms. Functions well in all respects.
Category 2. Functions well and without symptoms, but when stressed, shows occasional isolated signs of disturbance.
Category 3. Mild symptoms in nonstressing situations, or many symptoms in stressing situations.
Category 4. In nonstressing situations, symptoms that are troublesome. Is sometimes considered as deviant or sick by those around him/her. More or worse symptoms than in Category 3.
Category 5. Clear mental symptoms serious enough to occupy a dominant place in person's life. Normal functions interfered with or thrust aside.
Category 6. Grave psychiatric disturbances that completely dominate life for the present. Cannot adequately take care of him/herself.
Category 7. Very seriously ill, insight lacking, out of contact.

Active psychiatric disturbance. The mother's mental status both near the interview and during the entire pregnancy was judged by the interviewer based on information from the interview, with supplemental information from the second pregnancy interview regarding the later pregnancy period. This evaluation was expressed in terms of the 7-point general psychopathology scale (Table 3) used in previous research (McNeil, Persson-Blennow, & Kaij, 1974). As contrasted with controls, index women were significantly more often judged as disturbed at a Category 4–6 level, both near the time of the interview (35% for index versus 3% for control) and for the worst time during pregnancy (39% for index versus 4% for control). Disturbance at a Category 4–6 level (worst time) showed the following rates in the specific diagnostic groups: Schizophrenics, 65%; Psychogenics, 50%; Other Psychotics, 47%; Postpartum Psychotics, 39%; Cycloids, 20%; and Affectives, 13%. Most of the 13 different psychiatric symptoms or characteristics judged in the interview (e.g., anxiety, withdrawal, aggressiveness, suspiciousness, disordered thought, confusion, somatization, passivity, and irresponsibility toward the pregnancy) discriminated index subjects from controls quite clearly.

An entirely separate judgment of mental disturbance during pregnancy was obtained through the index subjects' psychiatric records, as judged by Kaij; 36% of the 88 index cases had been in contact with a psychiatric unit during pregnancy, 9% had been psychiatrically hospitalized sometime during pregnancy, and 15% were judged by Kaij to have been psychotic during pregnancy, about half of these latter representing Schizophrenics who were chronically psychotic. Based on psychiatric record information, 16 (18%) of the 88 index cases could be judged as disturbed at a Category 4–7 level during pregnancy; 14 of the 16 belonged to Endogenous Psychoses groups.

Health during pregnancy. A generic score representing extent and amount of usual pregnancy complaints (fatigue, nausea, sleep difficulties, dizziness, heartburn, varicose veins, etc.), as reported in the interview, was calculated both including and excluding typical psychological complaints of depression and uneasiness/anxiety. When these psychological complaints were excluded from the generic score, very little difference was found between the index and control subjects. With their inclusion, the Index group showed a nonsignificant trend toward reporting more typical pregnancy complaints. Heavy smoking during pregnancy was clearly related to index status and to degree of psychological disturbance.

The mothers were asked about any change experienced in their physical and in their mental health due to the pregnancy. Changes in physical health as a result of pregnancy showed little difference between Index and Control groups; about half of both total Index and Control groups experienced no change whereas one-third in each group felt a little worse than usual. The experience of the pregnancy's effect on mental health showed only a slight increase of much better health for index subjects (9%) as compared with controls (6%). If one looks at only those index subjects experiencing a change in mental status as a result of pregnancy, then more improvement than worsening was found for Cycloids (40% of the group improved versus 20% worsened) and for Affectives (33% better versus 20% worse). In contrast, worsening of mental health was more frequent in Schizophrenics (59% worse versus 29% better), Psychogenics (83% worse versus 17% better), Postpartum Psychotics (44% versus 22%), and Other Psychotics (47% versus 29%). These data do not confirm previous reports of improved mental condition during pregnancy for schizophrenics.

Follow-up interview. A shorter follow-up interview was conducted by research staff midwives in the third trimester in association with the study of fetal heart-rate responsivity. The purpose of the interview was to obtain information regarding the mother's attitude toward and experience of the pregnancy at its later stage. Again, the index subjects showed little difference from the controls on maternal report of physical health, but the index subjects still reported worse mental health and were judged by the interviewer as more often having active mental disturbance and as showing specific psychiatric symptoms such as anxiety, withdrawal, disordered thought, and confusion.

The results from both pregnancy interviews clearly support the conclusion that index women have an increased frequency of the characteristics that were hypothesized to constitute negative prognostic factors for later parent–child relations and child development, both psychologically and physically.

Postpartum psychiatric disturbance of the mothers

We evaluated psychiatric disturbance in the current postpartum period for women who had had psychiatric disturbance *prior* to entering the project during the current pregnancy. The Postpartum Psychosis diagnostic group thus had been psychotic in association with previous deliveries.

The standardized conduct of the research program during the postpartum period (defined as the first 6 months after birth) was often disturbed by psychiatric hospitalization of the mothers, and systematic study (by Kaij) of the psychiatric records of all 88 index subjects who began participation during pregnancy (Table 1) showed that 50% were either psychiatrically hospitalized or in contact with a psychiatric unit during the current postpartum period, this being true for more than 50% of each of the Schizophrenic, Cycloid, and Affective Index groups. Psychiatric hospitalization during this period was found for 26% of the total Index group, and was highest in the Cycloid (40%) and Affective (40%) groups, followed by the Schizophrenics (24%). The rate of psychiatric hospitalization was about 17% in each of the Psychogenic, Postpartum, and Other Psychoses groups.

Whether hospitalized or not, 32% of the total Index group were judged by Kaij to be psychotic during the postpartum period. These psychotic conditions represented acute episodes for all subjects except Schizophrenics, for whom seven of the eight psychotic conditions found after the delivery represented chronic conditions. Psychotic condition postpartum was found at high rates in the Schizophrenics (47%), Cycloids (47%), and Affectives (40%); lower rates were found for Other Psychotic (24%), Psychogenic Psychotic (0%), and (previous) Postpartum Psychotic (17%) groups.

Judgment of severity of disturbance after delivery was done for cases where sufficient psychiatric record information existed, and severity was expressed in terms of the 7-point general psychopathology scale (Table 3). In the total index sample, 27% were known to be disturbed at a Category 5–7 level, and 17% were known to be disturbed at a Category 6–7 level. The Cycloids represented the specific diagnostic type which showed the highest rate of serious postpartum disturbance, one-third of the Cycloid sample being at a Category 6–7 level.

In contrast, none of the 104 control cases was known to be psychotic or psychiatrically hospitalized during the postpartum period. The risk for psychosis during the postpartum period was thus much greater for women with histories of psychosis, the risk for postpartum episodes with acute onset being greatest for Cycloid and Affective Psychosis groups.

Neonatal functioning

Clear neurological abnormality was found infrequently. In the total sample, 69% of the neonates were clinically judged as having no neurological abnormality, 21% had suspicious but not certain deviation, and 10% were clearly neurologically abnormal. The total Index group was not significantly different from the total Control group in these evaluations. Similar comparisons showed only slight elevations in the rates of abnormality for offspring of Schizophrenics and Cycloids, but not among the other groups.

A rather coarse neurological deviation score (based on total points for simple and complex reflexes, motoric movement, activity level, and sensitivity to touch) showed that those neonates evidencing the most neurological deviation tended to be index cases (13%) rather than controls (6%).

These rates of deviation were also reflected in the frequency of clear neurological syndromes, which were found in 13% of index cases and 7% of controls. The most notable diagnostic group here was Cycloid Index, one-third of whose babies had at least one clear syndrome.

Although the sample sizes were rather small and the frequency of clear neurological abnormality rather low in the total sample, the results seem to point consistently in the same direction. True neurological abnormality, and especially that shown by the most deviant neonates in the total sample, was more frequent in the Index than in the Control groups; the Index diagnostic group that was most noteworthy for clear neurological abnormality was the offspring of the Cycloids, followed by the offspring of the Schizophrenics and the Other Psychotics. Neurological abnormality was not in any sense unique for index subjects, the Affectives' Controls showing a comparatively high rate of clear abnormality.

Interpretation of these results involves three important questions, which are being studied with the data which have been and are currently being collected: What is the real origin of these neurological abnormalities? What effect, if any, do they have on the neonate's immediate social environment? What do these neurological abnormalities indicate or signal for the later psychological and physical development of the individual neonates who were neurologically abnormal?

Temperament of the offspring. The total sample (index and control combined) generally showed very little difference from the previously studied demographically representative standardization sample (Persson-Blennow & McNeil, 1979; 1980) on the means and standard deviations for the nine temperament variables and on the frequency of temperament types (Difficult Child, Slow-to-Warm-up Child, etc.).

Comparison of the total Index versus Control groups on the temperament *variables* showed small and generally nonsignificant differences (two significant among 27 comparisons). Few statistically significant differences between specific diagnostic groups and their controls were found on group mean scores for the temperament variables, and these differences were inconsistent over the three measurement ages. A nonsignificant trend of theoretical interest was that, at every age, the offspring of Schizophrenics showed a lower stimulus threshold than did their matched Control group (based on group mean score).

In contrast, the comparison of specific diagnostic groups versus their controls on the frequency of the temperament *typologies* appeared to separate the offspring of the Schizophrenics and the Cycloids from those of the other diagnostic groups. Whereas the offspring of the other diagnostic groups evidenced no differences or even a somewhat lower rate of Difficult and Slow-to-Warm-up types, as compared with their controls, the offspring of the Schizophrenic and Cycloid mothers (as compared with their controls) showed differentially higher rates of the Difficult Child type and of the Slow-to-Warm-up type.

Stranger anxiety and attachment. The preliminary results showed no significant differences between the total Index and total Control groups either on scores for attachment or for stranger anxiety. In contrast, comparison of the specific diagnostic groups with their controls showed that the offspring of Schizophrenics and

Cycloids more often showed a low degree of reaction at separation (30% and 33% for Schizophrenic and Cycloid versus 10% and 17% for Controls), as well as no sign at all of stranger anxiety (70% and 67% for Schizophrenic and Cycloid versus 29% and 22% for Controls).

Language development. No significant differences were found between the Index groups and the Controls on group mean for size of the child's vocabulary. The standard deviation of scores was higher in the Endogenous Psychoses Index groups than in the matched Control groups, suggesting a greater range of scores within those Index groups. The six children who still said no words by 1 year of age were equally divided between Index and Control groups.

Results of the grammatic and semantic analysis showed that only seven children belonged to the Object-Oriented Language group. Of these seven, five (71%) were index cases (three offspring of Schizophrenics, one of a Cycloid, and one of an Other Psychotic). Index children also more often belonged to the Socially Expressive Language group than did control children, whereas control children more often belonged to the Action-Describing Language group. The hypothesis regarding differences between Index and Control groups in size of the children's vocabulary was thus not supported, but the hypothesis of differences in language group membership was supported.

DISCUSSION

The pregnancies of the index mothers, as compared with those of the controls, were considerably more negative and stressful. The diagnostic groups with especially stressful pregnancies were the Schizophrenics, the Psychogenics, and the Other Psychotics.

Index cases more often than controls were judged by interviewers as being actively mentally disturbed during pregnancy, the Schizophrenics, Psychogenics, and Other Psychotics showing the highest rates of disturbance. About 15% of the index subjects were independently classified from psychiatric records as psychotic at some time during the pregnancy.

Active mental disturbance during the postpartum period was highly frequent among the index mothers, with 26% of the total Index group psychiatrically hospitalized and 32% judged to be psychotic (from psychiatric records). Disturbance was most frequent among the Schizophrenics, Cycloids, and Affectives, with disturbance of a very serious degree most frequent among the Cycloids.

Regarding the characteristics of the offspring, neonatal neurological abnormality was more frequent in the total Index than in the Control group, and the Index group which was most noteworthy for clear neurological abnormality was the offspring of the Cycloids, followed by the offspring of the Schizophrenics and the Other Psychotics. Index offspring differed little from controls on most temperament characteristics, but the offspring of the Schizophrenics and the Cycloids (as compared with Controls) showed differentially higher rates of the Difficult Child and Slow-to-Warm-up types. Again, these same offspring groups showed a low degree of reaction to separation from the mother at 1 year of age and no sign of stranger anxiety.

Research context and future plans

Our current efforts in data analysis are aimed at comparing Index (High-Risk) and Control (Low-Risk) groups on the separate study areas described earlier, as well as on other areas included in the project's first phase. These comparisons may be put into perspective by remembering that results of the comparison of High-Risk and Low-Risk groups on personal and environmental variables are most appropriately interpreted as relevant to the characteristics, correlates and consequences of the risk criterion; observed differences between High-Risk and Low-Risk groups, like those reported, are thus not necessarily of etiological significance for the deviation and illness to develop in the subjects in the future (McNeil & Kaij, 1979).

The next analytic strategy to be employed concerns the study of relationships among different study areas, both those which are contemporaneous (e.g., the relationship between mother's experience of pregnancy and the existence of somatic pregnancy complications) and those which can be placed in a stepwise *developmental* sequence (e.g., maternal attitude toward the pregnancy, related to maternal response to the baby at birth, related to mother–child interaction at 6 months of age, related to the child's attachment to the mother at 1 year of age). These analyses can potentially yield theoretically relevant findings regarding both parental- and child-developmental phenomena. However, even when these sequences differ significantly between Index and Control groups, the differences are not necessarily of etiological relevance for disturbance which may develop in the subjects in the future.

Data of this kind, whether sequential or not, become potentially etiologically relevant when studied in relation to the subjects' health status after a subgroup has developed deviations and abnormality of interest to the study (McNeil & Kaij, 1979). Follow-up of the subjects to the age of breakdown is thus essential, if the purpose of the study is to yield information on etiological factors. Furthermore, although abnormality or disturbance of primary interest to such studies may lie far in the future, shorter follow-up periods may nevertheless be of considerable value in identifying the antecedents of specified intermediate disturbances developed by given age periods prior to the long-term follow-up of primary value.

37 *The early development of children born to mentally ill women*

ARNOLD J. SAMEROFF, RALPH BAROCAS, AND
RONALD SEIFER

Schizophrenia has generated over the years the largest body of research on functional mental disturbances. Where most other disorders can be viewed as extreme variations of some normal psychological characteristics, schizophrenia has been striking in its extreme divergence from typical modes of functioning.

Although broadly stated constitutional and environmental perspectives on schizophrenia have produced impressive statistics supporting their positions, they have not yielded the specific etiologies required to fully understand the disorder. Taken alone these two perspectives are not thought to have much explanatory power (Rosenthal, 1970). A variety of more complex models have been proposed by Sameroff and Zax (1978). Whether one conceives of a constitutional factor as producing some form of schizophrenia in every carrier or merely predisposing the carrier toward schizophrenia, one must be able to identify some unique difference between such individuals and their peers. Similarly, whether one considers an environmental factor as producing schizophrenia in any individual raised in that environment or merely acting as a predisposing agent, one must be able to identify some unique characteristic of that environment.

From a purely constitutional perspective the age at which the high-risk children are first studied is irrelevant, because the defect will be a developmental constant. The only purpose for beginning a study with young infants would be in the service of earlier detection. On the other hand, if one has concerns about environmental etiological factors, finding group differences in adolescence would reveal little about the development of those differences. Whether they were a function of some constitutional variable or the consequence of living with deranged parents for an extended time period would be unclear. In order to elucidate the relevant contributors of both constitution and environment one must begin the research effort when the children are as young as possible. In most cases this would be the period of infancy.

As younger and younger children are studied it becomes more difficult to make hypothesized connections between the behaviors that can be studied and the behaviors of mentally ill adult patients. For example, the thought disorder that characterizes a diagnosis of schizophrenia is difficult to assess in a child or infant who has not yet begun to think. Similarly, social competencies are difficult to assess in young children for whom parents provide the interface between the child and the rest of the environment.

482

Indeed, the last two decades have produced a variety of new measures and approaches for examining the behavior of young children. Many of the infant behaviors currently of interest were not recognized as being at all relevant until recently. Examples of such measures are the Neonatal Behavioral Assessment Scales (Brazelton, 1973), the "strange" situation of Ainsworth (1973), and new intellectual assessments such as the Ordinal Scales of Development (Uzgiris & Hunt, 1975). Family interaction variables had long been implicated in the study of schizophrenia (Goldstein & Rodnick, 1975), but it has only been recently that such studies have become common for young infants and their families (Moss, 1967; Osofsky & Connors, 1979). Even such areas as personality and adaptive behavior have been extended downward in work on temperament (Thomas, Chess, & Birch, 1968) and competency assessments (Jones, 1977; Seifer, Sameroff, & Jones, 1981).

These developments that enlarge the possibility for assessing early development of children offered unique opportunities for seeking the vulnerabilities in special populations such as the children-at-risk considered here. From these measures it was possible to examine characteristics of the child, the caretaking environment, and the interaction between the two throughout early development. The particular measures used in the study will be detailed in the methodology section to follow.

ROCHESTER LONGITUDINAL STUDY

The Rochester Longitudinal Study (RLS) was begun in 1970 to investigate the early development of children at risk for later mental disorder because of maternal psychopathology. Two features of this study set it apart from previous high-risk research. First, the study did not restrict itself to a comparison of Schizophrenic and Normal groups of parents; it also directly examined the effects of variables correlated with parental schizophrenia on the development of children. These variables included severity and chronicity of mental illness, independent of psychiatric diagnosis, and social status. Second, the study was a prospective longitudinal investigation, which began during the mother's pregnancy so that the child could be examined immediately after birth and then continuously through early childhood (Sameroff & Zax, 1973a, 1973b, 1978; Zax, Sameroff, & Babigian, 1977).

SUBJECTS

The names of women who were to deliver at a local hospital were checked against a psychiatric register (Gardner, Miles, Iker, & Romano, 1963). Potential subjects were identified from the register, particularly those who had been diagnosed as schizophrenic or neurotic depressive, and also those who had no evidence of prior mental illness. A stratified Control group was also recruited whose names did not appear on the psychiatric register. Women were selected from the obstetrical waiting list at the hospital who matched the psychiatric sample in age, race, SES, marital status, and number of children. Initial intake of the sample began in 1970 and extended over a 3 year period. The last infant was seen at the 48-month assessment in 1978.

Table 1. *Comparison of diagnostic makeup of Rochester Longitudinal Study sample with county psychiatric register*

Diagnosis	Rochester Longitudinal Study (%)[a]		1972 County psychiatric register (%)	
Schizophrenia	29	(16.4)	3834	(20.8)
Schizophrenic-Spectrum	9	(5.1)	419	(2.3)
Neurotic Depression	59	(33.3)	4860	(26.4)
Other Neuroses	17	(9.6)	2582	(14.0)
Personality Disorders	40	(22.6)	3717	(20.2)
Situational Reactions	23	(13.0)	3009	(16.3)
Total	177	(100)	18431	(100)

Note: The percentages for study subjects who appeared in the registry were virtually identical to the percentages of all subjects in the study.
[a]Based on information from prenatal interview only.
Source: Adapted from Zax et al., 1977.

Table 2. *Demographic characteristics of matched diagnostic groups*

	No Mental Illness (*N* = 57)	Schizophrenia (*N* = 29)	Depression (*N* = 58)	Personality Disorders (*N* = 40)
Socioeconomic status	4.01	4.20	3.87	4.02
Mother education (years)	11.74	11.24	11.47	11.48
Mother age (years)[a]	24.10	26.70	24.30	22.40
Race (% black)	.53	.28	.41	.43
Sex (% female)	.37	.52	.43	.48
Parity (% first child)	.23	.31	.22	.28
Mother married (%)	.79	.59	.57	.63

[a]ANOVA $p < .05$.

After recruitment into the study, diagnostic interviews, guided by the Current and Past Psychopathology Scales (CAPPS) of Spitzer and Endicott (1969), were given. Reliability checks of the diagnostic procedure revealed high agreement on major diagnostic category among the three experienced clinicians who interviewed all of the subjects (Sameroff and Zax, 1973a). All interviews were conducted without prior knowledge of whether the subject was listed in the psychiatric register.

Diagnostic determinations and group assignments were based on a combination of the prenatal clinical interview and a second interview when the infants reached 30 months of age, plus the data from the psychiatric registry both prenatally and during the ensuing 2.5 years. Data were collected on a total of 337 mothers. Diagnostically, they were distributed as described in Table 1. Note that besides schizophrenia and depression, several other diagnoses were represented in the total sample. Schizophrenic-spectrum cases were those diagnosed as schizoid or inadequate personality disorders. The personality disorders category included all personality disorders other than those falling on the schizophrenic spectrum. It will be noted in Table 1 that total figures for the local psychiatric register yield percentages in each diagnostic category that conform closely to the percentages in our sample. Thus, our sample of subjects seems quite representative of the total registry area population who sought help for emotional problems.

For diagnostic comparisons four groups, totaling 184 subjects, were identified: a Schizophrenic group (*N* = 29); a Neurotically Depressed group (*N* = 58); a Personality Disorder group (*N* = 40); and a Control group free of mental disorder of any kind (*N* = 57). The Control group was selected to match the psychiatric groups for the average values on the variables listed in Table 2. The diagnostic comparison was limited to the 184 women in these four groups. The remaining women received other diagnoses (none of which were frequent enough to comprise a comparison group), or they were No-Mental-Illness controls who did not match with the diagnostic groups on demographic factors. These remaining women were included in severity of illness, chronicity of illness, and social status comparisons described.

Severity and chronicity ratings

In addition to a diagnosis each woman in the study received a severity of illness and chronicity of illness rating. The severity score was based on information obtained at each of the two diagnostic interviews that resulted in rating of overall pathology. The final scale consisted of four points: (1) women who had no evidence of illness; (2) women who had low; (3) moderate; and (4) high severity of pathology. The chronicity rating was not based on any dimension of illness, but on the frequency of psychiatric contact. Again there were four groups: (1) those women who received no diagnosis by our clinicians and did not appear in the registry; (2) those who had one diagnosis by us or in the registry; (3) those who were diagnosed by us *and* appeared in the registry on one to three occasions; and (4) those who had four or more previous contacts and/or long hospitalization.

Social status

Information was collected from each mother concerning socioeconomic status (SES), race, age, marital history, and pregnancy and child-bearing history. SES was computed using a variation of the Hollingshead (1957) two factor index of social position. In addition to the original scoring that included only the father's occupation and education, we also used the mother's education in computing the SES level.

The SES was categorized in Hollingshead's five social classes with I being the highest and V the lowest. Whereas white subjects ranged across all SES levels, the black subjects fell predominantly into the two lowest SES groups. To control for this unequal distribution, race and SES were used to form three groups: (1) a High-SES White group from SES levels I, II, and III; (2) a Low-SES White group from levels IV and V; and (3) a Low-SES Black group from levels IV and V. Thus, SES effects could be tested by comparing the two white groups, and race effects by comparing the two lower SES groups.

PROCEDURES AND MEASURES

Prenatal assessment of mother

All mothers were interviewed while in their final month of pregnancy. In addition to undergoing diagnostic interviews described above, each subject filled out two pencil-and-paper test instruments: the anxiety scale from the IPAT (Cattell & Scheier, 1963) and the Maternal Attitudes to Pregnancy Instrument (MAPI; Blau, Welkowitz, & Cohen, 1964). The IPAT anxiety scale consists of 40 items reflecting current feelings of anxiety; each item is scored 0, 1, or 2 with high scores indicating high anxiety. The MAPI presents 48 statements with which the subject must express strong agreement, agreement, disagreement, or strong disagreement; items receive scores weighted from 1 to 4, depending upon whether the factor loading is positive or negative, with a high score reflecting positive attitudes.

A social incompetence score (Fox, 1975) was calculated for each mother based on the sum of six measures, taken from the CAPPS and hospital records, similar to those used by Zigler and Phillips (1962). These measures included: (1) highest level of adult heterosexual adjustment over a sustained period of time; (2) adult friendship pattern during the last 5 years; (3) an estimate of role impairment in relationship with a spouse or someone the subject had been living with in a housekeeping relationship; (4) age of first contact where a pathological diagnosis was applied; (5) age of first hospitalization where a pathological diagnosis was applied; and (6) total number of contacts and hospitalizations.

Birth process

The course of the mother's pregnancy, the delivery, and the condition of the newborn were assessed using the Research Obstetric Scale (ROS) developed at the University of Rochester (Zax et al., 1977). Earlier reviews of the long-term effect of prenatal and perinatal complications had found little evidence for specific complications leading to specific risks. Parmelee and Haber (1973) have argued that using multiple criteria combined into single scores would increase the predictive potential of perinatal variables. Parmelee and associates (Beckwith, Cohen, & Parmelee, 1973) revised an earlier Prechtl (1968) Scale for use in the United States, and the Rochester Research Obstetric Scale (ROS) was based on these two versions. The ROS consists of 27 items, 6 items in a Prenatal Scale evaluating the mother's pregnancy, 13 items in a Delivery Scale evaluating labor and delivery factors, and 8 items in an Infant Scale evaluating the condition of the newborn. The items were adjusted to United States standards of obstetrical treatment using norms derived from a collaborative study of 40,000 pregnancies (Niswander & Gordon, 1972).

During the last day in the hospital, when the infants were between 48 and 72 hours old, they were brought to a laboratory where assessments were made of autonomic functioning, that is, heart rate, respiratory rate, and sucking; and of behavioral responses using Brazelton's (1973) Neonatal Behavioral Assessment Scales, which consisted of items ranging from neurological reflexes to alertness. Finally, using a scale developed by Waldrop, Pederson, and Bell (1968), we examined the infants for minor physical anomalies that have been associated with chromosomal abnormalities, particularly Down syndrome.

Four-month assessment

At 4 months of age, intensive 4- to 6-hour naturalistic observations of the mother and infant interaction were undertaken in the home. Based on the work of Moss (1967), 64 variables were assessed at 60-second intervals for the 4-month observations; 73 variables were assessed every 20 seconds at the 12-month observation.

These variables described the state and position of both the infant and the mother, the background stimulation during the observation, and the spontaneous and interactive behaviors of both mother and child. This approach was chosen because it provided a comprehensive picture of the mother–child interaction that could be collected reliably in the widely varying home environments of the families in our study.

The data from each observation were summarized to provide the proportion of time the mother or infant engaged in any activity. Scales were created based on factor analyses that indexed, in the mother and infant, the degree of spontaneous behavior, responsive behavior, positive affect, negative affect, proximity, movement, and physical contact.

The child was then tested in the laboratory using the Bayley Scales of Infant Development that produced a Mental Development Index (MDI) and a Psycho-motor Developmental Index (PDI). In addition, the social and emotional behaviors of the infant were scored by the examiner on the Bayley Infant Behavior Rating Scale (IBR). The Bayley Scales represented the state of the art in developmental assessment during infancy at the time of this study.

The mother completed the Carey (1970) Infant Temperament Questionnaire. This instrument produces nine scales of infant behavior: activity, rhythmicity, adaptability, approach (versus withdrawal), threshold to stimulation, intensity of response, mood, distractibility (really soothability when upset), and persistence. Infant temperament was measured because it is an analog of later personality, and because it has been proposed as an important component in the development of parent–child relationships (Thomas et al., 1968).

Twelve-month assessment

Observations similar to those at 4 months were made in the home again when the infants were 12 months of age. In the laboratory, the psychometric testing was repeated as were the IBR observations of the testing session. We administered an additional test, the Uzgiris–Hunt (1975) Scale for Visual Pursuit and the Permanence of Objects, that measures development of the concept of a permanent object, as described by Piaget. Also during this laboratory session social differentiation and maternal attachment were evaluated using the procedures developed by Ainsworth (1973) in which the mother plays with her child, a stranger enters and leaves, the mother leaves and then returns for a final reunion episode. This procedure has been useful in differentiating styles of infant emotional response to disruptions in the normal flow of caretaking relations.

Thirty-month assessment

The mother and child were evaluated separately during the 30-month assessment, the child to be tested and the mother to be interviewed. The testing included the Bayley Scales and IBR observations, the Peabody Picture Vocabulary Test (PPVT), and the vocabulary scale from the Stanford–Binet. The mother's interview included the Rochester Adaptive Behavior Inventory (RABI), which is a detailed, behavior-specific, maternal report of the child's behavior (Seifer et al., 1981), and a social and medical history of the family covering the past 30 months. The mother completed the Parental Attitude Research Instrument (PARI), a measure of parenting attitudes (Schaefer & Bell, 1958) yielding scales for authoritarian control, hostility–rejection, and democratic attitude. She also completed the Parent Estimate of Development Scale, or PEDS (Heriot & Schmickel, 1967), yielding estimated IQ in terms of mental age, general description, occupation, education, and total, as well as the Vineland Social Maturity Scale (Doll, 1965). The mother returned alone for a second session that was a repeat of the initial prenatal clinical interview to determine if any changes had occurred in her emotional status.

Forty-eight-month assessment

The mother and child were again brought to the laboratory where we made a more elaborate assessment of the mother in terms of her orientation to child rearing and the world in general. She was interviewed with the RABI to assess the child's competence, and she completed a child temperament questionnaire that yielded the nine scales described for the questionnaire used at 4 months (Thomas & Chess, 1977). In addition to these reports of child behavior, the mother was assessed with a variation of the Rotter I–E scale (yielding scales pertaining to easy versus difficult world and predictability of events), the Kohn (1969) parental values measure (yielding a conformity score), the Eysenck and Eysenck (1969) personality scales (Neuroticism and Extraversion), the Crowne and Marlowe (1960) social desirability scale (yielding positive, negative, and total scales), and our Concepts of Development Questionnaire (Feil & Sameroff, 1979) that has (in order of developmental sophistication) symbiotic, categorical, compensating, and perspectivistic scales.

The child's performance was assessed with the verbal scales of the WPPSI IQ, the Peabody Picture Vocabulary Test, plus two experimental procedures. These procedures evaluated the child's attentional processes in a Delayed Match-to-Sample task (Ostrow, 1980), and self-regulation and attention in a Luria bulb-squeezing task (Barocas & Sameroff, 1982). The examiner for psychometric testing filled out the Bayley IBR form.

Other procedures were administered that are not discussed in this chapter because data have not been fully analyzed. These include social-medical histories of the family taken at 30 and 48 months, a maternal teaching task done with the child at 48 months, and the Cook–Gumperz (1973) assessment of parental control-style administered at 48 months. A summary of RLS procedures can be found in Table 3.

RESULTS

This report presents cross-sectional analysis of group differences for Diagnosis, Severity of Illness, Chronicity of Illness, and Social Status. The data from longitudinal analysis and intercorrelations among measures are still being analyzed and

Table 3. *Rochester Longitudinal Study measures*

Age	Mother	Child	Interaction
Prenatal	CAPPS—psychiatric interview IPAT—anxiety scale MAPI—pregnancy attitudes Psychiatric registry		
Newborn		NBAS—neonatal status Minor physical anomalies Autonomic levels ROS—obstetric records	
4 months		Bayley Scales Infant temperament questionnaire Infant behavior record	Home observations
12 months		Bayley Scales Mother–infant attachment Object Permanence Scale Infant behavior record	Home observations
30 months	CAPPS—psychiatric interview IPAT—anxiety scale PARI—parent attitudes PEDS—estimate of development Psychiatry registry	Bayley Scales Stanford–Binet Verbal RABI—adaptive behavior Vineland Social Maturity Infant behavior record	
48 months	Concepts of development Kohn–parental values Parenting styles Malaise Scale Social desirability Eysenck personality I–E Scale	WPPSI—verbal Peabody IQ Delayed Match-to-Sample Luria verbal regulation RABI Child temperament Verbal production	Teaching style

will not be presented here. Some of these analyses of portions of RLS data have been reported elsewhere (Sameroff, Seifer, & Elias, 1982; Seifer et al., 1981; Seifer & Sameroff, 1982).

Three analyses of variance were performed on each dependent measure: (1) one-way ANOVA for diagnosis; (2) two-way ANOVA for Severity of Illness and Social Status; and (3) two-way ANOVA for Chronicity of Illness and Social Status. The latter two indices of mental illness, Severity and Chronicity, were crossed with Social Status because they were not matched for SES and race, as was diagnosis.

The following effects among subsets of groups were examined. For the diagnosis ANOVAs the No-Mental-Illness group was contrasted with each of the three illness groups: Schizophrenia, Depression, and Personality Disorder. For the Severity and Chronicity factors in the two-way ANOVAs, two comparisons were made. First, the lowest Severity or Chronicity group was compared with the remaining three. Second, linear effects were examined. Finally, for the Social Status factor in the two-way ANOVAs, three comparisons were made: first, contrasting the Upper- and Lower-SES Whites; second, contrasting the Lower-SES Whites and Blacks; and third, contrasting the extreme groups – Upper-SES Whites with Lower-SES Blacks. SES effects from the Severity by Social Status and Chronicity by Social Status analyses were identical.

In general, interactions were not present in the two-way ANOVAs for Severity or Chronicity by Social Status at a level greater than expected by chance. The interpretation of the main effects were straightforward, even in the presence of the very few interactions found. Therefore, only the main effects and related group contrasts for Severity, Chronicity, and Social Status are presented in the tables and discussed in the text.

Adoption and foster placement

When the data from the newborn assessment were examined an interesting finding regarding adoption and foster placement emerged. Six of the infants in the study were given up by their mothers during the neonatal period for either adoption or foster placement. An analysis of these six cases was thought to be of interest for interpreting the studies that have shown higher rates of psychopathology in the adopted offspring of schizophrenic women when compared to the adopted offspring of normal women.

The six infants given up in our study all came from schizophrenic women. No mother in any of the other diagnostic groups gave up a child in the newborn period. Comparisons between the characteristics of the 23 schizophrenic mothers who kept their infants and the six mothers who gave up their infants for placement in either adoptive ($N = 3$) or foster homes ($N = 3$) are listed in Table 4.

The Placement group mothers were significantly older and of lower SES than those keeping their children. Neither birth order nor race were reliably different for the two groups. Not unexpectedly, a greater proportion of the Placement mothers were either single, separated, or divorced than Home-rearing group

Table 4. *Social and mental health characteristics of schizophrenic mothers*

	Home-rearing	Placement
Number	23	6
Age (years)***	25.0	33.2
Socioeconomic status**	4.0	5.0
Birth order		
First born	6 (26%)	3 (50%)
Late born	17 (74%)	3 (50%)
Race		
White	17 (74%)	4 (67%)
Nonwhite	6 (26%)	2 (33%)
Marital status*		
Married	16 (70%)	1 (17%)
Single, separated, or divorced	7 (30%)	5 (83%)
Social incompetency*	31.9	36.5
Severity (CAPPS)***	2.9	4.5
Anxiety (CAPPS)***	2.5	4.0
Anxiety (IPAT)	38.4	41.8
Chronicity*		
Hospitalized > 6 mo.	8 (35%)	5 (83%)
Hospitalized < 6 mo.	10 (43%)	1 (17%)
Not hospitalized	5 (22%)	0 (0%)

*$p < .05$.   **$p < .01$.   ***$p < .001$.

mothers. Comparisons of the Home-rearing and Placement groups on mental health measures indicate that the six Placement mothers were more socially incompetent, were judged to have been more anxious and severely disturbed when interviewed in their last month of pregnancy, and had longer histories of emotional disturbance than Home-rearing mothers.

The prenatal and newborn condition of the infants given up for placement was compared with the condition of the Home-reared infants (see Table 5). The course of the pregnancy and the condition of the infants was worse for the Placement group. Their mothers had significantly more illnesses during pregnancy, their infants had more problems after birth, and the infants were significantly lighter in birth weight. Not one of the six Placement babies was over 2,800 g at birth, and four of these six spent their newborn period in the special care nursery.

These findings indicate that schizophrenic mothers in our sample who gave up their infants for adoption or foster placement were not a random sample of schizophrenic mothers. This contradicts at least one basic assumption of adoption studies. These mothers were, instead, a selected sample of severely and chronically disturbed women, who were older and less likely to be in an intact marriage than those schizophrenic mothers who chose to rear their infants themselves. In this light, the proportion of placement offspring expected to show emotional disorder,

Table 5. *Newborn status and Research Obstetrical Scale (ROS) scores*

	Home-reared	Placement
Number	23	6
ROS prenatal score*	1.08	2.66
ROS delivery score	2.47	2.66
ROS infant score*	0.39	2.33
ROS total score*	3.94	7.65
Birth weight (g)*	3317	2394

Note: A high score indicates more complications.
*$p < .001$.

based on a diathesis model, should be higher than the proportion of home-reared offspring who will exhibit disturbance. Indeed, researchers in the Danish adoption studies have made a similar point about their own control sample. They have grown suspicious that there is a far higher degree of pathology among mothers giving their children up for adoption than among mothers in general (Wender, Rosenthal, Kety, Schulsinger, & Welner, 1974).

Not only were the schizophrenic mothers who gave up their infants for placement not a random sample of schizophrenic mothers, but their offspring were not a random sample of schizophrenic offspring. This contradicts another basic assumption of adoption studies. In our sample, these placement infants were more premature and had more physical problems than the home-reared sample. Wender et al. (1974) found that children who were somehow deviant prior to adoption, for example, weak, difficult, or small, showed higher incidence of later mental illness. Such findings highlight the need to document the joint status of mothers and infants in adoption research. The adopted *infant* of a schizophrenic biological parent has been assumed to bring nothing unique to its new family other than schizophrenic genes. Sameroff and Zax (1973b) suggested that the infant might bring other things along with him or her, such as a difficult temperament. The adoption data from the current study, although derived from a small sample, suggest that the infant may bring far more concrete evidence of deviancy than schizophrenic genes. He or she also may bring an underweight, tiny body, thus placing extra caretaking demands on the new adoptive parents. These extra caretaking demands and deviant physical appearance have been demonstrated to affect mother–infant interaction (Field, 1977), and have the potential of beginning a negative chain of transactions that could produce a deviant outcome regardless of whether the infant carried schizophrenic genes (Sameroff, 1975).

To summarize our adoption data, this report is a cautionary tale. From our small sample of six placement babies, one cannot generate strong conclusions despite the highly significant differences we found. What can be said is that generalizations from other studies of schizophrenia using adoptees must also limit their conclusions because both the mothers and children associated with adoption appear to be an unusual and special sample, a situation that may be unique to mentally ill mothers.

Prenatal and newborn measures

After psychiatric and demographic information was obtained during our prenatal interviews, the first assessments of mother and child were made during the neonatal period. Many obstetrical variables were collected during the delivery process, and the newborn infants were examined with extensive laboratory procedures during the lying-in period at the hospital.

Almost all of the variables measured during the delivery process showed effects for mental illness, with poorer obstetric status associated with maternal illness (see Table 6). In this diagnosis analysis, Neurotic Depression was more often associated with problems than Schizophrenia; the Depression group had more delivery, infant, and total birth complications, and lower Apgar scores compared with Controls, whereas the Schizophrenia group had more prenatal complications and lower birth weight than Controls. The difference in prenatal complications, however, is attributable to a single item – chronic medication of the mother. Thus, this finding is an artifact of the standard treatment for schizophrenia. No effects for Personality Disorder were found. All but one of the measures showing diagnosis differences also showed Severity and/or Chronicity effects. Prenatal, infant, and total complications, short labor, low Apgar scores, and low birth weight all were associated with more severe or chronic mental illness in the mothers.

Low social status was also associated with poorer obstetric status, although fewer measures showed significant effects than in the mental illness analyses. Both Low-SES groups, Whites and Blacks, had more prenatal and infant complications, and lower Apgar scores at 1 minute (but not at 5 minutes). As in other obstetric studies (Niswander & Gordon, 1972), the Black infants had lower birth weights than either High-SES or Low-SES Whites.

Laboratory measures of the infants during the lying-in period showed far fewer effects than did delivery measures. The only differences due to mental illness were found on the Brazelton NBAS Scales. Both effects were for diagnosis and showed illness to be associated with poorer status. The infants of Depressed group mothers had lower tonus and less self-quieting ability than Controls. The Personality Disorder group had lower self-quieting ability as well. No Schizophrenia effects were found.

There were also few effects for Social Status on these measures. The black infants had more minor physical anomalies and higher heart rate than either group of whites. In a reversal of the general trend, blacks showed more self-quieting ability than whites on the Brazelton Scales. However, they also showed lower motor maturity than High-SES Whites.

To summarize the prenatal and newborn measures, most significant effects were found for obstetric measures. Mental illness of the mother was more predictive of poor outcome than Social Status, and among the mental illness compari-

Table 6. *Summary of ANOVA effects for prenatal and newborn data*[a]

	Diagnosis	Severity	Chronicity	Social Status
Prenatal measures				
IPAT–anxiety	SX, ND, PD > NI	Ill > No illness	Ill > No illness	HW < LW < LB
MAPI–pregnancy attitude		Ill < No illness	Ill < No illness	HW > LW > LB
Social competence	SX, ND, PD < NI	Ill < No illness	Ill < No illness	HW > LW, LB
Delivery measures				
ROS–prenatal	SX > NI	Ill > No illness	Ill > No illness	HW < LW, LB
ROS–delivery	ND > NI			
ROS–infant	ND > NI	Ill > No illness	Ill > No illness	HW < LW, LB
Total	ND > NI	Ill < No illness	Ill > No illness	
Total labor		Ill < No illness	Ill > No illness	
Apgar–1 min	ND < NI	Ill < No illness	Ill < No illness	HW > LW, LB
Apgar–5 min	ND > NI	Ill > No illness		
Birth weight	SX < NI	Ill < No illness	Ill < No illness	HW, LW > LB
Newborn measures				
Minor physical anomalies				HW, LW > LB
Heart rate				HW, LW < LB
NBAS–orientation				
NBAS–arousal				
NBAS–tonus	ND < NI			
NBAS–quieting	ND, PD < NI			HW < LB
NBAS–motor maturity				HW > LB
NBAS–cuddliness				
NBAS–response decrement				

Note: All effects listed are significant, $p < .05$.
[a] SX = Schizophrenia; ND = Neurotic Depression; PD = Personality Disorder; NI = No Illness; HW = High-SES White; LW = Low-SES White; LB = Low-SES Black.

sons, Severity and Chronicity of illness were equally useful as diagnosis. Among diagnoses, Neurotic Depression, not Schizophrenia, was the major correlate of poor status. Although there were few significant differences in the infants following delivery, more of these were attributable to Social Status than to Mental Illness. For the significant mental illness effects, Depression was again the key diagnosis to the exclusion of Schizophrenia.

Four-month measures

At 4 months of age, the infants were tested in the laboratory, their mothers reported on their general behavior characteristics, and the mother–infant pairs were observed in the home environment. All of these procedures produced effects for Mental Illness and Social Status (see Table 7).

The Bayley Developmental Test scores at 4 months were one of the few measures in the study to show an unequivocal effect for schizophrenia for an entire experimental procedure; the infants in the Schizophrenia group were the only ones with lower scores than Controls on both the MDI and PDI. In addition, both Severity of Illness and Chronicity of Illness were associated with lower Bayley Test scores. No effect for Social Status was found.

The observations of the children's behavior during this testing session, using the infant behavior record (IBR), yielded a different pattern of effects. Like the test scores, the observation measures showed mental illness to be related to less optimal behavior, but no effects for Schizophrenia were found. The only diagnosis effect was that the Depression group was less responsive to people than Controls. More severe and chronic illness was related to poorer response to people as well. Further, higher severity of illness was associated with less happy mood during the testing session.

Two Social Status effects were found in the laboratory observations. Black infants were more responsive to objects than High-SES White infants. They were also more active during the testing session than the High-SES Whites.

On the mother reports of infant temperament, Severity of illness, Chronicity of illness, and Social Status were all more powerful predictors than diagnosis. In general, mental illness and low social status were related to poorer infant temperament ratings. None of the diagnostic differences were attributable to Schizophrenia. The Depressed mothers reported their infants to be more active and more distractible. The Personality Disordered mothers also reported their infants to be more active as well as more persistent.

Chronicity, in contrast, differentiated subjects on seven of the nine ITQ scales. Children of chronically ill mothers were reportedly more active, irregular, withdrawn, intense, and negative in mood, with lower levels of adaptability, and threshold to stimulation. In sum, they scored as having more difficult temperaments. Severity showed a similar, though less consistent, pattern of effects. Social Status showed effects on six of the scales in common with the Chronicity factor. Black children were reported by their mothers as being more irregular and withdrawn, with poorer mood and lower levels of adaptation. Lower-class children from both

Table 7. *Summary of ANOVA effects for four-month data*[a]

	Diagnosis	Severity	Chronicity	Social Status
Developmental test scores				
Bayley–MDI	SX < NI	III < No illness	III < No illness	
Bayley–PDI	SX < NI	III < No illness	III < No illness	
Infant behavior record				
Response to people	ND < NI	III < No illness	III < No illness	
Response to objects				
Reactivity				HW < LB
Activity				
Happy mood		III < No illness		HW < LB
Temperament scales				
Activity (low)	ND, PD < NI	III < No illness	III < No illness	
Rhythmicity (low)			III > No illness	HW, LW < LB
Adaptability (low)		III > No illness	III > No illness	HW, LW < LB
Approach (low)			III > No illness	HW, LW < LB
Threshold (low)		III > No illness	III > No illness	HW < LW, LB
Intensity (low)		III < No illness	III < No illness	HW > LW, LB
Mood (negative)		III > No illness	III > No illness	HW, LW < LB
Distractibility (low)	ND < NI			
Persistence (low)	PD < NI	III < No illness		

Table 7 (cont.)

	Diagnosis	Severity	Chronicity	Social Status
Home observation (mother)				
Spontaneous	SX, ND < NI	Ill < No illness		
Responsive				HW < LB
Happy	ND < NI	Ill < No illness		
Smiles				
Vocalizes	ND < NI	Ill < No illness	Ill < No illness	HW > LB
Proximity	SX, ND, PD < NI	Ill < No illness		
Negative				HW < LW < LB
En-face			Ill > No illness	
Home observation (infant)				
Spontaneous				
Responsive				
Happy				
Object orientation				
Cry				HW < LB
Negative				HW < LB

Note: All effects listed are significant, $p < .05$.

[a]SX = Schizophrenia; ND = Neurotic Depression; PD = Personality Disorder; NI = No Illness; HW = High-SES White, LW = Low-SES White, LB = Low-SES Black.

races had a lower threshold and higher intensity of responses. Again, low social status was associated with poorer temperament.

The observations made in the home produced many effects for mother behavior, but few effects for infant behavior. There were about as many diagnosis effects as Severity or Chronicity effects. All of the diagnosis effects involved the Depression group. The Depressed mothers were less spontaneous, less happy, less vocal, and less in proximity to their children than controls. For two of these variables, spontaneous and proximity, the Schizophrenic and Personality Disordered mothers differed as well in the same direction as the Depression group.

The Severity of illness effects exactly paralleled those for depression. The more severely ill mothers were less spontaneous, happy, vocal, and proximal. Chronicity showed fewer effects, but the more chronic mothers did exhibit more negative behavior during the observations.

Three effects for social status were found for mother behavior. Black mothers were more responsive to their infants than High-SES White mothers, but they vocalized less often. All three groups differed in their amount of negative behavior. The High-SES Whites had the least, the Blacks had the most, and the Low-SES Whites were in between.

The infant observation variables, in contrast, showed few effects. None of these were for mental illness, but two Social Status effects were found. Black infants cried more and were more negative than High-SES White infants. The Low-SES Whites were in between.

Summarizing the 4-month findings, a pattern similar to that during the newborn period is apparent for the mental illness effects. Neurotic Depression, not Schizophrenia is most often related to poor mother and infant status. The Severity and/or Chronicity dimensions were about equally powerful in detecting differences as the diagnosis variable. In contrast to the newborn period, the effects for Social Status were about equal to those for Mental Illness by 4 months of age.

Twelve-month measures

When the infants were 1 year of age they were brought to the laboratory for developmental testing and an assessment of infant–mother attachment. The mother–child pairs were also observed in their home environments (see Table 8).

The Schizophrenia group continued to perform most poorly on the Bayley Developmental Test. On the MDI and PDI the Schizophrenia group scored lower than the Depression group, but neither group differed from Controls. There were no differences on Severity or Chronicity of illness. The Social Status comparisons showed that High-SES Whites had higher MDI scores than Blacks, but no difference for PDI scores was detected. A second psychometric test used was the Uzgiris–Hunt Object–Permanence Scale. On this measure there was no effect for either diagnosis or severity, although higher chronicity was associated with poorer performance. Also, the High-SES Whites scored higher than Blacks.

There were few significant differences on the IBR observations made during the testing session. The only diagnosis effect was that children in the Depression

Table 8. *Summary of ANOVA effects for 12-month data*[a]

	Diagnosis	Severity	Chronicity	Social Status
Developmental test scores				
Bayley–MDI	SX < ND			HW > LB
Bayley–PDI	SX < ND			HW > LB
Object permanence			Ill < No illness	
Infant behavior record				
Response to mother				
Response to examiner	ND > NI			
Response to objects		Ill < No illness	Ill > No illness	
Reactivity		Ill < No illness		HW, LW > LB
Activity				HW > LB
Motor maturity				
Happy food				
Home observation (mother)				
Spontaneous		Ill < No illness		HW, LW > LB
Responsive		Ill < No illness		

Cuddle			HW, LW < LB
Passive			
Vocalizes		Ill < No illness	HW > LB
Smiles			HW < LW, LB
Negative	Ill < No illness		
Proximity			
Home observation (infant)			
Spontaneous	Ill < No illness		HW > LB
Responsive	Ill < No illness		
Happy			LW > LB
Cry			HW, LW < LB
Clings			HW, LW < LB
Whimpers			
Movement		Ill < No illness	LW < LB
Play			LW < LB

Note: All effects listed are significant, $p < .05$.

[a] SX = Schizophrenia; ND = Neurotic Depression; PD = Personality Disorder; NI = No illness; HW = High-SES White, LW = Low-SES White, LB = Low-SES Black.

group had better reactions to the examiner than Controls. The only Chronicity difference was for this variable as well; higher chronicity was related to better response to examiner. Two severity effects were found. Higher severity was related to poorer response to objects and lower reactivity. In Social Status comparisons, the Blacks showed lower reactivity than either High- or Low-SES Whites, and lower activity than High-SES Whites.

During observations in the home, we found very few differences in mother or infant behavior as a function of mental illness, a pattern similar to that for the 4-month home observations. In contrast, almost all of the infant behavior variables differed by social status, as well as about one-half of the mother behaviors. In the mental illness comparisons, there were no effects for diagnosis. More severely ill mothers were less spontaneous, less responsive, and less in proximity to their children, and their infants were less spontaneous. More chronically ill mothers smiled less, and their infants moved less.

For all of the social status effects for mother behavior, the High-SES Whites and Blacks were most discrepant and the Low-SES Whites were about halfway in between. The High-SES Whites were most spontaneous and least passive, they smiled more, and were least negative. In contrast, most of the differences in infant behavior were apparently more a function of race than SES, that is, Blacks differed from High-SES and Low-SES Whites. These black infants were less spontaneous, less happy, more clinging, more mobile, and fussed more than white infants. They also engaged in more play than Low-SES Whites.

In sum, the findings at 12 months were not unlike those of the previous year. Severity and/or chronicity of mental illness were of greater or equal power in detecting differences compared with diagnosis although none of these showed many effects. The only unique schizophrenia effect was, as at 4 months, for the Bayley Developmental Test scores. Following the trend from birth to 4 months, social status increased its effect on mother and child behavior relative to mental illness, so that by 12 months social status was a somewhat more powerful predictor than mental illness.

Thirty-month measures

During the 30-month assessment the children were given the Bayley, Peabody IQ, and Stanford–Binet Verbal IQ tests, and their mothers gave several reports of their child's development, and their views of child rearing. These reports included the Parent Attitude Research Instrument (PARI), Parent Estimate of Development Scale (PEDS), Vineland Social Maturity Scale, and the Rochester Adaptive Behavior Inventory (RABI) (see Table 9).

The pattern of Bayley and IQ test results changed dramatically from 12 to 30 months. The diagnosis effects (especially for schizophrenia), notable during the first year of life, were absent at 2.5 years. However, high severity and chronicity of illness were both related to poorer test performance. Most striking, however, was that social status began to show the powerful effect uniformly observed for IQ tests after about 2 years of age; the groups were clearly ordered from Blacks, to Low-SES Whites, to High-SES Whites.

A similar pattern held for the IBR observations made of the test session. Only one diagnosis effect was found: The Schizophrenia group showed lower reactivity than the Control group. Both higher severity and chronicity of illness were also related to lower reactivity, and high chronicity was associated with poorer response to the examiner. All but one of the IBR measures showed a social status effect. Black children were less responsive to the examiner and to objects, less reactive, less mature motorically, and less happy than High-SES Whites. The Low-SES Whites were about midway between the other groups.

The mothers' estimates of their children's development showed effects like those for their actual test scores. More severely ill mothers gave lower estimates of development, and their children scored lower on the developmental assessment. Likewise the Social Status groups were ordered on the PEDS the same way as on the test scores: Blacks followed by Low-SES Whites, then High-SES Whites. No differences were found on the parent reports of children's social maturity using the Vineland Scale.

A more detailed report of social behavior, the RABI, did produce many group differences. Five of the 10 scales showed diagnosis effects; the Depression group was less cooperative in the family, less cooperative with others, more bizarre, more depressed, and engaged in more imaginary play than controls. On one of these scales, the Schizophrenia group was also more depressed than Controls. Severity and Chronicity of illness was related to less cooperation in the family, less cooperation with others, more timidity, more fearfulness, more bizarre behavior, more whiny behavior, and more depression. The more Chronic and Severe groups also had poor global ratings of adjustment.

Social status was a powerful predictor on the RABI as well. Black children were less cooperative with nonfamily members, more timid, more fearful, more overactive, more bizarre, more whiny, more demanding, and more depressed than High-SES Whites. The Low-SES Whites were generally midway between the extreme groups. The blacks also had more friends and engaged in less imaginary play. Finally, the blacks received the poorest global ratings of adjustment, and the High-SES Whites the highest.

The final 30-month measure was of parent attitudes. There were no diagnosis effects on the PARI scales, but more severly ill mothers had more authoritarian, more hostile, and less democratic attitudes. Black mothers also had more authoritarian, more hostile, and less democratic attitudes than whites.

Summarizing the 30-month data, the pattern established at 12 months was repeated; there were few diagnosis effects, and more effects for severity, chronicity, and social status. The major change from 12 to 30 months involved IQ scores. The effects for schizophrenia disappeared, whereas social status became a powerful predictor. Group differences were found across the board; mental illness and social status were related to child behavior, mother reports of child behavior, and maternal attitudes.

Table 9. Summary of ANOVA effects for 30-month data[a]

	Diagnosis	Severity	Chronicity	Social Status
Developmental test scores				
Bayley–MDI		Ill < No illness		HW > LW > LB
Bayley–PDI				HW > LW, LB
Peabody IQ		Ill < No illness	Ill < No illness	HW > LW > LB
Stanford–Binet Verbal		Ill < No illness	Ill < No illness	HW > LW > LB
Infant behavior record				
Response to examiner			Ill < No illness	HW > LB
Response to objects				HW > LB
Reactivity	SX < NI	Ill < No illness	Ill < No illness	HW > LB
Activity				
Motor maturity				HW > LB
Happy mood				HW > LB
PEDS–estimate of IQ				
Mental age				
General description				HW > LB
Occupation		Ill < No illness		HW > LW > LB
Education		Ill < No illness		HW > LW > LB
Average		Ill < No illness		HW > LW > LB

PARI–Parent attitudes				
Authoritarian control		III > No illness	III > No illness	HW < LW < LB
Hostility–rejection		III > No illness		LW > LB
Democratic attitude		III < No illness		LW > LB
Vineland				
Social Maturity				
RABI–Adaptive Behavior				
Global rating		III < No illness	III < No illness	HW > LB
Cooperation – family	ND < NI	III < No illness	III < No illness	
Cooperation – others	ND < NI	III < No illness	III < No illness	HW > LB
Friendships				HW < LB
Timidity		III > No illness		HW < LB
Fearfulness		III > No illness	III > No illness	HW < LB
Activity				HW < LB
Bizarre behavior	ND > NI	III > No illness	III > No illness	HW < LB
Whiny behavior		III > No illness		LW < LB
Demanding				
Depression	SX, ND > NI	III > No illness	III > No illness	HW < LB
Imaginary play	ND > NI			HW > LB

Note: All effects listed are significant, $p < .05$.

[a] SX = Schizophrenia; ND = Neurotic Depression; PD = Personality Disorder; NI = No Illness; HW = High-SES White; LW = Low-SES White; LB = Low-SES Black.

Forty-eight-month measures

At 48 months the children were given the verbal scales from the WPPSI, the Peabody IQ test, laboratory measures of attention, and they were observed during the psychometric testing session. The mothers reported on their children's behavior in a temperament questionnaire and a RABI interview. They also responded to questionnaires about their own beliefs, attitudes, and personality, including the Kohn parental values, Concepts of Development Questionnaire, Marlowe-Crowne social desirability, and Eysenck neuroticism and extraversion (see Table 10).

Results of the child psychometric tests were similar to those at 30 months. In mental illness comparisons no effects for diagnosis were found, although both severity and chronicity of illness produced substantial differences; higher illness was associated with poorer performance. Social status continued to show very large effects with the groups ordered from Blacks to Low-SES Whites to High-SES Whites.

In contrast to the test scores, IBR observations of child behavior made during the testing session yielded only a few differences that were equally distributed among the mental illness and social status comparisons. In diagnosis comparisons, the poorest response to mothers was found in the Personality Disorder group, and the Schizophrenia group had lower motor maturity than the Personality Disorder group but neither group differed from Controls. In other mental illness comparisons, chronicity was associated with poor response to mother, and severity related to low motor maturity. Three social status differences were found. Blacks had poorer response to their mothers and less happy mood than High-SES Whites (with Low-SES Whites in between), and higher motor maturity than Low-SES Whites.

The pattern of results for the two laboratory measures of attention was similar to that for IQ scores. No diagnostic group effects were found for either the Luria or DMS procedures, but for the Luria procedure high severity of illness and chronicity of illness were associated with poorer performance. However, the largest differences were found for social status where High-SES Whites performed best followed by Low-SES Whites and Blacks on both the DMS and the Luria procedures.

The two sets of information about child behavior obtained from mother report revealed different patterns of effects. On the temperament questionnaire few mental illness effects were found for the nine scales. Children in the Schizophrenia group were rated as less approaching than Controls, and those in the Depression group more intense. Higher severity was associated with less rhythmicity, adaptability, and persistence, and lower threshold to stimulation. Higher chronicity of illness related to lower adaptability and threshold to stimulation. In the social status comparison, all temperament scales showed differences. The Blacks were least active, rhythmic, adaptable, approaching, and distractible, more intense and negative in mood, and had the lowest threshold to stimulate. Contrary

Table 10. *Summary of ANOVA effects for 48-month data*[a]

	Diagnosis	Severity	Chronicity	Social Status
Developmental test scores				
WPPSI–Verbal		Ill < No illness	Ill < No illness	HW > LW > LB
Peabody IQ		Ill < No illness	Ill < No illness	HW > LW > LB
Infant behavior record				
Response to mother	PD < NI		Ill < No illness	HW > LB
Response to examiner				
Response to objects				
Activity				
Motor maturity	SX < PD			LW < LB
Happy mood				HW > LB
Attention measures				
Luria		Ill < No illness	Ill < No illness	HW > LW > LB
Delayed Match-to-Sample				HW, LW > LB
Temperament scales				
Activity (low)		Ill > No illness		HW, LW < LB
Rhythmicity (low)		Ill > No illness		HW, LW < LB
Adaptability (low)			Ill > No illness	HW < LW, LB
Approach (low)	SX < NI			HW, LW < LB
Threshold (low)		Ill > No illness	Ill > No illness	HW < LW, LB
Intensity (low)	ND < NI			HW, LW < LB
Mood (negative)				HW, LW < LB
Distractibility (low)				LW > LB
Persistence (low)		Ill < No illness		HW, LB > LW

Table 10 (cont.)

	Diagnosis	Severity	Chronicity	Social Status
RABI – Adaptive Behavior				
Global rating	ND < NI	Ill < No illness	Ill < No illness	HW > LW, LB
Cooperative – family	ND < NI	Ill < No illness	Ill < No illness	
Cooperative – others	ND < NI	Ill < No illness	Ill < No illness	HW, LW > LB
Friendships				HW, LW < LB
Timidity		Ill > No illness	Ill > No illness	HW, LW < LB
Fearfulness		Ill > No illness	Ill > No illness	
Activity				
Bizarre behavior	SX, ND > NI	Ill > No illness	Ill > No illness	
Whiny behavior	ND > NI	Ill > No illness	Ill > No illness	
Demanding	SX < NI			
Depression	SX, ND > NI	Ill > No illness	Ill > No illness	HW, LW > LB
Persistence				
Family closeness				
Eysenck Scales				
Neuroticism	SX, ND, PD > NI	Ill > No illness	Ill > No illness	HW < LW, LB
Extraversion				

Social desirability				
Positive	ND < NI		III < No illness	HW < LW, LB
Negative	SX, ND < NI		III < No illness	LW < LB
Locus of control				
Easy world		III > No illness		HW < LW, LB
Predictable world			III > No illness	
Concepts of development				
Symbiotic	SX > NI			
Categorical		III > No illness	III > No illness	HW, LW < LB
Compensating		III < No illness		HW, LW > LB
Perspectivistic		III < No illness		
Kohn – parental values				
Conformity		III > No illness	III > No illness	HW < LW < LB

Note: All effects listed are significant, $p < .05$.

[a] SX = Schizophrenia; ND = Neurotic Depression; PD = Personality Disorder; NI = No Illness; HW = High-SES White; LW = Low-SES White; LB = Low-SES Black.

to this pattern of more difficult temperament, the Blacks were reported to be most persistent.

Unlike the temperament survey, the RABI produced more mental illness than social status effects. For diagnosis, children in the Depression group had poorer global ratings, they were less cooperative in the family and with others, and they showed more bizarre behavior, whiny behavior, and depression than Controls. Of these differences, the Schizophrenia group was also more bizarre, whiny, and depressed than Controls. In addition, they were less demanding of their mothers than Controls. Both severity of illness and chronicity of illness were related to poorer global ratings, less cooperative in the family and with others, and more timidity, bizarre behavior, whiny behavior, and depression. Only severity of illness was associated with more fearfulness. As noted above, fewer effects were detected for social status. High-SES Whites had better global ratings than either Low-SES Whites or Blacks. Both White groups were more cooperative with those outside the family, more persistent, less timid, and showed fewer friendships and more imaginary play than Blacks.

As might be expected, the mothers in this study showed many differences in measures of their personality and attitudes. On the Eysenck Personality Inventory there were no differences for introversion, but very strong differences for neuroticism; all three diagnostic groups were higher than Controls, as were High Severity, High Chronicity, and Low-SES White and Black groups. Social desirability was lower in the Schizophrenia, Depression, High Severity, and White (both High- and Low-SES) groups. Severity, Chronicity, and Low-SES were related to external locus-of-control on one scale.

There were also many differences in Concepts of Development levels. Schizophrenic mothers were more symbiotic on the CODQ. More severely ill mothers were more categorical and less compensating and perspectivistic; the more chronically ill women were more categorical. For social status, High-SES Whites were least categorical and most perspectivistic. In short, the mentally ill and Low-SES mothers had less advanced concepts of child development. On the Kohn Parental Values Measure severely and chronically ill mothers, as well as Low-SES and Black mothers, were most conforming.

Summarizing the 48-month data, there was only one measure on which schizophrenic offspring were uniquely worse: IBR – motor maturity. As at earlier ages, where diagnosis differences were found, so too were severity and/or chronicity differences, and these latter effects outnumbered the diagnosis differences. Further, the extent of social status effects was similar to that of severity and chronicity. Finally, there were effects found for all types of measures: psychometric tests, attention measures, maternal reports, mother personality, and maternal attitudes and beliefs.

DISCUSSION

Sources of risk in early childhood

The investigation we have reported here was cast as an attempt to identify variables that place a child at risk for the later development of schizophrenia. The target population was the offspring of schizophrenic women; they have been shown to have more than 10 times the risk for developing disorder than offspring of nonschizophrenic women. The variables that define risk were conceptualized in a series of models that differentially emphasized constitutional and environmental factors. From the constitutional perspective, we were interested in identifying characteristics of the child's behavior uniquely associated with a maternal diagnosis of schizophrenia. From the environmental perspective we were interested in identifying characteristics of the child's caretakers uniquely associated with a maternal diagnosis of schizophrenia. To these ends we examined the characteristics of both child and mother in a series of assessments from the prenatal period until the child was 4 years old.

To determine if these characteristics were unique to a maternal diagnosis of schizophrenia, we included a variety of Control groups to examine maternal factors highly correlated with schizophrenia. Because schizophrenia is a severe and chronic mental illness predominantly found in lower social status groups, we included as controls mothers who had severe and chronic mental illnesses other than schizophrenia and mothers with no evidence of mental illness who came from lower social status groups.

The present study was primarily focused on the etiology of risks leading to an outcome of schizophrenia. But, in the course of such an investigation, this question must be embedded in an analysis of the general risks to which young children are subject and the range of outcomes associated with such risks.

Our results specific to the issue of schizophrenia lead us to two conclusions. The first is that the offspring of schizophrenic women as a group have many developmental problems. The second is that these problems do not appear to be the simple result of maternal schizophrenia. If one compares the offspring of schizophrenic women in our study to a group of offspring of middle-class, white mothers with no mental illness at 4 years of age, the children of the schizophrenics have lower cognitive, linguistic, and motor performance scores, poorer adaptive behavior and emotional state, and worse behavior in the testing situation (see Table 11). However, when social status, severity, and chronicity of mental disturbance were taken into account in the analyses reported in the results section, most of the differences between the Schizophrenic group and matched controls disappeared.

The differences in Table 11 did not appear to be the result of the maternal diagnosis of schizophrenia, but rather the effect of suffering from a serious and chronic mental disorder. Moreover, a high proportion of these women lived in poor economic circumstances that would impede their own adaptive behavior. It would not be surprising to us that children from such backgrounds, who get off to a bad start, might eventually become emotionally disturbed themselves, including among these disturbances a small percentage of schizophrenics.

If one conceives of schizophrenia as the result of a *specific* deficit that colors the individual's behavior throughout development, then one would have difficulty with our data. Two explanations for our results can be offered that still posit a constitutional deficit in high-risk schizophrenic offspring. The first explanation is that the deficit is a latent one that will emerge later in development. The second explana-

Table 11. *Means and t-values of Schizophrenia and High-SES-White–No-Mental-Illness groups for selected 30- and 48-month measures*

	Schizophrenia	High-SES-White–No-Mental-Illness	t-Value
30-Month measures			
Bayley – MD1	93.9	108.4	4.10**
Bayley – PDI	92.7	104.7	2.83**
Peabody – IQ	88.1	114.7	3.54**
Stanford–Binet – Verbal	102.8	129.6	4.57**
RABI – Global rating	2.59	1.92	3.67**
RABI – Cooperative with others	2.74	2.97	3.06**
RABI – Timidity	2.09	1.68	3.00**
RABI – Bizarre behavior	1.33	1.21	2.32*
RABI – Depression	1.49	1.23	2.91**
IBR – Response to examiner	−.45	.12	2.14*
IBR – Reactivity	−.28	.15	3.07**
48-Month measures			
WPPSI – Verbal	94.7	116.4	5.23**
Peabody – IQ	92.9	113.9	5.80**
RABI – Global rating	2.67	2.07	2.59*
IBR – Motor maturity	−.43	.09	2.49*
Luria – Verbal regulation	22.8	26.47	2.26*
Delayed Match-to-Sample	1.93	2.54	2.06*

Note: High RABI global rating indicates poor social adaptation. IBR Scale scores are sums of z-scores; high scores indicate adaptive behavior; Higher Luria and Delayed Match-to-Sample scores indicate better attention.
*$p < .05$.   **$p < .01$.

tion is that the wrong variables were measured. Both of these explanations can be evaluated to some degree by examining the data from high-risk studies of older children (e.g., Fisher, Kokes, Harder, & Jones, 1980; Weintraub, Neale, & Liebert, 1975; Rolf, 1972; Beisser, Glasser, & Grant, 1967; Worland, Lander, & Hesselbrock, 1979; and El-Guebaly, Offord, Sullivan, & Lynch, 1978). Such studies have not found features uniquely associated with having a schizophrenic parent, that is, that were not associated with having parents with other diagnoses. Whether the right variables are being assessed will always remain an open question. However, these studies have utilized measures ranging from cognitive and social adaptation to subtle attentional processes, spanning the breadth of normative and pathological developmental variables.

The crux of the matter is to define what, indeed, constitutes a high-risk sample. The risk can be subdivided into two categories, either severe mental disturbance in general or schizophrenia in particular. The data from the Rochester Longitudinal

Study indicate that the offspring of schizophrenics are indeed a high-risk sample in accord with previous epidemiological research (Hanson et al., 1977). However, it appears that this risk is the result less of the schizophrenia diagnosis, than of the combination of prolonged emotional disturbance, unstable family organization, poor economic circumstance, and low social status that characterizes many of these families. The possibility of finding sick offspring will be reduced if one searches for clean samples of schizophrenics who come from middle or upper social classes and intact families. The possibility would be increased if one used samples of lower social status, disrupted families, with any severe and prolonged parental mental illness. In other words we have confirmed the obvious. The poorest social adaptation will be found for children coming from the worst social, psychological, and financial circumstance. If one is searching for populations with strong needs for intervention programs and a good possibility for payoff in better developmental outcomes, the target is relatively clear.

As to the study of schizophrenia itself, it may at best be an esoteric aspect of current high-risk approaches. The most positive outcome of these studies of the offspring of schizophrenic parents is to indicate that schizophrenia will not be understood within a simple genetic or constitutional model with clear-cut developmental indicators of the latent disorder. If such markers exist it may be more important to search for them in the families of the 90% of schizophrenics who do not have schizophrenic parents. It is our impression from watching our sample of chronic schizophrenics rearing their children for the first few years of life that among their many incompetencies is the incompetence to make their children crazy. These children have many developmental problems, but we see little evidence of severe disorders that might lead to psychosis. It may be that 4 years is not long enough for the family to have worked its evil or that 4-year-olds do not have the cognitive competence to assimilate the disturbances in their environment. In the Rochester Longitudinal Study we hope to have some more answers as more of our longitudinal data becomes available. Meanwhile, we are still left with the challenge of interpreting the etiology of developmental disorders of all forms. Our interim conclusion is that we have found the appropriate level of analysis, not in the discovery of singular environmental or constitutional factors, but in the interplay of both systems which have an inseparable role in producing all developmental outcomes, schizophrenic or otherwise.

SUMMARY

The ways in which personality might be passed from generation to generation, though long studied, are still little understood. An examination of the transmission of extreme patterns of behavior, such as found in mental illness, was thought to be a reasonable strategy for illuminating the transmission of more typical psychological characteristics as well. Most of the research in this area has centered on the offspring of schizophrenics, because this group offers a potential model for both biological and social heredity. The work we have reported has been in this area.

In the cognitive area early differences in development scores disappear by 30 months of age for the mental illness comparisons of diagnosis, severity, and chronicity of disturbance. However, when the same data are viewed from the perspective of socioeconomic status, completely opposite results appear. There are no differences during the early sensorimotor period, but during the third year, when language becomes relevant to IQ performance, the effects of social class differences are enormous, as one would expect. Other research has shown that these 30- and 48-month measures are the ones that correlate with later IQ scores. What we can conclude from the analysis of both cognitive and social emotional adaptiveness at 30 and 48 months of age is that the effects of social milieu appear to match the effects of maternal psychopathology in the social–emotional sphere, and to overpower it in the cognitive sphere.

To summarize the results of our longitudinal study to date, we have not found that offspring of schizophrenic women are a healthy, happy, intelligent lot. Our measures have shown that they have high levels of illness, fearfulness, sadness, retardation, and social maladaptiveness. However, this does not make them uniquely different from the offspring of women with other severe or chronic mental disorders, or even children of psychiatrically normal women from the lower socioeconomic strata of our society. Without the appropriate control groups built into our study, we might have been led into the error of attributing these differences to the effects of a schizophrenic heritage alone. One must question, then, theories that posit a *unique* constitutional deficit (often believed to be genetic in origin) associated with the development of schizophrenia. In short, caretaking environments in which high levels of stress exist, whether through economic or emotional instability, produce young children with high levels of incompetent behavior. Whether or not these early manifestations of aggressiveness or fearfulness will express themselves in later mental illness will only be determined by further longitudinal research. In the interim, our findings have identified a population of vulnerable children toward which early intervention studies might fruitfully be directed.

38 Pregnancy and delivery complications in the births of an unselected series of Finnish children with schizophrenic mothers: II

GUNNEL WREDE, SARNOFF A. MEDNICK,
MATTI O. HUTTUNEN, AND
CARL GUSTAF NILSSON

McNeil and Kaij (1978) have summarized the literature relating pregnancy and birth complications (PBCs) to schizophrenia. They divided the studies into two major types: (1) studies of the births of individuals who subsequently became schizophrenic; and (2) studies of the births of children with a schizophrenic parent. Their review suggests that schizophrenics tend to have suffered unusually high levels of PBCs; they found, however, that the results of research with children of schizophrenics were mixed, most studies indicating no differences between indexes and controls. Studies that have appeared since the McNeil and Kaij review either suggest no more complications among schizophrenic than among well mothers (Cohler, Gallant, Grunebaum, Weiss, & Gamer, 1975) or indicate lighter birth weight, lower Apgar scores, and more prematures among children born to severely mentally ill, though not necessarily schizophrenic, mothers (Zax et al., 1977). Reider et al. (1975) noted an increased incidence of fetal and neonatal deaths among offspring of schizophrenics.

This chapter examines the perinatal histories of a group of children whose mothers were diagnosed later as having schizophrenia. The study was conducted in Helsinki, Finland; this location offers certain advantages. Almost all hospitalizations for serious mental illness in Helsinki are centralized at Hesperia Hospital. The Finnish perinatal care system involves 95% of all pregnant women (Valvanne, 1977). A system of Well-Baby Clinics routinely gathers detailed information concerning conditions of pregnancy. Almost all deliveries in Helsinki take place in two hospitals. Together these conditions provide the opportunity for an accurate ascertainment of a total population of schizophrenic women and access to complete records of their pregnancies and deliveries.

METHOD

Our sample consists of all the children born between 1960 and 1964 in Helsinki to all of the women with a hospital diagnosis of schizophrenia who were born be-

This work was supported by a fellowship to Gunnel Wrede by Finland's National Academy and National Institute of Mental Health Grant No. 31433 to Sarnoff A. Mednick.

The chapter is a revised version of an article previously published in *Acta Psychiatrica Scandinavica 62*, 369–381, 1980.

515

Table 1. *Characteristics of the groups*

| | Mother's diagnostic status | | |
	Chronic (N = 54)	Mild (N = 117)	Control (N = 171)
Male children (%)	60.0	52.5	50.5
Mothers unmarried (%)	20.4	4.3	2.0
Mean mother's age in years at index delivery	26.0	27.4	26.5
Parity			
First born (%)	50.0	44.4	43.4
Second and third born (%)	37.0	42.7	45.5
Fourth to eighth born (%)	13.0	12.8	11.1
Social class[a]			
Upper middle and upper (%)	9.3	23.1	27.4
Middle (%)	53.7	63.2	61.0
Low and lower middle (%)	37.0	13.7	11.6

[a]Social class scale adopted from Rauhala (1966). Scale runs 0–8 with 8 representing highest class. Scores were pooled into three levels.

tween 1916 and 1948. We began by ascertaining all female hospital patients born 1916 to 1948 with a diagnosis involving schizophrenia (N = 3,243). From the population registers of the city of Helsinki we noted all patients (N = 192) who gave birth to children in Helsinki during the years 1960 to 1964. A total of 212 deliveries were found for these 192 schizophrenic women, including five twin births. We then checked the files of the two birth clinics in Helsinki, where we found records for 199 of 212 children. Three of the other children were born at home; 10 were born in small private clinics that do not keep adequate records. Controls were chosen by taking the hospital delivery immediately preceding that of the index child.

The data for this study were analyzed by chi-square analyses. Yates's correction for continuity was not applied to 2 × 2 contingency table analyses. Recent evidence has shown that this correction decreases the accuracy of probability statements (Camilli & Hopkins, 1978). In addition the Camilli and Hopkins paper suggests that with Ns over 20, accurate chi-square probability statements are obtained even when the expected frequencies in one or two cells are as low as one or two.

Diagnosis. The hospital records of the schizophrenic women were examined by a psychiatrist (M.O.H.) and classified as chronic schizophrenics (Chronics) with permanent social deficit (N = 54) or mild schizophrenics (Milds) with one to three admissions (N = 117). Twenty-eight cases were excluded as not being definitely

Table 2. *Pregnancy variables recorded*

Failure to attend Well-Baby Clinic during pregnancy	Prior abortions
	Bleeding including abortus imminens
Height of mother	Proteinuria
Weight of mother at time of delivery	Toxemia
Mother's weight increase during pregnancy	Hypertension
	Nephropathia
Mother's ABO type	Nausea
Mother's Rh type	Heartburn
Mother's venereal disease	Itching
Mother's temperature at time of delivery	Headache
Mother's pulse at time of delivery	Backache
Mother's blood pressure at time of delivery	Cramps
	Miscellaneous: insomnia, dizziness,
Previous illnesses of mother	heart complaint, digestion complaint,
Treatment for previous illness	tonsillitis, febris e causa ignota,
Age at first menstruation	pyelitis gravidarum, rubeola (in
Menstruation duration	second month)
Menstruation cycle duration	Medication during pregnancy
Prior deliveries	

Note: Where appropriate this information was coded separately for each trimester of the pregnancy.

schizophrenic; their controls were also dropped. Table 1 provides information about certain characteristics of the index groups and controls.

The chronic schizophrenic women tended more to be unmarried $\chi^2_2 = 28.4$, $p < .001$) and belonged to a lower social class at the time of the delivery of the child ($\chi^2_2 = 29.4$, $p < .001$). Social class was based on the spouse with the highest level in the family, typically the husband. The sex ratio, the mother's age, and parity did not differ significantly.

RESULTS

Pregnancy complications

A list of the pregnancy variables recorded from the Well-Baby Clinic records is given in Table 2. Abnormality on any of these items was considered a pregnancy complication. An unweighted count was made of the number of pregnancy complications for each subject. Over the course of the entire pregnancy the chronic, mild and control groups had 90%, 85%, and 88% of their members registered as having experienced at least one pregnancy complication. The number of complications was then analyzed separately by trimester of pregnancy. As can be seen in Table 3, the chronics suffered more complications than the mild or control subjects. This difference is significant in the first and third trimesters. Of the 46.8%

Table 3. *Number of pregnancy complications experienced by trimester of pregnancy*

	Percentage of women with more than two pregnancy complications					
	Chronic Schizophrenics	Mild Schizophrenics	Controls			
Trimester	($N = 54$)	($N = 117$)	($N = 171$)	χ^{2a}	df	p
1	31.8	9.6	17.0	13.0	2	<.001
2	22.7	14.9	15.9	2.7	2	n.s.
3	46.8	26.6	17.8	18.1	2	<.001

[a]Note that the χ^2s were computed on the basis of a division of the groups into the number with 0 or 1 complications and 2 or more complications.

of the Chronics suffering more than two complications in the third trimester, 29.8% suffered more than three; only 6.2% of the Mild and 12.4% of the Controls suffered more than three complications in the last trimester.

We then examined the frequencies with which the three groups suffered the pregnancy complications listed in Table 2 to determine whether any particular complications were especially contributing to the observed difference. Where the frequencies permitted, tabulations were made by trimester.

As mentioned above, almost all pregnant women in Finland attended the Well-Baby Clinics. Only 1.8% of the Controls and .9% of the Mild schizophrenics did *not* attend, whereas 9.6% of the Chronics did not attend ($\chi^2_2 = 12.8, p < .01$). We then stratified the diagnostic groups by SES and retested the difference using Mantel's generalization of the Mantel–Haentzel formula for chi square ($2 \times k$). The difference did not hold within SES levels ($p = .11$). In all diagnostic groups the mothers who did not attend the clinics tended to belong to the lowest SES groups.

Most of the women in all groups experienced nausea and heartburn during the early stages of pregnancy. In the case of nausea, this tended more frequently to persist in the third trimester for the Chronic schizophrenics (36.2%) and the Mild schizophrenics (20.4%) than for the Controls (9.4%) ($\chi^2_2 = 20.1, p < .001$). This was also true for heartburn in the third trimester (Chronics 25.5%, Mild schizophrenics 8%, Controls 12%); ($\chi^2_2 = 8.5, p < .05$). More Chronics (21.8%) than Mild schizophrenics (11.7%) and Controls (9.9%) suffered from proteinuria ($\chi^2_2 = 6.0, p < .05$). The proteinuria was diagnosed at the Well-Baby Clinics as well as at the mother's admission to the hospital for the delivery. This was especially true in the last trimester of the pregnancy. The number of women suffering illnesses prior to the pregnancy was greater for the Chronic schizophrenics (40.7%) and the Mild schizophrenics (37.1%) than for the Controls (20.4%) ($\chi^2_2 = 13.5, p < .01$). The Chronic (50.0%) and Mild (48.0%) schizophrenic groups also evidenced more cases of hypertension (systolic pressure) than did the Controls (30.9%).

Table 4. *Obstetrician's criteria for rating severity of delivery complications*

Severity	Criteria
(1) No complications	Birth weight at least 5½ lb
	Duration of delivery no more than 24 hours
	Fetal heart rate 100–180/min
	Apgar score 7–10
(2) Moderate complications	Birth weight at least 5½ lb
	Duration of delivery 25–36 hours
	Amniotic fluid meconium stained
	Fetal heart rate 100–180/min
	Heavy analgesic medication during the course of delivery
	Apgar score 4–6
	Abnormal presentation without acute distress (mainly breech presentation)
	Elective Cesarean section
(3) Severe complications	Birth weight under 5½ lb
	Duration of delivery more than 36 hours
	Fetal heart rate over 180/min or under 100/min
	Abnormal presentation with acute distress (mainly breech presentation)
	Instrumental delivery (elective Cesarean sections not included)
	Apgar score 0–3
	Hemorrhaging during the first and second stages of delivery

Note: A case was assigned to Group 3 if two or more of the complications listed in Group 2 occurred.

Whereas the Chronic schizophrenics tended more frequently to evidence complications in other pregnancy items, these other differences did not reach significance.

Delivery complications

An obstetrician (C.G.N.) examined the delivery records (which, of course, had no group identification). He classified them into groups with Severe, Moderate, and No complications. His criteria are given in Table 4. The distributions of judged severity by groups are given in Table 5. The number of cases with severe complications was significantly higher for the Schizophrenic groups than for the controls ($\chi^2_2 = 12.2$, $p < .01$). The Milds evidenced the most delivery difficulty, significantly more than the Controls ($\chi^2_2 = 13.0$, $p < .01$). The Chronic schizophrenics did not differ significantly from either group.

Table 5. *Distribution of delivery complications by severity for Schizophrenics and Controls*

	Chronic schizophrenic (%)	Mild schizophrenic (%)	Controls (%)
No complications	64.7	54.0	68.5
Moderate complications	19.6	21.2	22.4
Severe complications	15.7	24.8	9.1

Table 6. *Delivery complications significantly differentiating Schizophrenics and Controls*

	Chronic schizophrenics (%)	Mild schizophrenics (%)	Controls (%)	Chronic/ Mild/ Controls	All Schizophrenics/ Controls
Nurse's notes					
Mother's mental status deviant	9.6	10.4	3.5	n.s.	<.05
Mother's physical status deviant	15.4	18.3	7.1	<.05	<.01
Mother too thin/too fat	43.2	24.2	16.4	<.01	<.05
Massage points[a] (2 or more)	9.1	13.3	4.1	<.05	<.05
Fetus's heart sound affected	9.3	3.4	0.5	<.01	<.01
Delivery prior to 38th week	11.4	7.8	2.9	<.05	<.05
Quality of placenta abnormal	27.8	27.9	16.0	n.s.	<.05
Medication during delivery	46.3	42.7	31.4	n.s.	<.05

[a] A derived scores reflecting the amount of squeezing and tactile stimulation the fetus experienced during delivery. One point is given for each observed item.

We then examined the list of delivery complications to see what the sources of this overall difference might be. Table 6 presents the complications for which significant differences emerged among the groups.

Upon arrival at the obstetrical clinic the nurses more frequently noted mental or physical problems among the Schizophrenics than among the Controls. The mental problems included such items as tense, irritable, troubled, restless, suffering, shock state; the physical problems included tired, anemia, vomiting, influenza, fever. The nurses also noted that the constitution or physical build of the Schizophrenics was deviant, usually too thin. This is also reflected in the fact that the Schizophrenics tended to weigh less at admission than the Controls (Chronics 151

Table 7. *Postpartum variables significantly differentiating Schizophrenics and Controls*

	Chronic schizophrenics (%)	Mild schizophrenics (%)	Controls (%)	Chronic/ Mild/ Controls	All Schizophrenics/ Controls
Child unhealthy at birth (nurse's rating)	7.3	11.7	3.5	<.05	<.02
Child unhealthy 2nd–7th day of life (nurse's rating)	11.1	5.4	1.2	<.05	<.01
Medication required for mother	3.7	6.0	1.2	n.s.	<.05

lb., Milds 153 lb., and Controls 157 lb.) and tended to evidence a smaller weight increase during pregnancy (Chronics 25 lb., Milds 28 lb., and Controls 28 lb.). (Neither of these latter two differences was significant.) During the delivery, the Schizophrenics more frequently received medication ($\chi^2_2 = 5.9$, $p < .05$). The medications administered to the schizophrenics tended to be sedatives, analgesics, and labor-inducing drugs.

At the mother's first visit to the Well-Baby Clinics she reported the time of her last menstruation. At the time of delivery the period of pregnancy was calculated. As can be seen in Table 6 the Schizophrenic groups tended to have shorter pregnancy periods. This difference is also reflected in the fact that the Schizophrenics evidenced nonsignificant tendencies toward small birth weight, birth length, and head circumference. The groups differed significantly in their "massage points" (Table 6). High massage points mean risk for the baby to suffer extended squeezing and tactile stimulation during the delivery. It is worth noting that fetal heart sound was affected more frequently among the Chronic schizophrenics than among the Mild schizophrenics and the Controls ($\chi^2_2 = 12.2$, $p < .01$).

Although no other delivery complications reached statistical significance, in most cases the Schizophrenics evidenced more difficulties.

Postpartum status

Table 7 lists the items significantly distinguishing the Schizophrenics from Controls by chi-square tests. More Schizophrenic mothers required medication after the delivery and the health status of their children was questioned by the nurses more often. The nurses noted the following items for the children of the Schizophrenics: respiration difficulties, cyanosis, yellow jaundice, vomiting, crying, temperature, rash, dry, mucous skin, maternal hemorrhaging, asphyxia neonatorum, mongoloid, swollen, luxatio coxae congenitalis, and staphyloch albus. There was a nonsignificant tendency for the children of the Schizophrenics to receive hospital medical care beyond that usually given. Three of the Schizophrenic mothers removed their infants from the hospital against medical advice.

Eleven percent of the children of the Chronic schizophrenics were placed in institutional care (orphanages, adoption placement agencies, etc.), whereas none of the Mild schizophrenic group and only 1.5% of the Controls experienced this treatment. Significantly more perinatal deaths (8) occurred among the children born to the Mild schizophrenics. No perinatal deaths occurred to the Chronics; one control girl was stillborn. Four of the children of Mild schizophrenics were stillborn (two boys, two girls) and four boys suffered neonatal death ($\chi^2_2 = 12.5$, $p < .01$).

Influence of mental illness. If the women were schizophrenic at the time of the delivery and if this were known, it could conceivably influence the physicians and nurses describing the pregnancy and delivery in the clinic journals. As has previously been reported for high-risk studies (S. Mednick, 1972), the large majority of the women (94%) became schizophrenic at some time after the delivery. This factor is unlikely to have unduly influenced the findings.

Social class and sex differences

There are large social class (SES) differences among the groups. Perinatal difficulty is known to vary as a function of social class (Zachau-Christiansen & Ross, 1975). In view of this, the influence of SES on group differences was assessed by calculating the correlations between SES and important perinatal variables (see Table 8). No correspondence between SES and obstetrical variables was found. In this respect our Finnish material differs from that reported from other countries. The universally available excellent perinatal care may have reduced the usual deficit for lower social class groups. This finding has also been reported by Rantakallio (1969) concerning low birth-weight infants and Amnell (1974) concerning perinatal mortality. The higher level of perinatal difficulties among the Schizophrenics cannot be explained by their lower social class status.

In view of the greater difficulty male neonates have in pregnancy and delivery (Butler & Bonham, 1963; Zachau-Christiansen & Ross, 1975) the severity of pregnancy and delivery complications was calculated separately for males and females as a function of diagnostic group. The increased severity of complications among the Schizophrenics was maintained for both males and females. No sex interactions were observed.

Season of birth effects

It is now well known that schizophrenics have a disproportionately high number of births in winter months. Videbech, Weeke, and Dupont (1974), for example, have demonstrated that the increase of winter births of schizophrenics in Denmark is

Table 8. *Correlations between social class and selected important perinatal variables (N = 398)*

Failure to attend Well-Baby Clinic during pregnancy	.24*
Pregnancy complications (nausea, heartburn, cramps)	.05
Pregnancy complications (bleeding, hypertension, proteinuria, itching)	−.02
Pregnancy complications (headache, backache)	.05
Delivery complications (obstetrician's grading)	−.01
Fetal heart sound affected	−.02
Child unhealthy at birth (nurse's rating)	.08
Child unhealthy 2nd–7th day of life (nurse's rating)	.00

*$p < .01$.

paralleled by an increase in stillbirths. They suggest that perhaps both of these effects are produced by an increased level of perinatal problems during the winter. If this were the case for this Finnish population, we might expect that the increased perinatal problems observed would be concentrating among those children of schizophrenics born in the winter months. In keeping with the literature in this area the winter months were defined as being from November through February, and the summer as May through August. Spring (March and April) and fall (September, October) were pooled. This produced three categories of season: winter, summer, and spring/fall. Within each of these categories of season, frequencies of perinatal complications were tabulated by diagnostic groups.

The differential deficit of the Schizophrenic groups was indeed greatest for those born in the winter months. The relatively increased level of perinatal difficulties for the Schizophrenics born in the winter was especially noted in complaints of nausea and heartburn during the last trimester of pregnancy, in the increased number of preterm births, and in terms of the infants' poor health in the first week of life (see Table 9). The relative disadvantage of the Schizophrenic groups was intermediate during the spring-fall season. No significant differences between children of Schizophrenics and Controls were observed for summer births.

DISCUSSION

The differences observed in this study indicate that the births of the children of the Schizophrenic women were attended by more difficulties. A number of the

Table 9. *Season of birth and selected perinatal variables for Schizophrenics and Controls*

Perinatal Variable	Winter	Spring/fall	Summer
Nausea third trimester			
% Chronic	41.2	40.0	26.7
% Mild	37.0	11.6	18.6
% Control	5.1	5.9	20.9
χ^2	18.3***	13.7**	n.s.
Heartburn			
% Chronic	47.1	26.7	0
% Mild	11.1	4.7	9.3
% Control	13.8	11.8	13.9
χ^2	11.0**	n.s.	n.s.
Preterm births			
% Chronic	18.8	6.7	7.7
% Mild	13.6	5.0	7.5
% Control	1.7	2.9	4.7
χ^2	7.2*	n.s.	n.s.
Infant poor health first week of life			
% Chronic	11.1	21.0	0
% Mild	0	7.3	7.5
% Control	0	0	4.6
χ^2	9.9**	13.3**	n.s.

*$p < .05$.   **$p < .01$.   ***$p < .001$.

difficulties that occurred during pregnancy could be considered subjective: nausea and heartburn. On the other hand, bleeding during pregnancy, proteinuria, and hypertension are relatively objective measures recorded during the pregnancy and at the birth clinic.

The increased frequency of delivery complications for Schizophrenics, blindly judged by the obstetrician, was especially marked for *severe* rather than moderate complications. The greater frequency of stillborns and neonatal deaths and the nurses' notes reflecting the poor health during the first week of life of the children of the Schizophrenics do not contradict the cumulative impression of an increased number of serious perinatal problems associated with the pregnancies and deliveries of the schizophrenic women.

We know that 10% to 15% of these 199 high-risk children may be expected to become schizophrenic. In view of their relative temporal primacy, the perinatal difficulties we have described must be considered among the possible factors contributing to the vulnerability of these children.

As mentioned earlier, the McNeil and Kaij (1978) review concludes that the results of research on births to schizophrenic women were quite mixed. As usual, although it is possible to pinpoint methodological differences between the current study and previous research, it is not easy to attribute differences in results to specific methodological features. One possible difference between the method reported here and that of most earlier research is the representativeness of this group of Finnish, schizophrenic, fertile women. This should increase our confidence in the generalizability of these results. In this study we observed a higher frequency of pregnancy complications for the Chronic than for the Mild schizophrenics. This is certainly not contradictory to the results found by Sameroff and Zax (1973a), who attribute increased perinatal risk not specifically to diagnosis but to severity of mental illness. Because schizophrenia does not rank among the least severe mental illnesses, their view is certainly consonant with the findings of this research.

In view of the conclusions of the McNeil and Kaij review, it seems plausible that perinatal complications may be more common and more severe in the births of individuals later diagnosed schizophrenic than among those not so diagnosed. They may be considered among the possible etiological factors in schizophrenia. As such, their influence may result from some (as yet unspecified) neurological damage to the fetus or through some form of overstimulation of some endocrine function which produces lasting effects. This type of hypothesis can be examined by following up this high-risk cohort. Such follow-up is currently in progress by the first author.

The concentration of the perinatal difficulties for the high-risk children in those born in the winter months is an interesting finding. To our knowledge such results have not been reported before. The results suggest some special susceptibility on the part of schizophrenics (or those born to schizophrenics) to a condition or conditions temporally synchronized with winter deliveries. Perhaps schizophrenics are particularly prone to certain viral and/or bacterial infectious processes whose virulence is seasonally variable. Or perhaps pregnant schizophrenics are particularly sensitive to summer heat in the early months of pregnancy and/or winter cold in the later stages. Finland's winters certainly qualify as providing the latter conditions. The nurse's indication of the inferior health status of the schizophrenic women on admission to the delivery clinic would not contradict the second of these speculations.

39 Contrasting developmental risks in preschool children of psychiatrically hospitalized parents

JON E. ROLF, JANIS CROWTHER, LINDA TERI, AND
LYNNE BOND

The first step in describing the nature and findings of the Vermont Vulnerable Child Development Project is to place it in its proper historical and conceptual contexts. The project was designed in 1971 and implemented during the 4 years between 1972 and 1976. It was intended to be a second generation child-at-risk project that would test the feasibility of combining earlier identification of vulnerable children with preventive intervention.

The roots of the Vermont project grew from the Minnesota project (Garmezy, 1974) that incorporated Rolf's (1972) dissertation research on the academic and social competence of school-aged children at risk. At that time, risk research was focused on validating the greater susceptibility to developmental psychopathology of children with schizophrenic or depressive parents. The early findings of the Minnesota Project did confirm the true vulnerabilities of many of these school-aged children. The Vermont project then extended the Minnesota design to preschool children at risk, to assess whether their vulnerabilities could be identified at earlier ages when prevention efforts might be most appropriate (Rolf & Harig, 1974).

As a consequence of our interest in prevention, the Vermont project became as much applied as experimental in its research methodology. In addition to designing descriptive assessments of developmental competencies and deviations of the children, the project also undertook epidemiological surveys and therapeutic day-care programs (Rolf & Hasazi, 1977). These applied components actually came to consume most of the projects resources. The extensive epidemiological surveys were necessary to provide us with previously unavailable information concerning the rates of change in the patterns of developmental problems and skills that were prevalent among the normal and high-risk preschoolers living in our catchment county (Crowther, Bond, & Rolf, 1981). The survey data enabled us to contrast the normal growth curves with the rates of improvement of our subjects in our preventive intervention program (Rolf, Fischer, & Hasazi, 1981).

Our greatest involvement in the applied area came about as a function of the

This research was supported by Grant MH 24152 MHS from NIMH, J. Rolf and J. Hasazi, principal investigators. The authors express their sincere appreciation to Jeannette L. Johnson for preparing this chapter.

activist spirit of the early 1970s. It seemed more *relevant* to study preventive intervention if we first created, staffed, and managed our own community-based day-care center (Rolf, Bevins, Hasazi, & Crowther, 1982). This decision, although proving most difficult to implement, was more productive than anticipated, for the project directors found themselves running a large center that shaped the cognitive and social experiences of 75 children each day. Indeed, the center still survives as a separate corporation some 4 years after the end of the research project.

With this introduction to the background and scope of the Vermont project, we now wish to focus on its more traditional component, namely, our studies of preschool-aged children with a psychiatrically hospitalized parent. Before presenting the data, however, there are two remaining issues that need discussion. The first issue concerns the pragmatic limitations of Vermont's population. The second involves our decision to broaden the scope of parental disorders to be studied for their pathogenic effects on children.

When the study began, Vermont's population had just reached 400,000. Less than one-quarter of these persons were residing in our catchment county. This segment of the local population was less than one-tenth of that available to the Minnesota project; it was a foregone conclusion that a very small cohort of schizophrenic parents with preschool children would be available for study. Consequently, the conventional high-risk child design was not feasible.

In designing our study, we wanted to incorporate multiple risk factors in our subject selection, including severity of parental disorder, types and severity of the child's own developmental deviations, presence of sensorimotor handicaps, degree of economic or cultural deprivation, and so forth (see Rolf & Hasazi, 1977). With respect to types of parental disorder, recruitment of schizophrenic parents would remain our priority, but it was probable that psychotically and neurotically depressed ones would be more prevalent, given their higher population base rates. Therefore, whereas the Minnesota and Stony Brook projects chose to include depressed parents as control groups for the effects of hospitalization, family upset, and social stigma, the Vermont project would, by necessity, focus more on depressed parents of both sexes than on schizophrenic parents.

Given the expected recruitment of a nonspecific assortment of parental disorders of a mostly depressive type, there would be no possibility of testing any genetic risk hypothesis. However, it had already been demonstrated that children of mostly neurotically depressed parents were no less deviant than the offspring of schizophrenic parents. Based on teacher ratings (Rolf, 1972; Weintraub, Neale, & Liebert, 1973), peer ratings (Rolf, 1976), and other academic performance measures (Rolf & Garmezy, 1974), it was evident that during their grade-school years, children of either schizophrenic or depressed parents were equally vulnerable to more types of difficulties than their matched controls. However, with regard to risk for depressed affect, the school-aged children of depressed mothers appeared to be particularly vulnerable by showing such internalizing symptoms as excessive shyness, sadness, and/or social withdrawal. It seemed reasonable to hypothesize – as would Weissman and Paykel (1974) several years later – that the hostility, resentment, and instability characterizing the social and familial interactions of depressed women create potent environmental risks for psychopathology in their children. Even so, given the protracted development of affective skills in children and the dissimilarity of young children's affective disorders to adolescent depression, it was questionable that preschool children of depressed parents would show the internalizing symptoms which were common among older children.

The High Risk Family Studies component of the overall project (Rolf et al., 1977) was intended to provide some initial information in this area by answering the following research questions: (1) What is the extent of the developmental problems of children from families with a psychiatrically hospitalized parent as compared to those with nondisturbed parents? (2) Is there evidence of greater risks for affective disorders in children with parents hospitalized for depression? (3) Would these children from the independent sample of hospitalized parents be in as much need of our preventive intervention services as those disturbed preschoolers already referred to our therapeutic day-care programs? This last question was particularly relevant to Vermont's Office of Child Development in order to estimate the need for the development of primary prevention programs in our catchment county.

THE HIGH-RISK FAMILY STUDY

The data to be reported in this chapter are based on 52 parent–child pairs from families residing in a northwestern Vermont county. These 52 pairs represent a subsample of a larger cohort of families at risk. Although many families provided us with only the first step data (the behavior ratings on their children), these 52 provided us with complete data. The children were aged 2 through 6 and were assigned to Hospitalized ($N = 24$) or Nonhospitalized ($N = 28$) groups. The Hospitalized group was subdivided according to DSM-II parental diagnoses (N Schizophrenic $= 6$; N Depressive $= 18$) that were determined by the Current and Past Psychopathology Scales Interview (Endicott & Spitzer, 1972). The hospitalized parents were recruited by contacting all parents admitted to the Medical Center Hospital of Vermont's psychiatric unit and all those admitted to Vermont State Hospital who resided in our catchment county. Control parents were recruited by the secretary of a local pediatrician who contacted families with children of an approximate age to seek permission for our project staff to contact them about volunteering. Control parents were selected for a negative psychiatric history and were thus not given the extensive psychiatric diagnostic interview for current and past psychopathology.

The average demographic characteristics of the groups were equivalent for most variables: children's age (4.4 years), sex (half boys), mothers' and fathers' ages (29 and 32 years), mothers' education (12 years) and Hollingshead (1957) SES indices (mostly Class III). Statistically significant differences ($p < .05$) were obtained on three variables. Control families contained fathers with slightly more education (14.3 vs 12.8 years), fewer broken homes (0 vs. 21%, and a slightly lower average number of offspring (1.3 vs. 2.0). Overall, the groups were well matched and differences on the dependent variables would be expected to result largely from the effects of group membership.

After informed consent had been obtained from both parents, they were asked to complete the following measures: (1) the Vermont Behavior Checklist (Rolf & Hasazi, 1977), a 90-item checklist rating the frequency with which the child emits various motor, perceptual–motor, self-care, language, cognitive, and social behaviors; (2) the Family Background Information Form (Klemchuk, Rolf, & Hasazi, 1975), a 120-item questionnaire providing demographic information; (3) the Vineland Social Maturity Scale (Doll, 1947), a measure of the child's level of social development as seen by the parent; and (4) the Family Evaluation Form (FEF) (Spitzer, Gibbon, & Endicott, 1971), and the Marital Adjustment Test (Locke & Wallace, 1959), the Katz Adjustment Scale (KAS) (Lyerly, 1973) and the CAPPS (Endicott & Spitzer, 1972). The children were directly assessed using the Stanford–Binet Intelligence Test (Terman & Merrill, 1973) and the Peabody Picture Vocabulary Test (Dunn, 1965). For this chapter, the presentation of findings will not include the KAS data. To further integrate their presentation, the various measures will be clustered according to the domains of physical, intellectual, and social–emotional childhood competencies.

Two series of statistical comparisons are presented. The first contrasts the hospitalized versus the nonhospitalized groups for all variables except those from the FEF. The second series tests for differences among three subgroups (two Hospitalized parent diagnostic groups and the one Control group).

HOSPITALIZED VERSUS NONHOSPITALIZED CONTRASTS

Analyses of variance were performed on the interval data and chi squares on the ordinal data. On the Marital Adjustment Test (MAT) where both spouses report on the presence of stress, conflict, social and sexual satisfaction in their marriage, nonhospitalized parents obtained scores in the more adjusted ranges whereas those in the hospitalized group who were still married had scores that averaged in the maladjusted range ($t = 4.1, p < .05$). Overall, there were fewer (0 vs. 21%, $p < .05$) broken marriages (separations, divorces, and widowed) and, as expected, significantly fewer disclosures of parental anxiety and other emotional problems in the nonhospitalized group. With regard to the children's physical health, there were no significant differences in recollected birth problems. There was a tendency ($\chi^2 = 10.78, p = .056$) for hospitalized parents to report more child physical problems (sensory impairments, allergies, etc.), but there was no difference in rate of reported parent physical problems.

The Binet and Peabody assessments yielded no significant group differences. Both groups obtained average scores with the children of the hospitalized parents slightly lower (97 vs. 103 IQs). To further confirm the null hypothesis, analyses of covariance were performed using age as a covariate. We chose to use this conservative second step consistently in the Vermont project as most measures for preschoolers often show significant covariations with age. However, in this instance, the pattern and the nonsignificance of differences in intellectual function remained the same.

None of the social competence measures obtained from maternal reports yielded significant differences. These measures included: (1) the Vineland Social

Maturity Scale; (2) the Vermont Behavior Checklist's (VBC) Externalizing (anti-socially aggressive) and Internalizing (socially withdrawing) factor scores (Crow-ther et al., 1981); and (3) parental reports of any problems in their children that led to professional diagnosis or treatment. Instead, both groups of parents tended to rate their children as more shy than the average Vermont child (z-scores = 1.72 and 1.44, hospitalized and nonhospitalized, respectively) but both parent groups also judged their children more competent, as evidenced by Vineland Social Quo-tients which averaged in the Superior Range. As will be demonstrated shortly, subdividing the Hospitalized groups by parental diagnosis produced more striking differences between the risk groups.

In order to better understand the relationship between parental disturbances and patterns of competencies among offspring, the variables obtained from the Hospitalized parent group and their children were intercorrelated. The obtained correlations should be interpreted cautiously in light of the small numbers of subject pairs ($N = 24$) and the attendant probability of sampling errors. Even so, the results are suggestive of promising leads to be confirmed with larger samples from the other risk projects represented in this volume.

The results of the intercorrelations of parent and child variables for the Hospi-talized group are as follows: (1)Reports by parents on their child's Vermont Behav-ior Checklist of parental physical health problems are positively correlated with reports of birth problems for their children ($r = .40, p < .05$). (2) In the intellec-tual competence domain, there are the expected positive correlations with social class, and mother's and father's education (rs range from .41 to .68). More in-teresting are the correlations between IQ scores and well parent's scores on both the FEF Social Isolation factor (ps $< .05$) and the scores of Marital Adjustment [rs $= .51$ (spouse satisfaction) and $-.41$ (couple's average rating of adjustment)]. Thus it would seem that higher child IQ scores are positively associated with internalizing parental dissatisfaction with the marriage.

The correlations between the Hospitalized parent group scores and their chil-dren's scores relating to social competence are as follows: (1) The Vineland Social Quotient is, as anticipated, positively correlated with social class (i.e., higher com-petence for higher sociometric variables ($p < .05$). Similarly, children's social competence is positively related to good Marital Adjustment Scores ($r = -.40, p < .05$) and lack of adequate parental role functioning in the home ($r = -.45, p < .05$); (2) Social *incompetence* in the child, determined by the Vermont Behavior Checklist Factor scores, showed a significant positive correlation with parents' report of parent emotional problems and the child's internalizing symptoms ($r = .47, p < .05$). On the other hand, there were significant positive associations with good marital adjustment, social status, and mother's education for the *absence* of externalizing aggressive symptoms in the children. Furthermore, among the FEF factors the "child pathology due to the hospitalized parent" score was highly correlated to the hospitalized parent's subjective distress score ($r = .72, p < .001$), which might suggest a pathogenic path of negative influences from the hospitalized parent to the child.

Emerging from these correlations is a pattern suggesting that, in the disturbed parent family, higher social status serves as a protective influence to reduce the probability that the child at risk will show high externalizing symptoms or low scores on standard measures of intellectual and social competence. Of particular interest is the pattern of significant positive correlations between child social competence variables and the hospitalized parent's distress, reduced parent-role functioning, and report of poor marital adjustment. Thus, although there were no signs of serious psychopathology among these high-risk preschoolers when they are contrasted to the Control group, there appear to be some suggestions of meaningful associations between parent and child problems within the high-risk families themselves.

Analyses of variance were performed to investigate the effects of the sex of the disturbed parent (or conversely, the co-parent) on the child competence scores. In this Hospitalized group, the only significant main effect for sex was obtained on the Vineland Communication Scale score, $F(1, 17) = 6.4, p < .05$, with daughters and sons seemingly more adversely affected by hospitalized fathers.

CONTRASTS AMONG SCHIZOPHRENIC, DEPRESSED, AND NORMAL SUBGROUPS

Hospitalized parents were subdivided according to their CAPPS DSM-II diagnoses into Schizophrenic ($N = 6$) and Depressed ($N = 18$) groups. Of the Depressed group, half were rated as psychotic, including one manic-depressive case. Significant differences in demographic characteristics occurred only on fathers' education ($F = 3.41, p < .05$) indicating that the Depressed group fathers' 12th-grade status averaged 2 years less than the other groups. Also, the three groups were not equivalent in percentage of broken homes ($\chi^2 = 6.39, p < .05$). The Depressed group had most (25%), the Schizophrenic group slightly less (17%), and the Normal group least (0%).

One-way analyses of variance were run between diagnostic groups with Vineland Social Quotient, Stanford–Binet IQ and Peabody IQ, using the composite birth problems and composite child problems as dependent variables. On those variables which might be affected by small maturational differences one-way analyses of covariance with age as a covariate were run. As shown in Table 1, the results indicated that the only statistically significant differences among the three groups occurred on the VBC Composite Problem scores ($F(2, 44) = 4.53, p < .05$) and the Internalizing factor score ($F(2, 44) = 3.44, p < .05$).

Within the Depressed group ($N = 18$), two-way analyses of variance were run on sex of child and sex of hospitalized parent using the Vineland Social Quotient, Stanford–Binet IQ, and Peabody IQ as dependent variables. In a similar manner, analyses of covariance with age as a covariate were run using the two VBC factor scores and Vineland subscales as dependent variables. (The small N in the Schizophrenic group prevented similar analyses within that group.) Results yielded a single significant main effect for sex on the Communication subscale of the Vineland Social Maturity Scale, with female children of depressed parents scoring significantly lower than male children ($F(1, 12) = 5.98$), $p < .05$. However, the interaction of child's sex with parent's sex was not statistically significant.

The limited sample size of the Depressed parent group hinders a robust test of

Table 1. *Summary of selected independent and dependent variables for the Schizophrenic, Depressed, and Control groups*

Variable	Schizophrenic	Depressed	Control	F
N	6	18	28	
Age (in months)	61.2	56.3	51.9	n.s.
Sex[a]				
Boys	3	8	14	n.s.
Girls	3	10	14	
Mother's age	29.7	28.4	29.2	n.s.
Father's age	31.3	32.2	32.0	n.s.
Mother's education	11.4	11.8	12.8	n.s.
Father's education	13.8	12.1	14.3	3.41*
Number of siblings	2.2	2.1	1.2	5.02*
Marital status[a]				
Married	5	14	27	6.39*[b]
Separated or divorced	1	4	0	
Rating of marital adjustment[c]	80.0	91.3	112.2	6.41**
Composite parent physical problems	1.0	.38	.46	3.94*
Composite parent emotional problems	2.0	2.31	.12	74.91***
Composite birth problems	1.17	.56	.46	n.s.[a]
Composite child problems	2.50	.81	.88	4.53*[a]
Externalizing factor score	−.53	−.43	−.20	n.s.[a]
Internalizing factor score	−.61	−2.14	−1.44	3.44*[a]
Vineland Social Quotient	120.2	123.7	131.4	n.s.[a]
Stanford–Binet IQ	97.5	99.46	108.96	n.s.[a]
Peabody Picture Vocabulary Test IQ	107.67	95.08	104.52	n.s.[a]

[a]One-way ANOVA instead of analysis of covariance.
[b]Chi-square analysis instead of ANOVA.
[c]Average of both spouses MAT scores.
*$p < .05$.   **$p < .01$.   ***$p < .001$.

the differential risks between the Neurotic and Psychotic Depressed parent groups. However, the pattern of results for our subjects is intriguing, especially with respect to the FEF variables summarized in Table 2. The Neurotic Depressed reaction group members are in every comparison reporting the most family problems, followed in descending order by the Schizophrenic and the Psychotic Depressed group. This finding prompts one to speculate that these families with a neurotic depressive parent can provide intense (if perhaps short-lived and reality-oriented) stresses for their children.

To test this specualtion we created a table of all children of hospitalized parents and within each variable ranked the degree of competence and adjustment across all subjects. We than computed composite rank scores across variables for each individual child to discover which diagnostic group would have the children with

Table 2. *Summary of ANOVAs on Family Evaluation Form (FEF) variables between diagnostic parent subgroups*

Variable	Neurotic Depressed (N = 9)		Psychotic Depressed (N = 9)		Schizo-phrenic (N = 6)		F	p Value
	M	SD	M	SD	M	SD		
Subjective distress due to family	31.9	3.8	21.0	4.9	23.8	5.9	7.97	<.05
Family disorganization	14.1	1.1	9.0	0.0	10.2	1.1	60.70	<.001
Family belligerence	20.7	3.9	15.3	2.0	17.4	0.9	6.32	<.01
Child pathology due to family	30.4	4.8	23.7	4.5	24.8	4.8	3.91	n.s.
Well parent subjective distress	30.4	5.1	22.3	3.9	25.2	2.2	6.57	<.01
Well parent social isolation	10.0	1.5	9.7	1.1	.6	1.1	5.68	<.05
Disorganization due to parent	12.4	2.2	9.0	0.0	9.8	1.1	9.10	<.01
Social isolation due to patient	6.7	1.8	5.0	0.0	8.4	3.1	4.05	<.05
Belligerence due to patient	19.9	4.0	14.7	1.5	16.6	2.2	5.37	<.05
Child pathology due to patient	25.9	1.6	18.7	2.3	23.0	4.0	11.85	<.001

the highest average parent and child competence ranks. We were also interested in seeing if these rankings would disclose relatively more vulnerable and invulnerable children in each group. These rankings indicated that, at the time of our evaluation, the children of the Depressed groups appeared to be more vulnerable to their families' problems whereas the children of our small sample of Schizophrenics seemed to be the most competent in terms of their factor scores, IQs, and social quotients. However, it is important to remember that the data were obtained only at one time during the children's preschool years. Follow-up assessments might show a different pattern of rankings. Also, missing from these indicators of competence and risk are ratings by nonparents (e.g., peers, teachers, and neighbors) who could provide independent judgments of these children's competencies. Such multioccasion and multisource data were obtained in the preventive intervention section of the Vermont Project and they clearly demonstrated large intraindividual changes in competency scores within a span of a few months. These changes seemed to result from interactions with environmental stressors and internal developmental staging processes.

CONCLUSIONS

The small sample size involved in this study necessitates cautious interpretation of the results. Significant differences among parental diagnostic groups on Internalizing factor scores indicated children of depressed parents exhibited more withdrawn, shy, and socially unresponsive behaviors than either Schizophrenic or Control group children. Similarly, there was evidence to suggest greater family distress in the Depressed group. Children of this same group were also lower (although not significantly) than Controls on standard tests of intelligence. Female children of depressed parents scored significantly lower on the Communication subscore of the Vineland than did male children, suggesting that more research is needed to investigate the possibility of parent–child gender interaction. Will female children of female depressives and male children of male depressives exhibit more impairment than their opposite-sex counterparts after age 3, when children typically acquire sex roles?

The young age of these children makes it difficult to predict the cumulative effects of parental disorders during the rapid developmental period of preschool; it is also difficult to obtain independent sources of information regarding their children's social competencies. But as preschoolers, these children of hospitalized parents *as a group* are not demonstrating obvious signs of severe behavior problems that would indicate a need for large-scale planning for therapeutic intervention programs. This conclusion runs counter to our initial expectations of high-risk research based on data from older children, but suggests important directions for future research. As Garmezy (1971) has already suggested, some children may be invulnerable, or resistant, to the possible negative effects of parental psychopathology. When they would show these effects, how best to measure them and how to predict them remain unsolved problems. Without these technologies, primary prevention programs would be timely, but the positive program effects would be unprovable. Furthermore, analyses that compare essentially mean scores may always be inappropriate as they average the vulnerables and invulnerables together.

There are no simple solutions for moving from the experimental methodology of risk research to the applied methods of prevention research. We will need to follow these and similar young children at risk through their successive developmental stages to see if a vulnerable child at one stage either outgrows his/her vulnerability or breaks down at a later stage. Time and further research may tell us when early stress due to parental deviance is only a source of risk for psychopathology for certain types of children and when it may also be for other types a dynamic crucible in which to develop the ability to cope with stress later in life.

PART X

A Life-Span Study of Children at Risk

The longitudinal studies of schizophrenics and their families by Manfred Bleuler began many years before the other risk research programs reported in this volume. His research methods and findings have been reported in detail in his monumental volume published in German in 1972 and translated into English in 1978. His painstaking care in recording clinical observations is abundantly apparent in that volume. But what is unique in Bleuler's approach is his comprehensive and integrative personal viewpoint of the human drama in these families over a lifetime. He has found expectable tragedy, but, more surprisingly and importantly, he has found, as other programs are now starting to discover, remarkable evidence of strength, courage, and health in the midst of disaster and adversity.

40 *Different forms of childhood stress and patterns of adult psychiatric outcome*

MANFRED BLEULER

MANFRED BLEULER

SCHIZOPHRENIC PARENTAGE

In 1941–1942 I designated for long-term follow-up 208 unselected schizophrenics who were admitted to my clinic. The follow-up study (Bleuler, 1978) extended until the death of the patient or at least 22 years. In the context of this study I also pursued all of the children of these schizophrenics, including those born before 1941 as well as those born after 1942. Their ages varied. At the conclusion of the study the oldest was already over 60 years of age, while a few others had not yet reached 10 years. The children numbered 184 altogether. For comparison purposes we used data from 160 children of senile parents and from my psychiatric examinations of large samples from the average population.

Nine percent (9%) of the offspring of schizophrenics also became schizophrenic. (That is the age-corrected figure; the raw percentage was similar.) That rate is smaller than has been found in all previous studies taken together (13%). The principal difference from previous studies lies in the larger number of *healthy*, full-grown offspring (several over 50 or 60 years of age) than has been found in preceding studies. Nearly three-fourths of my sample are to be regarded as healthy, whereas earlier studies found only between one-third and, at most, one-half. The following observations illustrate the success of their life development: Eighty-four percent of the married offspring of schizophrenics had successful marriages, and the great majority achieved a higher social status than that corresponding to their parents' status or their own schooling. The basis for the contradiction in the findings lies in the manner of judgment. Previous authors inquired about morbid traits, but did not relate the results of their inquiry to the life situation of the person. For example, they presented the characterization *isolated and withdrawn* in the sense of schizoid psychopathology, whereas I found that such reactions were entirely normal under certain dreadful life circumstances and that the later mental health of the children confirmed their normalcy. Although morbid personality development is less frequent according to my studies than according to earlier ones, nevertheless it is more common than in the general population.

The majority of the completely normal children believe that the schizophrenic disorder of the father or the mother cast a perpetual shadow over their enjoyment of life, which left a dark remembrance that pains them constantly.

537

I conducted special investigations into the question of how living with a schizophrenic parent affected the children. On the average, the 184 offspring spent one-third of their first 20 years in the household with manifestly schizophrenic parents. *It could not be proven that living with manifestly schizophrenic parents occasioned greater pathology than the absence of such relationship.* It could also not be proven that living together with schizophrenic parents in the first years of life after birth created a special disposition to schizophrenia. In order to evaluate the significance of the interaction with manifestly schizophrenic parents, it is important to compare the psychiatric disturbance among siblings and children of my schizophrenic probands: (1) schizophrenic and personality disorders have equal frequency among the offspring and the siblings; but (2) the siblings almost never lived together with manifestly schizophrenic parents whereas the offspring very often did. This suggests that the human relationship with psychotic parents is not a pivotal determinant.

Two children of two schizophrenic parents lived for the greatest part of their childhood under the most horrible circumstances with both parents blatantly psychotic. Both offspring developed difficult, but not schizophrenic, personalities.

The schizophrenic probands themselves were reared in dreadful circumstances more often than is typical in the general population, but less often than occurs among alcoholics. It is important to point out that schizoid personality development in the premorbid history of a schizophrenic is closely associated with disorganized childhood circumstances. Such circumstances have significant effects on the development of a schizoid personality. The prognosis of schizophrenic psychoses in schizoid personalities is less favorable than in general. As disorganized childhood conditions predispose to schizoid personality development, they are also an unfavorable influence on course and outcome of schizophrenic psychoses. It has not been demonstrated, however, that disorganized childhood conditions are an essential disposition for the genesis of schizophrenic psychoses. Further details are available in my book (Bleuler, 1978).

EXTREME POLITICAL PERSECUTION: SUMMARY OF A
STUDY BY KEILSON

The relation of extreme childhood stress to the development of personality has recently been studied by Keilson (1979). The author examined 204 Jews who were born in the Netherlands between 1925 and 1944 and who had become orphans when their parents were deported and murdered by the Nazi troops. All of these Jews had lived under tremendous stress during the Nazi occupation – or in hiding places or in concentration camps. The author has known many of them during his professional career and he examined the subjects in this study about 30 years after the end of the war. The great majority of them had never become healthy and happy personalities. Neurotic character developments, anxiety neuroses, and chronic depressive moods were the most frequent disturbances. Schizophrenic disorders, however, were not significantly more frequent than in the general population.

The frequency of different disturbances of the personality showed some relationship to the age of the child when the tragedy began. Children who had been exposed before the age of 3 suffered particularly from character neuroses as adults. Children who were exposed between the ages of 11 and 14 suffered particularly from anxiety neuroses as adults, and those who were exposed after the age of 14 suffered from chronic depressive moods. The consequences of brutal psychological stress during the occupation period (when the children lived hidden with foster families or in concentration camps) were much influenced by their living conditions after the war.

Comparing the fate of these poor Jews with the fate of children of schizophrenics whom I studied, we note as the most evident fact the difference in incidence of character and anxiety neuroses. They were much more frequent among the Jews who had been under the stress of continual threats against their lives and of impoverished or disturbed relationships. The schizophrenics, on the other hand, lived mainly with one particular stress: the disturbed relationship with one parent.

In both groups the development in adult age did not depend only on early childhood conditions but was also influenced by the conditions in later childhood and adolescence. Adults of both groups frequently lack real happiness and suffer from a depressive mood even if they adapt themselves well socially and seem to be normal. A characteristic saying of an adult of my own group who had gone through hell in the care of psychotic parents was "One cannot laugh as other people laugh after having gone through this misery."

EXTREME FAMILY DEPRIVATION

The viewpoints and the results cited thus far offer no surprises. In recent decades much research has been done with the conception in mind that miserable childhood conditions create a disposition for morbid personality development. Research work, however, has shown more and more clearly that the contrary is also true in many cases: Many children who suffer from the most terrible conditions become normal adults, sometimes with outstanding intelligence and surprising stability of character, who successfully take over the care of others and assume great responsibilities. This fact has been known for centuries and many biographies exist of great men and women who endured a painful childhood.

How can we explain the paradoxical consequences of misery in childhood? We first think, of course, that the inborn disposition for personality development plays a role. Nobody denies that. Such an assumption, however, does not satisfy us. We look for other influences on successful or unsuccessful ego defense. And we would like to find influences that we can manipulate.

It has become usual to praise objective, statistical research and to hold anecdotal presentations up to ridicule. I think, however, that in the field in which we work both anecdotal and statistical research are necessary. One is hardly useful without the other. As I have done my part in statistical research in psychiatry you will certainly excuse me if I fall back on an anecdotal presentation in order to discuss one aspect of our common problem. The anecdote I shall present, however, is a story of facts, true in every detail.

A PARADOXICAL CASE STUDY: VRENI

On ward rounds in my clinic at an unusual hour one evening in 1958 I met a girl with a large bag. She told me that her name was Vreni and that she wanted to bring the washing to her mother. She asked me to show her the way to her mother, who had been my patient for a few weeks. I told her that the hospital takes care of the laundry for all the patients, but she gave me the unusual answer: "I know. However, my mother is pleased if I do her washing myself."

She was 14 years old and I asked her how she got along at school. She again gave a very astonishing reply, saying that she did not go to school as she had to take care of four younger brothers and sisters. In Switzerland the authorities are extremely strict about children going to school at her age, and I don't know of any exception if no chronic childhood diseases are in question.

I want to summarize the history of this girl. Her mother was a voluntary patient of the clinic who was addicted to headache drugs containing phenacetine. For several years she had taken up to 4 g of phenacetine and prophenazone and had spent about 200 francs a month on this drug – at that time an excessive amount for a family with a small income. Under the drug, her character had changed. She had become inactive and careless and took no interest in her household or her children for a long time. The youngest of them, twins, were 6 years old in 1958. The patient presented hematological findings and a mild cerebral organic syndrome, with flatness of emotions and morbid indifference to everything. It is particularly important that she did not care in the least what was going on at home during her stay in the hospital. She attributed her drug addiction to headache and the headache to her husband's morbid emotionality. As a matter of fact, the husband had fallen sick with a severe vascular disease (thrombangiitis obliterans Winiwarter) that led to gangrene of the toes and cerebro-vascular accidents. He had become emotional and unstable. Finally he had become an alcoholic and frequently left home to run around with strange women. At home he nagged and scolded his family during every meal. The mother became very tense and thought that her headaches were the consequence. She withdrew into drugs. When I heard of these facts I worried, of course, about the children. Vreni at 14 was alone in a most disturbed home with a brother of 13, a sister of 12, twins of 6, and an alcoholic, irresponsible, emotional, mentally and physically ill father. Enough is enough! This was a terrible and threatening situation for the children, and the misery had started when Vreni was 2 years old.

I immediately sent a welfare worker to the home located far away from the clinic in the country. She brought back sensational news: The household was kept in perfect order by Vreni, the smaller children were healthy, happy, well fed, well dressed, went regularly to school, and their teachers had no complaints about their behavior. From the age of 11 on, Vreni had managed to go to school less and less and when she was 13 years old she gave up school entirely. Under conditions in

Switzerland, this is almost a miracle. It is an interesting story how she had managed it but it is too long to be recounted here.

While her mother was in my clinic Vreni visited her regularly, brought her the washing regularly, and went for walks outside with her. In 1959 the mother had several cerebrovascular accidents and finally died in the Neurosurgical Clinic. Vreni continued unremarkably, with the exception of drunken episodes of the father. We tried to help Vreni, but she did not need much help; she did everything herself and never asked for money or anything else. As she wished to become a nurse I looked for a private teacher for her who helped to overcome her lack of schooling. Thanks to him she was accepted in a nursing school. Her greatest wish seemed to become reality. However, before entering school she came to me in tears. She told me that she had wished so much to become a nurse, but that she could not seize the opportunity she had to be trained as a nurse. She felt that it was her duty to continue the care of the younger siblings and her sick father, which I understood. I have remained in touch with her over the years since then.

In the following years her father died, the younger sister took care of the twins, and later on all three became independent, with the exception of one mentally retarded twin. Vreni married in 1965 at the age of 22. I am still in touch with her. Her husband is a modest laborer, a kind-hearted man who devotes all his free time to his family. The couple has two healthy children and the family is happy.

Why has Vreni become a very healthy and happy wife and mother – in spite of a childhood that became soon after babyhood so threatening? Or is the question to be asked the other way around? Why is she healthy and happy on account of a threatening childhood? To point to inherited disposition in this connection is far from satisfactory. She is certainly not a "superkid." Her IQ is average, she lacks particular interests or talents, she was not gifted in any particular way. One could point out the fact that the living conditions of the child only began to deteriorate after babyhood. From her case history we are tempted to say that life gave her a rare chance in her childhood: the chance just to do what she liked to do and what she was able to do. She loved and still loves children; she was proud to care better for the sick father and for the other children than her mother had; and she was able to take over her mother's duties with a good heart and a practical skill. On the other hand, she was not interested in school. It seems that stressful, difficult childhood conditions are not felt as too stressful or as too difficult if they offer the possibility to the child to fulfill a great task that the child genuinely enjoys and is able to fulfill.

Such a statement seems too simple and too self-evident to be interesting. However, it might have some importance. It might happen that we can help to manipulate the living conditions of a child in stressful and threatening circumstances in such a way that the child does find a great task appropriate to him or her. I could speak of experiences that suggest that such a manipulation might perhaps play a role in the prevention of schizophrenic psychoses; up to now, however, these experiences are merely anecdotal. The studies of high-risk children will perhaps contribute more to our understanding than anecdotal experience.

We can even go one step further: We all complain that living conditions for children have become unfavorable in modern civilization, in large cities, in small apartments, before a television set, distant from everything that is natural, distant from earth, distant from gardening and agriculture, distant from caring for each other. The case of Vreni suggests that stressful childhood experience does not always lead inexorably to abnormal adult outcome, especially if that experience – however grim it may appear to us as observers – offers the child a sense of purpose and a satisfying life task that is appropriate to her nature.

PART XI

Summary and Overview

It is understandable for the reader to suffer from acute information overload after absorbing more than 40 relentless chapters filled with relatively novel scientific research. The last part presents concise conceptual overviews that synthesize and integrate our knowledge to this point in specific domains of high-risk research. Chapter 41 by Richard Lewine places in perspective the research findings on attention, intellectual and cognitive functioning and raises an interesting issue about etiological theory. The next chapter by Lyman Wynne draws together the principal conclusions about communication patterns and family relations. Chapter 43 points out some important pitfalls in sampling for high-risk research. Then John Strauss offers some insights about issues of diagnostic classification that have emerged from our studies. Finally, Norman Watt presents a condensed summary of the whole book in a nutshell, offering some tentative general conclusions that can be drawn from two decades of high-risk research in schizophrenia. The reader should be forewarned that more questions are raised in this part than answers delivered. That's the way things stand in the present state of our knowledge.

543

41 *Stalking the schizophrenia marker: evidence for a general vulnerability model of psychopathology*

RICHARD R. J. LEWINE

INTRODUCTION

A substantial part of high risk research has been devoted to the discovery of a marker for schizophrenia. Many of the measures chosen in this endeavor have tended toward the biologically mediated, such as attentional and cognitive tasks and psychophysiological recording – measures that make up the bulk of this part. The simplest form of the argument goes as follows: Any task (ultimately mediated by a biochemical process) on which children at risk for schizophrenia consistently deviate from the norm reflects a predisposition for schizophrenia in the absence of overt psychosis. The data presented in the preceding chapters suggest the following modifications:

1. A marker, if it exists, may reflect a general vulnerability to psychosis, rather than a specificity to schizophrenia.
2. Change or process, rather than a traitlike marker, may be an important focus for future research.
3. Among children at risk for schizophrenia, only a subset (from 11% to 44%) stands out as deviant.

GENERAL VULNERABILITY

The studies presented in this volume have been divided into two groups: those that include a comparison sample of nonschizophrenic psychotics' offspring (Table 1) and those that do not include such a comparison sample (Table 2). Almost without exception, when significant findings are reported in the former studies both risk groups (i.e., Schizophrenics' and Nonschizophrenic Psychotics' Offspring) deviate from normal controls. This is true for psychological, attentional, intellectual, and

Preparation of this chapter was supported, in part, by Grant No. 30059 from the National Institute of Mental Health.

I would like to thank Sue Hagerman for pointing out the traitlike nature of the marker for schizophrenia, the members of the High-Risk Research Seminar at the University of Illinois at Urbana-Champaign for providing a forum for some of the ideas expressed in this chapter, and Charlotte Coles for her help in the preparation of the manuscript.

545

Table 1. *Summary of findings from studies including Affective Psychotic controls*[a]

Study	Major findings
Physiological	
Worland, Janes, & Anthony et al.	Race and age (of subject) effects on responsiveness; no parental diagnosis effect
	Irrespective of parental diagnosis, uniphasic responders performed more poorly on psychological testing than biphasic responders
Attentional	
Neale, Winters, & Weintraub	Both schizophrenics' and depressives' offspring were significantly slower than normal controls on a visual search task
	Distraction had a significantly stronger effect on schizophrenic and depressive high-risk groups than on normal controls
Intellectual	
Neale, Winters, & Weintraub	Schizophrenia- and depression-risk children had significantly lower IQs than normal controls
Worland et al.	Schizophrenics' and manic-depressives' offspring had significantly lower IQs than normal controls and offspring of parents with physical illness using repeated measures ANOVA
	Manic-depressives' offspring showed the largest decrement in IQ from the first to the second testing
	Schizophrenia-risk children had the lowest time 1/time 2 IQ correlation ($r = .59$); correlations for the offspring of manic-depressives, physically ill, and normals were .87, .87, and .83, respectively
Cognitive	
Neal, Winters, & Weintraub	Object Sorting Test: (a) schizophrenics' offspring made significantly fewer superordinate responses than normal controls, but no less than depressives' offspring; (b) schizophrenics' offspring made significantly more complexive responses than either depressive or normal controls
	Referential thinking: both risk groups (schizophrenia and depression) did significantly worse than normal controls
Worland, Janes, & Anthony et al.	No parental diagnosis effect on cognitive differentiation, egocentrism, Child's Embedded Figures Test, or Three Mountains Test
Worland et al.	Psychological disturbance (measured by eight factors derived from 89 cognitive variables) greater in both risk groups than in controls

Table 1. (*cont.*)

Study	Major Findings
Worland, Janes, & Anthony et al. Worland et al.	Schizophrenics' offspring had the highest, manic-depressive's offspring the lowest, primitive Rorschach content
	Schizophrenics' offspring had the lowest, manic-depressives' offspring the highest, TAT aggression scores
	Large overlap among all groups in distribution of scores
Wynne	No effect of parental diagnosis on discrimination learning of nonsense syllables
	Censure led to significantly more errors in schizophrenic and nonpsychotic psychiatric offspring than in affective psychotic and normal control offspring; similar (nonsignificant) trend for praise

[a]Studies are reported in this volume.

cognitive measures. This set of findings is consistent with the view that a general vulnerability to psychosis is genetically transmitted, but that the specific form is a function of environmental factors (Zubin & Spring, 1978). Until proven otherwise, such an interpretation of the studies summarized in Table 1 would seem to be the most parsimonious. This further suggests a cautious interpretation of those studies in Table 2 that do not include a psychotic control group. Indeed, we may conclude that we do not have any evidence of a marker specific to schizophrenia, but that there is strong evidence for a general vulnerability marker.

A TRAIT IN BIOLOGICAL CLOTHING

As discussed by Neuchterlein in his chapter on future research perspectives (Chapter 22, this volume), one conclusion to be drawn from this generation of risk studies is that more attention be given to the selection of age-approriate tasks with respect to difficulty and psychological meaning. One reason for the assumption of longitudinal consistency in tasks may be the belief in a marker as an immutable characteristic of the individual. However, as long as a potential marker relies on behavioral assessment, whether it be a response to the Continuous Performance Test or to a Rorschach blot, it is subject to all the difficulties encountered in the study of traits (Fiske, 1971). It would seem important, therefore, that future high-risk researchers turn to the assessment literature for guidelines in the selection and application of their measures.

Relevant to the issue of longitudinal consistency is Worland et al.'s report (Chapter 8, this volume) of a deterioration in the IQ of high-risk children, especially the offspring of manic-depressives and the low test–retest correlation of

Table 2. *Summary of findings from studies excluding Affective Psychotic controls*[a]

Study	Major findings
Physiological	
Friedman, Erlenmeyer-Kimling, & Vaughan	Failure to replicate early Mednick finding of fast recovery rate in high-risk children
Erlenmeyer-Kimling, Marcuse, Cornblatt et al.	High-risk children had significantly lower factor scales (reflecting psychological aspects of task measured by event-related potential) than normal controls
	25% of high-risk group had significantly longer event-related potential latency than normal controls and remainder of risk group
Mednick, Cudeck, & Griffith et al.	Sick high-risk groups' electrodermal responses are characterized by: (1) fast latency, (2) little habituation, (3) resistance to experimental extinction of conditioned electrodermal response, and (4) fast recovery following response peak
Attentional	
Cornblatt & Erlenmeyer-Kimling,[b] Erlenmeyer-Kimling, Marcuse, & Cornblatt et al.[b]	Evidence for lower sensitivity (d') on Continuous Performance Test (CPT) in high-risk than control children
	High-risk group significantly more affected than controls by distraction
	11% of high-risk group marked by deviance in sustained attention and susceptibility to distraction
Garmezy & Devine, Nuechterlein & Phipps-Yonas	Schizophrenics' offspring and externalizers showed deficit performance on reaction time task; only Schizophrenia-risk group not helped by high incentive condition. Failure to replicate results
	Schizophrenia-risk group worse than comparison groups on CPT, especially with degraded stimulus; not due to response bias
	29% of Schizophrenia-risk group extensively deviant in sensitivity (d'); Hyperactive group exhibited low response criteria
Mednick et al.	CPT "drift" in high-risk subsample eventually having a breakdown
Steffy et al.	High-risk group most sensitive to complex tasks
	44% of high-risk group identified as extreme responders on basis of cluster analysis; interpreted as perceptual overload problem
Weintraub & Neale	15% of schizophrenia risk group identified as extremely deviant

Table 2 (*cont.*)

Study	Major findings
Intellectual	
Garmezy & Devine	All target groups received significantly lower grades than controls
Mednick et al.	No effect of parental diagnosis on IQ
Cognitive	
Driscoll	No parental diagnosis effect on intentional or incidental learning
Mednick et al.	No premorbid associative response differences between Sick and Well high-risk group

[a]Although the New York City project includes the offspring of nonschizophrenic psychiatric patients, the results from this risk group are not reported.
[b]Studies are reported in this volume.

IQ in schizophrenic offspring. The former finding points to the importance of assessing change, a strategy suggested by Ricks (1980). The latter brings to mind an observation by Wishner (1964) that schizophrenia researchers should concentrate on the measurement of variability rather than absolute performance. If intraindividual variability is indeed an important aspect of schizophrenia, then there may well be a logical impasse to finding a marker. That is, any biological predisposition may be manifested as variable (rather than consistently poor) performance. For example, adult schizophrenics' WAIS vocabulary performances are often marked by a variable pattern (Wechsler, 1958). If the same were true for some behaviorally assessed predisposition, then standard deviations or configural analyses of responses might yield more information than analysis of means. In either case – longitudinal change or intraindividual variability – attention to process as well as structure might be incorporated into future risk research.

Even with these caveats, we can point to the consistency with which complex attentional tasks distinguish vulnerable children from normal controls. A susceptibility to distraction seems to be an especially promising area in which to uncover a predisposition to psychopathology. We might note here that the assessment of attention and psychophysiology has been far more consistent across research groups than the assessment of cognition. This is a striking shortcoming in that complex, more dynamically oriented cognitive processes play such an important role in our understanding of schizophrenia in adults. Thus, it may be fruitful to invest more effort in the assessment of, for example, cognitive strategies, assimilation/accommodation, and differentiation/integration.

SUBGROUPS

As seen in Table 2, a number of studies have tried to identify a particularly deviant subgroup among the high-risk children. Most of these attempts have yielded subgroups on the order of 11% to 25% of the total high-risk sample. However, none of these studies has included a nonschizophrenic psychotic control group, so we do not know if the extreme deviance is specific to schizophrenia or not. Hopefully, future studies will provide us with an answer to this question.

The identification of subgroups of high-risk children on the basis of behavioral measures does present one problem. It could be that these deviant high-risk children have already passed an *illness threshold* (Hanson, Gottesman, & Meehl, 1977). We may, in other words, be picking up those risk children who already are caught up in a psychopathological process. The more generally and extensively disturbed these children are, the more likely that this is the case. Therefore, it would be most informative to examine a group of risk children who are deviant in some important way (e.g., attention), but who do not otherwise exhibit any other problems.

OVERVIEW

There is converging evidence for a predisposition to attentional dysfunction (especially under complex conditions) among children at risk for serious psychopathology. The most parsimonious interpretation of the data to date is that this predisposition is a general vulnerability to psychosis. It is reasonable to expect that any attentional disturbance will influence intellectual performance and cognition, with increasing deficits showing up with increasing age as the demands placed upon the child are increased. The high-risk child, like all others, is constantly changing with age. Thus, as we turn more and more to the study of process and longitudinal change, we should be able to say more about the factors that interact with genetic predisposition to produce the many different faces of high risk we now see.

42 Communications patterns and family relations of children at risk for schizophrenia

LYMAN C. WYNNE

The risk research programs reported in this volume differ drastically in the degree to which they attend to family relationships. The most common model in these studies emphasizes a genetic risk transmitted dyadically from one parent to the offspring. It is well recognized that assortative mating, which can be evaluated through diagnosis of psychopathology in the spouses of index parents, can enhance or diminish estimates of risk for the offspring. This risk is both genetic and environmental. When one parent is psychotic, the quality of the functioning of the spouse exerts a significant influence on the adjustment of the children, a point well demonstrated by B. Mednick (1973). She found that most offspring who had breakdowns as adults and who had a schizophrenic mother also had a deviant father. Some of the high-risk programs, such as the Stony Brook project, have explicitly emphasized the importance of studying the psychopathology and personality of the spouses of the index parents. However, it is probably accurate to acknowledge that the risk research field as a whole has not been so vigorous as it should have been in systematically assessing patterns of health or disturbance in the spouses.

Conceptually, the marital couple needs to be assessed not only in terms of genetic transmission and the environmental impact of individual parental pathology and health, but also in terms of a hierarchy of *systems* of relationships – within the marriage, within the family as a whole, and within the broader social network in which the family is embedded. Some of the programs reported in this volume, most explicitly those at UCLA and Rochester, make heavy use of general systems theory as a framework for collecting variables (von Bertalanffy, 1968; Engel, 1980). In this view of systems, larger units cannot be reduced simplistically to their components lest one lose important information about the patterning of the relationships among the components. Thus, the personality is more than a collection of bodily organs, and the family is more than an aggregate of symptoms and personalities. Those programs interested in a systems viewpoint have endeavored to study families as functioning units, especially in home visits and observations of direct interaction of family members with one another. Most of the other programs have relied more fully on the study of individual functioning of parents and their offspring.

Five main classes of methods are relevant to the study of family relationships:

551

1. Retrospective reports. Traditionally, there are those methods that obtain retrospective reports from individual family members about the content of past family life. Early studies of the family background of schizophrenics relied heavily upon retrospective accounts. Part of the stimulus for the risk research field was the widespread doubt that such accounts can provide accurate or relevant data. Hence, risk research has emphasized prospective rather than retrospective data, which are inevitably biased by respondents to fit their later knowledge about outcome. Nevertheless, *some* use of retrospective methods characterizes all of the risk programs, necessarily beginning with information about events preceding the first time of study. Also, until follow-up data become available, the retrospective approach is the main practical means of starting to build a picture of developmental continuities and changes.

Both retrospectively and prospectively, the concept of development needs to be applied to the marriage and the family as systems that go through expectable transitions at such times as when the children start school and the adolescent leaves home. Both the offspring as a developing individual and the family as a whole may become disturbed and reorganized at these transitions in the life cycle.

Several of the risk research programs have used retrospective data about *major* family changes. Most notably, the Danish high-risk study has examined the effects of maternal and paternal separation on subsequent development. Although the use of path analysis by Sarnoff Mednick and his colleagues will be viewed with skepticism by some critics, the findings, at the very least, provide explicit hypotheses worthy of replication. They have shown that the effect of separation from the parents is more profoundly disturbing for male offspring than for female offspring. When institutionalization follows the separation, the effects are especially great for males, but are ameliorated if a grandparent or other relative takes over the rearing. The investigators have interpreted these findings in a framework of stimulus-overload theory. This view is consistent with the finding that an overstimulating family environment after onset of schizophrenia, for example, through high family Expressed Emotion, may precipitate relapse (Vaughn & Leff, 1976a). The gross retrospective data related to separation and institutionalization provide important hypotheses, which need to be illuminated by more detailed study of the actual events and relationship processes in family life before and after such separations.

The whole issue of the differences induced by a new family environment can still be studied in the present risk programs in the follow-up phases yet to come. Sometimes the children will have been transferred to a new family altogether, but, more often, there will have been a new step-parent, creating a new home environment – sometimes with the index parent now missing. It is to be hoped that details about the altered patterns of family relatedness can be examined before and after such changes in the family structure. The McMaster–Waterloo program has attempted to separate out the current impact of the biological parents by selecting samples of foster-reared children; the children in this project were tested at an average age of 15 and had left their biological parents at an average age of 9 years. However, the special stresses necessitating foster placement may well make such samples difficult to compare with other families and other offspring who become schizophrenic. Sameroff has described a subsample in his project in which he found that all six of the mothers who had given up their offspring for adoption or foster-home placement were schizophrenic. These mothers differed from other mothers who were schizophrenic, and their babies also differed as newborns from other offspring of schizophrenics. Such selectivity may well affect the interpretation of adoption studies. Nevertheless, the large-scale adoptive families program currently being carried out in Finland by Tienari and associates (1983) includes not only retrospective data about placement in the adoptive home but also many more detailed data on family communication and relationships that were not obtained in the smaller Danish adoption studies by Rosenthal, Wender, Kety, Schulsinger, Welner, and Ostergaard (1968).

2. Family communication styles. A second approach to the study of family relationships involves the examination of the form and quality, rather than the content, of communication of individual family members, especially the parents. This approach has been used in the UCLA and Rochester programs, and to a lesser extent in the St. Louis project. The concept underlying this approach is that an analog of parent-to-offspring communication can be established by asking the parents to talk about standard materials, especially Rorschach and TAT cards. The form in which the parents focus on the percept, remain task-relevant in their communication, and reason in an understandable manner, can be reliably scored from verbatim tape-recorded protocols (Singer & Wynne, 1966; Jones, 1977). A consideration of categories of communicational problems has been labeled *Communication Deviance*, and, more recently, the healthy counterpart of these difficulties also has been studied systematically in the individual Rorschach (Schuldberg, 1981). Although these methods have been used extensively in prior studies of families in which the offspring is already disturbed, the preliminary data from the Rochester risk research program suggest that studies of the communication of family members meeting directly with one another provide better predictors of offspring adjustment than do the individual parental measures.

3. Interpersonal perception methods. A third approach to the study of family relationships is to obtain parallel data from family members, with each member rating the quality of his or her current relationships with the others, for example, in their ability to confide in one another and to settle disagreements by mutual give-and-take. These methods involve the interpretation of relationships by family members rather than direct measures of their behavior with one another. The Stony Brook, Vermont, St. Louis, and Rochester programs use various forms of these interpersonal perception methods. Unfortunately, there has not been much overlap in these methods that would help evaluate their usefulness, nor has there yet been much comparison of these methods with other measures of family relationships. Nevertheless, a commonsense view of these data would suggest that they are of value and should be pursued in the future as comprehensively and systematically as possible.

4. Direct interaction methods. The fourth class of methods for the study of family communication and relationship moves to the direct observation of family members interacting with one another. Two settings have been used for this approach: observations during home visits and observations during a variety of procedures in the clinic or research laboratory. The most extensive use of the home visit approach was in the first phase of the St. Louis program when naturalistic observations during brief visits were supplemented, with certain families, by an anthropologist (Jules Henry) who lived in the house for as long as a week at a time. This work led to the concept of "unroofing," which refers to the story of a demon who unroofed houses to find out what was going on in the families underneath the roofs. One important observation was that families radically differed with respect to a psychosis that was "involving," in contrast to a noninvolving psychosis. Involving psychoses were observed to include features frequently described in the past literature on families of schizophrenics, including a tendency to "drive one another crazy" with confusing and negative interaction, a lack of reconciling power on the part of the adult, scapegoating processes, and so forth. Among the more recent studies, even in the St. Louis program, there has been a surprising failure to utilize the home visit method. One exception is the Stony Brook High-Risk Project, but reports about their findings are not yet available. Another exception is the Malmö study by McNeil and Kaij, in which the staff members made six home visits during the first year with each of 142 mother–child pairs. This study differed from the more anthropological home observations by emphasizing specific interactions at the points of the mother–infant separation and reunion. This study of attachment failed to reveal differences between the Index and Control groups. Probably a combination of open-ended, unstructured observations, which can pick up unanticipated information, should be combined during home visits with focused, hypothesis-testing observations of family interaction. Professor Bleuler, who for many years has made such rich observations of families in a variety of contexts, would presumably strongly endorse the inclusion of naturalistic observations that are not preoccupied with "counting" measures.

The risk research programs in Rochester and UCLA have made special use of observations of direct family interaction during selected procedures in the clinic. These studies have the advantage over home observations in that interactions can be videotaped and studied in detail and yield high interrater reliability. (Home videotaping has been tried on a small scale, but is uneconomical.) In the Free Play procedure used by the Baldwins and Cole in Rochester, an effort toward a naturalistic, unstructured procedure has been sought through providing age-appropriate toys in the room for the child (who is in the room with the parents, but without a staff member present). By having the setting standardized, families can more readily be compared with one another, although it cannot be proved that the setting is representative of their ordinary home life. Another approach, particularly used at UCLA by Goldstein and Rodnick, has been to have the family discuss together problems that are known to be controversial for them. This modification of Strodbeck's (1954) Revealed Differences approach generates considerable affectivity that has been rated in several forms, especially as Affective Style. Another method, emphasized in the Rochester program, is the Consensus Rorschach, in which the parents are asked to teach the children a task and then to reach agreement about what they all saw in the Rorschach inkblots. These various procedures can be scored with interaction codes, some of which were developed using a Revealed Differences method by Mishler and Waxler (1968), who emphasized such features as positive and negative relationship statements, ability to stay on a present task focus, and acknowledgment or nonacknowledgment of one another's communication. In addition, the Communication Deviance and Healthy Communication measures, first developed for individual Rorschachs and TATs, also have been scored in the consensus procedures and appear to be highly predictive of offspring adjustment.

In the Rochester and UCLA programs, family communication and relationship variables are treated as a class of independent, predictor variables, which then are linked to the dependent child variables. The Rochester program has particularly emphasized the concept of the family system variables as distinct from the parental psychopathology variables. Their recent data suggest strongly that these family system variables are in fact statistically separable from parental psychopathology, whereas both are significant independent predictors of child adjustment in the nonfamily setting of the school.

Both the Rochester and UCLA groups recently have produced some exciting, although preliminary, findings on the links between the Communication Deviance and affective domains. It is possible that their measures of affectivity tap qualities similar to the concept of Expressed Emotion (EE) that has attracted so much attention in recent years as a predictor of relapse in schizophrenia (Vaughn & Leff, 1976b). It may be that the risk research programs shall contribute to continuity of data from the premorbid phase of schizophrenia through the active illness and the course of remissions and relapses. In addition, the UCLA group has clarified other aspects of how affective and communicational variables interact with structural variables, such as whether the father or mother is central in family interaction. Both programs have found that multiple measures obtained with contrasting procedures are clearly superior to single measures that may provide unrepresentative data. Because the analyses of this multiplicity of family variables have scarcely begun, particularly in relation to long-term follow-up, it is highly desirable that the various preliminary findings be replicated and validated. Unfortunately, only a few of the risk programs have given systematic attention to these family communication and relationship variables.

5. Social context. Emphasis in most of the studies has been given to the family triad of parents and an index offspring. However, siblings may be at equal risk; also, the siblings clearly contribute to the intrafamilial context that affects development and outcome.

Additionally, the social context beyond the nuclear family includes a great diversity of variables that appear relevant, beginning with the extended family and moving outward to broader social networks. Methods are now available, though not fully validated, for study of networks (for example, Mitchell, 1974). However, in the risk programs presented in this volume, there has been almost no empirical investigation of these kinds of contextual variables. This omission seems unfortunate, particularly in light of the evidence that families of schizophrenics often are unable to function adequately because they lack appropriate social support networks (Beels, 1978).

Still more broadly, major social variables that affect families and their offspring at risk include social class and ethnicity. The most striking data relevant to social class reported in this volume are found in the Rochester Longitudinal Study of Sameroff, who reports that the functioning of children at risk could be accounted for by social class variability rather than by parental diagnosis. It is not clear to what extent family communication and relationship variables, or at least the mother–infant relationship, may have mediated the social class effects that Sameroff described. In the St. Louis study as well, strong social class effects were found, which interacted with race and with parental diagnosis, making it difficult to have adequate numbers in each cell of the study sample. In the University of Rochester Child and Family Study, an effort to minimize the social class effect was made by not selecting social class V families in the study. Nevertheless, the investigators have found subsequently that social class differences still contribute to the variance in measures such as Communication Deviance. The limited extent to which social class, ethnicity, and other contextual variables have been examined in the risk research programs to date can perhaps be justified in part on the grounds that variables of more immediate clinical relevance (anything that would affect the offspring's symptoms) should be studied first. On the other hand, more definitive interpretations about the generalizability of the findings will be in doubt until contextual variables are examined more fully.

43 *High-risk-for-schizophrenia research: sampling bias and its implications*

RICHARD R. J. LEWINE, NORMAN F. WATT, AND
TED W. GRUBB

It is generally agreed that if we are to understand the etiology of schizophrenia and to prevent its devastating impact, we must study its development before the onset of psychosis (Keith, Gunderson, Reifman, Buchsbaum, and Mosher, 1976). Mednick and McNeil (1968) formalized the rationale for risk research with their critique of etiological studies of adult schizophrenics. They offered the prospective, longitudinal investigation of high-risk children (e.g., the offspring of schizophrenic parents) as a solution to the impossible task of untangling cause and effect in adults.

The importance of genetic predisposition(s) to schizophrenia(s) has been well established (Gottesman, 1978). What we seek now are clues to ontogenesis. It is precisely because the high-risk strategy was adopted to improve etiological studies that we must state clearly and explicitly any factors that may affect our understanding of the development of schizophrenia.

In this chapter, we examine some inadvertent sampling biases that have resulted from the use of parental diagnosis as the risk criterion, and suggest ways in which to complement parental diagnosis in the definition of high risk. We do not intend to suggest the "perfect sample." It simply does not exist. However, through the study of samples with different, but well-defined biases, we can hope to attain a more complete picture of the schizophrenias. Furthermore, by pointing out the limits of generalizability of current risk research, we restate a conceptual lesson easily forgotten in our search for the genetic marker of schizophrenia. Although we study schizophrenia as if it were a – more or less – homogeneous disorder, it is probably best thought of as a group of disorders (E. Bleuler, 1950; M. Bleuler, 1978).

Reprinted from *Schizophrenia Bulletin* (vol. 7, No. 2, 1981, pp. 273–80), a publication of the U.S. Department of Health and Human Services, Public Health Service, Alcohol, Drug Abuse, and Mental Health Administration.

The research reported was supported, in part, by National Institute of Mental Health grants MH-28648 and MH-25935. The authors would like to thank Sharon Medlock and Marsha Healy for their help in the preparation of this article, and Drs. Erlenmeyer-Kimling and Cornblatt for their helpful suggestions.

SAMPLE BIASES AND THEIR CONSEQUENCES

Parent–child concordance

Bleuler (1978) has pointed out that while genetic data indicate that 10 to 15% of adult schizophrenics have a schizophrenic parent, they also show that some 80 to 85% of all adult schizophrenics do *not* have a schizophrenic parent. By the very nature of the genetic risk selection procedure, all of the risk children who eventually develop schizophrenia as adults will have a schizophrenic parent. These schizophrenics with a schizophrenic parent ". . . may represent a subgroup of all schizophrenics who have atypically strong genetic and environmental diatheses" (Hanson et al., 1977, p. 582). The data from research in which risk is defined by parental diagnosis may be applicable, therefore, only to adult schizophrenics with a schizophrenic parent – a minority of all schizophrenics.

Sex bias in index parents

Table 1 presents the sex distribution of schizophrenic index parents for 25 genetic risk research projects. Of the 25 projects, 14 (56%) study only the children of schizophrenic women. Among the remaining 11 studies, index mothers ($N = 606$) far outnumber index fathers ($N = 355$). The disproportion of the sexes in the sampling of index parents contrasts with what is commonly believed to be roughly equivalent prevalence rates of schizophrenia in adult females and males (Dohrenwend & Dohrenwend, 1976).

The overrepresentation of females among index parents is important not only for the introduction of bias with respect to prevalence rates, but also for what may be systematic sex differences in schizophrenic characteristics. Specifically, evidence has been presented that male schizophrenics may generally be characterized as having early onset, poor premorbid histories, and typical, negative symptoms. On the other hand, female schizophrenics may be characterized as having late onset, good premorbid histories, and atypical, positive symptoms (Lewine, 1979, 1980a, 1980b; Lewine, Strauss, & Gift, 1981).

The presence of atypical, affective symptoms in schizophrenia (schizoaffective schizophrenia) has been interpreted by some (Tsuang, Dempsey, & Rauscher 1976) as evidence for a third major psychosis between affective and thinking disorders. However, the symptoms were interpreted by others (Pope & Lipinski, 1978) as evidence of misdiagnosis. Consequently, the overrepresentation of females, with whom the schizoaffective characteristics largely are associated, introduces diagnostic and etiological heterogeneity into the index samples. This is not a problem of risk research per se, but rather of diagnostic procedures.

IMPLICATIONS OF SAMPLING BIAS

Table 2 summarizes the sample biases in the use of parental schizophrenia to define risk in offspring. Aside from the psychometric issue of sample represen-

Table 1. *Sex distribution of schizophrenic index parents in genetic risk research*

Index parent female only	Index parent of either sex		
Study	Study	Females	Males
Garmezy (1974)	Anthony (cited in Garmezy,		
Grunebaum et al. (1975)	1974)	27	19
Itil (cited in Garmezy, 1974)	Dehorn and Strauss (cited		
McNeil and Kaij (1973)[a]	in McNeil & Kaij, 1978)	35	23
McNeil, Persson-Blennow, and	Erlenmeyer-Kimling et al.		
Kaij (1974)	(1979)	44	23
Mednick and Schulsinger (1968);	Hanson, et al. (1976)	14	15
Mizrahi et al. (1974)[a]	Lane and Albee (1970)[a]	66	45
Paffenbarger et al. (1961)[a]	J. Marcus et al. (1979)	11[b]	3[b]
Sameroff and Zax (1973a,		5[c]	0[c]
1973b, 1978)	S. Mednick et al. (1971)	57	26
Schachter, et al. (1975, 1977)	Miller (cited in Garmezy,		
Sobel (1961)	1974)	191	93
Soichet (1959)	Rieder et al. (1975)	46[b]	33[b]
Weidorn (1954)[a]		24[c]	22[c]
Wynne (1968)	Rieder et al[a]	28	17
Yarden and Suranyi (1968)[a]	Weintraub and Neale		
	(1980)	58	36
	Total	606	355
		577[d]	333[d]

Note: Of the 25 genetic risk studies, 14 (56%) examine only female index parents and their children. This table was adapted in part from Garmezy (1974) and McNeil and Kaij (1978).
[a]Cited in McNeil and Kay (1978).
[b]Definite schizophrenics.
[c]Possible schizophrenics.
[d]Excluding possible schizophrenics.

tativeness, evidence of sex differences and the 100% concordance rate between affected target children and parents suggest genotypic and/or phenotypic heterogeneity.

Until the issue of genotypic and phenotypic heterogeneity in schizophrenia is resolved, any systematic bias in sampling needs to be stated clearly and analyzed carefully. To present a highly simplified example, our review of the sample characteristics of current high-risk research suggests that we are ultimately studying a form of schizophrenia transmitted largely through the mother (Lewine, 1979), accompanied by affective, atypical symptoms (Lewine, 1979, 1980a), and yielding a 100% concordance rate between an affected child and its parent (Hanson et al., 1977). The selection of schizophrenic fathers also biases the sample, since male schizophrenics have a lower fertility rate than other males. To the extent that schizophrenic males who become fathers are more competent than those who do

Table 2. *Some sample biases in current genetic risk research*

Sample	Bias
Index offspring who develop schizophrenia	100 percent with schizophrenic parent versus 10%–15% of all adult schizophrenics
Index parent	Overrepresentation of females versus roughly equal prevalence of schizophrenia in adult females and males
	Unknown contribution of misdiagnosis or schizoaffective psychosis
	More fertile (hence, more competent?) male schizophrenics

not, the selection of the former contributes further to a less serious, atypical form of the disorder. Thus, parental diagnosis as the risk criterion may necessarily limit research findings to atypically competent schizophrenics.

There are several consequences of the specific sample biases that we have reviewed:

1. Current risk research relies on theoretical concepts and assessment procedures based largely on adult male populations (Wahl, 1977). Without empirical evidence, we simply do not know the extent to which these measures and theories are applicable to female schizophrenics. Growing recognition of the effects of bias and methodology in the assessment of males and females (Maccoby & Jacklin, 1974; Williams, 1977; Frieze, Parsons, Johnson, Ruble, & Zellman, 1978) suggests a careful reassessment of risk research measurement procedures.

2. As a result of the suggested sex differences in schizophrenia, we must be cautious in generalizing any data from the offspring of schizophrenic women to those of schizophrenic men. We may conceptualize this problem as the need to determine external validity (Campbell & Stanley, 1963) for research findings by sampling across sex of index parent. We do not question that the risk for schizophrenia is the same for the offspring of schizophrenic fathers and mothers (Gottesman, 1978). Rather, by pointing to the evidence that schizophrenia may take different forms in men and women, we raise the possibility that important factors may differ in the ontogenesis of schizophrenia in their offspring. In other words, although the schizophrenic diathesis may be the same for the sexes, differences in onset, clinical manifestation, and course suggest that different psychosocial factors may influence the development of schizophrenia in men and women.

3. To the extent that women more often have a reactive, atypical, or schizoaffective form of schizophrenia, we might expect fewer differences between risk offspring and nonrisk offspring. For example, a frequent finding of risk research is that schizophrenic offspring do not differ substantially from those of depressed

parents, though both do differ from offspring of controls (e.g., Rolf, 1969, 1972). Our analysis suggests that careful diagnosis of index parents – especially mothers – and subsequent analysis of data by schizophrenic subtype of index parent may yield differences between typical and atypical schizophrenic offspring.

We do not intend to deny that selection of risk samples on the basis of parental diagnosis has been useful or to urge that it be abandoned. Rather, we suggest complementing the use of parental diagnosis with other types of risk identification strategies. The adoption of such strategies may help to counteract what Garmezy (1974) has described as "Current definitions [that] are already tending to stereotypy" (p. 93).

SUGGESTIONS FOR FUTURE RESEARCH

Genetic risk identification

One approach might be a prospective, longitudinal study of individuals at risk for schizophrenia – but not currently schizophrenic – by virtue of a full sibling or parental relationship to an identified schizophrenic. Although siblings and parents of schizophrenics have approximately the same rate of schizophrenia as the children of schizophrenics (Gottesman & Shields, 1972) three obstacles would be circumvented in sibling–parent (versus offspring) risk research: (1) Sex bias in the selection of identified schizophrenics; (2) the long interval between initiation of a prospective, longitudinal study in childhood and ultimate schizophrenic psychosis in adulthood; and (3) the reduced fertility of adult male schizophrenics.

Clearly, this strategy produces a biased sample on three counts. First, it would yield a sample of schizophrenics 100% of whom have a schizophrenic first-degree relative. Second, a large portion of the nonaffected relatives' developmental period would be inaccessible to study. Finally, the sample would be biased toward later onset schizophrenia among the target relatives.

Development of behavioral risk indices

The development of behavioral risk indices is a difficult and costly task. Nevertheless, the importance of its contribution and the promising work of predecessors (e.g., Cowen, Gardner, & Zax, 1967; Bower, 1969) suggest that behavioral risk research is a risk worth taking.

We have suggested, for example, the development of teacher-rating forms to assist in the identification of adolescents at behavioral risk for schizophrenia and other serious psychiatric disorders among general school populations. Such behavioral indices would have several major advantages.

1. The sample of adolescents who eventually develop schizophrenia would not be biased by the sampling characteristics of the genetic risk samples. The data collected from such samples would, therefore, be generalizable to a broader spectrum of schizophrenics.

Naturally, the most important question about behavioral risk identification is the hit rate – that is, is there any evidence that behavioral indices predict any better than base rate? In a detailed analysis of this issue, Grubb (1979) employed a measure of discriminative efficiency (Wiggins, 1973) to assess the predictive efficiency of genetic and behavioral indices of schizophrenia. He found that the behavioral prediction of schizophrenia does well enough relative to genetic prediction to encourage further development of behavioral indices. (Both domains of prediction suffer from a high false positive rate and, therefore, exhibit poor discriminative efficiency when applied to the total population.)

2. Because samples of youngsters generated through public school screening would not be preselected for their problem behavior, and school assessment procedures such as the Pupil Rating Form (Watt et al., 1979) assess general behavior rather than problem behavior, risk identification through school assessment can yield important data about normal development. There is no reason to restrict our thinking to psychopathology. As emphasized by Garmezy (1972) in his discussion of invulnerable children, disorder is only part of the story; we must also seek to understand "good outcomes." Furthermore, the emphasis on normal development places the study of psychopathology in a strong theoretical framework from which we can draw upon previously validated assessment techniques. We might also note the potential advantage of both characterizing and conceptualizing risk in terms of predictable *change,* as well as continuity, in personal style, coping patterns, and competence (Ricks, 1980).

3. Behavioral indices are flexible because they are continuous measures and tap different domains of function. Such flexibility allows us to refine our definitions of risk as we gather more empirical evidence. We can, therefore, work to improve the discriminative efficiency of behavioral risk measures.

4. Because of their complexity, any successful set of behavioral predictors may provide us with insight into the developmental paths of the schizophrenias.

A recent critique of behavioral indices made by Hanson et al. (1977) is relevant here. Specifically:

Any time a high-risk child is identifiable on behavioral measures as a candidate for adult schizophrenia, there is reason to suspect that an important threshold in the disease process has already been passed (p. 584).

The problem essentially is whether behavioral indices tap an already extant pathological process or the susceptibility to such a process. We cannot resolve this logical dilemma. However, screening a general school population rather than a child guidance clinic, and focusing on normal rather than "problem" behaviors, might identify subtle indices that may precede more serious disturbance.

Refinement of genetic risk definition

Genetic risk – that is, parental status – and behavioral indices used in combination have proved helpful in the identification of subsets of children at genetic risk (e.g., Hanson, et al., 1977; J. Marcus et al., 1979). Accordingly, there are increasing numbers of reports showing that some offspring of schizophrenics are distinguish-

Table 3. *The use of genetic and behavioral risk indices to study the development of schizophrenia*

Behavioral risk (teacher assessment)	Genetic risk (parental diagnosis)	
	Low	High
Scholastic	Low	
motivation	High	
Extraversion	Low	
	High	
Harmony	Low	
	High	
Emotional stability	Low	
	High	

able by various behavioral characteristics, such as poor motor skills, intraindividual variability, and schizoid withdrawal.

Table 3 presents an outline of one way in which behavioral indices (e.g., behavioral factors based on teacher ratings) may be combined with genetic ones to refine risk classification. The behavioral domains are based on retrospective research (Watt et al., 1979) and current factor analysis of recent pilot data. For example, high risk may be defined statistically by selecting the 5% most introverted children. The direction of deviance that defines risk is determined by past studies that indicate schizophrenia may be preceded by academic incompetence, introversion, disharmony, or emotional tension.

This sort of behavioral definition of risk allows us to refine our classification of risk subjects in two ways: (1) by tapping different domains of functioning (e.g., cognitive, emotional, and interpersonal); and (2) by assessing the effect of varying the cutoff scores for behavioral deviance. We note here that behavioral assessments in this conceptualization are *independent* variables in contrast to their current use as *dependent* variables. The dependent variables might be biochemical, physiological, and behavioral measures taken in the laboratory.

Refinement of parental diagnosis

Diagnostic criteria used to assess index parents should be refined to include age of onset, sex, and degree of emotional symptoms. While the diagnostic data are being collected, they have generally not been used as independent variables to classify schizophrenic index parents. Sample sizes restrict the amount of subclassification that is possible. Consequently, cross-study comparison and replication are essential.

As a simple example, consider the analysis of data by sex of index parent. Although that has been done by some investigators (e.g., Rieder et al., 1975; Erlenmeyer-Kimling et al., 1979), more systematic comparisons of sex differences across risk research programs are needed. For example, in one infant risk study (J. Marcus et al., 1979), schizophrenics' offspring were found to have a lower mean birth weight ($M = 2,976$ g) than did the infants of affectively disordered patients ($M = 3,290$ g), personality disordered patients ($M = 3,434$ g), and normals ($M = 3,137$ g). When we reanalyze the data by sex (omitting one dual-mated couple), however, it appears that lower birth weight is more characteristic of the offspring of definite schizophrenic women ($M = 2,923$) than of schizophrenic men ($M = 3,285$). In view of the small samples used in risk research, it is important to provide analyses by sex in order to determine the stability of such findings.

We have reviewed what we perceive as sampling biases that result from the use of parental diagnosis in the definition of high risk. For both psychometric and theoretical reasons, it seems best to clarify these sampling biases. We do not, in suggesting complementary risk definition strategies, intend to specify the perfect sample. Rather, we believe that by beginning to think in terms of genetic risk, diagnostic complexity, and behavioral indices, we may start to build into our conception and study of risk the rich intricacies that a complete theory of schizophrenic disorders assuredly requires.

44 Overview: adult diagnosis in the study of vulnerability to schizophrenia

Understanding vulnerability to schizophrenia involves two diagnoses. The first is the diagnosis of those offspring who develop the disorder. The second is the diagnosis of the parents, often considered a major clue to offspring vulnerability. Although making both diagnoses has often been considered to be relatively straightforward – even mechanical – that view has been a serious error. Rather, studies of vulnerability allow, and require, one to start with a highly reliable, symptom-based diagnosis, but then in a bootstrapping fashion, to move toward a second phase of discovering diagnostically important characteristics that may define underlying pathologic processes. In the research on vulnerability to schizophrenia, this second phase has already begun. But this more complex phase requires a model for organizing the information obtained to provide an improved basis for conceptualization and discovery.

Studies of children vulnerable to schizophrenia originally focused on the many leads regarding abnormalities thought to be important in such children. Thought disorder, psychophysiologic dysfunction, disorders of socialization or impulse control, egocentricity of perception, and problems with affect, all provided challenging and difficult areas of exploration. Because one major basis for deciding who was vulnerable was to identify a child of a parent who was schizophrenic, there was a tendency to feel that given a reasonably proficient symptom-based diagnosis of schizophrenia in the parent, diagnostic problems were over. It was sometimes thought that diagnosis was almost like a demographic characteristic, such as age: important, but once assessed, focus should be shifted to other areas.

Quickly, however, any such expectations were dashed, and the more complex realities surfaced. These realities have also been more informative than would have been possible with a more mechanical concept of diagnosis. First, it was recognized that even at the level of symptom-based diagnosis, several sets of reliable, generally cross-sectional, diagnostic criteria were available (APA, 1980; Astrachan, Harrow, Adler, et al., 1972; Carpenter, Strauss, & Bartko, 1973; Feighner et al., 1972; Spitzer et al., 1978). The question immediately arose, Which set of criteria should be used? Several studies carried out in the past few years have suggested that, fortunately, there is considerable overlap (Strauss & Gift, 1977; Kendell, Breckington, & Leff, 1979) among the populations identified as schizophrenic by the various diagnostic systems. Although this overlap contributes to methodologic problems in comparing diagnostic approaches, it also means that the concept of schizophrenia appears to have a roughly common, agreed upon core. Actually, there is evidence to suggest that a somewhat expanded core definition of schizophrenia may be the most valid from a genetic viewpoint (Gottesman & Shields, 1976). But in vulnerability studies and other research, it is not even essential to depend totally on one or another diagnostic system. One can consider several diagnostic systems by collecting information to make diagnoses according to them and then by determining empirically which is most valid.

But the problem of diagnosis in vulnerability research is far more complex and interesting than the simple choice among various diagnostic systems. In even the earliest vulnerability studies, some diagnostic issues arose that in retrospect seem obvious. If subjects are selected on the basis of the mother having previously been diagnosed schizophrenic, what does the investigator do when, on evaluation now, the mother is asymptomatic and appears to be functioning well? It is always possible, of course, to say that the original diagnosis was incorrect, but what seems more valid is to question the belief "once a schizophrenic, always a schizophrenic" that had crept into vulnerability studies, as it had into other areas of research and clinical practice.

If one accepts the growing body of data showing that the person with schizophrenia can improve, then the diagnostic criteria of schizophrenia can no longer rest entirely on assuming permanent symptoms or dysfunction. And it has been shown repeatedly that a significant number of persons diagnosed schizophrenic by even the most narrow symptom criteria recover completely in terms of measurable symptomatology and disability (M. Bleuler, 1974a; Ciompi, 1980).

Defining the index parent for vulnerability studies might require attention to more persistent and perhaps more subtle characteristics than symptoms. These other characteristics could help to define persisting underlying processes in schizophrenia more accurately than using symptoms alone. For example, one interpretation of the findings described by Wrede et al. (Chapter 38, this volume) is that the manifest disorder, schizophrenia, in the parent is not an adequate marker of the pathologic processes involved. If birth complications are higher for children of parents who will be diagnosed as schizophrenic several years later, perhaps there is some more basic long-standing problem in the parent yet to become schizophrenic than the symptoms themselves. The work of Klein and Salzman (Chapter 28, this volume), may suggest one such characteristic – psychophysiologic abnormality – that persists even after symptoms diminish or disappear. The premorbid adjustment literature showing higher rates of withdrawal and aggressiveness in people who later become schizophrenic (Watt, 1978) may also reflect a more persistent underlying process than do symptoms. The possibility, becoming clearer as vulnerability studies progress, is that many kinds of abnormal processes in schizophrenic persons, occurring before or after psychotic episodes, need to be considered as diagnostically relevant in the parents and to be considered in their offspring.

But not all parents go from sick to well. Some stay sick, and an opposite phenomenon occurs. Mothers who are normal controls for vulnerability studies, when followed over time, may develop psychopathology (Sameroff et al., Chapter 37, this volume). These findings indicate that parents from Control as well as Risk groups that are used as potential markers for child vulnerability are like moving targets, just as the work of Fisher et al. (Chapter 25, this volume) and other studies have shown is true for the children. Neither remains static, so that in the diagnostic assessment of parents, as with children, longitudinal variation and evolution need to be considered along with the cross-sectional, symptom-based, diagnostic criteria formerly often viewed as sufficient.

The issues noted above are important for considering the environmental as well as genetic impact of parent characteristics that may contribute to offspring vulnerability. If one focuses primarily on environmental impact on the child, the longitudinal variation in schizophrenic parents opens up a range of important questions that are complex but also may shed more light on the processes involved. For one thing, just as with symptoms, other parent characteristics that may contribute to vulnerability in their offspring may also shift over time. Patterns of thought disorder, affective expression, perhaps even psychophysiologic variables, might vary longitudinally.

And what if it is not the presence or absence of a parental characteristic, but the duration of the characteristic that is crucial? Perhaps a parent who is symptomatic for several years is more likely to have a vulnerable child than a parent who is symptomatic for only a brief period. Or perhaps there are crucial periods in child development during which dysfunction in the parent has a maximum impact. Of course, if there is a buffering effect by a healthy parent (Wynne & Singer, 1964) that offsets pathogenic contributions of the disordered parent, a diagnosis of the healthy parent should also be available.

The work of Sameroff et al. (Chapter 37, this volume), suggesting that different environments at specific times can influence the emergence of deviance together with Worland et al.'s, reporting (Chapter 7, this volume) the importance of parent involvement and shifts in parent status as major factors, and Rodnick and Goldstein's findings on mothering patterns of schizophrenic women (1974) further suggest the complexity of the processes involved and the limitations of only considering a parent's symptom-based diagnosis as the major indicator of offspring vulnerability.

Some investigators have attempted to reduce the problem of parent variability by only studying children of those narrowly diagnosed schizophrenic persons who also have long-standing, unremitting disorder. Information from such studies can certainly provide one important segment of data about schizophrenia. By themselves, however, such studies are not sufficient. Several investigators (e.g., Lewine et al., 1981) have raised the question of whether children of chronic schizophrenic parents who themselves become schizophrenic are really representative of schizophrenia generally. Almost all research groups, even those in the densely populated New York City area, have found that children of process schizophrenic parents are relatively hard to find. As has frequently been noted, persons with chronic schizophrenia are less likely to have children than others. In any case, the considerable proportion (about 85%–90%) of people who become schizophrenic who are not offspring of a schizophrenic parent diagnosed by any criteria makes it essential for vulnerability research to extend beyond the study of only process schizophrenic parents and their children. Thus as so often happens, the original idea of studying children of schizophrenic parents, although continuing to be extremely valuable, has become more complex as it has become better understood.

These diagnostic issues in vulnerability research remain fragmented unless we also note briefly the relationship of some of these problems to diagnosing the vulnerable child who has a disorder. In the study of children who may be developing schizophrenia, diagnosis involves many of the same questions as for their parents. For the children, too, not only is the selection of criteria for diagnosis important, identifying *partial* or *pre*-schizophrenic abnormalities and the evolution of disorder is essential as well.

All of these issues point to what is really the crucial question: How do the key processes in the parent relate to key processes in the child? Thus, the question of diagnosis, expanding in complexity but also in validity, has evolved from an apparent attempt to identify a relatively fixed independent variable, parent diagnosis, to the construction of a canonical correlation, where both sides of the equation (parent/child) may vary considerably, and the degree and the nature of the relationship between the variables on each side needs to be explored.

It should not come as a total surprise that the processes involved in the vulnerability to schizophrenia and their implications for diagnosis are complex. Nor should the mental health field be particularly apologetic about such findings. There are over 20 interacting processes that determine something as comparatively simple as normal blood pressure. Recent findings on the function of the cerebral cortex indicate that there are hundreds of thousands of neurons involved, some of which function in coordinated bundles, many of which interact in diverse ways with other parts of the brain, and many of which, besides their basic excitatory function, have sets of inhibitory fibers and inhibitors of inhibitory fibers. There is no reason why vulnerability to schizophrenia should not also be complex.

Although empirical studies have led to new levels of diagnostic complexity in terms of methodology and conceptualization, they have also helped to bring us from a state of rather naïve theoretical bliss to a comprehension of the realistic possibilities that seems far more likely to be fruitful. The question, of course, is how to handle this complexity. Fortunately, several approaches to a solution are possible. The first is the Risk Research Consortium itself. Given the complexities of the field, it would be unrealistic to believe that any single group could study effectively the offspring of enough types of parents, have the expertise to make the necessary assessments in all areas, or have the longitudinal structure studying children and parents of various ages to explore the range of groups, variables, and processes that might be important. By bringing together several investigative groups with different but overlapping samples, assessment techniques, and areas of expertise, a much broader range of cause–effect relationships related to vulnerability can be explored effectively. This collaborative structure combines the efficiency of having research groups of limited size with the availability of a wide range of findings and methods, even at early stages of study. As Garmezy and

Streitman (1974) noted early in the development of the consortium, the sharing of methods and findings across investigative groups magnifies the value of all the projects.

Certain methodologic strategies applied within the structure of the consortium increase still further the potential for discovering even relatively complex factors important for improved parent and offspring classification. Several of these strategies were discussed in depth at the consortium statistical conferences held at UCLA and Yale. One of the more traditional approaches involves using control or comparison groups. The difficulties in applying even such a basic approach in vulnerability research are considerable because certain classification variables not often considered as essential are repeatedly found to have extremely important key relationships. Two variables most commonly associated with a wide range of other variables – and thus providing problems in establishing controls – are social class and IQ. Repeatedly, these characteristics correlate more highly with child performance in many areas, even certain areas originally considered as representative of psychopathology, than do many of the variables more specific to schizophrenia that are being employed. Techniques such as analysis of variance and of covariance have been used to provide statistical comparison groups, but there is the recurrent danger, as noted by Rolf (personal communication; 1975), that if too much is altered by the use of statistical (or sampling) controls, one is in the position of the person who tried to compare moose and bears. In order to get a comparable group in each sample, he picked only those moose who had no antlers. The comparison is possible, but may not be particularly informative.

A diagnostic approach to managing complexity, as demonstrated, for example, in the work of Wrede et al. (Chapter 38, this volume), is to focus on homogeneous subgroups of the population. Such an approach is important and needs to be pursued, but it can also create significant problems by reducing group size available in a given cell, by possibly selecting misleading subgrouping criteria, and by obscuring possible important dimensions in favor of selecting narrowly defined types (Cudeck et al., Chapter 3, this volume).

Multivariate statistical techniques have often been used to establish improved classifications of parent and offspring. These techniques include cluster analysis, multidimensional scalogram analysis (Marcus et al., Chapter 35, this volume), and path analysis (Mednick et al., Chapter 2, this volume). Another method of potential value that has not yet been applied for this purpose is stratification analysis (Feinstein, 1972), which is particularly helpful with discontinuous relationships. Although these various techniques are valuable for handling complex multivariate data, they are often more effective for hypothesis-generating than for hypothesis testing. Because of the number of choices that need to be made in using these approaches, the investigator must specify the basic hypotheses, weighting of variables, paths, and models, or these will be chosen, perhaps in an irrelevant fashion, by the method itself.

Finally, there is an approach that Bleuler has suggested and we have pursued for dealing with the complex processes that must be the basis for diagnosis; namely, to focus considerable effort on hypothesis generating and development through the

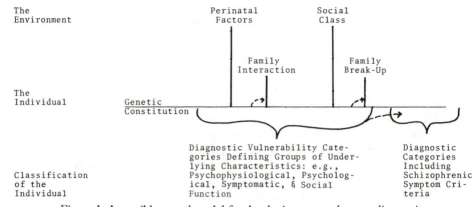

Figure 1. A possible causal model for developing more adequate diagnostic concepts for vulnerability research.

use of intensive research design with a limited number of subjects (Bleuler, Chapter 40, this volume; Strauss et al., 1981). Such an approach may work best when it combines both clinician and investigator input either by the participation of clinician–investigators, or by including persons with each type of skill as members of the research group.

If the complexities of classification in the vulnerability field appear to be overwhelming, it will be valuable to focus not so much on how far we have to go, but on how far we have come. The original model – explicit or implicit – of much etiologic research in schizophrenia was a simple causal model; either a genetic trait or an environmental factor (e.g., schizophrenogenic mother) caused schizophrenia. When empirical research began to demonstrate how difficult it was to validate these models and how incomplete were the definitions of the antecedents and the consequences (schizophrenia), a second generation of models was born. The concept of diathesis (genetic) and stress (environmental) provided a useful next step for investigating and conceptualizing cause–effect relationships. However, this model, although valuable, has also appeared to be insufficient (Strauss & Carpenter, 1981).

The work of this consortium demonstrates both the incompleteness of the earlier models and suggests the kinds of model that we may need for the next generation of conceptualization and classification. One such model, in a simple form, is depicted in Figure 1. Genetic characteristics start the process. These are modified by perinatal phenomena (McNeil & Kaij, Chapter 36, this volume; Wrede et al., Chapter 38, this volume), influencing the infant to have certain characteristics that may make him or her vulnerable to the development of schizophrenia as well as to having other possible evolutions. Family interaction patterns, family breakup, social class, interacting in an evolving way with the individual's psychophysiologic and other biologic variables, further shape the developing child and its environment. These characteristics, reflected in and perhaps further influenced by, behavior in school and its consequences, and perhaps finally triggered by life events to which the individual may have become specifically vulnerable, may complete the pathway that is the true representation of vulnerability to schizophrenia. Identification of groups at each stage is necessary, but no single cross-sectional characteristic or characteristics in this pathway seem likely to be sufficient. Although some may be necessary, even this has not yet been demonstrated.

As many, such as Bleuler, Wynne, Anthony, and others, have suggested, the evolution of vulnerability to schizophrenia appears to be a complex process reflecting the basic longitudinal processes of the disorder itself. Concepts of adult assessment and diagnosis to be useful must progress from depending primarily on symptom criteria to reflecting these processes and their evolution. The work of the consortium, including further development and revision of a causal model and related classificatory concepts, and the placing of each project at a specified point or points within that model, will greatly promote continued progress in this effort.

45 In a nutshell: the first two decades of high-risk research in schizophrenia

NORMAN F. WATT

Professor Bleuler observed accurately that longitudinal investigation – lasting decades – of the fate of children at risk for psychosis is a task of gigantic scope. Synthesizing the results of 15 such programs in a few pages is ambitious at the very least; some might say it is preposterous. There are some observations about method and design that are important to underline. These will be dealt with first. There are abundant research findings that represent what we have learned about schizophrenic disorders, and several more that show what we must unlearn about these enigmatic conditions. Several large questions remain unanswered, including some of the most important ones. The second part of this review will summarize these results. Finally, every research group has formulated some conceptual rationale to make theoretical sense of its observations and inferences about the manifestations, causes, course, and outcome of schizophrenic illness. The last part of the chapter will highlight these theoretical formulations.

Ideas and findings featured in this review will sometimes cite the name of the project as it is listed in the table of contents and sometimes the first author. Abbreviations will seldom be used, except that HR shall stand for High Risk or children of schizophrenic parents, PC for Psychiatric Controls or children of nonschizophrenic psychiatric patients, NC for Normal Controls or children of two normal parents, and RRC for Risk Research Consortium.

METHOD

The basic logic of the high-risk approach has been emphasized throughout this volume: to study prospectively children believed to have greater risk for schizophrenia than the average person. The issue of employing shotguns or rifles for this purpose has clearly weighed in favor of rifles. The Mauritius Project is the only large-scale attempt to study a whole population of children by any criterion of risk. There have been no population surveys with follow-up that have *not* selected research subjects by some specific criterion of risk. Hence we have not followed the suggestion of a sociologist to pursue large stratified samples in order to offset the scientific restrictions imposed by studying narrowly defined risk groups. The

This chapter was supported, in part, by NIMH Grant No. MH00340.

572

overwhelming majority in the RRC have concentrated on children of schizophrenic parents, perhaps reflecting the urgent need, felt by most, to exceed population base rates for schizophrenic prevalence in our research samples. Except for the UCLA and Mauritius programs, and to a lesser extent the Minneapolis program, selection criteria other than genetic ones have been neglected. There is, however, a growing research base within the RRC for developing prospective studies based on behavioral, familial, cognitive, and sociocultural indices of risk.

We have paid a strategic price for that preference. Lewine et al. (Chapter 43) remind us that we have concentrated on quite unrepresentative samples, in effect targeting only 10% to 15% of the ultimate spectrum of schizophrenic adults, namely those with schizophrenic parents. Moreover, our samples contain an overwhelming predominance of schizophrenic mothers over fathers, and selective sampling of the fathers because schizophrenic men usually do not marry and have families. It is also likely that the schizophrenic parents we have studied are unrepresentative of schizophrenics generally, for example, being less chronic or tending more toward schizoaffective forms of the disorder. We must be circumspect about these sampling restrictions, recognizing that we may learn a great deal about some schizophrenic people that does not apply to others.

Diagnostic issues

How do we classify schizophrenic people? Garmezy (Chapter 1) points out that distinctions between process and reactive forms, paranoid versus nonparanoid syndromes, and acute versus chronic course of illness have been useful in past research, but these subclassifications have not been featured systematically by most of the studies in this volume. Dramatic changes in the diagnostic criteria for schizophrenic disorders recently published in DSM-III have sensitized us to the large differences in diagnostic practice here and in Europe, and narrowed the gap substantially. Increasing diagnostic rigor has revealed how many of the patients considered schizophrenic by hospital personnel, even employing relatively conservative criteria, later must be reclassified, usually among the affective psychoses. Agonizing reclassifications of index parents to bring the diagnoses into line with DSM-III have been time-consuming and costly, with the general result of shrinking the size of the schizophrenic samples, displacing many of those subjects into the psychiatric control groups. One can plausibly ask if the striking similarities in the behavior and performance of the high-risk (HR) offspring and the psychiatric control (PC) offspring are attributable, in part, to similarities among the index parent groups on dimensions such as chronicity and affectivity.

The University of Rochester Child and Family Study (URCAFS) team has probably taken the greatest effort to evaluate the clinical diagnosis of the index parents and to incorporate diagnostic variability into the fabric of their research program. According to Kokes, almost half of their index parents were diagnosed as chronic patients and more than half were unequivocally psychotic, but the average length of total hospitalization was only 20 weeks, spread over less than three admissions. Their subjects came from intact, mostly middle-class families with middle-aged parents of above-average intelligence, whose social and work functioning were not severely impaired. Two things are noteworthy about this description, which is not atypical of most of the samples in the consortium. First, it is remarkable to compare the 20 weeks of total hospitalization for these patients with the median of several years recorded for mental patients hospitalized in 1955. Clearly, times (and practices) have changed! The description also raises a serious concern about sampling. The cross-fostering studies in Copenhagen (Kety, Rosenthal, Wender, Schulsinger, & Jacobsen, 1975) indicate clearly that schizophrenia is more prevalent among the offspring of chronic schizophrenic parents than among those with more benignly affected schizophrenic parents. If our selection procedures yield samples of index schizophrenic parents with predominantly mild impairments, the payoff in the proportion of their offspring who become schizophrenic may therefore be reduced.

Strauss (Chapter 44) raises the interesting issue that schizophrenic disorder, defined in traditional terms of clinical symptoms, is not constant over time. Schizophrenics do improve, some recover completely, and others get worse. In all cases, a dynamic model incorporating possibilities for change is required for the diagnosis of parents, just as dynamic models of development are required for characterizing their children. The findings in this volume that show significant deviance at times before or after the emergence of clinical symptoms in schizophrenics – whether the objects of study are parents or offspring – reflect continuing underlying processes that may be causally important but *not directly related* to the symptoms that have traditionally defined the disorder. Many kinds of abnormal processes in schizophrenic persons, occurring before, during, or after psychotic episodes, need to be considered as diagnostically relevant.

Mednick (Chapter 2) presents a very thoughtful argument for *dimensionalizing* the clinical manifestations of disorder in place of the currently accepted practice of discrete classification by syndrome or type. He makes a pitch for path analysis and causal modeling as useful new techniques for analyzing such dimensional variables. The example cited concluded that institutional child care is a common precursor of adult schizophrenic clinical symptoms in HR males. The analysis further suggested that rearing by more benign agents than a schizophrenic mother may reduce psychiatric risk, a disputable point for environmental protection.

Working in the same shop, Cudeck (Chapter 3) decries the limitations of clinical symptoms for classifying schizophrenic disorders in a meaningful way. On the other hand, despite the exhortations of Szasz and other antipsychiatry enthusiasts, the consensus of specialists in this volume is that a valid schizophrenic pattern of abnormal behavior actually exists, although the exact boundaries of the condition are elusive and the behavioral pattern is variable between persons and over time. Experts feel that they know schizophrenia when they see it, although it's hard to prove they know it or to describe what they know. The extraordinary heterogeneity among schizophrenic people, both prior to and after the onset of psychosis, is repeatedly emphasized in the investigations reported here. In an effort to deal constructively with such heterogeneity, Cudeck presented an elaborate multidimensional analysis of clinical symptoms that yielded seven reliable factors, in terms of which schizophrenic disorder was depicted as a combination of very poor cognitive functioning, salient interpersonal avoidance, and a low level of depression.

Considering the controversial history of psychiatric diagnosis, it is encouraging to see how much progress has been made by RRC teams toward achieving precision and reliability of classification, but it remains one of our greatest and most complex problems.

Variables studied

The variables chosen for study in HR children focus primarily on social, cognitive, emotional, neurophysiological, and sociocultural factors that have some plausible relation to the signs and symptoms commonly associated with schizophrenic disorders. Interpersonal evaluations have centered on extraversion, harmony, popularity, assertiveness, and general competence, obviously expecting bad news to emerge early among HR children who eventually become schizophrenic. Cognitive assessments have examined attention deployment, problem solving, intelligence, and cognitive styles. Emotional appraisals have looked for stability, integrity of emotions, and temperamental styles. Neurophysiological investigations have examined electrodermal functions, such as autonomic lability and arousal, and hard or soft signs of brain damage or neurointegrative defects. Related to this are the studies of pregnancy and birth complications, which obviously seek reproductive abnormalities that might contribute to neonatal or developmental deviations. Sociocultural investigations have featured family dynamics, social class, and communication styles.

Notably lacking in the research reported are developmental studies of belief systems and neuropathological studies of ventricular size in the brain which have been implicated in adult schizophrenia. The latter omission can be attributed to its recent emergence in the research literature since the inception of these high-risk projects. Nevertheless, both areas deserve some attention in future studies.

Transsituational pervasiveness in behavior patterns has been emphasized clearly by the RRC teams, which indicates a strong commitment to search for persisting traits with both contemporary and longitudinal stability. Cynics might write this search off as wishful thinking, especially in view of the diversity and variability already observed in schizophrenic people. Nevertheless, it is noteworthy that most of these investigators expect to find at least some dependable regularities that cut across situations and/or persons.

Research designs and procedures

Collectively, the consortium teams have clearly favored longitudinal, rather than cross-sectional, research designs. Several limitations derive from that choice. When the span of a research program stretches over decades, the developmental variables chosen for study and the psychological measures for them may become somewhat obsolete. Even for a span as short as 2 or 3 years, performance on a particular measure may hold very different psychological significance in a 10-year-old than in that same person at 13. Not only do variables or measures erode with time, so also do investigators. Virtually every research group has experienced some turnover in personnel. URCAFS, the largest group, started with 22 professional investigators in 1972, but only a handful of the original team remains in Rochester a decade later. Some investigators retire before their research subjects grow up; others move to new areas of research interest or other institutions; still others leave research altogether and take up new professional challenges. Some, notably the team leaders who initially conceived the projects, persist with steadfast determination. It is these, obviously, who carry out the follow-up studies and draft the progress reports.

Garmezy (Chapter 18) makes the strongest claims for cross-sectional studies of developmental issues. A strong feature of the URCAFS program, largely influenced by consultation with Garmezy, is the *convergence* design for accelerating longitudinal research: studying different cohorts of research subjects at 3-year age gates, in order to piece together the whole developmental sequence of behavior. In many respects, Wynne's introductory overview of the URCAFS program (Chapter 23) provides an instructive conceptual model for planning a systematic longitudinal project. Recently, the St. Louis project has also added some features of the convergence design, but the majority of the consortium teams have held firmly to the prospective, high-risk model originally exemplified in the Danish project.

Longitudinal designs do not establish causal relations. All of us recognize that fact, and Sameroff (Chapter 37) emphatically reminds us of it. They do, however, offer unique vantage points for viewing development and for making inferences about causal relations. There seems to be an implicit concession by most in the RRC that careful, systematic longitudinal description of developmental patterns is sufficient at this point, in view of our ignorance about the developmental precursors of schizophrenic disorders. There has been no neglect of the importance of control comparisons and of psychological theory, but much has been wagered on the instruction to be anticipated from prospectively tracing the childhood development of the few subjects that ultimately will become schizophrenic.

Hopefully, the reader has not overlooked the importance of the methodological innovations that have formed the groundwork for these projects, such as the Baldwins' creative employment of Free Play as a medium for measuring family relations (Chapter 29), Marcus's use of Guttmann's scalogram techniques (Chapter 35), Cudeck's sophisticated multidimensional analysis of clinical symptoms (Chapter 3), and Munson's unique (in the RRC) adaptation of the Q-sort for classifying children psychiatrically (Chapter 26). Countless assessment devices have been created and painstakingly developed for these projects, and their recognition is often slighted in the rush to learn about project findings and conclusions.

Sex differences have been studied by some research groups, but the salience of those differences has not been impressive. Most of the sex differences observed in the samples at risk have paralleled differences found in the control groups, thus offering little leverage to advance our knowledge in this area of psychopathology.

Problems of method and inference

All of the research groups have contended with powerful forces of attrition in their samples: family disintegration, withdrawal from study participation, geographic migration, diagnostic reclassification, further hospitalizations, and so on. It is a tribute to the stubborn persistence of dedicated research staffs that the great majority of the samples have been followed throughout the childhood of the subjects.

The problem of sample attrition is related to the question of the optimal age to begin the study of children at risk, which has been resolved pluralistically. Various projects have focused on the parental period, birth, early infancy, preschool age, school age, and adolescence. It is not surprising that the findings with the most transparent relevance to the ontogenesis of schizophrenic disorders have been drawn from the later age-group studies, but plausible and promising leads have derived from investigations at all developmental periods. Moreover, it is too early to evaluate the relevance of the findings from the earliest age periods because few of those subjects have yet reached the age of maximum risk for disorder. Youngsters followed from middle childhood and adolescence have entered young adulthood only recently, so the jury is still out on the question of when to begin high-risk studies.

Most RRC groups have included appropriate contrast groups for study, frequently children of psychiatrically hospitalized (but not schizophrenic) parents. Intelligence and social class have proven to be pervasive and troublesome sources of confusion in interpreting research results. Should they be controlled as "sources of contamination" in analyzing statistical results, or should they be considered as important precursors of schizophrenic disorders worthy of study in their own right? Social class plays a powerful role in the family lives and in the individual functioning of both children and their parents, indeed a greater role in Sameroff's project than parental diagnosis (Chapter 37). We should confess that social class has received inadequate attention, either methodologically or conceptually, from most RRC groups. It remains a continuing source of ambiguity in regard to interpreting our data.

Teachers and parents clearly have been entrusted with much responsibility for evaluating children's behavior, notwithstanding the heavy skepticism from decades past regarding the reliability and validity of their judgments. Asarnow's methodological study (Chapter 33), using systematic classroom observations of attending behavior as a criterion, strongly validated teacher ratings of competence, as did Watt's validity studies with sociometric procedures and systematic observation (Chapter 13). The breadth of their employment as referees, in Copenhagen, New York, Stony Brook, Rochester, Minneapolis, Waterloo, and St. Louis, speaks both for the confidence in them as observers and for the lack of alternative sources of observation. More than was envisioned in 1972, peers have been similarly employed, especially in Stony Brook, Minneapolis, Rochester, and Waterloo.

There has been an appreciable swing during the last decade from linear analyses of group differences to more diversified searches for *outliers* that may plausibly include the subjects most likely to become schizophrenic. This may, in part, reflect some frustration in seeking monolithic markers that distinguish high-risk samples from controls, for such have decidedly *not* been found. It also reflects increasing sophistication and appropriate disillusionment with simplistic conceptions about very complex disorders. It is unrealistic to expect breakthroughs in treatment and etiological theory along the lines of the Salk vaccine for polio and the discovery of chromosomal damage in Down's syndrome. The adjustments in statistical approach take account of the subtlety and complexity of the disorders under study.

The St. Louis team has been more willing than most to conduct and report qualitative clinical studies, with anecdotal evidence and frankly intuitive analysis. Very revealing, for example, is the description of the exasperating task of making home visits to families with a psychotic parent, an experience to which many in the RRC surely resonate. Though most groups have refrained from such qualitative studies, many have videotaped interviews, conducted case studies, and incorporated anecdotes to illustrate their more traditional research reports.

Ethical safeguards

How does one protect research subjects from unethical exposure or stigmatization – either in their own minds or in the view of others – regarding a possible eventuality that probably will never occur? On the other hand, how does one present a compelling invitation to participate in high-risk research without creating unethical exposure or stigmatizing awareness? The answers are that one treads many fine lines and straddles several fences to achieve the worthy aims of the research and still protect the subjects from harm or unnecessary anxiety.

The consortium has set and maintained a standard of ethical safeguards that is truly impressive. Most have obtained written, informed consent from subjects and their parents repeatedly, sometimes every year. This has been accomplished with little deception, usually on the grounds of needing to know more about the children and families of hospitalized psychiatric patients. "Screens" have been created and maintained carefully to protect children from harmful stigmatization at school, while still offering plausible explanations to teachers and others for their cooperation in the research. Despite enormous strains imposed by longitudinal research designs, unavoidable involvements with many public and social service agencies, the psychiatric condition of the parents, and many others, most of the research groups have maintained successful research alliances with the great majority of their subjects and their families. Many teams, notably the St. Louis and New York groups, have provided clinical or referral services for their subjects, either directly or indirectly. When dealing with populations as severely disturbed as our index parents, some legal complications are unavoidable, but to our knowledge there have not been more than minor legal or ethical complaints raised by our subjects against the investigators for their conduct of the research. Bill Curran, an expert on legal and ethical issues in mental health research, considered the investigations we planned in 1972 as comparatively "benign." It seems fair to judge the studies, in retrospect, both benign in their effects and tenaciously persistent in their execution. In view of social sensitivities about the subject of schizophrenia, that is encouraging news for other areas of mental health research where high-risk approaches might be contemplated.

RESULTS

The findings of the various research programs will be reviewed here in roughly chronological sequence of development, starting with studies of pregnancy and birth, then infancy and early development, and later childhood next. After that we shall discuss family relations, followed by cognitive functions, and the premorbid picture in cases of early clinical breakdown. Finally, we shall touch on three relatively neglected areas of research: biopsychological functions, intervention, and the adaptive strengths of children at risk.

Pregnancy and birth

The studies of pregnancy and delivery present a grim picture of schizophrenic mothers, but one that hardly differs from the plight of mothers with other psychiatric disturbance. Wrede (Chapter 38) found that the deliveries of schizophrenic women, most of which occurred *before* the onset of psychosis, were attended by more difficulties than average. Similarly, Sameroff (Chapter 37) found more prenatal complications and lower birth weight in HR infants than in NCs, but these were attributed to chronic antipsychotic medications. (This implies that most of Sameroff's deliveries occurred *after* the onset of psychosis.) According to McNeil (Chapter 36), mothers with previous psychiatric disturbances of *all* kinds reported more stressful pregnancies than average, which was visibly reflected in their psychological status during the pregnancy interviews.

Severity and chronicity of psychiatric disability were associated strongly with socioeconomic deprivation in Wrede's and Sameroff's samples. It is not clear which caused which, but from the work of Strauss and Carpenter (1981) showing the importance of social competence and work history for shaping the long-term course of schizophrenic disorder, it is plausible to infer that external social and economic factors in early development are powerful determinants of the potential for recovery from acute schizophrenic disorder, conceivably greater in power than intrinsic diatheses for the disorder. We cannot clearly relate social class to reproductive problems, however, because of conflicting findings. Sameroff found reproductive abnormalities of many kinds were associated with socioeconomic deprivation, but Wrede reported they were not. Wrede found that Chronic schizophrenics experienced the most pregnancy complications, but Mild schizophrenics registered the most severe complications at delivery. She also discovered that reproductive complications were most frequent among winter deliveries and least frequent among summer deliveries, a replicated finding in Scandinavia of obscure significance at present.

It is not surprising that many schizophrenic mothers give up their babies for adoption or foster-home placement, and Sameroff studied them closely. Those who gave up their babies were older and from lower class backgrounds than those who kept their babies; they were also more likely to be unmarried currently, socially incompetent, anxious, severely disturbed, and to have longer histories of emotional disturbance. The course of the pregnancy and the condition of the infants were also worse, which indicates that schizophrenic mothers who relinquish their babies are not a random sample of schizophrenic mothers in general. On the contrary, they are severely and chronically disturbed, older, poorer, and so forth. Hence, their offspring might be expected to have a more malignant disposition for emotional disorder. A higher degree of pathology has likewise been suspected in the Danish adoption studies (Wender et al., 1974).

Infancy and early development

Most of Fish's HR infants (Chapter 34) were relinquished by severely and chronically disturbed schizophrenic mothers, like those described by Sameroff. About half of these infants showed temporary delays and disorganization of motor and sensorimotor development and physical growth. These were not associated with pregnancy or birth complications in this small sample. Fish believes that this *pandysmaturation* reflects an inherited neurointegrative defect in schizotypal infants who may compensate or break down, depending on their environments. However, proof of specificity would require a large scale replication including PCs.

In the Israeli study (Chapter 35), Marcus found about two-thirds of the HR infants performed poorly in the motor and sensorimotor tasks during the first year of life (with two extreme outliers) and discounted the potential explanation of causation by reproductive complications. He speculated that the findings may reflect some genetically determined neurointegrative defect, which is consistent with the findings and formulations of Fish regarding pandevelopmental retardation. However, Marcus's theory glides over a parsimonious interpretation of his results, namely, that low birth weight per se may account for most of the sensorimotor deficiencies observed, independently of any genetic mediation.

The HR infants observed by McNeil (Chapter 36) showed slightly more evidence of neurological abnormality, which corroborates results of both Marcus and Fish, but they differed very little from controls temperamentally. Especially the babies of cycloid and schizophrenic psychotics displayed little reaction to separation from their mothers and no sign of stranger anxiety, which suggests early disturbance in the emotional bonding of these babies. McNeil warns us, however, not to leap too quickly from such preliminary results to inferences about the etiology of psychiatric disorders. That is prudent advice, considering that few results clearly distinguish HR cases from psychiatric controls.

Sameroff (Chapter 37) found no behavioral abnormalities at birth among HR infants, and the only deficiencies observed at 4 months and 12 months were in psychomotor development. This corroborates the findings of Marcus, Fish, and McNeil, but the motoric immaturity observed by Sameroff in the first year of life was absent at 30 months (except as compared with white controls from high social class families). At 30 months the HR infants were only "less reactive" than NC infants, which seems consistent with McNeil's finding a possible disturbance of emotional bonding at about the same age. Sameroff departs sharply from Fish and Marcus in interpreting the significance of his findings. He concludes that HR children have many developmental problems, but these do not appear to be the simple result of schizophrenic parentage. When compared to the offspring of white, normal, middle-class mothers, HR children have lower cognitive, linguistic, and motor performance scores, poor adaptive behavior and emotional state, and worse behavior in the testing situation. However, social class and severity and chronicity of the mother's psychiatric condition accounted for most of these differences, not schizophrenia per se. It might be argued, on the other hand, that such extreme environmental circumstances restrict the range of behavioral variability expressed or observed. In less oppressive circumstances greater genetic variation might be more observable.

Sameroff reinforces his viewpoint in interpreting the findings for HR babies given up for adoption. Placement infants were more premature and had more physical problems than the home-reared sample, which challenges the assumption that such HR babies bring nothing unique to their new families other than "schizophrenic genes." The extra caretaking demands for prematurity, as well as predictable temperamental abnormalities, may contribute to a negative chain of interpersonal transactions that could produce a deviant outcome regardless of the infant's genetic inheritance.

From the studies of pregnancy, birth, and infant development we can draw several general conclusions. Schizophrenic mothers have unusually frequent and serious complications of pregnancy and delivery that may threaten the development of their children. Such complications are more extreme if the mother's psychiatric disturbance is severe and chronic, and in such cases the mothers are more likely to give up their babies for adoption or foster-home placement. It is not clear which reproductive complications may be specific to schizophrenic disorders or characteristic of psychiatric disorders generally. Infants of schizophrenic mothers are not extremely deviant in most respects, but some do show deficiencies in psychomotor development early and in emotional attachment later in the preschool period. Again it is problematic to attribute these developmental abnormalities to a genetically inherited diathesis for schizophrenia because they could plausibly result from socioeconomic deprivation and/or the damaging effects of reproductive complications.

Later childhood development

The studies of school-aged children have focused mainly on competence, interpersonal style, and temperament. The picture of early childhood in children at risk is not very distinctive. Rolf (Chapter 39) reports that, as preschoolers, the children of psychotic parents in Vermont did not show signs of severe behavior problems. Worland (Chapter 7) found that the St. Louis groups did not differ behaviorally in elementary school. Weintraub's (Chapter 15) overall impression of the HR children in the Stony Brook project was that they were not grossly deviant as young children.

Behavioral differences did begin to emerge in the middle childhood years. Rolf's dissertation results in Minneapolis generally showed that teachers and peers rated competence lowest in externalizing, HR, and internalizing children, whereas PC children were considered to be the most competent. The follow-up of 540 subjects in the Minneapolis project several years later (including Rolf's sample) located only 356 (66%) in the same school system, which underlies the logistical difficulties of longitudinal research. The HR children had migration rates twice as high as their controls (48% vs. 26%), probably reflecting greater instability in the family lives of schizophrenic parents. Academic grades were highest for PC children, then internalizers, HR children, and externalizers. Reaction-time performance of the HR children was the poorest of the four groups, which brings to mind the findings of retarded psychomotor development in infancy reported by Fish, Marcus, McNeil, and Sameroff. Externalizing children displayed the poorest citizenship in school, and HR children the best. All target groups except the HR group had poorer intermediate outcomes than their controls, although the high migration rate for HR children may have masked negative outcomes for them. Externalizing children generally showed the poorest outcomes.

Fisher (Chapter 25) developed an interesting profile of school behavior combining teacher and peer ratings in the URCAFS Project. Initial comparisons showed teachers and peers in close agreement judging sons of affective psychotics strikingly above average in competence, sons of schizophrenics even more than that *below* average, and sons of nonpsychotic psychiatric controls slightly below average. On the other hand, children of depressed parents in Stony Brook resembled HR offspring in most respects, including that both groups were less competent than their respective control groups. In contrast to both the Rochester and Stony Brook patterns, Worland (Chapter 7) found that offspring of manic-depressives in St. Louis were rated lowest on social competence and total competence in high school, whereas HR offspring were not different from normal controls. The teacher ratings of competence remained stable over time in St. Louis, which implies temporal constancy throughout development.

Yu (Chapter 27) examined relationships among various sources of evaluation for the URCAFS children. Psychiatric ratings correlated strongly with parental reports at ages 4 and 7, presumably because parents were an important source of information for the early psychiatric evaluations, but that correlation was lower at age 10. On the other hand, psychiatric ratings correlated only modestly with teacher ratings at 7 but very highly at 10, when both clinicians and teachers could obtain more information directly from the children themselves. The psychiatric ratings related strongly to other evaluations with cognitive components and with salient expressive or compliance features. Social class correlated significantly with the psychiatric ratings and substantially with parental, teacher, and peer evaluations. Discounting the social class contributions, however, did not weaken the relations among the various sources of child evaluation. In the main, evaluations of child competence by different observers in various settings concurred substantially, but each added unique variance, thus broadening the overall perspective on the child's behavior. The general presumption in seeking diverse evaluations is that children with poor evaluations across settings may have the greatest risk for psychological disorder.

Janes (Chapter 9) found that scholastic motivation and emotional stability were lower among HR adolescents in St. Louis than among NC adolescents. Watt (Chapter 13) corroborated these findings in the New York sample, but was not able definitively to rule out social class or intelligence as explanations for his findings. Janes offers the suggestion that intelligence and psychophysiological functioning may mediate these relationships to some extent, although the difference in emotional stability appeared to be independent of such mediation. She speculates that schizophrenic parentage, intelligence, and electrodermal activity may all be functionally related to future schizophrenia, but the functional mechanisms are not spelled out precisely.

Greater uniformity emerges in the descriptions of interpersonal style. The HR children in Stony Brook were rated by teachers more aggressive/disruptive, less cognitively competent, and less socially competent than NC children, but not significantly different from PC children, who were rated less socially competent and less anxious about achievement than NC children. Peer ratings showed HR children more aggressive and more unhappy/withdrawn than NC children. HR girls were less likeable than NC girls. The Stony Brook results showed no differences in social behavior among the offspring of the two patient groups. School assessments of the New York sample reported by Watt showed strong evidence of interpersonal disharmony, but little indication of introversion among HR subjects at about age 15. Similarly, Rolf (Chapter 39) found children of schizophrenic mothers in Minneapolis to resemble externalizing children the most, and in Vermont to be *less* withdrawn, shy, and socially unresponsive than children of depressed parents. Convergent results were found in Rodnick's follow-up of four adolescent risk groups (Chapter 5). Among the eight subjects classified in the schizophrenic-spectrum outcome group in young adulthood, only three had been characterized as passive negative or withdrawn and socially isolated adolescents, whereas five had been antisocially aggressive or had active family conflict.

The follow-up study of the Danish HR sample located 15 eventual schizophrenics, who had been described by schoolteachers as prone to be angered and upset, disturbing in class with inappropriate behavior, violent, aggressive, and frequently subject to disciplinary action. Clearly, the results of all of these studies conform more to Arieti's (1975) characterization of the *stormy* prepsychotic personality than of the *introverted* type.

In this connection it is interesting to note that the lowest psychiatric evaluation scores in the URCAFS project reported by Munson (Chapter 26) were obtained by eight boys clustered as disobedient and overactive. Their ratings were appreciably lower than those for constricted, depressed boys or shy, anxious ones, which suggests that assertively antagonistic behavior elicits the greatest concern from clinicians in contemporary evaluations.

Asarnow (Chapter 33) presents a group of basic studies on interpersonal style of young school-aged children, which shed some light on the association between aggressive behavior and peer rejection. Children with negative peer ratings were more often than usual the targets of assertive actions from classmates, to which they responded with playful aggression that was somewhat inappropriate. Asarnow suggests that abrasive or hostile behavior in such situations may represent poorly implemented efforts to be assertive. Unpopular boys, in particular, tended most often to respond to playful aggression from peers by backing down, being atypically unassertive. Thus, they seemed to have difficulty integrating normal assertiveness in their daily interactions with peers. Possibly as a partial consequence of this, children with negative peer ratings initiated and received more negative interactions with peers and with teachers than did positively rated boys. From such beginnings one can easily imagine a pattern evolving that leads to progressive alienation and social isolation.

Intellectual functions

Neale (Chapter 16) found lower verbal and performance IQs among HR subjects in the Stony Brook sample than among NC subjects. The lower verbal intelligence replicates a finding of Mednick (Chapter 2) in the Danish project. However, IQs of the Stony Brook HR group did not differ from the PC group. In the St. Louis sample Worland (Chapter 8) found that HR and PC children also had lower verbal IQs than NC subjects, but there were not performance IQ differences. Relative to their controls, the IQs of the HR children were lower in adolescence than in early childhood. Worland implies that the drop in intelligence may be attributed to the cumulative *psychological* impact of parental psychosis on their children, but the epigenetic change observed could equally plausibly reflect an incipient intellectual deterioration that is *not* mediated by the psychological relationship with an ill parent. (Note that the drop was not found in the PC group.)

More than any other project in the consortium the St. Louis study implemented the traditional approach to psychological testing for psychodynamic evidence of development. In many respects their negative findings were among the most instructive. Franklin (1977) did not find differences among groups in cognitive or perceptual differentiation, nor differences in egocentrism. Spatial egocentrism was not found to be associated with severity of parental illness, which contradicts findings by Strauss, Harder, and Chandler (1979), and children later treated or hospitalized were not more egocentric or less differentiated psychologically as young children than untreated comparison children. Children of schizophrenic and of manic-depressive parents were more clinically disturbed than the children of normal or physically ill parents. HR children also gave the most primitive Rorschach responses and the *least* aggressive TAT stories, whereas children of manic-depressive parents gave the least primitive Rorschachs and the most aggressive TATs. Worland concluded that preadolescent children of psychotic parents are not noticeably impaired in either cognitive or intellectual development. By adolescence, children of both schizophrenic and depressed parents have lower verbal intelligence, with the greatest decline in the former group.

In an object-sorting task, HR children at Stony Brook made fewer superordinate responses than the NC group (though not more than the PC group), but more *complexive* errors than either control group, which implies more disjointed conceptualization in HR children. Except for cognitive slippage, deficits in most areas of cognitive functioning among HR children were matched in the offspring of depressed parents, raising doubts whether the findings are specific to risk for schizophrenic disorder.

Studies of attention were featured prominently in the New York, Minneapolis, and Waterloo projects. In the New York study (Chapter 12), Cornblatt found deficits in sustained and focused attention and greater susceptibility to distraction among HR subjects. Composite measures of such deviance and stability of these scores over time permitted her to isolate a particularly deviant subgroup expected to include some preschizophrenics. Early attentional dysfunction was correlated with behavioral deviance in adolescence, which was interpreted as support for the hypothesis that attentional deviance is a precursor of later psychopathology. However, no evidence is presented to show that attention is a *discriminantly* better predictor than other (e.g., behavioral) indicators. Some corroboration was presented from the McMaster–Waterloo project, which was unique in sampling HR children raised in foster homes. Steffy (Chapter 32) reported that four of five subjects with extreme attentional deficits recorded significant elevations on the Schizophrenia scale of the MMPI. HR children with both attentional problems and high MMPI scores for Schizophrenia and Psychasthenia also showed role difficulties as students at school, some social isolation, and difficulty in modulating anger. Asarnow's dissertation study (1980) of randomly selected schoolchildren indicates that wandering attention at school is associated with aversive and avoidant interaction patterns with peers and teachers. This does not offer direct causal explanations related to schizophrenia, but does describe a pattern of maladjustment not unusual in high-risk samples that might well jeopardize a school career.

The experimental studies in Minneapolis yielded largely negative findings. Phipps-Yonas (Chapter 20) found no differences between HR and Control groups on speed of reactions, variability in individual performance, extraneous behaviors, or attentional deficits. Neither was it possible for her to identify a deviant subset within the sample. The HR children were rated as average by their peers, and achievement test scores were on par with general norms. In Nuechterlein's analysis (Chapter 19) the HR children scored lower than matched controls on sustained attention, corroborating Cornblatt's results. Hyperactive children, by contrast, were impatient to see relevance among stimuli, even with meagre evidence to support it. Driscoll (Chapter 21) found the HR children remarkably able, with high levels of incidental learning. They were rated by peers as being no different from normal controls. The only deficit she found was that they were more susceptible than average to distraction, which is consistent with Cornblatt's results. The general conclusion from the three Minneapolis studies was that there was no major attentional dysfunction in these HR children.

In his overview of the attentional, intellectual, and cognitive research presented (Chapter 41), Lewine draws appropriately conservative conclusions. Among children at risk for schizophrenia, only a modest subset (11%–44%) stands out as deviant. Almost without exception, significant deviance found in HR children is found likewise in psychiatric controls. A parsimonious inference to draw from this is that a general vulnerability to psychosis may be transmitted genetically, with the specific form of the psychosis largely determined environmentally (Zubin & Spring, 1978). Furthermore, Lewine makes an excellent observation about *instability of deviance*. Early markers for schizophrenia may be more distinguished by variability than by constancy. Hence, we may be mistaken to expect future schizophrenics to be permanently branded by stigmata as visible and as stable as neon lights announcing their vulnerability. The early evidence may be much more subtle, fluctuating, and erratic. That possibility behooves us to search as patiently and as persistently for patterns of variation and change as for constant, structural precursors of psychopathology.

Family relations and communication

Wynne (Chapter 42) points out that even the most ardent genetic theorists concede that environmental experience plays a significant role in determining the occurence, course, and outcome of schizophrenic disorder. As a consequence, the unafflicted spouses of schizophrenic parents are pivotal persons who exert important formative influence on their children. The family, which constitutes the "soil" in which the developing organisms grow, must be regarded as an interactive system, not as a collection of independent individuals that interact occasionally. Mednick's path analysis (Chapter 2) suggests that separation from parents may affect HR children significantly, for example, augmenting antisocial tendencies, and subsequent institutionalization may exacerbate that disturbance further.

Some appreciation of the family system of children at risk is necessitated by the large number of families that have disintegrated since our studies of them began. As investigative intruders we have also been directly exposed to the self-protective maneuvers of these vulnerable family systems. Early reports of home visits in the St. Louis project indicated that families vary quite widely in the extent to which the psychological disturbance of a parent infiltrates and involves the family system. The evidence about the families and their impact on the children is mostly "bad news," although it should be acknowledged that mostly bad news was expected from the beginning.

In Stony Brook marital adjustment was found to be better in the PC families than in the HR families, and best in the NC families. Marital discord was reflected in parental disagreements over demonstrations of affection, sex relations, and propriety of conduct. As compared with the normal controls, spouses in both patient groups were less conciliatory toward one another, less happy, less engaged in mutual outside interests, and less inclined to confide in their mates or to marry the same partner again. Depressives rated their marriages even less happy than schizophrenics. These extremely negative marital evaluations, especially among the depressives, reveal emphatically how conflictual their marriages must be. Weintraub (Chapter 15) expresses uncertainty about how to interpret these results, but it seems no mystery that spouses who argue chronically, have few common interests, and have serious difficulties in expressing affection and in sexual relations would dislike one another.

Family functioning in the Stony Brook sample was also more disturbed among the two patient groups in several areas: family solidarity, children's relations, household facilities, and financial circumstances. The two patient groups did not differ from one another in these respects. The parenting characteristics, as viewed by their children, are instructive. Schizophrenic mothers were considered more accepting and child-centered than were normal mothers. Depressed mothers were also more child-centered. Schizophrenics were more lax in discipline than depressives. Schizophrenic fathers were perceived more negatively (i.e., unaccepting and uninvolved) than normal fathers, whereas depressed fathers were not different from the normals. Husbands of schizophrenic and depressed mothers controlled their offspring covertly through inducing anxiety or guilt. (It should be remembered that *lack* of control by these mothers was criticized by the offspring.)

From a methodological viewpoint the most impressive work in this area is the research on Free Play among families, inspired mainly by Clara and Al Baldwin (Chapter 29). Not surprisingly, interactions between a child and a parent are reciprocal: Frequent actions directed to one person are matched by frequent actions in return. Interestingly, a hydraulic principle seems to apply to the general family ecology: Initiatives directed to one person in the family are "subtracted" from initiatives to another. Hence we can surmise that the relationship to a nonpatient parent has important compensating potential for healthy development of the offspring.

It is important to observe that expressive warmth is contagious within the family. Affection expressed by one family member is generally shared among others in the family. Conversely, emotional detachment generally begets detachment elsewhere in the family. The amount of interaction initiated by parents toward a child declines with the child's increasing age from 4 to 10, probably reflecting the growth of independence. The decline is greatest for boys from 4 to 7, and for girls from 7 to 10, perhaps showing a preference to shelter girls a little longer.

URCAFS patients interacted less with their children than healthy spouses did, presumably reflecting a depletion in the patients' emotional resources for family living that can be attributed to their illness. As expected, schizophrenic parents were the least active in Free Play participation and nonpsychotic patients were the most active, with affectively disordered patients in between. Also as predicted, patients rated as most disturbed psychiatrically interacted least with their children, and their families displayed the least warmth.

What are the effects on children of relating to, and communicating with, psychiatrically disturbed parents? Worland (Chapter 7) reported there was some evidence that family skew was predictive of later need for psychological treatment in the offspring. Klein (Chapter 28) found that censure or praise from mothers seemed to disrupt learning in the children of schizophrenic or nonpsychotic parents. The authors reasoned that the results may reflect the disruptive influence of chronicity in parental illness (whether schizophrenic or nonpsychotic). On the other hand, affective psychosis often runs an episodic course, exposing the chil-

dren to intermittent periods when the affected parent is free from clinical disturbance, hence exerting a (cumulatively) less disruptive effect on their communications and relationships with their children.

Also reporting on the URCAFS sample, Cole (Chapter 30) found that transactional style and warmth of family interaction were correlated positively with teacher and peer ratings of children's competence at school. Active, warm, and balanced
communication among family members in the Family Rorschach Test likewise
related positively to teacher ratings (in one sample) and to peer ratings of children's competence. A refinement of sorts can be discerned in Jones's finding
(Chapter 31) that a composite measure of parental Communication Deviance
(CD) predicted children's competence in school at 10 years of age but not at 7. No
explanation is offered for this result, but it is plausible (because of similar findings
in other areas) to infer that some developmental changes emerge by 10 that are
premature at 7, conceivably changes that relate to long-term prognosis for the
children. Alternatively, it might reflect episodic emergence of behaviors that are
unstable over time, with no consistent longitudinal trends.

The UCLA Family Project yielded results that were quite independent but
highly convergent with the URCAFS findings. Rodnick (Chapter 5) found that
level of parental CD was strongly related to schizophrenia-spectrum disorders in
the offspring. Similarly, rejecting style in parental affective expression toward the
offspring was also significantly related to later schizophrenic outcome. Communication Deviance was stronger than Affective Style in predictive power, but both
were significant. Parents of later schizophrenics seemed disinclined to acknowledge their children in direct interactions, implying either indifference or hostility.
They also did not impose the required structure when discussions drifted off
target. When both parents were high in CD, they exerted a dominant force in the
family interaction, which might explain their apparent pathogenic impact on the
development of their children. High CD in parents was associated with avoidance
of eye contact and with unchanging facial expression, which obviously could lead
to a sense of disconfirmation in the children.

Doane (Chapter 6) pursued Rodnick's research with configural analysis of
parental styles, concluding that families who are *not* affectively rejecting in either
what they say or how they say it produce offspring with benign outcomes. Conversely, if parents say harshly negative things and deliver them in a hostile, angry,
or challenging tone of voice, the result is often (eight of nine cases!) an outcome in
the schizophrenic spectrum.

The rationale emerging gradually from these two projects is that the transactional style of children is shaped (for better or worse) by the transactional style of
the family's interactions. Children reared in families with active, warm, and responsive interpersonal style are likely to be outgoing and friendly and successful in
engaging their social environment outside the home. By contrast, children reared
in rejecting or detached family environments are likely to reflect that style in their
approach to others outside the home, and thus be seriously handicapped. For this
reason, accurate assessment of the modal pattern of interaction within the family
may help to identify those children with the highest risk for serious behavioral or
emotional disorders.

The premorbid picture in cases of early breakdown

Mednick's 1967 follow-up (Chapter 2) found that HR children with poor intermediate outcomes (the Sick group) experienced frequent pregnancy and birth complications, were separated from their mothers early in life, showed volatile electrodermal patterns and attentional drift in their associative functioning, and were disruptive at school rather than retiring. The 1972 follow-up yielded 15 diagnosed schizophrenics who also had frequent perinatal problems, were placed early in children's homes, recorded volatile autonomic functions, and were disruptive in school. Nothing was reported about attentional drift, but their mothers experienced severe courses of illness. Mothers of borderline schizophrenics, on the other hand, showed late onset of schizophrenic disorder, high frequency of paranoid syndromes, somewhat less severe clinical symptoms, and relatively good social, vocational, and personal adjustment, providing therefore a comparatively stable rearing environment for their children. Mednick suggests that there may be a gradient of potency in the genetically transmitted disposition for psychopathology, the diathesis for chronic schizophrenia being the strongest, for borderline disorders weaker, and for normal or neurotic conditions weakest of all. However, by his own reasoning, the severity of the maternal syndrome also shapes the quality of the home environment, which in turn influences the development of the child *psychologically*. Both patterns of causation may be important.

By an average of 17.5 years, five of Erlenmeyer-Kimling's HR subjects, two PC subjects, and one normal control were hospitalized for psychiatric disorders, most of them with schizophrenic hospital diagnoses (Chapter 14). Fifteen others required some form of psychological treatment outside the hospital. Global assessments by psychiatrists at 7 to 12 years of age were poorest for those subsequently hospitalized, highest for those that functioned well, and intermediate for the treated subjects, indicating that early clinical appraisals can identify the most vulnerable youngsters. Reviewing the early performance deficits of the hospitalized HR children, she found significantly lower IQs (mean of 93 vs. 104 for other HR subjects) and a relative deficit in Verbal IQ (mean of 88 vs. 99 for Performance IQ). This suggests that low (especially verbal) intelligence may be an early marker for clinical breakdown or for early onset of psychiatric disorder. In contrast, the hospitalized PC subjects both achieved high IQs (117 and 109). The hospitalized HR group also performed poorly on the Bender–Gestalt Test, the Lincoln–Oseretsky Test of Motor Impairment, and on several attentional measures, but their electrodermal responding was not deviant.

Worland (Chapter 7) examined the *precursors* of schizophrenia and borderline schizophrenia, primarily in terms of interpersonal style and temperament. Among the boys, preschizophrenics were anxious, lonely, and restrained, having discipline problems at school (the latter corroborating Mednick's results). The preborderline boys were simply described as isolated and distant. Both female groups were anhedonic, withdrawn, disengaged, and isolated, but the preschizophrenic girls were poorly controlled, whereas the preborderline girls were overly restrained. Contrary to Mednick's finding, the precursors of schizophrenia did *not* include verbal associative disturbance. Childhood intelligence was *not* lower than average overall and verbal IQ was higher than performance IQ, contradicting Erlenmeyer-Kimling's results.

It is noteworthy that few of the findings reported in this area by one research group have been replicated by other groups. This might be attributed to the very small samples with detectable clinical outcomes thus far. However, it is also consistent with Cudeck's observation (Chapter 3) that the early patterns of clinical symptoms that emerge among high-risk subjects in young adulthood are extremely diverse, including a broad range of familiar syndromes: psychosis, personality disorders, psychopathy, antisocial disorders, depression, and various (rather ill-defined) neurotic disorders. Both the precursive childhood patterns and the adult clinical outcomes for children of schizophrenic parents may show such diversity.

Neglected research issues

Several concepts have received theoretical attention in the risk research field, but either been neglected empirically or yielded confusing results. They merit further consideration in future research.

Biopsychological functions. Methodological difficulties in psychophysiological techniques precluded effective testing of research hypotheses in the St. Louis project. The New York project failed to replicate Mednick's (Chapter 2) findings on psychophysiological deviance in HR subjects (i.e., short response latency, increased response amplitude, fast recovery, and lack of habituation). Further analysis also disconfirmed the hypothesis that fast recovery is associated with severity of the mother's illness. On the hopeful side, Friedman (Chapter 11) observed reduced response amplitudes in electrodermal functioning of HR children following perceptual stimulation, which is consistent with results on adult schizophrenics and may be an early indicator of vulnerability to the disorder. Promising leads in the areas of cortical evoked-potential response and neuromotor functioning may take on significance mainly as evidence accumulates regarding outcomes. For the most part, the evidence and conclusions about biopsychological functioning are ambiguous, at best.

Adaptive strengths of children at risk. There has been much speculation and enthusiastic support for studying adaptive strengths in children of schizophrenic parents, but little programmatic pursuit of this intriguing idea. Many have paid lip service to the concept of the *invulnerable,* or resistant, child at risk. Bleuler (Chapter 40) found that 84% of his HR subjects who married had successful marriages, and the great majority achieved higher social status than their parents, which implies adaptive and relationship skills. A strong new emphasis on stress and coping in the theoretical literature and in research funding programs (e.g., the Grant Foundation's new program direction) promises some headway along these lines in the near future.

Early intervention. There is an obvious natural alliance between high-risk research and practical efforts at preventive intervention. All of the research groups in the consortium have been conscious of this connection and many have taken concrete steps to offer treatment referral services for their subjects and/or their families. With NIMH support, one of the first intervention research clinics in this field was created at St. Louis. The only systematic intervention project reported in this volume took place on the island of Mauritius, off the coast of East Africa (Chapter 4). Children were selected on the basis of deviant skin conductance patterns and placed in nursery schools for special enrichment in their learning experience. Follow-up studies after 3 years showed that the nursery school training channeled the children into constructive modes of play, displacing watching behavior with more positive interactions of a social nature. An 11-year follow-up of their school progress since that time is currently underway.

The dilemma for investigations of early intervention is plain to see. It is difficult to know what to treat in children at risk until we know what is "wrong" or abnormal about them. The primary objective of this first phase of risk research is precisely to determine how such children differ from others. Until the answers to this question are well established, intervention efforts will have to grope in the dark.

DISCUSSION

Formulations of etiology

One of the most important objectives of high-risk research is to develop an understanding of the causes of schizophrenic and other serious emotional disorders. Let us first observe the theoretical partisanship of the investigators in the RRC projects. Mednick (Chapter 4) concentrates on electrodermal evidence of the early precursors of schizophrenic disorder, chooses the HR sample on that basis in Mauritius, and develops an etiological model that emphasizes reproductive causalties and hinges on psychophysiological dysfunction as a primary causal factor. Erlenmeyer-Kimling (Chapter 10) espouses explicitly a genetic theory of etiology, looks primarily for early indicators in cognitive processes and evoked brain potentials, and expects biophysiological abnormalities to precede the appearance of social and emotional deviance in schizophrenic people. Similarly, Steffy (Chapter 32) focuses on attentional disturbances and hypothesizes that they will precede and give rise to subsequent behavioral deviance.

In sharp contrast, the URCAFS program, the UCLA Family Project, and the St. Louis study endorse psychodynamic conceptions of etiology for schizophrenic disorders, and develop theoretical formulations that emphasize the potential causal primacy of distortions in family communication and relationship. Along these lines there is a broad consensus of support for *transactional* models of development that emphasize relationship and coping procedures, as illustrated by the research of Rodnick, Steffy, Watt, and the Baldwins. Transactional conceptions represent an important advance beyond traditional disease models based on epigenetic principles, which tend to stereotype developmental processes. The early results from these projects do not resoundingly confirm our wishful (and plausible) hypothesizing along such traditional lines. For example, Mednick found that malignant parental schizophrenia does *not* yield a high frequency of schizophrenia (at least with early onset) among offspring. Hence we must look toward more complex and less monolithic models to explain the transmission and development of schizophrenic disorders.

Similar observations can be made about the etiological parochialism of Fish and Marcus (Chapters 34 and 35, respectively) with regard to neurological functions, Watt (Chapter 13) and Lewine (Chapter 43) with regard to school behavior, and McNeil and Wrede (Chapters 36 and 38, respectively) regarding reproductive casualties. This, of course, does not make their research less important, but we need more interactive models for formulations about etiology.

The Minneapolis group and the Stony Brook group show the most theoretical eclecticism in this regard. Both groups staunchly pursue cognitive–perceptual studies and social–familial studies with about equal commitment, and both refrain from postulating causal hegemony for either the genetic–constitutional or the environmental–social domain.

There is an interesting contrast in the conceptual treatment of developmental events. Environmentalists look for "pathogenic" life experiences to explain schizophrenic vulnerability, whereas geneticists look for "buffering" life experiences to explain the suppression of such vulnerability. It is tempting to point out that a rose, by any other name, smells just as sweet, but horticulturists will still disagree about where it should be placed in the garden.

Steffy (Chapter 32) draws a distinction between schizophrenic disorder, which is usually manifested episodically, and vulnerability to the disorder, which is relatively enduring. His work on attentional functions seeks to find markers for vulnerability, which admittedly may be quite subtle. The rationale is that attentional dysfunctions may account, in part, for deviance in transactional style. In other words, social or behavioral manifestations of schizophrenic disorder may be caused by disturbances of attention.

The URCAFS project takes an interesting approach to the problem of causal reasoning: pitting the deviance of family relations against the severity of parental psychopathology as competing explanations for functioning in the offspring. Chronicity of parental illness is another plausible causal contributor. The UR-CAFS results presented in this volume do not address this issue very explicitly, but the space given to family relations seems to predominate. As mentioned, severity of parental disorder has not yet proved to be a powerful explanatory factor in their data.

The Stony Brook program is explicitly based on a diathesis–stress model of etiology, which seems to be the most popular approach. Weintraub (Chapter 15) argues that it is unjustified to search for a single cause, in view of the obvious heterogeneity of the disorders. Research is therefore focused primarily on a wide variety of factors that may potentiate the diathesis, that is, trigger the manifest disorder. For this reason, much of the Stony Brook work attempts to describe the general ecology of the HR children and their families. The project has been quite successful in providing many such provocative descriptions.

Sameroff (Chapter 37) is the most outspoken about etiological theory, frankly doubting that a *specific* deficit can account for the predisposition to schizophrenia.

He concedes that some latent constitutional deficit might emerge later in development, or that the wrong variables were measured to reveal such a deficit. On the basis of the published research thus far, he concludes that risk in the offspring of schizophrenic mothers can be attributed more to prolonged emotional disturbance in the mothers, unstable family organization, poor economic circumstances, and low social status than to the schizophrenic disorders of the mothers per se. He also doubts that many of the HR children will become schizophrenic. Bleuler (Chapter 40) found, after all, that only 9% of the HR offspring in his sample became schizophrenic in their lifetimes. Sameroff concludes that social milieu at least matches the effects of maternal psychopathology on social and emotional development of children, and overpowers it in the cognitive sphere. This leads him to question theories that posit a unique constitutional deficit, usually inferred to be transmitted genetically, as the cause of schizophrenia. Caretaking environments with high levels of stress, whether through economic or emotional instability of the caregivers, produce young children with high levels of incompetent behavior. Hence they deserve primary attention as potential causes of schizophrenic disorders. For balance, we should point out, on the other hand, that adoptive studies that have matched for social class show that genetic loading does, in fact, make a difference.

The question of specificity

This volume reports hundreds of significant findings about children at risk for schizophrenia. This usually means that they differ in some respects from children of normal parents or from children otherwise considered unlikely to become schizophrenic adults. It is vitally important to know whether such findings signal specific precursors of schizophrenic disorders or markers for psychopathology in general. The answer to this question has been complicated by recent advances in the DSM-III diagnostic system, which have virtually dictated changes in the sampling of the schizophrenic spectrum and in the combinations of genetic loading studied. For example, many subjects previously diagnosed as schizophrenic are now considered schizoaffectives or affective psychotics. Lewine concludes that the evidence thus far weighs against specificity, because most findings that distinguish HR subjects from normal controls also characterize psychiatric controls as well. High-risk samples, of course, include relatively few future schizophrenics, so the conceptual significance of findings may change as psychological outcomes unfold. For the present, Mednick concludes that there may be no monolithic schizophrenic disorder that follows predictable rules of genetic transmission, as phenylketonuria and Huntington's chorea do. Consequently, he recommends that we look for "degrees of schizophrenicity" or schizophrenic vulnerability, which obviously calls for subtle and complex conceptions of the disorder.

Behavioral continuity

A thorny problem confronts any longitudinal investigation covering an extensive period of time. It is obviously advantageous for purposes of prediction to establish developmental continuities in the behavior of subjects being studied, but how should that be tested and proved if the concrete performance and actions that reflect psychological constructs are expected to change with age? Nuechterlein (Chapter 22) emphasizes this problem and proposes specific procedures to deal with it in the realm of cognitive research. Most teams in the consortium seem to operate on the assumption that broad continuities in behavior over time can be found. Children with early attentional deficits are expected to have problems deploying attention later, and abrasive, antisocial children are expected to have conduct problems in adolescence. For the most part, these theoretical expectations are accommodated by making *operational* adjustments in measurement to account for age differences. For example, the behavior defined as competent at 4 years of age may differ from the actions considered competent at 13, but it is generally assumed that a child's *relative* position in a sample on the competence dimension will not change substantially in the interim. In point of fact, some rather large changes have been observed, leading Lewine to conclude that change or process may be a more important focus for future research and conceptual formulation than stable traits. However, enough evidence of modest temporal stability has emerged to sustain the general expectation that stable traits can be found.

A special problem in this regard arises in longitudinal research on psychoses. Considering that typical signs and symptoms of schizophrenic and affective disorders seldom occur prior to adolescence, even in those destined to be afflicted as adults, what are the logical precursors to look for in childhood? Here the bootstraps of risk research are most prominent to view. We have looked for early aberrations in thinking, interpersonal style, mood, intelligence, temperament, psychophysiological functions, and competence, but we have also studied pregnancy and birth complications, parental communication deviance, socioeconomic deprivation, and family relations, which might contribute to such aberrations. We still do not know what the key variables are. We do know that children at risk are different from normal children in many respects, some of which seem to be associated with the earliest signs of psychological disruption in adolescence or young adulthood. But we cannot yet judge how much developmental continuity will be found ultimately.

CONCLUSION

The tantalizing challenge of risk research in schizophrenia is captured by a fairy tale called "The Field of Boliauns" (Jacobs, 1968). It tells of Tom Fitzpatrick's chance meeting with a leprechaun, who refuses to reveal a secret recipe for brewing beer that has been in his family for many years. Tom loses his temper and threatens to kill the leprechaun unless he shows where his money is. The leprechaun leads him to a great field all full of boliauns and points to one of the big flowers, under which he assures Tom there lies a great crock of gold. Having no spade with him, Tom ties one of his red garters around the boliaun and makes the leprechaun swear not to touch it before he returns.

So Tom ran for dear life, til he came home and got a spade, and then away with him, as hard as he could go, back to the field of boliauns; but when he got there, lo and behold! Not a boliaun in the field but had a red garter, the very model of his own, tied about it; and as to digging up the whole field, that was all nonsense, for there were more than forty good Irish acres in it. So Tom came home again with his spade on his shoulder, a little cooler than he went, and many's the hearty curse he gave the leprechaun every time he thought of the neat turn he had served him [p. 29].

The parallel to the identification of children vulnerable to schizophrenia is obvious. The acute awareness of the low prevalence of schizophrenia has, for the most part, immobilized predictive efforts on the pragmatic gound that "you'd have to dig up 40 good Irish acres to find that crock of gold." Perhaps even more inhibiting is the suspicion that most of the "right" flowers display no garters at all; that is, there may be no prodromal signs that can be identified and relied on. The intrepid members of the Risk Research Consortium have begun to plow that field, risking the curses of many leprechauns. It is still too soon to evaluate our chances to find that crock of gold or to estimate precisely its worth, but few of us have sold our shovels.

References

Achenbach, M. 1977. *Child behavior checklist.* Bethesda, Md.: National Institute of Mental Health.

Achenbach, T. M. 1966. The classification of children's psychiatric symptoms: A factor analytic study. *Psychological Monographs, 80*(7), Whole No. 615.

Achenbach, T. M. 1978. Psychopathology of childhood: Research problems and issues. *Journal of Consulting and Clinical Psychology, 46,* 759–776.

Ainsworth, M. D. S. 1964. Patterns of attachment behavior shown by the infant in interaction with his mother. *Merrill-Palmer Quarterly, 10,* 51–58.

Ainsworth, M. D. S. 1973. The development of infant–mother attachment. In B. M. Caldwell and H. N. Ricciutti (eds.), *Review of child development research* (vol. 3). Chicago: University of Chicago.

Al-Khayyal, M. 1980. "Healthy parental communication as a predictor of child competence in families with a schizophrenic and psychiatrically disturbed non-schizophrenic parent." Doctoral dissertation, University of Rochester.

Alkire, A. A., Goldstein, M. J., Rodnick, E. H., and Judd, L. L. 1971. Social influence and counterinfluence within families of four types of disturbed adolescents. *Journal of Abnormal Psychology, 77,* 32–41.

Altman, H. 1980. "Family schism and skew and their relation to psychiatric treatment in children at risk." Unpublished doctoral dissertation, St. Louis University.

American Psychiatric Association. 1968. *Diagnostic and statistical manual of mental disorders* (2nd ed.). Washington, D.C.: American Psychiatric Association.

American Psychiatric Association. 1980. *Diagnostic and statistical manual of mental disorders* (3rd ed.). Washington, D.C.: American Psychiatric Association.

Ames, L. B., Learned, J., Metraux, R., and Walker, R. 1957. *Child Rorschach responses: Developmental trends from two to ten years.* New York: Hoeber.

Amnell, G. 1974. *Mortality and chronic morbidity in childhood. A cohort study of children born in 1955 in Helsinki.* Helsingfors: Samfundet Folkhalsan.

Andrews, D. F., Bickel, P. J., Hampel, F. R., Huber, P. J., Rogers, W. H., and Tukey, J. W. 1972. *Robust estimates of location.* Princeton, N.J.: Princeton University Press.

Anthony, B. J. 1978a. Piagetian egocentrism, empathy, and affect discrimination in children at high risk for psychosis. In E. J. Anthony and C. Chiland (eds.), *The child in his family: Vulnerable children* (vol. 4). New York: Wiley.

Anthony, B. J. 1978b. The development of empathy in high risk children. In E. J. Anthony, C. Koupernik, and C. Chiland (eds.), *The child in his family: Vulnerable children* (vol. 6). New York: Wiley.

597

Anthony, E. J. 1966. Piaget et le clinicien. In F. Bresson and M. de Montmollin (eds.), *Psychologie et épistémologie génétique. Thèmes Piaget.* Paris: Dunod.

Anthony, E. J. 1968a. The developmental precursors of adult schizophrenia. *Journal of Psychiatric Research, 6*(1), 293–361.

Anthony, E. J. 1968b. A clinical evaluation of children with psychotic parents. *Psychiatric Progress, 3*(4), 3.

Anthony, E. J. 1969a. Folie à deux: A developmental failure in the process of separation–individuation. In J. B. McDevitt, P. Elkisch, and D. Settlage (eds.), *Studies in the separation–individuation process. Festschrift in honor of Margaret Mahler.* New York: International Universities Press.

Anthony, E. J. 1969b. The mutative impact on family life of serious mental and physical illness in a parent. *Canadian Psychiatric Association Journal, 14,* 433–453.

Anthony, E. J. 1969c. The influence of maternal psychosis on children – a folie à deux. In E. J. Anthony and T. Benedek (eds.), *Parenthood, its psychology and psychopathology.* Boston: Little, Brown.

Anthony, E. J. 1970a. The impact of mental and physical illness on family life. *American Journal of Psychiatry, 127*(2), 138–146.

Anthony, E. J. 1970b. The mutative impact of serious mental and physical illness in a parent on family life. In E. J. Anthony and C. Koupernik (eds.), *The child in his family* (vol. 1). New York: Wiley.

Anthony, E. J. 1971. A clinical and experimental study of high-risk children and their schizophrenic parents. In A. R. Kaplan (ed.), *Genetic factors in schizophrenia.* Springfield, Ill.: Thomas, pp. 380–406.

Anthony, E. J. 1972. The contagious subculture of psychosis. In C. J. Sager and H. S. Kaplan (eds.), *Progress in group and family therapy.* New York: Brunner/Mazel.

Anthony, E. J. 1973a. Living-in experiences with disturbed families. *Symposium on community and family psychiatry.* Montreal: McGill University Press.

Anthony, E. J. 1973b. Mourning and psychic loss of the parent. In E. J. Anthony and C. Koupernik (eds.), *The child in his family: The impact of disease and death* (vol. 2). New York: Wiley.

Anthony, E. J. 1974a. The syndrome of the psychologically vulnerable child. In E. J. Anthony and C. Koupernik (eds.), *The child in his family: Children at psychiatric risk* (vol. 3). New York: Wiley.

Anthony, E. J. 1974b. A risk-vulnerability intervention model for children of psychotic parents. In E. J. Anthony and C. Koupernik (eds.), *The child in his family: Children at psychiatric risk* (vol. 3). New York: Wiley.

Anthony, E. J. 1975a. The use of the "serious" experiment in child psychiatric research. In E. J. Anthony (ed.), *Explorations in child psychiatry.* New York: Plenum.

Anthony, E. J. 1975b. The influence of a manic-depressive environment on the developing child. In E. J. Anthony and T. Benedek (eds.), *Depression and human existence.* Boston: Little, Brown.

Anthony, E. J. 1975c. Naturalistic studies of disturbed families. In E. J. Anthony (ed.), *Explorations in child psychiatry.* New York: Plenum.

Anthony, E. J. 1976. How children cope in families with a psychotic parent. In E. N. Rexford, L. W. Sander, and T. Shapiro (eds.), *Infant psychiatry: A new synthesis.* New Haven, Conn.: Yale University Press.

Anthony, E. J. 1977. Preventive measures for children and adolescents at high risk for psychosis. In G. W. Albee and J. M. Joffe (eds.), *Primary prevention of psychopathology.* Hanover, N.H.: University Press of New England.

Anthony, E. J., and Cytryn, L. 1977. Discussion of childhood depression: A clinical and behavioral perspective. In J. Schulterbrandt and A. Raskin (eds.), *Depression in childhood: Diagnosis, treatment and conceptual models.* New York: Raven Press.

Anthony, E. J., and McGinnis, M. 1978. Counselling very disturbed parents. In L. E. Arnold (ed.), *Helping parents help their children.* New York: Brunner/Mazel.

Anthony, E. J., and Rizzo, A. 1971. The effect of drug treatment on the patient's family. In C. Shagass (ed.), *The role of drugs in community psychiatry: Modern problems in pharmacopsychiatry* (vol. 6). Basel: Karger.

Arieti, S. 1975. *Interpretation of schizophrenia.* New York: Basic Books.

Armstrong, J. S., and Soelberg, P. 1968. On the interpretation of factor analysis. *Psychological Bulletin, 70,* 361–364.

Asarnow, J. R. 1980. "Interpersonal competence in preadolescent boys: An analysis of peer assessment measures and social interaction." Unpublished doctoral dissertation, University of Waterloo, Ontario.

Asarnow, R. F., and Asarnow, J. R. 1982. Attention–information processing dysfunction and vulnerability to schizophrenia: Implications of preventive intervention. In M. J. Goldstein (ed.), *Preventive intervention in schizophrenia.* Washington, D.C.: National Institute of Mental Health.

Asarnow, R. F., and MacCrimmon, D. J. 1978. Residual performance deficit in clinically remitted schizophrenics: A marker of schizophrenia? *Journal of Abnormal Psychology, 87,* 597–608.

Asarnow, R. F., and MacCrimmon, D. J. 1980. "Span of apprehension deficits during the post-psychotic stages of schizophrenia: A replication and extension." Unpublished manuscript, University of California at Los Angeles.

Asarnow, R. F., MacCrimmon, D. J., Cleghorn, J. M., and Steffy, R. A. 1978. The McMaster-Waterloo Project: An attentional and clinical assessment of foster children at risk for schizophrenia. In L. C. Wynne, R. L. Cromwell, and S. Matthysse (eds.), *The nature of schizophrenia: New approaches to research and treatment.* New York: Wiley, pp. 339–358.

Asarnow, R. F., Steffy, R. A., Cleghorn, J. M., and MacCrimmon, D. J. 1979. The McMaster-Waterloo studies of children at risk for severe psychopathology. In J. Shamie (ed.), *New directions in children's mental health.* New York: Spectrum Press.

Asarnow, R. F., Steffy, R. A., MacCrimmon, D. J., and Cleghorn, J. M. 1977. An attentional assessment of foster children at risk for schizophrenia. *Journal of Abnormal Psychology, 86,* 267–275. Reprinted in L. C. Wynne, R. L. Cromwell, and S. Matthysse (eds.), *The nature of schizophrenia: New approaches to research and treatment.* New York: Wiley.

Astrachan, B. M., Harrow, M., Adler, D., et al. 1972. A checklist for the diagnosis of schizophrenia. *British Journal of Psychiatry, 121,* 529.

Atkinson, R. L., and Robinson, N. M. 1961. Paired-associate learning by schizophrenic and normal subjects under conditions of personal and impersonal reward and punishment. *Journal of Abnormal and Social Psychology, 62,* 322–326.

Ax, A. F., and Bamford, J. L. 1970. The GSR recovery limb in chronic schizophrenia. *Psychophysiology, 7,* 145–147.

Baar, D. E. September, 1979. "Interaction patterns in families of normal and aggressive adolescent males." Paper presented at the annual meeting of the American Psychological Association, New York City.

Bakeman, R., and Dabbs, J. M., Jr. 1976. Social interaction observed: Some approaches to the analysis of behavior streams. *Personality and Social Psychology Bulletin, 2,* 335–345.

Baldwin, A. L. 1960. The study of child behavior and development. In P. H. Mussen (ed.), *Handbook of research methods in child development.* New York: Wiley, pp. 3–35.

Baldwin, A. L., Baldwin, C. P., and Cole, R. E. 1982. Family Free-Play interaction: Setting and methods. *Parental pathology, family interaction, and the competence of the child in school. Monographs of the Society for Research in Child Development, 47*(5), 36–44.

Bannister, D. 1968. The logical requirements of research into schizophrenia. *British Journal of Psychiatry, 114,* 181–188.

Bannister, D., and Fransella, F. 1967. *Grid test of schizophrenic thought disorder.* Pilton, England: Psychological Test Publications.

Barocas, R., and Sameroff, A. J. 1982. Social class, maternal psychopathology, and mediational processes in young children. In J. J. Steffen and P. Karoly (eds.), *Autism and severe psychopathology: Advances in child behavioral analysis and therapy* (vol. 2). Lexington, Mass.: Lexington Books.

Bayley, N. 1969. *Bayley Scales of Infant Development.* New York: Psychological Corp.

Beardslee, W. R., Bemporad, J., Keller, M. B., and Klerman, G. L. 1983. Children of parents with major affective disorder: A review. *American Journal of Psychiatry, 140,* 825–832.

Beavers, R. W., Blumberg, S., Timken, K. R., and Weiner, M. F. 1965. Communication patterns of mothers of schizophrenics. *Family Process, 4,* 95–104.

Beck, A. G. 1967. *Depression: Clinical, experimental, and theoretical aspects.* New York: Hoeber.

Beck, S., Beck, A., Levitt, E., and Molish, H. 1961. *Rorschach's test: I. Basic processes.* New York: Grune & Stratton.

Becker, J. 1977. *Affective disorders.* Morristown, N.J.: General Learning Press.

Becker, W. C. 1956. A genetic approach to the interpretation and evaluation of the process–reactive distinction in schizophrenia. *Journal of Abnormal and Social Psychology, 47,* 489–496.

Becker, W. C. 1959. The process–reactive distinction – a key to the problem of schizophrenia? *Journal of Nervous and Mental Disease, 129,* 442–449.

Beckwith, L., Cohen, S., and Parmalee, A. H. August, 1973. "Risk, sex, and situational influences in social interactions with premature infants." Paper presented at the meetings of the American Psychological Association, Montreal.

Beels, C. C. 1978. Social networks, the family, and the schizophrenic parent: Introduction to the issue. *Schizophrenic Bulletin, 4*(4), 512–521.

Beery, K. E. 1967. *Developmental test of visual–motor integration: Administration and scoring manual.* Chicago: Follett.

Behrens, M. I., Rosenthal, A. J., and Chodoff, P. 1968. Communication in lower-class families of schizophrenics: 2. Observations and findings. *Archives of General Psychiatry, 18,* 689–696.

Behrens, M. L., Goldfarb, W., Meyers, D., Goldfarb, N., and Fieldsteel, N. 1969. The Henry Ittleson Center Family Interaction Scales (Behrens–Goldfarb). *Genetic Psychology Monographs, 80,* 203–295.

Beisser, A., Glasser, N., and Grant, M. 1967. Psychosocial adjustment in children of schizophrenic mothers. *Journal of Nervous and Mental Disease, 145,* 429–440.

Bell, B., Gottesman, I. I., Mednick, S. A., and Sergeant, J. 1977. Electrodermal parameters in young, normal male twins. In S. A. Mednick and K. O. Christianson (eds.), *Biosocial bases of criminal behavior.* New York: Gardner Press, pp. 227–228.

Bell, R. Q. 1953. Convergence: An accelerated longitudinal approach. *Child Development, 24,* 145–152.

Bell, R. Q. 1968. A reinterpretation of the direction of effects in studies of socialization. *Psychological Review, 75,* 81–95.

Bell, R. Q., Weller, G. M., and Waldrop, M. F. 1971. Newborn and preschooler: Organization of behavior and relations between periods. *Monographs of the Society for Research in Child Development, 36,* 1–2.

Bellack, L., Hurvich, M., and Gediman, H. K. 1973. *Ego functions in schizophrenics, neurotics and normals.* New York: Wiley.

Bellissimo, A., and Steffy, R. A. 1972. Redundancy-associated deficit in schizophrenic reaction time performance. *Journal of Abnormal Psychology, 80,* 299–307.

Bellissimo, A., and Steffy, R. A. 1975. Contextual influence on crossover in the reaction time performance of schizophrenics. *Journal of Abnormal Psychology, 84,* 210–220.

Bender, L. 1937. Behavior problems in the children of psychotic and criminal parents. *Genetic Psychology Monographs, 19,* 229–239.

Bender, L. 1947. Childhood schizophrenia. *American Journal of Orthopsychiatry, 17,* 40–56.

Bender, L., and Freedman, A. M. 1952. A study of the first three years in the maturation of schizophrenic children. *Quarterly Journal of Child Behavior, 1,* 245–272.

Bene, E., and Anthony, E. J. 1957. *Manual for the Family Relations Test: An objective technique for exploring attitudes in children.* Slough, England: National Foundation for Educational Research.

Bentler, P. M. 1980. Multivariate analysis with latent variables: Causal modeling. *Annual Review of Psychology, 31,* 419–456.

Beuhring, T., Cudeck, R., Mednick, S. A., Walker, E. F., and Schulsinger, F. 1982. Susceptibility to environmental stress: High-risk research on the development of schizophrenia. In R. W. J. Neufeld (ed.), *Psychological stress and psychopathology.* New York: McGraw-Hill.

Birley, J. L. T., and Brown, G. W. 1970. Crises and life changes preceding the onset or relapse of acute schizophrenia: Clinical aspects. *British Journal of Psychiatry, 116,* 327–333.

Blau, A., Welkowitz, J., and Cohen, J. 1964. Maternal attitude to pregnancy instrument. *Archives of General Psychiatry, 10,* 324–331.

Blennow, G., and McNeil, T. F. 1980. "Offspring of women with nonorganic psychoses: Neonatal neurological assessment: Preliminary report." Unpublished manuscript.

Bleuler, E. 1950. [*Dementia praecox or the group of schizophrenias*] (J. Zinkin, trans.). New York: International Universities Press. (Originally published, 1911.)

Bleuler, M. 1974a. The long-term course of the schizophrenic psychoses. *Psychological Medicine, 4,* 244–254.

Bleuler, M. 1974b. The offspring of schizophrenics. *Schizophrenia Bulletin, 1*(8), 93–109.

Bleuler, M., 1976. An approach to a survey of research results on schizophrenia. *Schizophrenia Bulletin, 2,* 356–357.

Bleuler, M. 1978. [*The schizophrenic disorders: Long-term patients and family studies*] (S. Clemens, trans.). New Haven: Yale University Press. (Originally published as *Die schizophrenen Geistesstoerungen im Lichte langjaehriger Kranken-und Familiengeschichten.* Stuttgart: Thieme, 1972.)

Block, J. H. 1961. *The Q-sort method in personality assessment and psychiatric research.* Springfield, Ill.: Thomas.

Block, J. H. 1973. Conceptions of sex roles: Some cross-cultural and longitudinal perspectives. *American Psychologist, 28,* 512–529.

Block, J. H. 1978. Another look at differentiation in the socilization behaviors of mothers and fathers. In F. Denmark and J. Sherman (eds.), *Psychology of women: Future directions of research.* New York: Psychological Dimensions.

Blum, J. D. 1978. On changes in psychiatric diagnosis over time. *American Psychologist, 33,* 1017–1031.

Boulding, K. E. 1980. The human mind as a set of epistemological fields. *American Academy of Arts and Sciences Bulletin, 33*(8), 14–30.

Bower, E. M. 1960. *Early identification of emotionally handicapped children in school* (1st ed.). Springfield, Ill.: Thomas.

Bower, E. M. 1969. *Early identification of emotionally handicapped children in school* (2nd ed.). Springfield, Ill.: Thomas.

Bowlby, J. 1970. *Attachment and loss* (vol. 1): *Attachment.* London: Hogarth.

Bowlby, J. 1973. *Attachment and loss* (vol. 2): *Separation.* New York: Basic Books.

Braine, M. D., Heimer, C., Wortis, H., and Freedman, A. M. 1966. Factors associated with impairment of the early development of prematures. *Monographs of the Society for Research in Child Development, 31*(4, Serial No. 106).

Brazelton, T. B. 1973. *Neonatal Behavioral Assessment Scale,* No. 50. Philadelphia: Lippincott. Also London: Heinemann.

Brill, N. Q., and Glass, J. F. 1965. Hebephrenic schizophrenic reactions. *Archives of General Psychiatry, 12,* 545–551.

Broadbent, D. E. 1958. *Perception and communication.* London: Pergamon Press.

Broadbent, D. E. 1971. *Decision and stress.* London: Academic Press.

Brockington, I. R., and Leff, J. P. 1979. Schizo-affective psychosis: Definitions and incidence. *Psychological Medicine, 9,* 91–99.

Broen, W. E., Jr. 1968. *Schizophrenia: Research and theory.* New York: Academic Press.

Broen, W. E., Jr., and Storms, L. H. 1967. A theory of response interference in schizophrenia. In B. A. Maher (ed.), *Progress in experimental personality research* (vol. 4). New York: Academic Press.

Broman, S. H., Nichols, P. L., and Kennedy, W. A. 1975. *Preschool IQ: Prenatal and early developmental correlates.* New York: Erlbaum.

Brown, G. W., Birley, J. L. I., and Wing, J. F. 1972. Influence of family life on the course of schizophrenic disorders: A replication. *British Journal of Psychiatry, 121,* 241–258.

Browne, M. W. 1979. The maximum-likelihood solution in interbattery factor analysis. *British Journal of Mathematical and Statistical Psychology, 32,* 75–86.

Buchsbaum, M. S. 1977. The middle evoked response components and schizophrenia. *Schizophrenia Bulletin, 3,* 93–104.

Buchsbaum, M. S., Murphy, D. L., Coursey, R. D., Lake, C. R., and Ziegler, M. G. 1978. Platelet monoamine oxidase, plasma dopamine-beta-hydroxylase and attention in a "biochemical high risk sample." *Journal of Psychiatric Research, 14,* 215–224.

Buchsbaum, M. S., and Rieder, R. O. 1979. Biologic heterogeneity and psychiatric research: Platelet MAO activity as a case study. *Archives of General Psychiatry, 36,* 1163–1172.

Burger, G. K., and Armentrout, J. A. 1971. A factor analysis of 5th and 6th graders' reports of parental child-rearing behavior. *Developmental Psychology, 4,* 483.

Burket, G. B. 1964. A study of reduced rank models for multiple predictions. *Psychometric Monographs,* No. 12.

Butler, L. 1979. "Interpersonal problem-solving skills, peer acceptance and social behavior in preadolescent children." Unpublished master's thesis, University of Waterloo, Ontario.

Butler, N. R., and D. G. Bonham. 1963. *Perinatal mortality. The first report of the British perinatal mortality survey.* London: Livingston.

Camilli, G., and D. D. Hopkins. 1978. Applicability of chi-square to 2×2 contingency tables with small expected cell frequencies. *Psychological Bulletin, 85*(1), 163–167.

Campbell, D. T., and Fiske, D. W. 1959. Convergent and discriminant validation by the multitrait–multimethod matrix. *Psychological Bulletin, 56,* 81–105.

Campbell, D. T., and Stanley, J. C. 1963. *Experimental and quasi-experimental designs for research.* Chicago: Rand McNally.

Campbell, J. D., and Yarrow, M. R. 1961. Perceptual and behavioral correlates of social effectiveness. *Sociometry, 24,* 1–20.

Cancro, R., Sutton, S., Kerr, J., and Sugerman, A. A. 1971. Reaction time and prognosis in acute schizophrenia. *Journal of Nervous and Mental Disease, 153,* 351–359.

Carey, W. B. 1970. A simplified method for measuring infant temperament. *Journal of Pediatrics, 77,* 188–194.

Carpenter, W. T., Bartko, J. J., Carpenter, C. L., and Strauss, J. S. 1976. Another review of schizophrenia subtypes. *Archives of General Psychiatry, 33,* 508–516.

Carpenter, W. T., Strauss, J. S., and Bartko, J. J. 1973. Flexible system for the identification of schizophrenia: A report from the International Pilot Study of Schizophrenia. *Science, 182,* 1275–1278.

Carpenter, W. T., Strauss, J. S., and Bartko, J. J. 1974. The diagnosis and understanding of schizophrenia: Part 1. Use of signs and symptoms for the identification of schizophrenic patients. *Schizophrenia Bulletin, 11,* 37–49.

Carson, R. C. 1969. *Interaction concepts of personality.* Chicago: Aldine.

Cass, L. 1973. *Manual for ratings from psychological evaluation.* St. Louis: Unpublished manuscript.

Cass, L., Franklin, L., and Bass, L. 1973. "The use of psychological test battery in the study of disturbance in children of psychotic parents as compared with children of nonpsychotic parents." St. Louis: Unpublished manuscript.

Cattell, R. B. 1966. The scree test for the number of factors. *Multivariate Behavioral Research, 1,* 245–276.

Cattell, R. B., and Scheier, I. H. 1963. *Handbook for the IPAT Anxiety Scale Questionnaire* (2nd ed.). Champaign, Ill.: Institute for Personality and Ability Testing.

Cavanaugh, D. K., Cohen, W., and Lang, P. J. 1960. The effect of "social censure" and "social approval" on the psychomotor performance of schizophrenics. *Journal of Abnormal and Social Psychology, 60,* 213–218.

Chapman, J. S., and McGhie, A. 1962. A comparative study of disordered attention in schizophrenia. *Journal of Mental Science, 108,* 487–500.

Chapman, L. J., and Chapman, J. P. 1973. *Disordered thought in schizophrenia.* New York: Appleton-Century-Crofts.

Chapman, L. J., and Chapman, J. P. 1978. The measurement of differential deficit. *Journal of Psychiatric Research, 14,* 303–311.

Chapman, L. J., Chapman, J. P., and Miller, G. 1964. A theory of verbal behavior in schizophrenia. In B. A. Maher (ed.), *Progress in experimental personality research* (vol. 1). New York: Academic Press.

Chapman, L. J., Chapman, J. P., and Raulin, M. L. 1976. Scales for physical and social anhedonia. *Journal of Abnormal Psychology, 85,* 374–382.

Charlesworth, R., and Hartup, W. W. 1967. Positive social reinforcement in the nursery school peer group. *Child Development, 38,* 993–1002.

Ciompi, L. 1980. Catamnestic long-term study on the course of life and aging of schizophrenics. *Schizophrenia Bulletin, 6,* 606–618.

Clack, G. S. 1970. "Effects of social class, age and sex on tests of perception, affect discrimination and deferred gratification in children." Unpublished doctoral dissertation, Washington University.

Cliff, N. 1966. Orthogonal rotation to congruence. *Psychometrika, 31,* 33–42.

Cliff, N. 1982. What is and isn't measurement? In G. Keren (ed.), *Issues in quantitative psychology.* New York: Erlbaum.

Cloninger, C. R., Christiansen, K. O., Reich, T., and Gottesman, I. I. 1978. Implications of sex differences in the prevalences of antisocial personality, alcoholism, and criminality for familial trasmission. *Archives of General Psychiatry, 35,* 941–951.

Cobb, J. A. 1969. "The relationship of observable classroom behaviors to achievement of fourth grade pupils." Unpublished doctoral dissertation, Eugene, Ore.: University of Oregon.

Cohen, B. D., and Camhi, J. 1967. Schizophrenic performance in a word communication task. *Journal of Abnormal Psychology, 72,* 240–246.

Cohen, B. D., Nachmani, G., and Rosenberg, S. 1974. Referent communication disturbances in acute schizophrenia. *Journal of Abnormal Psychology, 83,* 1–14.

Cohen, J. A. 1960. A coefficient of agreement for nominal scales. *Educational and Psychological Measurement, 20,* 37–46.

Cohler, B. J., Gallant, D. H., Grunebaum, H. U., Weiss, J. L., and Gamer, E. 1975. Pregnancy and birth complications among mentally ill and well mothers and their children. *Social Biology, 22,* 269–278.

Cohler, B. J., Grunebaum, H. U., Weiss, J. L., Gamer, E., and Gallant, D. H. 1977. Disturbance of attention among schizophrenic, depressed and well mothers and their young children. *Journal of Child Psychology and Psychiatry, 18,* 115–135.

Cole, R., and Al-Khayyal, M. 1979. "A model for studying whole family interaction with special attention to task and family configuration." University of Rochester, unpublished manuscript.

Cole, R., and Al-Khayyal, M. 1980. "Family interaction and warmth: A study of high-risk families working together." University of Rochester, unpublished manuscript.

Coleman, R. E., and Miller, A. G. 1975. The relationship between depression and marital adjustment in a clinic population. *Journal of Consulting and Clinical Psychology, 43,* 647–651.

Collins, W. E. 1963. Manipulation of arousal and its effects on human vestibular nystagmus induced by caloric irrigation and angular acceleration. *Aerospace Medicine, 54,* 124–129.

Conger, J. J., and Miller, W. C. 1966. *Personality, social class, and delinquency.* New York: Wiley.

Cook-Gumperz, J. 1973. *Social control and socialization: A study of class differences in the language of maternal control.* London: Routledge & Kegan Paul.

Cooley, W. W., and Lohnes, P. R. 1971. *Multivariate data analysis.* New York: Wiley.

Cooper, J. E., Kendell, R. E., Gurland, B. J., Sharpe, L., Copeland, J. R. M., and Simon, R. 1972. *Psychiatric diagnosis in New York and London: A comparative study of mental hospital admissions.* Institute of Psychiatry, Maudsley Monographs, No. 20. London: Oxford University Press.

Corning, W. C., and Steffy, R. A. 1979. Taximetric strategies applied to psychiatric classification. *Schizophrenia Bulletin, 5,* 294–305.

Corning, W. C., Steffy, R. A., and Chaprin, I. C. 1981. "EEG slow frequency and WISC-R correlates." Unpublished manuscript, University of Waterloo.

Cowan, P. A. 1966. Cognitive egocentrism and social interaction in children. *American Psychologist, 21,* 623.

Cowen, E. L., Gardner, E. A., and Zax, M. 1967. *Emergent approaches to mental health problems.* New York: Appleton-Century-Crofts.

Cowen, E. L., Pederson, A., Babigian, H., Izzo, L., and Trost, M. A. 1973. Long-term follow-up of early detected vulnerable children. *Journal of Consulting and Clinical Psychology, 41,* 438–446.

Croft, R. G. F. 1977. "The relationship of maternal teaching style and socioeconomic status to four-year-old children's locus of control orientation." Unpublished doctoral dissertation, University of Rochester.

Cromwell, R. L. 1975. Assessment of schizophrenia. *Annual Review of Psychology, 26*, 593–619.

Cromwell, R. L., Rosenthal, D., Shakow, D., and Zahn, T. P. 1961. Reaction time, locus of control, choice behavior, and descriptions of parental behavior in schizophrenic and normal subjects. *Journal of Personality, 29*, 363–379.

Cronbach, L. J. 1951. Coefficient alpha and the internal structure of tests. *Psychometrika, 16*, 297–334.

Crowne, D. P., and Marlowe, D. 1960. A new scale of social desirability independent of psychopathology. *Journal of Consulting Psychology, 24*, 349–354.

Crowther, J. H., Bond, L. A., and Rolf, J. E. 1981. The incidence, prevalence, and severity of behavior disorders among preschool-aged children in day care. *Journal of Abnormal Child Psychology, 9*(1), 23–42.

Csapo, E. E. 1977. "A comparison of measurement instruments in scoring communication deviance." Senior honors thesis, Department of Psychology, Washington University.

Daut, R. L., and Chapman, L. J. 1974. Object-sorting and the heterogeneity of schizophrenia. *Journal of Abnormal Psychology, 83*, 581–584.

Dawes, R. M., and Meehl, P. E. 1966. Mixed group validation: A method for determining the validity of diagnostic signs without using criterion groups. *Psychological Bulletin, 66*, 63–67.

DeAmicis, L. A., and Cromwell, R. L. 1979. Reaction time crossover in process schizophrenic patients, their relatives, and control subjects. *The Journal of Nervous and Mental Disease, 167*, 593–600.

DePree, S. 1966. "Time perspective, frustration–failure, and delay of gratification in middle-class and lower-class children from organized and disorganized families." Unpublished doctoral dissertation, Minneapolis: University of Minnesota.

Deutsch, J. A., and Deutsch, D. 1963. Attention: Some theoretical considerations. *Psychological Review, 70*, 80–90.

Devine, V., and Tomlinson, J. R. 1975. "Teachers' ratings of children's adaptation and attentional adequacy as exhibited in the classroom." Unpublished manuscript, University of Minnesota.

Dixon, W. E. 1975. *The BMDP Biomedical Computer Programs.* Los Angeles: University of California Press.

Dixon, W. J., and Massey, F. J., Jr. 1969. *Introduction to statistical analyses* (3rd ed.). New York: McGraw-Hill.

Doane, J. A. 1977. "Parental communication deviance as a predictor of child competence in families with a schizophrenic and nonschizophrenic parent." Doctoral dissertation, University of Rochester.

Doane, J. A., Jones, J. E., Fisher, L., Ritzler, B., Singer, M. T., and Wynne, L. C. 1982. Parental communication deviance as a predictor of competence in children at risk for adult psychiatric disorder. *Family Process, 21*, 211–223.

Doane, J. A., West, K. L., Goldstein, M. J., Rodnick, E. H., and Jones, J. E. 1981. Parental communication deviance and affective style: Predictors of subsequent schizophrenia spectrum disorders in vulnerable adolescents. *Archives of General Psychiatry, 38*, 679–685.

Dohrenwend, B. P., and Dohrenwend, B. S. 1974. Social and cultural influences on psychopathology. *Annual Review of Psychology, 25*, 417–452.

Dohrenwend, B. P., and Dohrenwend, B. S. 1976. Sex differences and psychiatric disorders. *American Journal of Sociology, 81*, 1447–1454.

Doll, E. A. 1947. *Vineland Social Maturity Scale.* Minneapolis: Educational Test Bureau, Educational Publishers.

Doll, E. A. 1965. *Vineland Social Maturity Scale: Condensed manual of directions* (1965 ed.). Circle Pines, Minn.: American Guidance Service.

Donchin, E., and Heffley, E. F. 1978. Multivariate analysis of ERP data: A tutorial review. In D. Otto (ed.), *Multidisciplinary perspectives in event-related brain potential research.* Washington, D.C.: U.S. Government Printing Office, pp. 556–572.

Douglas, V. I. 1972. Stop, look, and listen. The problem of sustained attention and impulse control in hyperactive and normal children. *Canadian Journal of Behavioral Science, 4,* 259–282.

Draguns, J. G., Haley, E. M., and Phillips, L. 1967. Studies of Rorschach content: A review of the research literature. Part 1: Traditional content categories. *Journal of Projective Techniques and Personality Assessment, 31,* 3–32.

Driscoll, R. M. September, 1979. "Incidental and intentional learning and social competence in high-risk children." Paper presented at the 87th annual convention of the American Psychological Association in New York.

Driscoll, R. M. June, 1980. "Incidental and intentional learning as measures of selective attention in children vulnerable to psychopathology." Unpublished doctoral dissertation, Minneapolis: University of Minnesota.

Druker, J. F., and Hagen, J. W. 1969. Developmental trends in the processing of task relevant and task irrelevant information. *Child Development, 40,* 371–382.

Dunn, L. M. 1965. *The Peabody Picture Vocabulary Test.* Minneapolis, Minn.: American Guidance Service.

Ebel, R. I. 1951. Estimation of reliability of ratings. *Psychometrika. 16,* 407–424.

Edelberg, R. 1970. The information content of the recovery limb of the electrodermal response. *Psychophysiology, 6*(5), 527–539.

Edwards, J. H. 1960. The stimulation of Mendelism. *Acta Genetic and Statistical Medicine, 10,* 63.

El-Guebaly, N., Offord, D. R., Sullivan, K. T., and Lynch, G. W. 1978. Psychosocial adjustment of the offspring of psychiatric patients. *Canadian Psychiatric Association Journal, 23,* 281–289.

Emde, R. N. 1978. Commentary on organization and stability of newborn behavior: A commentary on the Brazelton Neonatal Behavior Assessment Scale. *Monographs of the Society for Research in Child Development,* Serial No. 177, *43*(5–6), 135–138.

Emde, R. N., Gaensbauer, T. J., and Harmon, R.J. 1976. Emotional expression in infancy: A biobehavioral study. *Psychological Issues,* Monograph 37, *10*(1).

Eme, R. F. 1979. Sex differences in childhood psychopathology: A review. *Psychological Bulletin, 86,* 574–595.

Endicott, J., and Spitzer, R. L. 1972. Current and past psychopathology scales (CAPPS): Rationale, reliability and validity. *Archives of General Psychiatry, 27,* 678–687.

Endicott, J., Spitzer, R. L., Fleiss, J. L., and Cohen, J. 1976. The Global Assessment Scale: A procedure for measuring overall severity of psychiatric disturbance. *Archives of General Psychiatry, 33,* 766–771.

Engel, G. L. 1980. The clinical application of the biopsychosocial model. *American Journal of Psychiatry, 137*(5), 535–544.

Epley, D., and Ricks, D. R. 1963. Foresight and hindsight in the TAT. *Journal of Projective Techniques, 27,* 51–59.

Erlenmeyer-Kimling, L. 1968. Studies on the offspring of two schizophrenic parents. *Journal of Psychiatric Research, 6,* 65–83. Reprinted in D. Rosenthal and S. S. Kety (eds.), *The transmission of schizophrenia.* New York: Pergamon Press.

Erlenmeyer-Kimling, L. 1972a. Comments on past and present in genetic research on schizophrenia. *Psychiatric Quarterly, 46*(4), 363–370.

Erlenmeyer-Kimling, L. 1972b. Gene environment interactions and the variability of behavior. In L. Ehrman, G. S. Omenn, and E. Caspari (eds.), *Genetics, environment and behavior.* New York: Academic Press.

Erlenmeyer-Kimling, L. 1975. A prospective study of children at risk for schizophrenia: Methodological considerations and some preliminary findings. In R. D. Wirt, G. Winokur, and M. Roff (eds.), *Life history research in psychopathology* (vol. 4). Minneapolis: University of Minnesota Press.

Erlenmeyer-Kimling, L. 1976. "Distractibility in children at risk for schizophrenia." Paper presented at the second Rochester Conference on Schizophrenia, Rochester, New York.

Erlenmeyer-Kimling, L. 1977. Issues pertaining to prevention and intervention in genetic disorders affecting human behavior. In G. W. Albee and J. M. Joffee (eds.), *Primary prevention in psychopathology.* Hanover, N.H.: University Press of New England.

Erlenmeyer-Kimling, L. 1978. Genetic approaches to the study of schizophrenia: The genetic evidence as a tool in research. In D. Bergsma and A. L. Goldstein (eds.), *Neurochemical and immunologic components in schizophrenia.* New York: Liss.

Erlenmeyer-Kimling, L., and Cornblatt, B. 1978. Attentional measures in a study of children at high-risk for schizophrenia. In L. C. Wynne, R. L. Cromwell, and S. Matthysse (eds.), *The nature of schizophrenia: New approaches to research and treatment.* New York: Wiley, pp. 359–365. Also in *Journal of Psychiatric Research, 114,* 93–98, 1978.

Erlenmeyer-Kimling, L., and Cornblatt, B. 1980. Children at risk for schizophrenia: Cognitive and clinical assessments at early ages. In Y. P. Altukhov (ed.), *Problems in general genetics: Proceedings of the 14th International Congress of Genetics* (vol. 2, book 2). Moscow: MIR, pp. 91–101.

Erlenmeyer-Kimling, L., Cornblatt, B., and Fleiss, J. 1979. High-risk research in schizophrenia. *Psychiatric Annals, 9,* 79–111.

Erlenmeyer-Kimling, L., and Paradowski, W. 1966. Selection and schizophrenia. *American Naturalist, 100,* 651–665.

Estes, W. K. 1978. Perceptual processing in letter recognition and reading. In E. C. Carterette and M. P. Friedman (eds.), *Handbook of perception* (vol. 9): *Perceptual processing.* New York: Academic Press.

Eysenck, H. J., and Eysenck, S. B. G. 1969. *Personality structure and measurement.* San Diego: Knapp.

Faschingbauer, T. 1976. Substitution and regression models, base rates, and the clinical validity of the Mini-Mult. *Journal of Clinical Psychology, 32,* 70–74.

Feighner, J. P., Robins, E., Guze, S. B., Woodruff, R. A., Winokur, G., and Munoz, R. 1972. Diagnostic criteria for use in psychiatric research. *Archives of General Psychiatry, 26,* 57–63.

Feil, L. A., and Sameroff, A. J. 1979. "Mother's conception of child development: Socioeconomic status, cross-cultural, and parity comparisons." Paper presented at the meeting of the American Psychological Association, New York.

Feinstein, A. R. 1972. Clinical biostatistics XIV: The purposes of prognostic stratification. *Clinical Pharmacology and Therapeutics, 13*(2), 285–297.

Field, T. M. 1977. Effects of early separation, interactive deficits, and experimental manipulations on infant–mother face-to-face stimulation. *Child Development, 48,* 763–771.

Finn, S. November, 1975. "Involvement of male offspring in families with a psychiatrically ill parent." Paper presented at the 27th annual meeting of the American Association for Psychiatric Services for Children, New Orleans.

Fish, B. 1957. The detection of schizophrenia in infancy. *Journal of Nervous and Mental Disease, 125,* 1–24.

Fish, B. 1959. Longitudinal observations of biological deviations in a schizophrenic infant. *American Journal of Psychiatry, 116,* 25–31.

Fish, B. 1960. Involvement of the central nervous system in infants with schizophrenia. *Archives of Neurology, 2,* 115–121.

Fish, B. 1963. The maturation of arousal and attention in the first months of life: A study of variations in ego development. *Journal of the American Academy of Child Psychiatry, 2,* 253–270.

Fish, B. 1971a. Contributions of developmental research to a theory of schizophrenia. In J. Hellmuth (ed.), *Exceptional infant, Vol. 2: Studies in abnormalities.* New York: Brunner/Mazel, pp. 473–482.

Fish, B. 1971b. Discussion: Genetic or traumatic developmental deviation? *Social Biology, 18,* S117–S119.

Fish, B. 1975. Biologic antecedents of psychosis in children. In D. X. Freedman (ed.), *The biology of the major psychoses: A comparative analysis. Association for Research in Nervous and Mental Disease* (vol. 54). New York: Raven Press, pp. 49–80.

Fish, B. 1976a. An approach to prevention in infants at risk for schizophrenia: Developmental deviations from birth to 10 years. *Journal of the American Academy of Child Psychiatry, 15,* 62–82.

Fish, B. 1976b. The maturation of arousal and attention in the first months of life: A study of variations in ego development. *Journal of the American Academy of Child Psychiatry,* 1963, *2,* 253–270. Reprinted in E. N. Rexford, L. W. Sander, and T. Shapiro (eds.), *Infant psychiatry: A new synthesis.* New Haven: Yale University Press, pp. 207–219.

Fish, B. 1977. Neurobiologic antecedents of schizophrenia in children: Evidence for an inherited, congenital neurointegrative defect. *Archives of General Psychiatry, 34,* 1297–1313.

Fish, B. 1982. Attempts at intervention with high-risk children, from infancy on. In M. J. Goldstein (ed.), *Preventive intervention in schizophrenia: Are we ready?* Washington, D.C.: U.S. Government Printing Office.

Fish, B., and Alpert, M. 1962. Abnormal states of consciousness and muscle tone in infants born to schizophrenic mothers. *American Journal of Psychiatry, 119,* 439–445.

Fish, B., and Alpert, M. 1963. Patterns of neurological development in infants born to schizophrenic mothers. In J. Wortis (ed.), *Recent advances in biological psychiatry.* New York: Plenum, pp. 37–42.

Fish, B., and Dixon, W. J. 1978. Vestibular hyporeactivity in infants at risk for schizophrenia: Its association with critical developmental disorders. *Archives of General Psychiatry, 35,* 963–971.

Fish, B., and Hagin, R. 1973. Visual–motor disorders in infants at risk for schizophrenia. *Archives of General Psychiatry, 28,* 900–904.

Fish, B., and Ritvo, E. R. 1979. Psychoses of childhood. In J. D. Noshpitz (ed.), *Basic handbook of child psychiatry* (vol. 2). New York: Basic Books, pp. 249–304.

Fish, B., Shapiro, T., Halpern, F., and Wile, R. 1965. The prediction of schizophrenia in infancy: 3. A ten-year follow-up report of neurological and psychological development. *American Journal of Psychiatry, 121,* 768–775.

Fish, B., Shapiro, T., Halpern, F., and Wile, F. 1966. The prediction of schizophrenia in infancy: 2. A ten-year follow-up of predictions made at one month. In P. Hoch and J. Zubin (eds.), *Psychopathology of schizophrenia.* New York: Grune & Stratton, pp. 335–353.

Fisher, L. 1980. Child competence and psychiatric risk: 1. Model and method. *Journal of Nervous and Mental Disease, 168,* 323–331.

Fisher, L., Harder, D. W., and Kokes, R. F. 1980. Child competence and psychiatric risk: 3. Comparisons based on diagnosis of hospitalized parent. *Journal of Nervous and Mental Disease, 168,* 338–342.

Fisher, L., and Jones, J. E. 1980. Child competence and psychiatric risk: 2. Areas of relationship between child and family functioning. *Journal of Nervous and Mental Disease, 168,* 332–337.

Fisher, L., Kokes, R. F., Harder, D. W., and Jones, J. E. 1980. Child competence and psychiatric risk: 6. Summary and integration of findings. *Journal of Nervous and Mental Disease, 168,* 353–355.

Fiske, D. 1971. *Measuring the concepts of personality.* Chicago: Aldine.

Flavell, J. H., Botkin, P. T., Fry, C. L., et al. 1968. *The development of role-taking and communication skills in children.* New York: Wiley.

Flor-Henry, R. 1976. Lateralized temporal–limbic dysfunction and psychopathology. *Annals of the New York Academy of Sciences, 280,* 770–795.

Fowler, R. C., Tsuang, M. T., and Cadoret, R. J. 1977. Psychiatric illness in the offspring of schizophrenics. *Comprehensive Psychiatry, 18*(2), 127–134.

Fox, B. A. 1975. "Socioeconomic status, psychopathology, and socialization." Unpublished master's thesis, University of Rochester.

Franklin, L. 1977. "A study of psychological differentiation in children of psychotic parents." Doctoral dissertation, St. Louis University.

Franklin, L., Worland, J., Cass, L., Bass, L., and Anthony, E. J. 1978. Study of children at risk: Use of psychological test batteries. In E. J. Anthony, C. Koupernik, and C. Chiland (eds.), *The child in his family: Vulnerable children* (vol. 4). New York: Wiley.

Friedman, D., Frosch, A., and Erlenmeyer-Kimling, L. 1979. Auditory evoked potentials in children at high risk for schizophrenia. In H. Begleiter (ed.), *Evoked brain potentials and behavior.* New York: Plenum, pp. 385–400.

Friedman, D., Vaughan, H. G., Jr., and Erlenmeyer-Kimling, L. 1978. Stimulus and response related components of the late positive complex in visual discrimination tasks. *Electroencephalography and Clinical Neurophysiology, 45,* 319–330.

Friedman, D., Vaughn, H. G., Jr., and Erlenmeyer-Kimling, L. 1979a. Event-related potential investigations in children at high risk for schizophrenia. In D. Lehmann and E. Callaway (eds.), *Human evoked potentials: Applications and problems.* New York: Plenum.

Friedman, D., Vaughn, H. G., Jr., and Erlenmeyer-Kimling, L. 1979b. "The late positive complex to unpredictable auditory events in children at high risk for schizophrenia." Paper presented at the annual meeting of the Society for Psychophysiological Research, Cincinnati, Ohio.

Friedman, H. 1952. Perceptual regression in schizophrenia: An hypothesis suggested by the use of the Rorschach Test. *Journal of Genetic Psychology, 81,* 63–98.

Frieze, I., Parsons, J., Johnson, P., Ruble, D., and Zelman, G. 1978. *Women and sex roles: A social psychological perspective.* New York: Norton.

Gallant, D. H. 1972. "Selective and sustained attention in young children of psychotic mothers." Unpublished doctoral dissertation, Boston University.

Gamer, E., Gallant, D. H., Grunebaum, H. U., and Cohler, B. J. 1977. Children of psychotic mothers: Performance of three-year-old children on tests of attention. *Archives of General Psychiatry, 34,* 592–597.

Garai, J., and Scheinfeld, A. 1968. Sex differences in mental and behavioral traits. *Genetic Psychology Monographs, 77,* 169–199.

Gardner, E. D., Miles, H. C., Iker, H. P., and Romano, J. A. 1963. A cumulative register of psychiatric services in a community. *American Journal of Public Health, 53,* 1269–1277.

Gardner, G. G. 1967. The role of maternal psychopathology in male and female schizophrenics. *Journal of Consulting Psychology, 31,* 411–413.

Garmezy, N. 1952. Stimulus differentiation by schizophrenic and normal subjects under conditions of reward and punishment. *Journal of Personality, 20,* 243–276.

Garmezy, N. 1966. The prediction of performance in schizophrenia. In P. Hoch and J. Zubin (eds.), *Psychopathology of schizophrenia.* New York: Grune & Stratton, pp. 129–181.

Garmezy, N. 1967. "The origins of schizophrenia." Paper presented at the Proceedings of the first Rochester International Conference, Rochester.

Garmezy, N. 1970. Vulnerable children: Implications derived from studies of an internalizing–externalizing symptom dimension. In J. Zubin and A. M. Freedman (eds.), *Psychopathology of adolescence.* New York: Grune & Stratton.

Garmezy, N. 1971. Vulnerability research and the issue of primary prevention. *American Journal of Orthopsychiatry. 41,* 101–116.

Garmezy, N. 1972. Models of etiology for the study of children at risk for schizophrenia. In M. Roff, L. Robins, and M. Pollack (eds.), *Life history research in psychopathology* (vol. 2). Minneapolis: University of Minnesota Press, pp. 9–34.

Garmezy, N. 1973. Competence and adaptation in adult schizophrenic patients and children at risk. In S. R. Dean (ed.), *Schizophrenia: The first ten Dean Award Lectures.* New York: M.S.S. Information Corp., pp. 168–204.

Garmezy, N. 1974. Children at risk: The search for the antecedents of schizophrenia. Part 2: Ongoing research programs, issues and intervention. *Schizophrenia Bulletin, 9,* 55–125.

Garmezy, N. 1975a. The study of competence in children at risk for severe psychopathology. In E. J. Anthony and C. Koupernik (eds.), *The child in his family: Children at psychiatric risk* (vol. 3). New York: Wiley.

Garmezy, N. 1975b. The experimental study of children vulnerable to psychopathology. In A. Davids (ed.), *Child personality and psychopathology: Current topics* (vol. 2). New York: Wiley Interscience, pp. 171–216.

Garmezy, N. 1977. The psychology and psychopathology of attention. *Schizophrenia Bulletin, 3,* 360–369.

Garmezy, N. 1978. Attentional processes in adult schizophrenia and in children at risk. *Journal of Psychiatric Research, 14,* 3–34.

Garmezy, N. 1981. The current status of research with children at risk for schizophrenia and other forms of psychopathology. In D. A. Regier and G. Allen (eds.), *Risk factor research in the major mental disorders.* Washington, D.C.: U.S. Government Printing Office, pp. 23–41.

Garmezy, N., Masten, A., Ferrarese, N., and Nordstrom, L. 1978. The nature of competence in normal and deviant children. In M. W. Kent and J. E. Rolf (eds.), *The primary prevention of psychopathology: Promoting social competence and coping in children* (vol. 3). Hanover, N.H.: University Press of New England.

Garmezy, N., and Rodnick, E. H. 1959. Premorbid adjustment and performance in schizophrenia: Implications for interpreting heterogeneity in schizophrenia. *Journal of Nervous and Mental Disease, 129,* 450–466.

Garmezy, N., and Streitman, S. 1974. Children at risk: The search for the antecedents of schizophrenia. Part 1: Conceptual models and research methods. *Schizophrenia Bulletin, 1*(8), 14–90.

Geismar, L. L., and Ayres, B. 1960. *Measuring family functioning: A manual on a method for evaluating the social functioning of disordered families.* St. Paul, Minn.: Family Centered Project, Greater St. Paul Community Chest and Councils, Inc.

Gerard, R. 1973. The nosology of schizophrenia: A cooperative study. In S. Dean (ed.), *Schizophrenia: The first ten Dean Award Lectures.* New York: M.S.S. Information Corp.

Gesell, A. 1947. *Developmental diagnosis* (2nd ed.). New York: Hoeber.

Gibson, E. J. 1969. *Principles of perceptual learning and development.* New York: Appleton-Century-Crofts.

Gilberstadt, H., and Dukes, J. 1965. *A handbook for clinical and actuarial MMPI interpretation.* Philadelphia: Saunders.

Ginsburg, B. E. 1967. Genetic parameters in behavioral research. In J. Hirsch (ed.), *Behavior–genetic analysis.* New York: McGraw-Hill.

Glazer, J. A. 1928. The association value of nonsense syllables. *Journal of Genetic Psychology, 35,* 255–263.

Glidewell, J., Domke, H., and Kantor, H. 1963. Screening in school for behavior disorders: Use of mother's report of symptoms. *Journal of Educational Research, 36,* 508–515.

Gnanadesikan, R. 1977. *Methods for statistical data analysis of multivariate observations.* New York: Wiley.

Goldfried, M. R., Stricker, G., and Weinert, I. B. 1971. *Rorschach handbook of clinical and research applications.* Englewood Cliffs, N.J.: Prentice-Hall.

Goldschmidt, M. L. 1967. Different types of conservation and nonconservation and their relation to age, sex, IQ, MA, and vocabulary. *Child Development, 38,* 1229–1246.

Goldstein, M. J. 1975. *Psychotherapeutic intervention with families of adolescents at risk for schizophrenia.* Copenhagen: World Health Organization.

Goldstein, M. J. 1980. The course of schizophrenic psychosis. In O. G. Brim, Jr., and J. Kagan (eds.), *Constancy and change in human development.* Cambridge, Mass.: Harvard University Press, pp. 325–358.

Goldstein, M. J., Judd, L. L., Rodnick, E. H., Alkire, A. A., and Gould, E. 1968. A method for the study of social influence and coping patterns in the families of disturbed adolescents. *Journal of Nervous and Mental Disease, 147,* 233–251.

Goldstein, M. J., and Rodnick, E. H. 1975. The family's contribution to the etiology of schizophrenia: Current status. *Schizophrenia Bulletin, 14,* 48–63.

Goldstein, M. J., Rodnick, E. H., Jones, J. E., McPherson, S. R., and West, K. L. 1978. Familial precursors of schizophrenia spectrum disorders. In L. C. Wynne, R. L. Cromwell, and S. Matthysse (eds.), *The nature of schizophrenia: New approaches to research and treatment.* New York: Wiley, pp. 487–498.

Goldstein, M. J., Rodnick, E. H., Judd, L. L., and Gould, E. 1970. Galvanic skin reactivity among family groups containing disturbed adolescents. *Journal of Abnormal Psychology, 75,* 57–67.

Goodenough, F. 1926. *Measurement of intelligence by drawings.* New York: Harcourt, Brace.

Goodman, L. A. 1970. The multivariate analysis of qualitative data: Interaction among multiple classifications. *Journal of the American Statistical Association, 65,* 226–256.

Gorsuch, R. L. 1974. *Factor analysis.* Philadelphia: Saunders.

Gottesman, I. I. 1978. Schizophrenia and genetics: Where are we? Are you sure? In L. C. Wynne, R. L. Cromwell, and S. Matthysse (eds.), *The nature of schizophrenia: New approaches to research and treatment.* New York: Wiley, pp. 59–69.

Gottesman, I. I. 1979. Schizophrenia and genetics: Toward understanding uncertainty. *Psychiatric Annals, 9,* 26–37.

Gottesman, I. I., and Shields, J. 1966. Schizophrenia in twins: 16 years' consecutive admissions to a psychiatric clinic. *British Journal of Psychiatry, 112,* 809–819.

Gottesman, I. I., and Shields, J. 1972. *Schizophrenia and genetics: A twin study vantage point.* New York: Academic Press, 1972.

Gottesman, I. I., and Shields, J. 1973; 1976. Genetic theorizing and schizophrenia. *British Journal of Psychiatry, 122,* 15–30. Reprinted in R. Cancro (ed.), *Annual review of the schizophrenic syndrome* (vol. 4). New York: Brunner/Mazel, pp. 261–286.

Gottesman, I. I., and Shields, J. 1976. A critical review of recent adoption, twin and family studies of schizophrenia: Behavior genetics perspectives. *Schizophrenia Bulletin, 2,* 360–401.

Gottfried, A. W. 1973. Intellectual consequences of perinatal anoxia. *Psychological Bulletin, 80,* 231–242.

Gottman, J., Gonso, J., and Rasmussen, B. 1975. Social interaction, social competence, and friendship in children. *Child Development, 46,* 709–718.

Gottman, J., Markman, H., and Notarius, C. 1977. The topography of marital conflict: A sequential analysis of verbal and nonverbal behavior. *Journal of Marriage and Family, 39,* 461–477.

Green, D. M., and Swets, J. A. 1966. *Signal detection theory and psychophysics.* New York: Wiley.

Griffith, J. J., Mednick, S. A., Schulsinger, F., and Diderichsen, B. 1980. Verbal associative disturbances in children at high-risk for schizophrenia. *Journal of Abnormal Psychology, 89,* 125–131.

Grinker, R. R., and Holzman, P. S. 1973. Schizophrenic pathology in young adults. *Archives of General Psychiatry, 28,* 168–175.

Gronlund, N. E., and Holmlund, W. S. 1958. The value of elementary school sociometric status scores for predicting pupils' adjustment in high school. *Educational Administration and Supervision, 44,* 225–260.

Grubb, T. W. 1979. "Early prediction of adult schizophrenia." Unpublished manuscript, University of Massachusetts.

Grunebaum, H. U., Cohler, B. J., Kauffman, C., and Gallant, D. H. 1978. Children of depressed and schizophrenic mothers. *Child Psychiatry and Human Development, 8*(4), 219–228.

Grunebaum, H. U., Weiss, J. L., Cohler, B. J., Hartman, C., and Gallant, D. H. 1975. *Mentally ill mothers and their children.* Chicago: University of Chicago Press.

Grunebaum, H. U., Weiss, J. L., Gallant, D. H., and Cohler, B. J. 1974. Attention in young children of psychotic mothers. *American Journal of Psychiatry, 131,* 887–891.

Gruzelier, J. H., and Hammond, N. V. 1976. Schizophrenia: A dominant hemisphere temporal–limbic disorder? *Research Communications in Psychology, Psychiatry, and Behavior, 1,* 33–72.

Gruzelier, J. H., and Venables, P. H. 1972. Skin conductance orienting activity in a heterogeneous sample of schizophrenics. *Journal of Nervous and Mental Disease, 155,* 277–287.

Gunderson, J. G. 1975. "Borderline evaluation schedule. Differential diagnosis of borderline disorders and schizophrenia." Unpublished manuscript.

Gunderson, J. G. 1977. Characteristics of borderlines. In P. Hartocollis (ed.), *Borderline personality disorders: The concept, the syndrome, the patient.* New York: International Universities Press, pp. 173–192.

Gunderson, J. G., Autry, J. H., Mosher, L. R., and Buchsbaum, S. 1974. Special report: Schizophrenia. *Schizophrenia Bulletin, 9*(Summer), 15.

Gur, R. E. 1977. Motoric laterality imbalance in schizophrenia: A possible concomitant of left hemisphere dysfunction. *Archives of General Psychiatry, 34*, 33–37.

Guttman, L. 1954. Some necessary conditions for common factor analysis. *Psychometrika, 19*, 149–161.

Hagen, J. W., and Sabo, R. A. 1967. A developmental study of selective attention. *Merrill-Palmer Quarterly, 13*, 159–172.

Hamburg, D. A. 1967. Genetics of adrenocortical hormone metabolism in relation to psychological stress. In J. Hirsch (ed.), *Behavior–genetic analysis.* New York: McGraw-Hill.

Hampel, F. R. 1974. The influence curve and its role in robust estimation. *Journal of the American Statistical Association, 69*, 383–393.

Hanson, D. R., Gottesman, I. I., and Heston, L. L. 1976. Some possible childhood indicators of adult schizophrenia inferred from children of schizophrenics. *British Journal of Psychiatry, 129*, 142–154.

Hanson, D. R., Gottesman, I. I., and Meehl, P. E. 1977. Genetic theories and the validation of psychiatric diagnoses: Implications for the study of children of schizophrenics. *Journal of Abnormal Psychology, 86*, 575–588.

Harder, D. W., Kokes, R. F., Fisher, L., Cole, R. E., and Perkins, P. 1982. Parent psychopathology and child functioning among sons at risk for psychological disorder. *Monographs of the Society for Research in Child Development, 47*, (5, Serial No. 197), 25–35 (Chapter IV).

Harder, D. W., Kokes, R. F., Fisher, L., and Strauss, J. S. 1980. Child competence and psychiatric risk: 4. Relationships of parent diagnostic classifications and parent psychopathology severity to child functioning. *Journal of Nervous and Mental Disease, 168*, 343–347.

Harris, C. W. 1967. On factors and factor scores. *Psychometrika, 32*, 363–379.

Harris, D. 1963. *Goodenough–Harris Drawing Test manual.* New York: Harcourt, Brace and World.

Hartman, G., and Robertson, M. 1972. Comparison of the Mini-Mult and the MMPI in a community mental health agency. *Proceedings of the Annual Convention of the American Psychological Association, 7*, 33–34.

Hartup, W. W. 1970. Peer interaction and social organization. In P. H. Mussen (ed.), *Carmichael's manual of child psychology* (3rd ed., vol. 2). New York: Wiley.

Hartup, W. W., Glazer, J., and Charlesworth, R. 1967. Peer reinforcement and sociometric status. *Child Development, 38*, 1017–1024.

Harvey, P., Winters, K., Weintraub, S., and Neale, J. M. 1981. Distractibility in children vulnerable to psychopathology. *Journal of Abnormal Psychology, 90*(4), 298–304.

Hase, H. D., and Goldberg, L. R. 1967. Comparative validity of different strategies of constructing personality inventory scales. *Psychological Bulletin, 67*, 231–248.

Hathaway, S. R., and McKinley, J. C. 1942. *The Minnesota Multiphasic Personality Inventory.* Minneapolis: University of Minnesota Press.

Hawk, A. B., Carpenter, W. T., and Strauss, J. S. 1975. Diagnostic criteria and five-year outcome in schizophrenia. *Archives of General Psychiatry, 32*, 343–347.

Heise, D. R. 1975. *Causal analysis.* New York: Wiley Interscience.

Held, J. M., and Cromwell, R. L. 1968. Premorbid adjustment in schizophrenia: An evaluation of a method and some general comments. *Journal of Nervous and Mental Disease, 146*, 246–272.

Hemsley, D. R., and Zawada, S. L. 1976. "Filtering" and the cognitive deficit in schizophrenia. *British Journal of Psychiatry, 128,* 456–461.

Henrysson, J. 1962. The relation between factor loadings and biserial correlations in factor analysis. *Psychometrika, 27,* 419–422.

Herbert, S. H. 1977. "Vulnerable children growing older: A follow-up study of children at risk for adult psychopathology." Unpublished summa cum laude thesis: University of Minnesota.

Heriot, J., and Schmickel, C. A. 1967. Maternal estimate of intelligence in children evaluated for learning potential. *American Journal of Mental Deficiency, 71*(6), 920–924.

Herman, J., Mirsky, A. F., Ricks, N. L., and Gallant, D. H. 1977. Behavioral and electrographic measures of attention in children at risk for schizophrenia. *Journal of Abnormal Psychology, 86,* 27–33.

Hertz, M. 1961. *Frequency tables for scoring Rorschach responses* (4th ed.). Beverly Hills, Calif.: Western Psychological Services.

Heston, L. L. 1966. Psychiatric disorders in foster home reared children of schizophrenic mothers. *British Journal of Psychiatry, 112,* 819–825.

Heston, L. L., and Denney, D. 1968. Interactions between early life experience and biological factors in schizophrenia. In D. Rosenthal and S. S. Kety (eds.), *The transmission of schizophrenia.* Oxford: Pergamon Press, pp. 363–376.

Higgins, J. 1974. Effects of child rearing by schizophrenic mothers. In S. A. Mednick, F. Schulsinger, J. Higgins, and B. Bell (eds.), *Genetics, environment and psychopathology.* New York: North Holland.

Hinrichs, J. V., and Craft, J. L. 1971. Verbal expectancy and probability in two-choice reaction time. *Journal of Experimental Psychology, 88,* 367–371.

Hirschi, T. 1969. *Cause of delinquency.* Berkeley: University of California Press.

Hollingshead, A. B. 1957. "The two factor index of social position." Unpublished manuscript, Yale University.

Hollingshead, A. B. 1968. The two factor index of social position. In J. Myers and Y. L. Bean (eds.), *A decade later: A follow-up of social class and mental illness.* New York: Wiley.

Hollingshead, A. B. 1978. "Four factor index of social status." Unpublished manuscript.

Holmes, T. H., and Masuda, M. 1973. Life change and illness susceptibility. *Separation and depression,* AAAS, *94,* 161–186.

Holmes, T. H., and Rahe, R. H. 1967. The Social Readjustment Scale. *Journal of Psychosomatic Research, 11,* 213–218.

Holzman, P. S., Levy, D. L., and Proctor, L. R. 1976. Smooth pursuit eye movements, attention, and schizophrenia. *Archives of General Psychiatry, 33,* 1415–1420.

Hopper, S. 1976. "Family climate in families of psychotic parents." Unpublished master's thesis, St. Louis University.

Huston, P. E., Shakow, D., and Riggs, L. A. 1937. Studies of motor function in schizophrenia. 2. Reaction time. *Journal of General Psychology, 16,* 39–82.

Hymel, S., and Asher, S. March, 1977. "Assessment and training of isolated children's social skills." Paper presented at the biennial meeting of the Society for Research in Child Development, New Orleans.

Itil, T. M., Hus, W., Saletu, B., and Mednick, S. A. 1974. Auditory evoked potential investigations in children at high risk for schizophrenia. *American Journal of Psychiatry, 131,* 892–900.

Jackson, D. N. 1970. A sequential strategy for personality scale construction. In C. Spielberger (ed.), *Current topics in clinical and community psychology.* New York: Academic Press.

Jackson, D. N. 1971. *The Personality Research Form-E.* Palo Alto, Calif.: Research Psychologists Press.

Jackson, D. N., and Skinner, H. A. 1975. Univocal varimax: An orthogonal factor rotation program for optimal simple structure. *Educational and Psychological Measurement, 35,* 663–665.

Jacobs, J. (ed.). 1968. *Celtic fairy tales.* New York: Dover.

Jacobs, T. 1975. Family interaction in disturbed and normal families: A methodological and substantive review. *Psychological Bulletin, 82,* 33–65.

Janes, C. L. 1974. "Psychiatric and psychological correlates of electrodermal responding in children of psychotic parents." Paper presented at the Congress of the International Association for Child Psychiatry and the Allied Professions, Philadelphia.

Janes, C. L. November, 1975. "Parent–child relations in families with a psychiatrically ill parent." Paper presented at the American Association of Psychiatric Services for Children, New Orleans.

Janes, C. L. September, 1976. "Perceived family environment and school adjustment of children of schizophrenics." Paper presented at the 84th convention of the American Psychological Association, Washington, D.C.

Janes, C. L., Hesselbrock, V., Myers, D. G., and Penniman, J. 1979. Problem boys in young adulthood: Teachers' ratings and 12-year follow-up. *Journal of Youth and Adolescence, 8,* 453–472.

Janes, C. L., Hesselbrock, V., and Stern, J. 1978. Parental psychopathology, age and race as factors in electrodermal activity of children. *Psychophysiology, 15,* 24–34.

Janes, C. L., Hudson, W., Hesselbrock, V., and Anthony, E. J. September, 1975. "How much intra-family involvement when a parent is schizophrenic?" Paper presented at the 83rd annual convention of the American Psychological Association, Chicago.

Janes, C. L., and Stern, J. 1973. Personality and psychopathology. In D. C. Raskin and W. F. Prokasy (eds.), *Electrodermal activity in psychological research.* New York: Academic Press.

Janes, C. L., and Stern, J. 1976. Electrodermal response configuration as a function of rated psychopathology in children. *Journal of Nervous and Mental Disease,* 184–194.

Janes, C. L., Worland, J., and Stern, J. 1971. Racial differences in skin potential responses. *Psychophysiology, 8,* 254.

Janes, C. L., Worland, J., and Stern, J. 1976. Skin potential and vasomotor responsiveness of black and white children. *Psychophysiology, 13,* 523–527.

Jaspers, K. 1965. *Allgemeine Psychopathologie,* 8th ed. Berlin: Springer.

Jastak, J. F., Bijou, S. W., and Jastak, S. R. 1965. *The wide range achievement test.* Wilmington: Guidance Associates.

Johannsen, W. J. 1964. Motivation in schizophrenic performance: A review. *Psychological Reports, 15,* 839–870.

John, E. R., Karmel, B. Z., Corning, W. C., Easton, P., Brown, D., Ahn, H., John, M., Harmony, T., Prichep, L., Toro, A., Gerson, I., Bartlett, F., Thatcher, R., Kaye, H., Valdes, P., and Schwartz, E. 1977. Neurometrics: Numerical taxonomy identifies different profiles of brain functions within groups of behaviorally similar people. *Science, 196,* 1393–1410.

John, R. S., Mednick, S. A., and Schulsinger, F. 1982. Teacher reports as a predictor of schizophrenia and borderline schizophrenia: A Bayesian decision analysis. *Journal of Abnormal Psychology, 91,* 399–413.

Johnson, S. C. 1967. Hierarchical clustering scheme. *Psychometrika, 32,* 241–254.

Jones, F. H. 1974. A four-year follow-up of vulnerable adolescents: The prediction of outcomes in early adulthood from measures of social competence, coping style and overall level of psychopathology. *Journal of Nervous and Mental Disease, 159,* 20–39.

Jones, F. H. 1977. The Rochester Adaptive Behavior Inventory: A parallel series of instruments for assessing social competence during early and middle childhood and adolescence. In J. Strauss, H. Babigian, and M. Roff (eds.), *The origins and course of psychopathology: Methods of longitudinal research.* New York: Plenum.

Jones, J. E. 1977. Patterns of transactional style deviance in the TAT's of parents of schizophrenics. *Family Process, 16*(3), 327–337.

Jones, J. E., Rodnick, E. H., Goldstein, M. J., McPherson, S. R., and West, K. L. 1977. Parental transactional style deviance in families of disturbed adolescents as an indicator of risk for schizophrenia. *Archives of General Psychiatry, 34,* 71–74.

Jöreskog, K. G. 1971. Simultaneous factor analysis in several populations. *Psychometrika, 36,* 409–426.

Jöreskog, K. G. 1978. Structural analysis of covariance and correlational matrices. *Psychometrika, 43,* 443–477.

Kagan, J., Moss, H. A., and Sigel, I. E. 1963. Psychological significance of styles of conceptualization. In J. C. Wright and J. Kagan (eds.), *Basic cognitive processes in children.* Monographs of the Society for Research in Child Development, *28,* No. 2 (Serial No. 86), 73–112.

Kahana, B., Stern, J., and Clack, J. 1969. Age related differences in logical responses to the Word Association Test. *Proceedings of the American Psychological Association,* Washington, D.C.

Kahana, B., and Sterneck, R. October, 1969. The effects of age, sex and instructional set on children's Word Association responses. *Journal of Genetic Psychology, 120.*

Kahneman, D. 1973. *Attention and effort.* Englewood Cliffs, N.J.: Prentice-Hall.

Kaiser, H. F. 1970. A second generation little jiffy. *Psychometrika, 35,* 401–415.

Kantor, R., Wallner, J., and Winder, C. 1953. Process and reactive schizophrenia. *Journal of Consulting Psychology, 17,* 157–162.

Karp, S. A., and Konstadt, N. 1963. "Manual for the Children's Embedded-Figures Test: Cognitive tests." Unpublished manuscript.

Katz, M. M., Cole, J. D., and Lowery, H. A. 1964. Non-specificity of diagnosis of paranoid schizophrenia. *Archives of General Psychiatry, 11,* 197–202.

Katz, M. M., and Lyerly, S. G. 1963. Methods for measuring adjustment and behavior in the community. 1. Rationale, description, discrimination validity and scale development. *Psychological Reports, 13,* 503–535.

Keele, S. W., and Neill, W. T. 1978. Mechanisms of attention. In E. C. Carterette and M. P. Friedman (eds.), *Handbook of perception* (vol. 9): *Perceptual processing.* New York: Academic Press.

Keilson, H. 1979. *Sequentielle Traumatisierung bie Kindern.* Stuttgart: Enke.

Keith, S. J., Gunderson, J. G., Reifman, A., Buchsbaum, S., and Mosher, L. R. 1976. Special report: Schizophrenia, 1976. *Schizophrenia Bulletin, 2,* 510–565.

Kelly, P. 1976. The relation of infant's temperament and mother's psychopathology to interaction in early infancy. In K. F. Riegel and J. A. Meacham (eds.), *The developing individual in a changing world* (vol. 2): *Social and environmental issues.* The Hague: Mouton.

Kendell, R. E., Brockington, I. F., and Leff, J. P. 1979. Prognostic implications of six alternative definitions of schizophrenia. *Archives of General Psychiatry, 36,* 25–31.

Kenney, D. A. 1979. *Correlation and causality.* New York: Wiley.

Kessen, W. 1960. Research design in the study of developmental problems. In P. H. Mussen (ed.), *Handbook of research methods in child development.* New York: Wiley, pp. 36–70.

Kestenbaum, C. J., and Bird, H. R. 1978. A reliability study of the mental health assessment form for school age children. *Journal of the American Academy of Child Psychiatry, 17,* 338–347.

Kety, S. S. 1978. Genetic and biochemical aspects of schizophrenia. In A. M. Nicholi, Jr. (ed.), *The Harvard guide to modern psychiatry.* Cambridge, Mass.: Harvard University Press, pp. 93–102.

Kety, S. S., Rosenthal, D., Schulsinger, F., and Wender, P. H. 1968. The types and prevalance of mental illness in the biological and adoptive families of adopted schizophrenics. *Journal of Psychiatric Research, 1* (supplement), 345–362. Reprinted in D. Rosenthal and S. S. Kety (eds.), *The transmission of schizophrenia.* New York: Pergamon Press.

Kety, S., Rosenthal, D., Wender, P., and Schulsinger, F. 1971. Mental illness in the biological and adoptive families of adopted schizophrenics. *American Journal of Psychiatry, 128*(3), 82–86.

Kety, S. S., Rosenthal, D., Wender, P. H., and Schulsinger, F. 1974. The types and prevalence of mental illness in the biological and adoptive families of adopted schizophrenics. In S. A. Mednick, F. Schulsinger, J. Higgins, and B. Bell (eds.), *Genetics, environment and psychopathology.* Amsterdam: North Holland/Elsevier.

Kety, S. S., Rosenthal, D., Wender, P. H., Schulsinger, F., and Jacobsen, B. 1975. Mental illness in the biological and adoptive families of adopted individuals who have become schizophrenic: A preliminary report based upon psychiatric interviews. In R. Fieve, D. Rosenthal, and H. Brill (eds.), *Genetic research in psychiatry.* Baltimore: Johns Hopkins University Press.

Kidd, K. K. 1978. A genetic perspective on schizophrenia. In L. C. Wynne, R. L. Cromwell, and S. Matthysse (eds.), *The nature of schizophrenia: New approaches to research and treatment.* New York: Wiley, pp. 70–75.

Kidd, K. K., and Matthysse, S. 1978. Research designs for the study of gene–environment interactions in psychiatric disorders. *Archives of General Psychiatry, 35,* 925–932.

Kim, J., and Mueller, C. W. 1978. *Factor analysis: Statistical methods and practical issues.* Beverly Hills: Sage.

Kincannon, J. C. 1968. Prediction of the standard MMPI scale scores from 71 items: The Mini-Mult. *Journal of Consulting and Clinical Psychology, 32,* 319–325.

King, H. E. 1954. *Psychomotor aspects of mental disease.* Cambridge, Mass.: Harvard University Press.

Klein, R. H., and Salzman, L. F. 1977. Habituation and conditioning in high-risk children: A preliminary report. *Psychophysiology, 14,* 105.

Klein, R. H., and Salzman, L. F. 1978. Censure–praise learning of children at risk. *Journal of Nervous and Mental Disease, 166,* 799–804.

Klemchuk, H., Rolf, J. E., and Hasazi, J. September, 1975. "Preschool children at risk: A multi-level approach to developmental psychopathology." Paper presented at the meeting of the American Psychological Association, Chicago.

Klerman, G. L., Endicott, J., Spitzer, R., and Hirschfeld, R. M. A. 1979. Neurotic depressions: A systematic analysis of multiple criteria and meanings. *American Journal of Psychiatry, 136,* 57–61.

Klorman, R., Strauss, J., and Kokes, R. 1977. The relationship of demographic and diagnostic factors to measures of premorbid adjustment. *Schizophrenia Bulletin, 3*, 214–225.

Knight, R. G., and Russell, P. N. 1978. Global capacity reduction and schizophrenia. *British Journal of Social and Clinical Psychology, 17*, 275–280.

Kohlberg, L., LaCrosse, J., and Ricks, D. 1972. The predictability of adult mental health and childhood behavior. In B. B. Wolman (ed.), *Manual of child psychopathology*. New York: McGraw-Hill, pp. 1217–1284.

Kohn, M. L. 1969. *Class and conformity: A study in values*. Homewood, Ill.: Dorsey.

Kokes, R. F., Harder, D. W., Fisher, L., and Strauss, J. S. 1980. Child competence and psychiatry risk: 5. Sex of patient parent and dimensions of psychopathology. *Journal of Nervous and Mental Disease, 168*, 348–352.

Kolata, G. B. 1978. Behavioral teratology: Birth defects of the mind. *Science, 202*, 732–734.

Kopfstein, J. H., and Neale, J. M. 1972. A multivariate study of attention dysfunction in schizophrenia. *Journal of Abnormal Psychology, 80*, 294–298.

Koppitz, E. M. 1963. *The Bender Gestalt Test for young children*. New York: Grune & Stratton.

Koppitz, E. M. 1968. *Psychological evaluation of children's human figure drawings*. New York: Grune & Stratton.

Koppitz, E. M. 1973. Visual aural digit span test performance of boys with emotional and learning problems. *Journal of Clinical Psychology, 29*, 463–466.

Kornetsky, C. 1972. The use of a simple test of attention as a measure of drug effects in schizophrenic patients. *Psychopharmacologia, 24*, 99–106.

Kornetsky, C., and Mirsky, A. 1966. On certain psychopharmacological and physiological differences between schizophrenic and normal persons. *Psychopharmacology* (Berlin), *8*, 309–318.

Kornetsky, C., and Orzack, M. 1978. Physiological and behavioral correlates of attention dysfunction in schizophrenic patients. *Journal of Psychiatric Research, 14*, 69–79.

Kringlen, E. 1967. *Heredity and environment in the functional psychoses: An epidemiological–clinical twin study*. London: Heinemann.

Kupietz, S. S., Camp, J. A., and Weissman, A. D. 1976. Reaction time performance of behaviorally deviant children: Effects of prior preparatory interval and reinforcement. *Journal of Child Psychology and Psychiatry, 17*, 123–131.

LaBerge, D. L., VanGelder, P., and Yellott, J., Jr. 1970. A cueing technique in choice reaction time. *Perception and Psychophysics, 7*, 57–62.

Lacks, P. 1970. Further investigation of the Mini-Mult. *Journal of Consulting and Clinical Psychology, 35*, 126–127.

Lambert, N., and Bower, E. 1961. *Technical report on in-school screening of emotionally handicapped children*. Princeton, N.J.: Educational Testing Service.

Landau, R., Harth, P., Othnay, N., and Sharfhertz, C. 1972. The influence of psychotic parents on their children's development. *American Journal of Psychiatry, 129*(1), 70–75.

Lander, H., Anthony, E. J., Cass, L., Franklin, L., and Bass, L. 1978. A measure of vulnerability to risk of parental psychosis. In E. J. Anthony, C. Koupernik, and C. Chiland (eds.), *The child in his family: Vulnerable children* (vol. 4). New York: Wiley.

Lane, E. A., and Albee, G. W. 1964. Early childhood intellectual differences between schizophrenic adults and their siblings. *Journal of Abnormal Social Psychology, 68*, 193–195.

Lane, E. A., Albee, G. W., and Doll, L. 1970. The intelligence of children of schizophrenics. *Developmental Psychology, 2*(3), 315–317.

Lang, P. H., and Buss, A. H. 1965. Psychological deficit in schizophrenia, 2. Interference and activation. *Journal of Abnormal Psychology, 70,* 77–106.

Lawson, J. S., McGhie, A., and Chapman, J. 1967. Distractibility in schizophrenia and organic brain disease. *British Journal of Psychiatry, 113,* 527–535.

Lehman, E. B. 1972. Selective strategies in children's attention to task-relevant information. *Child Development, 43,* 197–209.

Leonhard, K. 1961. Cycloid psychoses – endogenous psychoses which are neither schizophrenic nor manic-depressive. *Journal of Mental Science, 107,* 633–648.

Lerner, P. M. 1965. Resolution of intrafamilial role conflict in families of schizophrenic patients: 1. Thought disturbance. *Journal of Nervous and Mental Disease, 141,* 342–351.

Lerner, P. M. 1968. Correlation of social competence and level of cognitive perceptual functioning in male schizophrenics. *Journal of Nervous and Mental Disease, 146,* 412–416.

Lerner, P. M. 1975. The genetic level score: A review. In P. M. Lerner (ed.), *Handbook of Rorschach scales.* New York: International Universities Press.

Lerner, S., Bie, I., and Lehrer, P. 1972. Concrete-operational thinking in mentally ill adolescents. *Merrill-Palmer Quarterly of Behavior and Development, 18,* 287–291.

Levit, R. L., Sutton, S., and Zubin, J. 1973. Evoked potential correlates of information processing in psychiatric patients. *Psychological Medicine, 3,* 487–494.

Lewine, R. R. J. 1979. Sex differences in schizophrenia: A commentary. *Schizophrenia Bulletin, 5*(1), 4–7.

Lewine, R. R. J. 1980a. Sex differences in the age of symptom onset and first hospitalization in typical schizophrenia, schizophreniform psychosis, and paranoid psychosis. *American Journal of Orthopsychiatry, 50,* 316–322.

Lewine, R. R. J. 1980b. "Review of theoretical implications of sex differences in schizophrenia." Unpublished manuscript.

Lewine, R. R. J. 1981. Sex differences in schizophrenia: Timing or subtype? *Psychological Bulletin, 90,* 432–444.

Lewine, R. R. J., Strauss, J. S., and Gift, T. 1981. Sex differences in age at first hospital admission for schizophrenia: Fact or artifact? *American Journal of Psychiatry, 138,* 440–444.

Lewine, R. R. J., Watt, N. F., and Grubb, T. W. March, 1980. "The role of school assessment in the identification of adolescents at behavioral risk for schizophrenia." Paper presented at the Risk Research Consortium Plenary Conference, San Juan, Puerto Rico.

Lewine, R. R. J., Watt, N. F., and Grubb, T. W. 1981. High risk for schizophrenia research: Sampling bias and its implications. *Schizophrenia Bulletin, 7,* 273–280. (Reprinted as Chapter 43, this volume.)

Lewinsohn, P. M. 1975. The behavioral study and treatment of depression. In M. Hersen, R. M. Eisler, and P. M. Miller (eds.), *Progress in behavior modification.* New York: Academic Press.

Lewis, J. M. 1979. "Disorder index of risk for schizophrenia." Doctoral dissertation, University of California, Los Angeles.

Lewis, M., and Rosenblum, L. A. (eds.). 1975. *Friendship and peer relations.* New York: Wiley (Interscience).

Lidz, T., Fleck, S., and Cornelison, A. 1965. *Schizophrenia and the family.* New York: International Universities Press.

Lieber, D. J. 1977. Parental focus of attention in a videotape feedback task as a function of hypothesized risk for offspring schizophrenia. *Family Process, 16,* 467–475.

Lingoes, J. C. 1973. *The Guttman–Lingoes nonmetric program series.* Ann Arbor, Mich.: Mathesis Press.

List, M. 1980. "The development of attention–information processing abilities and their relationship to cognitive tempo, general mental ability, and behaviour engaged in during task performance in 7, 10, and 13 year-old boys." Unpublished thesis, University of Waterloo, Ontario.

Locke, H. J., and Wallace, K. M. 1959. Short marital adjustment and prediction tests: Their reliability and validity. *Marriage and Family Living, 21,* 251–255.

Loevinger, J. 1971. Measurement in clinical research. In A. E. Bergin and S. L. Garfield (eds.), *Handbook of psychotherapy and behavior change: An empirical analysis.* New York: Wiley.

Lord, F. M. 1967. A paradox in the interpretation of group comparisons. *Psychological Bulletin, 68,* 304–305.

Lord, F. M., and Novick, M. N. 1968. *Statistical theories of mental test scores.* Reading, Mass.: Addison-Wesley.

Losen, S. M. 1961. The differential effects of censure on the problem solving behavior of schizophrenic and normal subjects. *Journal of Personality, 29,* 258–272.

Loveland, N. T., Wynne, L. C., and Singer, M. T. 1963. The Family Rorschach: A method for studying family interaction. *Family Process, 2,* 187–215.

Lyerly, S. 1973. *Handbook of psychiatric rating scales* (2nd ed.). Washington, D.C.: U.S. Government Printing Office, DHEW Publication No. (HSM) 73–9061, pp. 36–40.

McCabe, M. S. 1975. Reactive psychoses. *Acta Psychiatrica Scandinavica,* Suppl. 259.

Maccoby, E. E. 1969. The development of stimulus selection. In J. P. Hill (ed.), *Minnesota symposium on child psychology* (vol. 3). Minneapolis: University of Minnesota Press.

Maccoby, E. E., and Hagen, J. W. 1965. Effects of distraction upon central versus incidental recall: Developmental trends. *Journal of Experimental Child Psychology, 2,* 280–289.

Maccoby, E. E., and Jacklin, C. 1974. *The psychology of sex differences.* Stanford: Stanford University Press.

MacCrimmon, D. J., Cleghorn, J. M., Asarnow, R. F., and Steffy, R. A. 1980. Children at risk for schizophrenia: Clinical and attentional characteristics. *Archives of General Psychiatry, 37,* 671–674.

McGhie, A. 1969. *Pathology of attention.* Middlesex, England: Penguin Books.

McGhie, A., and Chapman, J. 1961. Disorders of attention and perception in early schizophrenia. *British Journal of Medical Psychology, 34,* 103–117.

McGhie, A., Chapman, J., and Lawson, J. S. 1965a. The effect of distraction on schizophrenic performance. 1. Perception and immediate memory. *British Journal of Psychiatry, 111,* 383–390.

McGhie, A., Chapman, J., and Lawson, J. S. 1965b. The effect of distraction on schizophrenic performance. 2. Psychomotor ability. *British Journal of Psychiatry, 111,* 391–398.

McGinnis, M., and Sumer, E. 1978. Certain interaction patterns among members of high risk families with implications for possible deviant development in the children. In E. J. Anthony, C. Koupernik, and C. Chiland (eds.), *The child in his family: Vulnerable children.* New York: Wiley.

McKnew, D., Cytryn, L., Efron, A., Gershon, E., and Bunney, W. 1979. Offspring patients with affective disorders. *British Journal of Psychiatry, 134,* 148–152.

Mackworth, J. F. 1970. *Vigilance and attention: A signal detection approach.* Baltimore: Penguin Books.

McNally, W. J., and Stuart, E. A. 1953. *Examination of the labyrinth in relation to its physiology and nonsuppurative diseases.* Omaha: Douglas.

McNeil, T. F., and Kaij, L. 1978. Obstetric factors in the development of schizophrenia: Complications in the births of preschizophrenics and in reproduction by schizophrenic parents. In L. C. Wynne, R. L. Cromwell, and S. Matthysse (eds.), *The nature of schizophrenia: New approaches to research and treatment.* New York: Wiley, pp. 401–429.

McNeil, T. F., and Kaij, L. 1979. Etiological relevance of comparisons of high-risk and low-risk groups. *Acta Psychiatrica Scandinavica, 59,* 545–560.

McNeil, T. F., Persson-Blennow, I., and Kaij, L. 1974. Reproduction in female psychiatric patients: Severity of mental disturbance near reproduction and rates of obstetric complications. *Acta Psychiatrica Scandinavica, 50,* 23–32.

McNicol, D. 1972. *A primer of signal detection theory.* London: Allen & Unwin.

Marcus, J. 1970. Neurological findings in offspring of schizophrenics. In *Proceedings of the Seventh Congress of the International Association of Child Psychiatry and Allied Professions,* Jerusalem.

Marcus, J. 1974. Cerebral functioning in offspring of schizophrenics: A possible genetic factor. *International Journal of Mental Health, 3,* 57–73.

Marcus, J., Auerbach, J., Wilkinson, L., and Burack, C. M. 1981. Infants at risk for schizophrenia: The Jerusalem Infant Development Study. *Archives of General Psychiatry, 38,* 703–713. (Reprinted as Chapter 35, this volume.)

Marcus, J., Auerbach, J., Wilkinson, L., Maier, S., Mark, A., and Pelis, V. 1979. "Infants born to parents with serious mental disorders: The Jerusalem Infant Development Study." Unpublished manuscript.

Marcus, J., Hans, S. L., Mednick, S. A., Schulsinger, F., and Mikkelson, N. 1983. "Neurological functioning in offspring of schizophrenics in Israel and Denmark: A replication study." Unpublished manuscript.

Marcus, L. M. 1972. "Studies of attention in children vulnerable to psychopathology." Unpublished doctoral dissertation. University of Minnesota.

Marcuse, Y., and Cornblatt, B. In press. Children at high risk for schizophrenia: Predictions from infancy to childhood functioning. In L. Erlenmeyer-Kimling and N. Miller (eds.), *Life span research on the prediction of psychopathology.* New York: Columbia University Press.

Margolies, P. J., and Weintraub, S. 1977. The revised 56 item CRPBI as a research instrument: Reliability and factor structure. *Journal of Clinical Psychology, 33,* 472–476.

Marks, P. A., Seeman, W., and Haller, D. 1974. *The actuarial use of the MMPI with adolescents and adults.* Baltimore, Md.: Williams & Wilkins.

Maruyama, G., and McGarvey, B. 1980. Evaluating causal models: An application of maximum-likelihood analysis of structural equations. *Psychological Bulletin, 87,* 502–512.

Masten, A., and Morison, P. 1981. *The measurement of interpersonal competence: The Class Play.* Technical Report. Project Competence: Studies of stress-resistant children. Minneapolis: University of Minnesota.

Matthysse, S. 1974. The new research strategies – a critique. *Neuro-Sciences Research Progress Bulletin, 14,* 80–86.

Matthysse, S. 1977. The biology of attention. *Schizophrenia Bulletin, 3,* 370–372.

Matthysse, S., and Kidd, K. K. 1976. Estimating the genetic contribution to schizophrenia. *American Journal of Psychiatry, 133,* 185–191.

Mednick, B. R. 1973. Breakdown in high-risk subjects: Familial and early environmental factors. *Journal of Abnormal Psychology, 82,* 469–475.

Mednick, B. 1977. Intellectual and behavioral functioning of 10–11-year-old children who showed certain transient neurological symptoms in the neonatal period. *Child Development, 48,* 844–853.

Mednick, S. A. 1958. A learning theory approach to research in schizophrenia. *Psychological Bulletin, 55,* 316–327.

Mednick, S. A. 1960. The early and advanced schizophrenic. In S. A. Mednick and J. Higgins (eds.), *Current research in schizophrenia.* Ann Arbor, Mich.: Edwards.

Mednick, S. A. 1962. Schizophrenia: A learned thought disorder. In G. Nielsen (ed.), *Clinical Psychology.* Proceedings of the XIV International Congress of Applied Psychology. Copenhagen: Munksgaard.

Mednick, S. A. 1970. Breakdown in individuals at high risk for schizophrenia: Possible predispositional perinatal factors. *Mental Hygiene, 54,* 50–63.

Mednick, S. A. 1972. The predisposition of schizophrenia. In M. Roff and D. Ricks (eds.), *Life history research in psychopathology.* Minneapolis: University of Minnesota Press.

Mednick, S. A. 1978. Bergson's fallacy and high-risk research. In L. Wynne, R. L. Cromwell, and S. Matthysse (eds.), *The nature of schizophrenia: New approaches to research and treatment.* New York: Wiley, pp. 442–452.

Mednick, S. A., and Garfinkel, R. 1975. Children at risk for schizophrenia: Predisposing factors and intervention. In M. Kietzman (ed.), *Experimental approaches to psychopathology.* New York: Academic Press.

Mednick, S. A., and McNeil, T. 1968. Current methodology in research on the etiology of schizophrenia. *Psychological Bulletin, 70,* 681–693.

Mednick, S. A., Mura, E., Schulsinger, F., and Mednick, B. 1971. Perinatal conditions and infant development in children with schizophrenic parents. *Social Biology* (Suppl.), *18,* S103–S113.

Mednick, S. A., and Schulsinger, F. 1968. Some premorbid characteristics related to breakdown in children with schizophrenic mothers. *Journal of Psychiatric Research* (Suppl. 1), *6,* 354–362. Reprinted in D. Rosenthal and S. S. Kety (eds.), *The transmission of schizophrenia.* Oxford: Pergamon Press, 1968, pp. 267–291.

Mednick, S. A., and Schulsinger, F. 1973. Studies of children at high-risk for schizophrenia. In S. R. Dean (ed.), *Schizophrenia: The first ten Dean Award Lectures.* New York: M.S.S. Information Corp.

Mednick, S. A., and Schulsinger, F. 1974. A longitudinal study of children with a high risk for schizophrenia: A preliminary report. In S. A. Mednick, F. Schulsinger, J. Higgins, and B. Bell (eds.), *Genetics, environment and psychopathology.* Amsterdam: North-Holland/Elsevier.

Mednick, S. A., Schulsinger, F., Higgins, J., and Bell, B. (eds.). 1974. *Genetics, environment and psychopathology.* Amsterdam: North-Holland/Elsevier.

Mednick, S. A., Schulsinger, H., and Schulsinger, F. 1975. Schizophrenia in children of schizophrenic mothers. In A. Davids (ed.), *Childhood personality and psychopathology: Current topics, 2.* New York: Wiley.

Mednick, S. A., Schulsinger, F., Teasdale, T. W., Schulsinger, H., Venables, P. H., and Rock, D. R. 1978. Schizophrenia in high-risk children: Sex differences in predisposing factors. In G. Serban (ed.), *Cognitive defects in the development of mental illness.* New York: Brunner/Mazel.

Mednick, S. A., and Witkin-Lanoil, G. H. 1977. Intervention in children at high risk for schizophrenia. In G. W. Albee and J. M. Joffee (eds.), *Primary prevention of psychopathology.* Hanover, N.H.: University Press of New England.

Meehl, P. E. 1962. Schizotaxia, schizotypy, schizophrenia. *American Psychologist, 17,* 824–838.

Meehl, P. E. 1970. Nuisance variables and the ex post facto design. In M. Radner and S. Winokur (eds.), *Minnesota studies in the philosophy of science* (vol. 4). Minneapolis: University of Minnesota Press.

Meehl, P. E. 1971. High school yearbooks: A reply to Schwarz. *Journal of Abnormal Psychology, 77*, 143–147.

Meehl, P. E. 1972a. A critical afterwork. In I. I. Gottesman and J. Shields (eds.), *Schizophrenia and genetics: A twin study vantage point.* New York: Academic Press, pp. 367–415.

Meehl, P. E. 1972b. Specific genetic etiology, psychodynamics and therapeutic nihilism. *International Journal of Mental Health* (Spring/Summer), *1*, 10–27.

Meltzer, H. Y. 1979. Biology of schizophrenia subtypes: A review and proposal for method of study. *Schizophrenia Bulletin, 5*, 460–479.

Mendelson, W., Johnson, N., and Stewart, J. H. 1971. Hyperactive children as teenagers: A follow-up study. *Journal of Nervous and Mental Disease, 153*, 273–279.

Miller, R. G., Jr. 1966. *Simultaneous statistical inference.* New York: McGraw-Hill.

Miller, W. R. 1975. Psychological deficits in depression. *Psychological Bulletin, 82*, 238–260.

Minturn, M., and Lewis, M. 1968. Age differences in peer ratings of socially desirable and socially undesirable behavior. *Psychology Reports, 23*, 783–791.

Mishler, E. G., and Waxler, N. E. 1968. *Interaction in families: An experimental study of family processes and schizophrenia.* New York: Wiley.

Mitchell, J. C. 1974. Social networks. In B. J. Siegel, A. R. Beals, and S. A. Tyler (eds.), *Annual review of anthropology.* Palo Alto, Calif.: Annual Reviews.

Moos, R. 1974. *Family Environment Scale: Preliminary manual.* Unpublished manuscript, Palo Alto, California.

Moray, N. 1969. *Attention: Selective processes in vision and hearing.* New York: Academic Press.

Morris, G. O., and Wynne, L. C. 1965. Schizophrenic offspring and styles of parental communication: A predictive study using family therapy excerpts. *Psychiatry, 28*, 19–24.

Morris, H. H., Jr., Escoll, P. J., and Wexler, R. 1956. Aggressive behavior disorders of childhood: A follow-up study. *American Journal of Psychiatry, 112*, 991–997.

Morrison, J. R., Hudgens, R. W., and Barchha, R. G. 1968. Life events and psychiatric illness. A study of 100 patients and 100 controls. *British Journal of Psychiatry, 114*, 423–432.

Mosher, L. R., and Gunderson, J. 1973. Special report: Schizophrenia, 1972. *Schizophrenia Bulletin, 7*, 12–52.

Mosher, L. R., and Wynne, L. C. 1970. Methodological issues in research with groups at high risk for the development of schizophrenia. *Schizophrenia Bulletin, 2*, 4–8.

Moss, H. A. 1965. Methodological issues in studying mother–infant interaction. *American Journal of Orthopsychiatry, 35*, 482–486.

Moss, H. A. 1967. Sex, age, and state as determinants of mother–infant interaction. *Merrill-Palmer Quarterly, 13*, 19–36.

Munoz, R. A., Kulak, G., Marten, S., and Tuason, V. B. 1972. Simple and hebephrenic schizophrenia: A follow-up study. In M. Roff, L. N. Robins, and M. Pollack (eds.), *Life history research in psychopathology* (vol. 2). Minneapolis: University of Minnesota Press, pp. 228–235.

Murray, H. 1943. *Thematic Apperception Test manual.* Los Angeles, Calif.: Western Psychological Services.

Nameche, G. F., Waring, M., and Ricks, D. F. 1964. Early indicators of outcome in schizophrenia. *Journal of Nervous and Mental Disease, 139*, 232–240.

Näslund, B., and Persson-Blennow, I. 1979. *Mor–barninteraktion och barnutveckling. 1. Ettariga barns ordkunskap* [Mother–child interaction and child development. 1. One-year-olds' vocabulary]. Unpublished manuscript.

Naslund, B., Persson-Blennow, I., and McNeil, T. F. 1974. "A pilot study of mother–infant interaction during the infant's first six months of life." Unpublished manuscript.

Neale, J. M. 1966. Egocentrism in institutionalized and noninstitutionalized children. *Child Development, 37*, 97–101.

Neale, J. M. 1971. Perceptual span in schizophrenia. *Journal of Abnormal Psychology, 77*, 196–204.

Neale, J. M., and Cromwell, R. L. 1970. Attention and schizophrenia. In B. A. Maher (ed.), *Progress in experimental personality research* (vol. 5). New York: Academic Press.

Neale, J. M., McIntyre, C. W., Fox, R., and Cromwell, R. L. 1969. Span of apprenhension in acute schizophrenics. *Journal of Abnormal Psychology, 74*, 593–596.

Nelson, K. 1973. Structure and strategy in learning to talk. *Society for Research in Child Development*, Monograph No. 149, *38*(1–2), pp. 1–137.

Nesselroade, J. R., and Baltes, P. B. (eds.). 1979. *Longitudinal research in the study of behavior and development.* New York: Academic Press.

Niswander, K., and Gordon, M. 1972. *The collaborative perinatal study of the National Institute of Neurological Disease and Stroke: The women and their pregnancies.* Philadelphia: Saunders.

Norman, D. A. 1968. Toward a theory of memory and attention. *Psychological Review, 75*, 522–536.

Norman, D. A., and Bobrow, D. G. 1975. On data-limited and resource-limited processes. *Cognitive Psychology, 7*, 44–64.

Norman, W. T. 1963. Toward an adequate taxonomy of personality attributes: Replicated factor structure in peer nomination personality ratings. *Journal of Abnormal and Social Psychology, 66*, 574–583.

Nuechterlein, K. H. 1977a. Reaction time and attention in schizophrenia: A critical evaluation of the data and theories. *Schizophrenia Bulletin, 3*, 373–428.

Nuechterlein, K. H. 1977b. Refocusing on attentional dysfunctions in schizophrenia. *Schizophrenia Bulletin, 3*, 457–469.

Nuechterlein, K. H. 1978. On the fallacy of "undivided attention" in an attentional task: The PPI–PI effect. *Schizophrenia Bulletin, 4*, 157–159.

Nuechterlein, K. H. 1979. "Sustained attention and social competence among offspring of schizophrenic mothers." Paper presented at the annual convention of the American Psychological Association, New York.

Nuechterlein, K. H. 1983. Signal detection in vigilance tasks and behavioral attributes among offspring of schizophrenic mothers and among hyperactive children. *Journal of Abnormal Psychology, 92*, 4–28.

Nuechterlein, K. H., Phipps-Yonas, S., Driscoll, R., and Garmezy, N. March, 1980. "Attentional functioning among children vulnerable to adult schizophrenia: Vigilance, reaction time, and incidental learning." Paper presented at the Risk Research Consortium Plenary Conference, San Juan, Puerto Rico.

Nunnally, J. C. 1967. *Psychometric theory.* New York: McGraw-Hill.

Nyman, G. E., Nyman, A. K., and Nylander, B. I. 1978. Non-regressive schizophrenia. 1. A comparative study of clinical picture, social prognosis, and heredity. *Acta Psychiatrica Scandinavica, 57*, 165–192.

Offord, D. R., and Cross, L. A. 1969. Behavioral antecedents of adult schizophrenia. *Archives of General Psychiatry, 21*, 267–283.

Ogilvie, P., Kotkin, J., and Stanley, D. 1976. Comparison of the MMPI and the Mini-Mult in a psychiatric outpatient clinic. *Journal of Consulting and Clinical Psychology, 3*, 497–498.

Oltmanns, T. F., and Neale, J. M. 1975. Schizophrenic performance when distractors are present: Attentional deficit or differential task difficulty? *Journal of Abnormal Psychology, 84*(3), 205–209.

Oltmanns, T. F., and Neale, J. M. 1977. Abstraction and schizophrenia. In B. Maher (ed.), *Progress in experimental personality research,* vol. 8. New York: Academic Press.

Oltmanns, T. F., O'Hayon, J., and Neale, J. M. 1978. The effect of anti-psychotic medication and diagnostic criteria on distractibility in schizophrenia. *Journal of Psychiatric Research, 14,* 81–92. Reprinted in L. C. Wynne, R. L. Cromwell, and S. Matthysse (eds.), *The nature of schizophrenia: New approaches to research and treatment.* New York: Wiley.

Oltmanns, T. F., Weintraub, S., Stone, A. A., and Neale, J. M. 1978. Cognitive slippage in children vulnerable to schizophrenia. *Journal of Abnormal Child Psychology, 6,* 237–245.

Olver, R. R., and Hornsby, J. R. 1966. On equivalence. In J. S. Bruner, R. R. Olver, and P. M. Greenfield (eds.), *Studies of cognitive growth.* New York: Wiley.

O'Neal, P., and Robins, L. N. 1958. Childhood patterns predictive of adult schizophrenia: A 30-year follow-up study. *American Journal of Psychiatry, 115,* 385–391.

Orvaschel, H., Mednick, S., Schulsinger, F., and Rock, D. 1979. The children of psychiatrically disturbed parents: Differences as a function of the sex of the sick parent. *Archives of General Psychiatry, 36,* 691–695.

Orvaschel, H., Weissman, M. M., and Kidd, K. K. 1980. Children and depression: The children of depressed parents; the childhood of depressed patients; depression in children. *Journal of Affective Disorders, 2,* 1–16.

Orzack, M. H., and Kornetsky, C. 1966. Attention dysfunction in chronic schizophrenia. *Archives of General Psychiatry, 14,* 323–326.

Osofsky, J. D., and Connors, K. 1979. Mother–infant interaction: An integrative view of a complex system. In J. D. Osofsky (ed.), *Handbook of infant development.* New York: Wiley.

Ostrow, E. 1980. "Maternal teaching style and delayed match-to-sample performance in four-year-old children." Unpublished doctoral dissertation, University of Rochester.

Overall, J. C. 1972. Empirical approaches to classification. In J. A. Jacques (ed.), *Computer diagnosis and diagnostic methods.* Springfield, Ill.: Thomas.

Overbey, G. 1979. "Competence and psychopathology at two periods in the childhood of children at risk." Doctoral dissertation, University of Texas.

Paine, R. S., and Oppe, T. E. 1966. *Neurological examination of children.* London: Spastics Society Medical and Information Unit, Heinemann.

Parasuraman, R. 1979. Memory load and event rate control sensitivity decrements in sustained attention. *Science, 205,* 924–927.

Parmalee, A., and Haber, A. 1973. Who is the "risk" infant? *Clinical Obstetrics and Gynecology, 16,* 376–387.

Parnas, J., Schulsinger, F., Teasdale, T. W., Schulsinger, H., Feldman, P. M., and Mednick, S. A. 1982. Perinatal complications and clinical outcome within the schizophrenia spectrum. *British Journal of Psychiatry, 140,* 416–420.

Pass, H. L., Klorman, R., Salzman, L. F., Klein, R. H., and Kaskey, G. B. 1977; 1980. The late positive component of the evoked response in acute schizophrenics during a test of sustained attention. *Society for Psychophysiologic Research Abstracts,* 1977. Also in *Biological Psychiatry, 15,* 10–20.

Patterson, G. R., Littman, R. A., and Bricker, W. 1967. Assertive behavior in children: A step toward a theory of aggression. *Monograph of the Society for Research in Child Development, 32,* 5–6.

Pekarik, E., Prinz, R., Liebert, D., Weintraub, S., and Neale, J. M. 1976. The pupil evaluation inventory. *Journal of Abnormal Child Psychology, 4,* 83–97.

Pendleton, M. E., and Paine, R. S. 1961. Vestibular nystagmus in human infants. *Neurology, 2,* 450–458.

Perris, C. 1973. The genetics of affective disorders. In J. Mendels (ed.), *Biological psychiatry.* New York: Wiley.

Persson-Blennow, I., and McNeil, T. F. 1979. A questionnaire for measurement of temperament in six-month-old infants: Development and standardization. *Journal of Child Psychology and Psychiatry, 20,* 1–13.

Persson-Blennow, I., and McNeil, T. F. 1980. Questionnaire for measurement of temperament in one- and two-year-old children: Development and standardization. *Journal of Child Psychology and Psychiatry, 21,* 37–46.

Persson-Blennow, I., and McNeil, T. F. 1981. Temperament characteristics of children in relation to gender, birth order and social class. *American Journal of Orthopsychiatry, 51,* 710–714.

Phillips, L. 1968. *Human adaptation and its failures.* New York: Academic Press.

Phillips, L., and Draguns, J. G. 1971. Classification of the behavioral disorders. *Annual Review of Psychology, 22,* 447–482.

Phipps-Yonas, S. R. 1978. "Visual and auditory reaction time in children vulnerable to psychopathology." Unpublished doctoral dissertation, University of Minnesota.

Phipps-Yonas, S. R. September, 1979. "Reaction time, peer assessment, and achievement in vulnerable children." Paper presented at the 87th convention of the American Psychological Association, New York, New York.

Piaget, J. 1932. *The moral judgment of the child.* London: Kegan Paul.

Piaget, J., and Inhelder, B. 1956. *The child's conception of space.* London: Routledge & Kegan Paul.

Pick, A. D., Christy, M. D., and Frankel, G. W. 1972. A developmental study of visual selective attention. *Journal of Experimental Child Psychology, 14,* 165–175.

Pick, A. D., and Frankel, G. W. 1974. A developmental study of strategies of visual selectivity. *Child Development, 45,* 1162–1165.

Pimm, J. B. 1972. "The performance of the emotionally disturbed child on Piaget's conservation tasks." Paper presented at Jean Piaget Conference, William James College, Michigan.

Plenderleith, M., and Postman, L. 1956. Discriminative and verbal habits in incidental learning. *American Journal of Psychology, 69,* 236–243.

Pope, W. R., and Lipinski, J. 1978. Diagnosis in schizophrenia and manic-depressive illness: A reassessment of the specificity of "schizophrenic" symptoms in the light of current research. *Archives of General Psychiatry, 35,* 811–828.

Postman, L. 1964. Short-term memory and incidental learning. In A. W. Melton (ed.), *Categories of human learning.* New York: Academic Press.

Prechtl, H. 1968. Neurological findings in newborn infants after pre- and perinatal complications. In J. Jonxis, H. Vissern, and J. Trodstran (eds.), *Aspects of prematurity and dysmaturity: Nutricia symposium.* Leiden: Stenfert Kroese.

Prentky, R. 1979. "Index to analysis of the Rochester Adaptive Behavior Inventory." Unpublished document, University of Rochester.

Prentky, R., Salzman, L., and Klein, R. 1981. Habituation and conditioning of skin conductance responses in children at risk. *Schizophrenia Bulletin, 7,* 281–291.

Prinz, R., Swan, G., Liebert, D., Weintraub, S., and Neale, J. M. 1978. ASSESS: Adjustment scales for sociometric evaluation of secondary-school students. *Journal of Abnormal Child Psychology, 6*, 493–501.

Procci, W. R. 1976. Schizo-affective psychosis: Fact or fiction? A survey of the literature. *Archives of General Psychiatry, 33*, 1167–1178.

Quitkin, F., Rifkin, A., and Klein, D. 1976. Neurologic soft signs in schizophrenia and character disorders: Organicity in schizophrenia with premorbid asociality and emotionally unstable character disorders. *Archives of General Psychiatry, 33*, 845–853.

Ragins, N., Schachter, J., Elmer, E., Preisman, R., Bowes, A., and Harway, V. 1975. Infants and children at risk for schizophrenia. *Journal of the American Academy of Child Psychiatry, 14*, 150–177.

Rantakallio, P. 1969. Groups at risk in low birth weight infants and perinatal mortality. *Acta Paedopsychiatrica Scandinavica* (Suppl. 193).

Rao, C. R. 1973. *Linear statistical inference and its applications.* New York: Wiley.

Rappaport, M. 1967. Competing voice messages: Effects of message load and drugs on the ability of acute schizophrenics to attend. *Archives of General Psychiatry, 17*, 97–103.

Rappaport, M. 1968. Attention to competing voice messages by nonacute schizophrenic patients. Effects of message load, drugs, dosage levels and patient background. *Journal of Nervous and Mental Disease, 146*, 404–411.

Rattan, R. B., and Chapman, L. J. 1973. Associative intrusions in schizophrenic verbal behavior. *Journal of Abnormal Psychology, 82*, 169–173.

Rauhala, U. 1966. Suomalaisen yhteiskunnan sosiaalinen kerrostuneisuus. 1960-luvun suomalaisen yhteiskunnan sosiallinene kerrostuneisuus ammattien arvostuksen valossa [The social stratification of the Finnish society. The social stratification of the Finnish society in the decade of 1960 in the light of the evaluation of occupations.] 9. Porvoo-Helsinki: *Research Reports from the Society of Social Policy.*

Rawlins, M. 1979. Unpublished doctoral dissertation, University of Rochester.

Reich, T., Cloninger, C. R., and Guze, S. B. 1975. The multifactorial model of disease transmission: 1. Description of the model and its use in psychiatry. *British Journal of Psychiatry, 127*, 1–10.

Reisby, N. 1967. Psychosis in children of schizophrenic mothers. *Acta Psychiatrica Scandinavica, 43*, 8–20.

Reitan, R. M., and Davison, L. A. 1974. *Clinical neuropsychology: Current status and applications.* Washington, D.C.: Winston.

Ricks, D. F. 1980. Discussion of Watt–Prentky–Lewine–Fryer paper. In S. B. Sells, R. Crandall, M. Roff, J. S. Strauss, and W. Pollin (eds.), *Human functioning in longitudinal perspective.* Baltimore: Williams & Wilkins, pp. 29–31.

Ricks, D. F., and Berry, J. C. 1970. Family and symptom patterns that precede schizophrenia. In M. Roff and D. F. Ricks (eds.), *Life history research in psychopathology* (vol. 1). Minneapolis: University of Minnesota Press, pp. 31–50.

Rieder, R. O., Broman, S. H., and Rosenthal, D. 1977. The offspring of schizophrenics: 2. Perinatal factors and IQ. *Archives of General Psychiatry, 34*, 789–799.

Rieder, R. O., and Nichols, P. L. 1979. The offspring of schizophrenics. 3. Hyperactivity and neurological soft signs. *Archives of General Psychiatry, 36*, 665–674.

Rieder, R. O., Rosenthal, D., Wender, P., and Blumenthal, H. 1975. The offspring of schizophrenics: Fetal and neonatal deaths. *Archives of General Psychiatry, 32*, 200–211.

Rigney, J. C. 1962. "A developmental study of cognitive equivalence transformations and their use in the acquisition and processing of information." Unpublished honors thesis, Radcliffe College.

Robins, L. N. 1966. *Deviant children grown up.* Baltimore: Williams & Wilkins.

Robins, L. N. 1972. Follow-up studies of behavior disorders in children. In H. C. Quay and J. S. Werry (eds.), *Psychopathological disorders of childhood.* New York: Wiley.

Rochford, J. M., Detre, T., Tucker, G. J., and Harrow, M. 1970. Neuropsychological impairments in functional psychiatric diseases. *Archives of General Psychiatry, 22,* 114–119.

Rodnick, E., and Garmezy, N. 1957. An experimental approach to the study of motivation in schizophrenia. In M. R. Jones (ed.), *Nebraska symposium on motivation.* Lincoln, Neb.: University of Nebraska Press, 109–184.

Rodnick, E. H., and Goldstein, M. J. 1974. Premorbid adjustment and the recovery of mothering functioning in acute schizophrenic women. *Journal of Abnormal Psychology, 83,* 623–628.

Rodnick, E. H., and Shakow, D. 1940. Set in the schizophrenic as measured by a composite reaction time index. *American Journal of Psychiatry, 97,* 214–225.

Roff, J., Knight, R., and Wertheim, E. 1976. A factor–analytic study of childhood symptoms antecedent to schizophrenia. *Journal of Abnormal Psychology, 85,* 543–549.

Roff, M., and Sells, S. 1968. Juvenile delinquency in relation to peer acceptance–rejection and socioeconomic status. *Psychology in the Schools, 5,* 3–18.

Roff, M., Sells, S. B., and Golden, M. 1972. *Social adjustment and personality development in children.* Minneapolis: University of Minnesota Press.

Rolf, J. E. 1969. "The academic and social competence of school children vulnerable to behavior pathology." Unpublished doctoral dissertation, University of Minnesota.

Rolf, J. E. 1972. The social and academic competence of children vulnerable to schizophrenia and other behavior pathologies. *Journal of Abnormal Psychology, 80,* 225–243.

Rolf, J. E. 1975. Personal communication.

Rolf, J. E. 1976. Peer status and the directionality of symptomatic behavior: Prime social competence predictors of outcome for vulnerable children. *American Journal of Orthopsychiatry, 46,* 74–87.

Rolf, J. E., Bevins, S., Hasazi, J., and Crowther, J. 1982. Prospective research with vulnerable children and the risky arts of preventive intervention. *Journal of Prevention in Human Services, 1*(Fall).

Rolf, J. E., Crowther, J., Teri, L., and Bond, L. 1977. "Contrasting developmental risks of young children of psychiatric patients and normal parents." Eighty-fifth Annual Convention of the American Psychological Association, San Francisco.

Rolf, J. E., Fischer, M., and Hasazi, J. E. 1981. Assessing preventive interventions for multi-risk preschoolers. *NIMH Science Monographs* in M. Goldstein (ed.), *The prevention of schizophrenia,* (ADM), pp. 81–111.

Rolf, J. E., and Garmezy, N. 1974. The school performance of children vulnerable to behavior pathology. In D. F. Ricks, A. Thomas, and M. Roff (eds.), *Life History research in psychopathology* (vol. 3). Minneapolis: University of Minnesota Press, pp. 87–107.

Rolf, J. E., and Harig, P. T. 1974. Etiological research in schizophrenia and the rationale for primary intervention. *American Journal of Orthopsychiatry, 44*(4), 538–554.

Rolf, J. E., and Hasazi, J. 1977. Identification of preschool children at risk and some guidelines for primary intervention. In J. Joffe and G. Albee (eds.), *The issues: The primary prevention of psychopathology* (vol. 1). Hanover, N.H.: University of New England Press.

Rose, R. J. 1976. "In search of schizotaxia: Heritable variation in susceptibility to auditory distraction." Paper presented at the annual meeting of the Behavior Genetics Association, Austin, Texas.

Rosenthal, D. (ed.). 1963. *The Genain quadruplets*. New York: Basic Books.

Rosenthal, D. 1970. *Genetic theory and abnormal behavior*. New York: McGraw-Hill.

Rosenthal, D. 1971. A program of research on heredity in schizophrenia. *Behavioral Science*, *16*, 191–201.

Rosenthal, D. 1972. Hereditary nature of schizophrenia. *Neurosciences Research Program Bulletin*, *10*(4), 397–403.

Rosenthal, D. 1975a. Discussion: The concept of subschizophrenic disorders. In R. R. Fieve, D. Rosenthal, and H. Brill (eds.), *Genetic research in psychiatry*. Baltimore: Johns Hopkins University Press.

Rosenthal, D. 1975b. The spectrum concept in schizophrenic and manic-depressive disorders. In D. X. Freedman (ed.), *Biology of the major psychoses: A comparative analysis. Research publications for Association for Research in Nervous and Mental Disease* (vol. 54). New York: Raven Press, pp. 19–25.

Rosenthal, D., Lawlor, W. G., Zahn, T. P., and Shakow, D. 1960. The relationship of some aspects of mental set to degree of schizophrenic disorganization. *Journal of Personality*, *28*, 26–38.

Rosenthal, D., Wender, P. H., Kety, S. S., Schulsinger, F., Welner, J., and Ostergaard, L. 1968. Schizophrenics' offspring reared in adoptive homes. In D. Rosenthal and S. S. Kety (eds.), *The transmission of schizophrenia*. Oxford: Pergamon Press, pp. 377–391.

Rosenthal, D., Wender, P. H., Kety, S. S., Schulsinger, F., Welner, J., and Ostergaard, L. 1968. Schizophrenics' offspring reared in adoptive homes. *Journal of Psychiatric Research*, *6*, 377–391.

Rosenthal, D., Wender, P., Kety, S., Schulsinger, F., Welner, J., and Rieder, O. 1975. Parent–child relationships and psychopathological disorder in the child. *Archives of General Psychiatry*, *32*, 466–476.

Rosenthal, D., Wender, P., Kety, S., Welner, J., and Schulsinger, F. 1971. The adopted-away offspring of schizophrenics. *American Journal of Psychiatry*, *128*, 307–311.

Rosvold, H. E., Mirsky, A., Sarason, I., Bransome, E. D., Jr., and Beck, L. H. 1956. A continuous performance test of brain damage. *Journal of Consulting Psychology*, *20*, 343–350.

Roth, W. T. 1977. Late event-related potentials and psychopathology. *Schizophrenia Bulletin*, *3*, 105–120.

Roth, W. T., and Cannon, E. H. 1972. Some features of the auditory evoked response in schizophrenics. *Archives of General Psychiatry*, *27*, 466–471.

Roth, W. T., Pfefferbaum, A., Horvath, T. B., and Kopell, B. S. 1980. P300 and reaction time in schizophrenics and controls. In H. H. Kornhuber and L. Deecke (eds.), *Motivation, motor and sensory processes of the brain: Electrical potentials, behavior and clinical use. Progress in brain research* (vol. 54). Amsterdam: North-Holland/Elsevier, pp. 522–525.

Roth, W. T., Pfefferbaum, A., Horvath, T. B., Berger, P. A., and Kopell, B. S. 1980. P3 reduction in auditory evoked potentials of schizophrenics. *Electroencephalography and Clinical Neurophysiology*, *49*, 497–505.

Rubenstein, G., and Fisher, L. 1974. A measure of teachers' observations of student behavior. *Journal of Consulting and Clinical Psychology*, *42*, 310.

Rubenstein, G., Fisher, L., and Iker, H. 1975. Peer observations of student behavior in elementary school classrooms. *Developmental Psychology*, *11*, 867–868.

Rutschmann, J., Cornblatt, B., and Erlenmeyer-Kimling, L. 1977. Sustained attention in children at risk for schizophrenia. *Archives of General Psychiatry*, *34*, 571–575.

Rutschmann, J., Cornblatt, B., and Erlenmeyer-Kimling, L. 1980. Auditory recognition memory in adolescents at risk for schizophrenia: Report on a verbal continuous recognition task. *Psychiatry Research, 3,* 151–161.

Rutter, M. R. 1966. Children of sick parents: An environmental and psychiatric study. *Maudsley Monograph* (No. 16). London: Oxford University Press.

Rutter, M. R. 1970. Sex differences in children's responses to family stress. In E. J. Anthony and C. Koupernik (eds.), *The child in his family.* New York: Wiley.

Rutter, M. R. 1972. Relationships between child and adult psychiatric disorders. *Acta Psychiatrica Scandinavica, 48,* 3–21.

Rutter, M. R. (ed.). 1980. *Scientific foundations of developmental psychiatry.* London: Heinemann.

Rutter, M. R., and Garmezy, N. 1983. Childhood psychopathology. In M. Hetherington and P. H. Mussen (eds.), *Carmichael's Manual of Child Psychology,* vol. 4 (4th ed.). New York: Wiley.

Rutter, M. R., Shaffer, D., and Shepherd, M. 1973. An evaluation of the proposal for a multiaxial classification of child psychiatric disorders. *Psychological Medicine, 3,* 244–250.

SAS users guide, 1979 edition. Raleigh, N.C.: SAS Institute, p. 157.

Sackett, G. P. 1977. The lag sequential analysis of contingency and cyclicity in behavioral interaction research. In J. Osofsky (ed.), *Handbook of infant development.* New York: Wiley.

Saletu, B., Saletu, M., Marasa, J., Mednick, S., and Schulsinger, F. 1975. Acoustic evoked potentials in offspring of schizophrenic mothers ("High Risk" children for schizophrenia). *Clinical Electroencephalography, 6,* 92–102.

Salzman, L. F., and Klein, R. H. 1978. Habituation and conditioning of electrodermal responses in high-risk children. *Schizophrenia Bulletin, 4,* 210–222.

Sameroff, A. J. 1975. Early influences on development: Fact or fancy? *Merrill-Palmer Quarterly, 21,* 267–294.

Sameroff, A. J. 1978a. Infant risk factors in developmental deviancy. In E. J. Anthony, C. Koupernik, and C. Chiland (eds.), *The child in his family: Vulnerable children* (vol. 4). New York: Wiley.

Sameroff, A. J. (ed.). 1978b. Organization and stability of newborn behavior: A commentary on the Brazelton Neonatal Behavior Assessment Scale. *Monographs of the Society for Research in Child Development,* Ser. No. 177, *43*(5–6).

Sameroff, A. J. 1979. The etiology of cognitive competence: A systems perspective. In I. Sigel and R. Kearsley (eds.), *Premature and small for date babies: The assessment of cognitive competence among a population at risk.* New York: Erlbaum.

Sameroff, A. J., Bakow, H. A., McComb, N., and Collins, A. 1978. Racial and social class differences in newborn heart rate. *Infant Behavior and Development, 1,* 199–204.

Sameroff, A. J., Seifer, R., and Elias, P. K. 1982. Socio-cultural variability in infant temperament ratings. *Child Development, 53,* 164–173.

Sameroff, A. J., and Zax, M. 1973a. Perinatal characteristics of the offspring of schizophrenic women. *Journal of Nervous and Mental Disease, 157,* 191–199.

Sameroff, A. J., and Zax, M. 1973b. Schizotaxia revisited: Model issues in the etiology of schizophrenia. *American Journal of Orthopsychiatry, 43,* 744–754.

Sameroff, A. J., and Zax, M. 1978. In search of schizophrenia: Young offspring of schizophrenic women. In L. C. Wynne, R. L. Cromwell, and S. Matthysse (eds.), *The nature of schizophrenia: New approaches to research and treatment.* New York: Wiley, pp. 430–441.

Sameroff, A. J., and Zax, M. 1979. The child of psychotic parents. In S. Wolkind (ed.),

Medical aspects of adoption and foster care. London: Spastics International Medical Publications.

Sarason, I., Johnson, J., and Siegel, J. 1078. Assessing the impact of life changes: Development of the Life Experiences Survey. *Journal of Consulting and Clinical Psychology, 40,* 932–946.

Saunders, E. B., and Isaacs, S. 1929. Tests of reaction time and motor inhibition in the psychoses. *American Journal of Psychiatry, 9,* 79–112.

Schachter, J., Elmer, E., Ragins, N., and Wimberly, F. 1977. Assessment of mother–infant interaction: Schizophrenic and non-schizophrenic mothers. *Merrill-Palmer Quarterly, 23*(23), 193–206.

Schaefer, E. S. 1965a. Children's reports of parental behavior: An inventory. *Child Development, 36,* 413–424.

Schaefer, E. S. 1965b. A configurational analysis of children's reports of parent behavior. *Journal of Consulting Psychology, 29,* 552–557.

Schaefer, E. S., and Bell, R. Q. 1958. Development of a parental attitude research instrument. *Child Development, 29*(3), 339–361.

Schaffer, D., and O'Connor, P. A. N.D. "Columbia Psychiatric Interview for Children and Adolescents (COLPICA-C Form)." Unpublished manuscript.

Schaffer, H. R., and Emerson, P. E. 1964. The development of social attachments in infancy. *Society for Research in Child Development,* Monograph No. 94, *29*(3), 1–77.

Schaie, K. W., and Strother, C. R. 1968. A cross-sequential study of age changes in cognitive behavior. *Psychological Bulletin, 70,* 671–680.

Schless, A. P., Schwartz, G., Goetz, C., and Mendels, J. 1974. How depressives view the significance of life events. *British Journal of Psychiatry, 125,* 406–410.

Schuldberg, D. 1981. "Healthy features in the individual Rorschach transactions of parents of children at risk for severe mental disorders." Doctoral dissertation, University of California at Berkeley.

Schulsinger, F., Mednick, S. A., Venables, P. H., Ramon, A. C., and Bell, B. 1975. Early detection and prevention of mental illness: The Mauritius Project. *Neuropsychobiology, 1,* 166–179.

Schulsinger, H. 1976. A ten-year follow-up of children of schizophrenic mothers: Clinical assessment. *Acta Psychiatrica Scandinavica, 53,* 371–386.

Scripture, E. W. 1916. Reaction time in nervous and mental disease. *Journal of Mental Science, 62,* 698–719.

Seifer, R., and Sameroff, A. J. 1982. A structural equation model analysis of competence in children at risk for mental disorder. *Prevention in Human Services, 1,* 64–77.

Seifer, R., Sameroff, A. J., and Jones, F. H. 1981. Adaptive behavior in young children of emotionally disturbed women. *Journal of Applied Developmental Psychology, 1*(4), 251–276.

Seligman, M. E. 1974. Depression and learned helplessness. In R. J. Friedman and M. M. Katz (eds.), *The psychology of depression: Contemporary theory and research.* New York: Wiley.

Shabad, P., Worland, J., Lander, H., and Dietrich, D. 1979. A retrospective analysis of the TATs of children at risk who subsequently broke down. *Child Psychiatry and Human Development, 10*(1), 49–59.

Shagass, C. 1976. An electrophysiological view of schizophrenia. *Biological Psychiatry, 11,* 3–30.

Shagass, C. 1977. Early evoked potentials. *Schizophrenia Bulletin, 3,* 80–92.

Shakow, D. 1946. The nature of deterioration in schizophrenic conditions. *Nervous and Mental Disease Monographs, 70,* 1–88.

Shakow, D. 1962. Segmental set: A theory of the formal psychological deficit in schizophrenia. *Archives of General Psychiatry, 6,* 1–17.

Shakow, D. 1963. Psychological deficit in schizophrenia. *Behavioral Science, 8,* 275–305.

Shakow, D. 1979. *Adaptation in schizophrenia: The theory of segmental set.* New York: Wiley Interscience.

Shaw, M. 1976. *Group dynamics: The psychology of small group behavior.* New York: McGraw-Hill.

Shay, J. J. 1978. "A methodological investigation of reliability, validity, and factor structure of the Amherst Pupil Rating Form." Unpublished doctoral dissertation, University of Massachusetts at Amherst.

Shea, M. J. 1972. "A follow-up study into adulthood of adolescent psychiatric patients in relation to internalizing and externalizing symptoms, MMPI configurations, social competence and life history variables." Unpublished doctoral dissertation, Minneapolis: University of Minnesota.

Shimkunas, A. 1978. Hemispheric asymmetry and schizophrenic thought disorder. In S. Schwartz (ed.), *Language and cognition in schizophrenia.* New York: Halstead Press.

Shye, S. (ed.). 1978. *Theory construction and data analysis in the behavioral sciences.* San Francisco: Jossey-Bass.

Simeonsson, R. J. 1973. Egocentric responses of normal and emotionally disturbed children in different treatment settings. *Child Psychiatry and Human Development, 3,* 179–186.

Simmons, J. 1974. *Psychiatric examination of the child* (2nd ed.). Philadelphia: Lea & Febiger.

Singer, M. T. 1967. Family transactions and schizophrenia: 1. Recent research findings. In J. Romano (ed.), *The origins of schizophrenia.* Amsterdam: Excerpta Medica Foundation, pp. 147–164.

Singer, M. T. 1973. "Scoring manual for communication deviances seen in individually administered Rorschachs." Mimeograph, Berkeiey.

Singer, M. T., and Wynne, L. C. 1966. Principles for scoring communication defects and deviances in parents of schizophrenics: Rorschach and TAT scoring manuals. *Psychiatry, 29,* 260–288.

Singer, M. T., Wynne, L. C., and Toohey, M. L. 1978. Communication disorders and the families of schizophrenics. In L. C. Wynne, R. L. Cromwell, and S. Matthysse (eds.), *The nature of schizophrenia: New approaches to research and treatment.* New York: Wiley, pp. 499–511.

Skinner, H. A. 1977. Exploring relationships among multiple datasets. *Multivariate Behavioral Research, 12,* 199–220.

Skinner, H. A. 1979. Dimension and clusters: A hybrid approach to classification. *Applied Psychological Measurement, 3,* 327–341.

Smith, G. 1967. Usefulness of peer ratings of personality in education research. *Education and Psychological Measurement, 24,* 967–984.

Sobel, D. E. 1961. Children of schizophrenic patients: Preliminary observations on early development. *American Journal of Psychiatry, 118,* 512–517.

Soichet, S. 1959. Emotional factors in toxemia of pregnancy. *American Journal of Obstetrics and Gynecology, 77,* 1065.

Soli, S. D., Nuechterlein, K. H., Garmezy, N., Devine, V. T., and Schaefer, S. M. 1981. A classification system for research in childhood psychopathology: Part 1. An empirical approach using factor and cluster analyses and conjunctive decision rules. In B. A.

Maher (ed.), *Progress in experimental personality research* (vol. 10). New York: Academic Press.

Sorbom, D. 1974. A general method for studying differences in factor means and factor structure between groups. *British Journal of Mathematical and Statistical Psychology, 27,* 229–239.

Spitzer, R. L., Andreasen, N., Endicott, J., and Woodruff, R. 1978. Proposed classification of schizophrenia in DSM-III. In L. C. Wynne, R. Cromwell, and S. Matthysse (eds.), *The nature of schizophrenia: New approaches to research and treatment.* New York: Wiley, pp. 670–685.

Spitzer, R. L., and Endicott, J. 1968. *Current and past psychopathology scale (CAPPS).* New York: Evaluations Unit, Biometrics Research, New York State Department of Mental Hygiene.

Spitzer, R. L., and Endicott, J. 1969. DIAGNO II: Further developments in a computer program for psychiatric diagnosis. *American Journal of Psychiatry, 125*(suppl. 7), 12–21.

Spitzer, R. L., and Endicott, J. 1975. *Schedule for affective disorders and schizophrenia – Lifetime version (SADS-L).* New York: Biometrics Research, New York State Psychiatric Institute.

Spitzer, R. L., and Endicott, J. 1979. *Schedule for affective disorders and schizophrenia (SADS)* (3rd ed.). New York: Biometrics Research, New York State Psychiatric Institute.

Spitzer, R. L., Endicott, J., Cohen, J., and Fleiss, J. 1974. Constraints on the validity of computer diagnosis. *Archives of General Psychiatry, 31,* 197–203.

Spitzer, R. L. Endicott, J., Fleiss, J. L., and Cohen, J. 1970. The Psychiatric Status Schedule: A technique for evaluating psychopathology and impairment in role functioning. *Archives of General Psychiatry, 23,* 41–55.

Spitzer, R. L., Endicott, J., and Robins, E. 1975. *Research diagnostic criteria (RDC) for a selected group of functional disorders* (2nd ed.). New York: Biometrics Research, New York State Psychiatric Institute.

Spitzer, R. L., Endicott, J., and Robins, E. 1977. *Research diagnostic criteria (RDC) for a selected group of functional disorders* (3rd ed.). New York: Biometrics Research, New York State Psychiatric Institute.

Spitzer, R. L., Endicott, J., and Robins, E. 1978. Research diagnostic criteria: Rationale and reliability. *Archives of General Psychiatry, 35,* 773–782.

Spitzer, R., Gibbon, M., and Endicott, J. 1971. *The family evaluation form.* New York: Biometrics Research, New York State Psychiatric Institute.

Spivack, G. S., and Spotts, J. 1966. *The Devereux Child Behavior Rating Scale Manual.* Devon, Pa.: Devereux Foundation.

Spivack, G. S., and Swift, M. 1967. *Devereux Elementary School Behavior Rating Scale Manual.* Devon, Pa.: Devereux Foundation.

Spivack, G. S., and Swift, M. 1971. *Hahnemann High School Behavior (HHSB) Rating Scale.* Philadelphia, Pa.: Hahnemann Medical College and Hospital.

Spivack, G. S., and Swift, M. 1972. *Hahnemann High School Behavior Rating Scale (HHSB): Manual.* Philadelphia, Pa.: Hahnemann Medical College and Hospital.

Spivack, G. S., and Swift, M. 1973. The classroom behavior of children: A critical review of teacher administered rating scales. *Journal of Special Education, 7,* 55–89.

Spivack, G. S., and Swift, M. 1977. The Hahnemann High School Behavior (HHSB) Rating Scale. *Journal of Abnormal Child Psychology, 5,* 299–307.

Spivack, G., Swift, M., and Prewitt, J. 1972. Syndrome of disturbed classroom behavior: A behavioral diagnostic system for elementary schools. *Journal of Special Education, 5,* 269–293.

Squires, K. C., Donchin, E., Herning, R. I., and McCarthy, G. 1977. On the influence of task relevance and stimulus probability on event-related potential components. *Electroencephalography and Clinical Neurophysiology, 42,* 1–14.

Squires, N., Squires, K. C., and Hillyard, S. A. 1975. Two varieties of long-latency positive waves evoked by unpredictable auditory stimuli in man. *Electroencephalography and Clinical Neurophysiology, 38,* 387–401.

Steffy, R. A. 1977. Issues in the study of schizophrenic reaction time: A review of the K. H. Nuechterlein paper. *Schizophrenia Bulletin, 3,* 445–451.

Steffy, R. A. 1978. An early cue sometimes impairs process schizophrenic performance. *Journal of Psychiatric Research, 14,* 47–57.

Steffy, R. A. 1980a. "The discriminative and predictive utility of latency and redundancy-deficit reaction time indexes in process schizophrenia." Unpublished manuscript, University of Waterloo.

Steffy, R. A. 1980b. "Tools of the trade: A study of measures used in investigation of children at risk for schizophrenia." Unpublished manuscript, University of Waterloo.

Steffy, R. A., and Becker, W. C. 1961. Measurement of the severity of disorder in schizophrenia by means of the Holtzman Inkblot Test. *Journal of Consulting Psychology, 25,* 555.

Steffy, R. A., and Galbraith, K. J. 1974. A comparison of segmental set and inhibitory deficit explanations of the crossover pattern in process schizophrenic reaction time. *Journal of Abnormal Psychology, 83,* 227–322.

Steffy, R. A., and Galbraith, K. J. 1975. Time-linked impairment in schizophrenic reaction time performance. *Journal of Abnormal Psychology, 84,* 315–324.

Steffy, R. A., and Galbraith, K. J. 1980. Relationship between latency and redundancy-associated deficit in schizophrenic reaction time performance. *Journal of Abnormal Psychology, 89,* 419–427.

Stephens, J. H. 1978. Long-term prognosis and follow-up in schizophrenia. *Schizophrenia Bulletin, 4,* 25–47.

Stiffman, A. 1976. "Congruence–incongruence between parent and child scores on the Bene-Anthony Family Relations Test." Washington University: Practicum paper.

Stone, A. A., Weintraub, S., and Neale, J. M. August, 1977. "Using information processing tasks to form groups of vulnerable and invulnerable children of schizophrenic parents." Paper presented at the 85th annual convention of the American Psychological Association, San Francisco.

Strauss, J. S. 1973. Diagnostic models and the nature of psychiatric disorder. *Archives of General Psychiatry, 29,* 445–449.

Strauss, J. S. 1975a. A comprehensive approach to psychiatric diagnosis. *American Journal of Psychiatry, 132,* 1193–1197.

Strauss, J. S. 1975b. Untangling the antecedents of schizophrenic behaviors. In D. V. Siva Sankar (ed.), *Mental health in children.* New York: PJD Publications.

Strauss, J. S., and Carpenter, W. T. 1972. The prediction of outcome in schizophrenia: 1. Characteristics of outcome. *Archives of General Psychiatry, 27,* 739–746.

Strauss, J. S., and Carpenter, W. T. 1974a. The prediction of outcome in schizophrenia: 2. Relationships between predictor and outcome variables: A report from the WHO International Pilot Study of Schizophrenia. *Archives of General Psychiatry, 31,* 37–42.

Strauss, J. S., and Carpenter, W. T. 1974b. Evaluation of outcome in schizophrenia. In M. Roff and D. Ricks (eds.), *Life history research in psychopathology* (vol. 3). Minneapolis: University of Minnesota Press, pp. 313–335.

Strauss, J. S., and Carpenter, W. T. 1978. The prognosis of schizophrenia: Rationale for a multidimensional concept. *Schizophrenia Bulletin, 4,* 56–67.

Strauss, J. S., and Carpenter, W. T. 1981. *Schizophrenia.* New York: Plenum.

Strauss, J. S., and Gift, T. E. 1977. Choosing an approach for diagnosing schizophrenia. *Archives of General Psychiatry, 34,* 1248–1252.

Strauss, J. S., and Harder, D. W. 1974. "The case record rating scale: A method for rating symptom and social data from case records." Unpublished manuscript.

Strauss, J. S., Harder, D. W., and Chandler, M. 1979. Egocentrism in children of parents with a history of psychotic disorders. *Archives of General Psychiatry, 36,* 191–196.

Strauss, J. S., Loevsky, L., Glazer, W., et al. 1981. Organizing the complexities of schizophrenia. *Journal of Nervous and Mental Disease, 169*(2), 120–126.

Strauss, M. 1973. Behavioral differences between acute and chronic schizophrenics: Course of psychosis, effects of institutionalization, or sampling bias? *Psychological Bulletin, 79,* 271–279.

Strodbeck, F. L. 1954. The family as a three-person group. *American Sociological Review, 19,* 23–29.

Stroh, C. M. 1971. *Vigilance: The problem of sustained attention.* Oxford: Pergamon Press.

Sutcliffe, J. P. 1957. A general method of analysis of frequency data for multiple classification designs. *Psychological Bulletin, 54,* 134–137.

Sutton, S., Braren, M., Zubin, J., and John, E. R. 1965. Evoked-potential correlates of stimulus uncertainty. *Science, 150,* 1187–1188.

Sutton, S., Hakerem, G., Zubin, J., and Portnoy, M. 1961. The effects of shift of sensory modality on serial reaction time: A comparison of schizophrenics and normals. *American Journal of Psychology, 74,* 224–232.

Sutton, S., Spring, B., and Tueting, P. May, 1976. "Modality shift at the crossroads." Paper presented at the Scottish Rite Schizophrenia Research Program Conference on Attention and Information Processing in Schizophrenia, Rochester, New York.

Sutton, S., and Zubin, J. 1965. Effects of sequence on reaction time in schizophrenia. In A. F. Welford and J. E. Buren (eds.), *Behavior, aging, and the nervous system.* Springfield, Ill.: Thomas.

Swets, J. A. 1973. The relative operating characteristic in psychology. *Science, 182,* 990–1000.

Swift, M., and Spivack, G. 1969. Achievement related classroom behaviors of secondary school normal and disturbed students. *Exceptional Children, 35,* 677–684.

Sykes, D. H., Douglas, V. I., and Morgenstern, G. 1972. The effects of methylphenidate (Ritalin) on sustained attention in hyperactive children. *Psychopharmacologia, 25,* 262–274.

Talovic, S. A., Mednick, S. A., Schulsinger, F., and Falloon, J. R. H. 1980. Schizophrenia in high risk subjects: Prognostic maternal characteristics. *Journal of Abnormal Psychology, 89,* 501–504.

Tatsuoka, M. M. 1971. *Multivariate analysis: Techniques for educational and psychological research.* New York: Wiley.

Taylor, M. 1972. Schneiderian first-rank symptoms and clinical prognostic features in schizophrenia. *Archives of General Psychiatry, 26,* 64–67.

Terman, L., and Merrill, M. 1973. *The Stanford–Binet Intelligence Scale* (3rd ed.). New York: Houghton Mifflin.

Thomas, A., Birch, H. G., Chess, S., Hertzig, M. E., and Korn, S. 1963. *Behavioral individuality in early childhood.* London: University of London Press.

Thomas, A., and Chess, S. 1977. *Temperament and development.* New York: Brunner/Mazel.

Thomas, A., Chess, S., and Birch, H. G. 1968. *Temperament and behavior disorders in children.* New York: New York University Press.

Thomas, A., Chess, S., Birch, H. G., Hertzig, M. E., and Korn, S. 1963. *Behavioral individuality in early childhood.* New York: New York University Press.

Tienari, P., Sorri, A., Naarala, M., Lahti, I., Pohjola, J., Bostrom, C., and Wahlberg, K-E. 1983. The Finnish adoptive family study: Adopted-away offspring of schizophrenic mothers. In H. Stierlin, M. Wirshing, and L. C. Wynne (eds.), *Psychosocial interventions in schizophrenia: An international view.* Berlin/New York: Springer-Verlag, pp. 21–34.

Timsit-Berthier, M., and Gerono, A. 1979. Late components of the auditory evoked response in schizophrenics. In D. Lehmann and E. Callaway (eds.), *Event-related potentials in man: Applications and problems.* New York: Plenum, p. 476 (Abstract).

Torgerson, W. 1965. Multidimensional representation of similarity structures. In M. Katz, J. Cole and W. Barton (eds.), *The role and methodology of classification in psychiatry and psychopathology.* Washington, D.C.: U.S. Public Health Service (No. 1584).

Tsuang, M. T., Dempsey, G. M., and Rauscher, F. 1976. A study of "atypical schizophrenia": Comparison with schizophrenia and affective disorder by sex, age of admission, precipitant, outcome and family history. *Archives of General Psychiatry, 33,* 1157–1160.

Tucker, G. J., Campion, E. W., and Silverfarb, P. M. 1975. Sensorimotor functions and cognitive disturbance in psychiatric patients. *American Journal of Psychiatry, 132,* 17–21.

Tucker, L. R. 1958. An inter-battery method of factor analysis. *Psychometrika, 23,* 111–136.

Tutko, T. A., and Spence, J. T. 1962. The performance of process and reactive schizophrenics and brain injured subjects on a conceptual task. *Journal of Abnormal and Social Psychology, 65,* 387–394.

Uzgiris, I., and Hunt, J. McV. 1975. *Assessment in infancy: Ordinal scales of psychological development.* Urbana, Ill.: University of Illinois Press.

Valvanne, L. 1977. "Family health service in rural areas. A joint Finland–ICC international course." Unpublished manuscript.

Van Dyke, J. L., Rosenthal, D., and Rasmussen, P. V. 1974. Electrodermal functioning in adopted-away offspring of schizophrenics. *Journal of Psychiatric Research, 10,* 199–215.

Van Dyke, J. L., Rosenthal, D., and Rasmussen, P. V. 1975. Schizophrenia: Effects of inheritance and rearing on reaction time. *Canadian Journal of Behavioral Science, 7,* 223–236.

Vartanyan, M. E., and Gindillis, V. M. 1972. The role of chromosomal aberrations in the clinical polymorphism of schizophrenia. *International Journal of Mental Health, 1,* 93–106.

Vaughn, C. E., and Leff, J. P. 1976a. The influence of family and social factors on the course of psychiatric illness. *British Journal of Psychiatry, 129,* 125–137.

Vaughn, C. E., and Leff, J. P. 1976b. The measurement of expressed emotion in the families of psychiatric patients. *British Journal of Social and Clinical Psychology, 15,* 157–165.

Venables, P. H. 1964. Input dysfunction in schizophrenia. In B. A. Maher (ed.), *Progress in experimental personality research* (vol. 1). New York: Academic Press.

Venables, P. H. 1977. The electrodermal psychophysiology of schizophrenics and children at risk for schizophrenia: Controversies and developments. *Schizophrenia Bulletin, 3,* 28–48.

Venables, P. H. 1978. Psychophysiology and psychometrics. *Psychophysiology, 15,* 302–315.

Videbech, T. H., Weeke, A., and Dupont, A. 1974. Endogenous psychoses and season of birth. *Acta Psychiatrica Scandinavica, 50,* 202–218.

von Bertalanffy, L. 1968. *General systems theory.* New York: Braziller.

Wagner, E. 1978. "The interpersonal behavior of preadolescent boys with high and low peer status." Unpublished master's thesis, University of Waterloo, Waterloo, Ontario.

Wagner, S., and Krus, D. M. 1960. Effects of lysergic acid diethylamide, and differences between normals and schizophrenics on the Stroop color/word test. *Journal of Neuropsychiatry, 2,* 76–81.

Wahl, O. F. 1977. Sex bias in schizophrenia research: A short report. *Journal of Abnormal Psychology, 86,* 195–198.

Wainer, H., and Schacht, S. 1978. Gapping. *Psychometrika, 43,* 203–212.

Wainer, H., and Thissen, D. 1976. Three steps towards robust regression. *Psychometrika, 41,* 9–34.

Waldrop, M. F., Pederson, F. A., and Bell, R. Q. 1968. Minor physical anomalies and behavior in preschool children. *Child Development, 39,* 391–400.

Walker, E. F., Cudeck, R., Mednick, S. A., and Schulsinger, F. 1981. Effects of parental absence and institutionalization on the development of clinical symptoms in high-risk children. *Acta Psychiatrica Scandinavica, 63,* 95–109.

Walker, E. F., Hoppes, D., Mednick, S. A., and Schulsinger, F. 1981. Premorbid intellectual functioning of subjects at high-risk for schizophrenia. *Journal of Abnormal Psychology, 90,* 313–320.

Ward, P. T. 1971. "LANAL II: A computer system for the programmable content analysis of behavior." Unpublished manuscript, Cornell University.

Watkins, J. G., and Stauffacher, J. C. 1952. An index of pathological thinking in the Rorschach. *Journal of Projective Techniques, 16,* 276–286.

Watt, N. F. 1972. Longitudinal changes in the social behavior of children hospitalized for schizophrenia as adults. *Journal of Nervous and Mental Disease, 155,* 42–54.

Watt, N. F. 1974. Childhood and adolescent routes to schizophrenia. In D. F. Ricks, A. Thomas, and M. Roff (eds.), *Life history research in psychopathology* (vol. 3). Minneapolis: University of Minnesota Press, pp. 194–211.

Watt, N. F. 1978. Patterns of childhood social development in adult schizophrenics. *Archives of General Psychiatry, 35,* 160–165.

Watt, N. F. 1979. The longitudinal research base for early intervention. *Journal of Community Psychology, 7,* 158–168.

Watt, N. F., Fryer, J. H., Lewine, R. R. J., and Prentky, R. A. 1979. Toward longitudinal conceptions of psychiatric disorder. In B. A. Maher (ed.), *Progress in experimental personality research* (vol. 9). New York: Academic Press, pp. 202–283.

Watt, N. F., Grubb, T. W., and Erlenmeyer-Kimling, L. 1982. Social, emotional and intellectual behavior at school among children at high risk for schizophrenia. *Journal of Consulting and Clinical Psychology, 50,* 171–181.

Watt, N. F., and Lubensky, A. 1976. Childhood roots of schizophrenia. *Journal of Consulting and Clinical Psychology, 44,* 363–375.

Watt, N. F., Stolorow, R. D., Lubensky, A. W., and McClelland, D. C. 1970. School adjustment and behavior of children hospitalized for schizophrenia as adults. *American Journal of Orthopsychiatry, 40,* 637–657.

Webb, W. W. 1955. Conceptual ability of schizophrenics as a function of threat failure. *Journal of Abnormal and Social Psychology, 50,* 221–224.

Wechsler, D. 1949. *The Wechsler Intelligence Scale for Children.* New York: The Psychological Corp.

Wechsler, D. 1955. *Manual for the Wechsler Adult Intelligence Scale.* New York: The Psychological Corp.

Wechsler, D. 1958. *The measurement and appraisal of adult intelligence* (4th ed.). Baltimore: Wilkins.

Wechsler, D. 1967. *Manual for the Wechsler Preschool and Primary Scale of Intelligence.* New York: The Psychological Corp.

Wechsler, D. 1974. *Manual for the Wechsler Intelligence Scale – Revised.* New York: The Psychological Corp.

Weintraub, S. 1973. Self-control as a correlate of an internalizing and externalizing symptom dimension. *Journal of Abnormal Child Psychology, 1,* 292–307.

Weintraub, S., Margolis, P., and Neale, J. M. 1980. *Schizophrenic patients and their spouses as parents: Their children's perceptions.* Stony Brook, N.Y.: State University of New York at Stony Brook.

Weintraub, S., and Neale, J. M. 1978. The Stony Brook high-risk project. In B. Feingold and C. Bank (eds.), *Developmental disabilities of early childhood.* Springfield, Ill.: Thomas.

Weintraub, S., and Neale, J. M. March, 1980. "The Stony Brook High Risk Project." Paper presented at the Risk Consortium Plenary Conference, San Juan, Puerto Rico.

Weintraub, S., Neale, J. M., and Liebert, D. E. 1975. Teacher ratings of children vulnerable to psychopathology. *American Journal of Orthopsychiatry, 43,* 838–845.

Weintraub, S., Prinz, R., and Neale, J. M. 1978. Peer evaluations of the competence of children vulnerable to psychopathology. *Journal of Abnormal Child Psychology, 4,* 461–473.

Weiss, G., Minde, K., Werry, J. S., Douglas, V., and Nemeth, E. 1971. Studies on the hyperactive child. 8. Five-year follow-up. *Archives of General Psychiatry, 24,* 409–414.

Weissman, M. M. 1979. Depressed parents and their children: Implications for prevention. In J. D. Noshpitz (ed.), *Basic handbook of child psychiatry* (vol. 4; vol. eds.: I. M. Berlin and L. A. Stone). New York: Basic Books, pp. 292–299.

Weissmann, M. M., and Paykel, E. S. 1974. *The depressed woman.* Chicago: University of Chicago Press.

Weissman, M. M., Paykel, E. S., and Klerman, G. L. 1972. The depressed woman as a mother. *Social Psychiatry, 7,* 98–108.

Welford, A. T. 1959. Evidence of a single channel decision mechanism limiting performance in a serial reaction task. *Quarterly Journal of Experimental Psychology, 11,* 193–210.

Wells, F. L., and Kelley, C. M. 1922. The simple reaction in psychoses. *American Journal of Psychiatry, 2,* 53–59.

Welner, Z., Welner, A., McCrary, B., and Leonard, M. 1977. Psychopathology in children of inpatients with depression: A controlled study. *Journal of Nervous and Mental Disease, 164,* 408–413.

Wender, P. H., Rosenthal, D., and Kety, S. S. 1968. A psychiatric assessment of the adoptive parents of schizophrenics. In D. Rosenthal and S. S. Kety (eds.), *The transmission of schizophrenia.* Oxford: Pergamon Press.

Wender, P. H., Rosenthal, D., Kety, S. S., Schulsinger, F., and Welner, J. 1974. Crossfostering: A research strategy for clarifying the role of genetic and experiential factors in the etiology of schizophrenia. *Archives of General Psychiatry, 30,* 121–128.

Werner, H. 1948. *Comparative psychology of mental development.* New York: International Universities Press.

Werner, H. 1957. The concept of behavior from a comparative and organismic point of view. In D. Harris (ed.), *The concept of development: An issue in the study of human behavior.* Minneapolis, Minn.: University of Minnesota Press.

Wetzel, N. C. 1946. The baby grid. *Journal of Pediatrics, 29,* 439–454.

White, B. L., and Held, R. 1967. Plasticity of sensori-motor development in the human infant. In J. Hellmuth (ed.), *Exceptional infant: The normal infant* (vol. 1). New York: Brunner/Mazel.

White, B. L., and Watts, J. C. 1973. *Experience and environment: Major influence on the development of the young child.* Englewood Cliffs, N.J.: Prentice-Hall.

Wiggins, J. S. 1973. *Personality and prediction: Principles of personality assessment.* New York: Addison-Wesley.

Wiggins, J. S., and Winder, C. L. 1961. The peer nomination inventory: An empirically derived sociometric measure of adjustment in pre-adolescent boys. *Psychological Reports, 9* (Monograph Suppl. 5–v9), 643–677.

Wild, C., Singer, M. T., Rosman, B., Ricci, J., and Lidz, T. 1965. Measuring disordered styles of thinking. *Archives of General Psychiatry, 13,* 471–476.

Wilkinson, L. 1979. Permuting a matrix to a simple pattern. In *Proceedings of the American Statistical Association.* Washington, D.C.: American Statistical Association, pp. 409–412.

Williams, J. 1977. *Psychology of women: Behavior in a biosocial context.* New York: Norton.

Winder, C. L., and Wiggins, J. S. 1964. Social reputation and behavior: A further validation of the Peer Nomination Inventory. *Journal of Social Psychology, 68,* 681–684.

Winer, B. J. 1971. *Statistical principles in experimental design.* New York: McGraw-Hill.

Wing, J. K., Birley, J. L. T., Cooper, J. E., Graham, P., and Isaacs, A. 1967. Reliability of a procedure for measuring and classifying present psychiatric state. *British Journal of Psychiatry, 113,* 499–515.

Wing, J. K., Cooper, J. E., and Sartorius, N. 1974. *The measurement and classification of psychiatric symptoms.* Cambridge: Cambridge University Press.

Winokur, G., Clayton, P., and Reich, T. 1969. *Manic depressive illness.* St. Louis: Mosby.

Winters, K., Stone, A., Weintraub, S., and Neale, J. 1980. *Cognitive and attentional deficits in children vulnerable to psychopathology.* Stony Brook, N.Y.: State University of New York at Stony Brook.

Winters, K., Weintraub, S., and Neale, J. 1979. "The validity of MMPI codetypes in identifying DSM-III schizophrenics." Paper presented at the annual convention of the American Psychological Association, New York, New York.

Wishner, J. August 3, 1964. *Efficiency in schizophrenia.* Paper presented at the 15th International Congress of Applied Psychology, Ljubljana, Yugoslavia.

Witkin, H. H. 1965. Psychological differentiation and forms of pathology. *Journal of Abnormal Psychology, 70,* 317–336.

Witkin, H. W., Dyk, R. B., Faterson, H. F., Goodenough, D. R., and Karp, S. A. 1962. *Psychological differentiation.* New York: Wiley.

Wittman, P. 1941. A scale for measuring prognosis in schizophrenic patients. *Elgin State Hospital Papers, 4,* 20–33.

Wohlford, P. 1966. Extension of personal time, affective states, and expectation of personal death. *Journal of Personal and Social Psychology, 3*(5), 559–566.

Wohlberg, G. W., and Kornetsky, C. 1973. Sustained attention in remitted schizophrenics. *Archives of General Psychiatry, 28,* 533–537.

Worland, J. 1979. Rorschach developmental level in children of patients with schizophrenia and affective illness. *Journal of Personality Assessment, 43,* 591–594.

Worland, J., and Hesselbrock, V. 1980. The intelligence of children and their parents with

640 *References*

schizophrenia and affective illness. *Journal of Child Psychology and Psychiatry, 21,* 191–201.

Worland, J., Lander, H., and Hesselbrock, V. 1979. Psychological evaluation of clinical disturbance in children at risk for psychopathology. *Journal of Abnormal Psychology,* *88*(1), 13–26.

Worland, J., Weeks, D., Weiner, S., and Schechtman, J. 1982. Longitudinal, prospective evaluation of intelligence in children at risk. *Schizophrenia Bulletin, 8*(1), 135–141.

World Health Organization. 1973. *The international pilot study of schizophrenia* (vol. 1). Geneva: World Health Organization Press.

Wyatt, R. J., Potkin, S. G., and Murphy, D. L. 1979. Platelet monomine oxidase activity in schizophrenia: A review of the data. *American Journal of Psychiatry, 136*(4A), 377–386.

Wynne, L. C. 1968. Methodologic and conceptual issues in the study of schizophrenics and their families. In D. Rosenthal and S. S. Kety (eds.), *The transmission of schizophrenia.* Oxford: Pergamon Press, pp. 185–199.

Wynne, L. C., Jones, J. E., and Al-Khayyal, M. 1982. Healthy family communication patterns: Observations in families "at risk" for psychopathology. In F. Walsh (ed.), *Normal family processes: Implications for clinical practice.* New York: Guilford Press, pp. 142–164.

Wynne, L. C., and Singer, M. T. 1964. Thought disorder and family relations of schizophrenics. 4. *Archives of General Psychiatry, 12,* 201–212.

Wynne, L. C., Singer, M. T., Bartko, J. J., and Toohey, M. L. 1977. Schizophrenics and their families: Recent research on parental communication. In J. M. Tanner (ed.), *Developments in psychiatric research.* London: Hodder & Stoughton, pp. 254–286.

Zachau-Christiansen, B., and Ross, E. M. 1975. *Babies.* London: Wiley.

Zahn, T. P. 1977. Autonomic nervous system characteristics possibly related to a genetic predisposition to schizophrenia. *Schizophrenia Bulletin, 3,* 49–60.

Zahn, T. P. October, 1979. "Heart rate, hyperactivity and schizophrenia." Paper presented at the 19th annual meeting of the Society for Psychophysiological Research.

Zax, M., Cowen, E., Izzo, L., and Trost, M. 1964. Identifying emotional disturbances in the school setting. *American Journal of Orthopsychiatry, 34,* 446–454.

Zax, M., Sameroff, A. J., and Babigian, H. M. 1977. Birth outcomes in the offspring of mentally disordered women. *American Journal of Orthopsychiatry, 47,* 218–230.

Zerbin-Rudin, E. 1972. Genetic research and the theory of schizophrenia. *International Journal of Mental Health, 1,* 42–62.

Zigler, E., and Phillips, L. 1960. Social competence and symptomatic behaviors. *Journal of Abnormal and Social Psychology, 62,* 231–238.

Zigler, E., and Phillips, L. 1961. Social competence and outcome in psychiatric disorder. *Journal of Abnormal and Social Psychology, 63,* 264–271.

Zigler, E., and Phillips, L. 1962. Social competence and the process-reactive distinction in psychopathology. *Journal of Abnormal Psychology, 65,* 215–222.

Zigler, E., and Trickett, P. K. 1978. IQ, social competence, and evaluation of early childhood intervention programs. *American Psychologist, 33,* 789–798.

Zubin, J. 1975. Problem of attention in schizophrenia. In M. L. Kietzman, S. Sutton, and J. Zubin (eds.), *Experimental approaches to psychopathology.* New York: Academic Press, pp. 139–166.

Zubin, J., and Spring, B. 1978. Vulnerability – a new view of schizophrenia. *Journal of Abnormal Psychology, 86,* 103–126.

Author index

641

Subject index

645